USP — the standard of quality.

You may have seen the initials "USP" on the label of a drug product. They assure that legal standards of strength, quality, purity, packaging, and labeling exist for the medicine inside the package. What lies behind those initials is the United States Pharmacopeial Convention, Inc. (USP), a nongovernmental, not-for-profit, unbiased scientific organization dedicated to quality health care.

The USP is made up of representatives from colleges, national and state organizations of medicine and pharmacy, U.S. government agencies, consumer organizations, and foreign countries that recognize USP standards. Since 1820 it has established the drug standards in the U.S. The USP standards are recognized as official by the Federal Food, Drug, and Cosmetic Act and are enforced by the U.S. Food and Drug Administration (FDA).

USP publishes the drug standards in the *United States Pharmacopeia* and the *National Formulary*. Additionally, the USP maintains a vast data base of drug use information for both health care professionals and consumers, which is published as *USP DI*.® The information included in the "About Your Medicines" books is derived from the *USP DI* data base.

For more information about USP see page xxvii.

About Your MEDICINES

By authority of the
United States Pharmacopeial Convention, Inc.

NOTICE AND WARNING

Concerning U. S. Patent or Trademark Rights

The inclusion in *About Your Medicines* of a monograph on any drug in respect to which patent or trademark rights may exist shall not be deemed, and is not intended as, a grant of, or authority to exercise, any right or privilege protected by such patent or trademark. All such rights and privileges are vested in the patent or trademark owner, and no other person may exercise the same without express permission, authority, or license secured from such patent or trademark owner.

The listing of selected brand names is intended only for ease of reference. The inclusion of a brand name does not mean the USPC has any particular knowledge that the brand listed has properties different from other brands of the same drug, nor should it be interpreted as an endorsement by the USPC. Similarly, the fact that a particular brand has not been included does not indicate that the product has been judged to be unsatisfactory or unacceptable.

Concerning Use of *About Your Medicines*

NOTICE: The information about the drugs contained herein is general in nature and is intended to be used in consultation with your health care providers. It is not intended to replace specific instructions or directions or warnings given to you by your physician or other prescriber or accompanying a particular product. The information is selective and it is not claimed that it includes all known precautions, contraindications, effects, or interactions possibly related to the use of a drug. The information may differ from that contained in the product labeling which is required by law. The information is not sufficient to make an evaluation as to the risks and benefits of taking a particular drug in a particular case and is not medical advice for individual problems and should not alone be relied upon for these purposes. Since the inclusion or exclusion of particular information about a drug is judgmental in nature and since opinion as to drug usage may differ, you may wish to consult additional sources. Should you desire additional information or if you have any questions as to how this information may relate to you in particular, ask your doctor, nurse, pharmacist, or other health care provider.

For permission to copy or utilize portions of this text, address inquiries to the Secretary of the USPC Board of Trustees, 12601 Twinbrook Parkway, Rockville, Maryland 20852.

First printing 1993 edition, distributed in Canada by Pharmasystems, Inc.— April 1993

Contents

The United States Pharmacopeial Convention 1990–1995

Judy P. Boehlert, Ph.D.
Nutley, NJ

James C. Boylan, Ph.D.
Abbott Park, IL

Lynn R. Brady, Ph.D.
Seattle, WA

R. Edward Branson, Ph.D.
Andover, MA

William H. Briner, CAPT., B.S.
Durham, NC

Stephen R. Byrn, Ph.D.
West Lafayette, IN

Peter R. Byron, Ph.D.
Richmond, VA

Herbert S. Carlin, D.Sc.
Chappaqua, NY

Dennis L. Casey, Ph.D.
Raritan, NJ

Lester Chafetz, Ph.D.
Kansas City, MO

Virginia C. Chamberlain, Ph.D.
Rockville, MD

Wei-Wei, Chang, Ph.D.
(1992–)
Rockville, MD

Mary Beth Chenault, B.S.
Rockville, MD

Zak T. Chowhan, Ph.D.
Palo Alto, CA

Sebastian G. Ciancio, D.D.S.
Buffalo, NY

Murray S. Cooper, Ph.D.
Islamorada, FL

Lloyd E. Davis, Ph.D., D.V.M.
Urbana, IL

Leon Ellenbogen, Ph.D.
Clifton, NJ

R. Michael Enzinger, Ph.D.
(1990–1992)
Kalamazoo, MI

Clyde R. Erskine, B.S., M.B.A.
Newtown Square, PA

Edward A. Fitzgerald, Ph.D.
Bethesda, MD

Everett Flanigan, Ph.D.
Kankakee, IL

Klaus G. Florey, Ph.D.
Princeton, NJ

Thomas S. Foster, Pharm.D.
Lexington, KY

Joseph F. Gallelli, Ph.D.
Bethesda, MD

Robert L. Garnick, Ph.D.
So. San Francisco, CA

Douglas D. Glover, M.D., R.Ph.
Morgantown, WV

Alan M. Goldberg, Ph.D.
Baltimore, MD

Burton J. Goldstein, M.D.
Miami, FL

Dennis K. J. Gorecki, Ph.D.
Saskatoon, Saskatchewan,
Canada

Michael J. Groves, Ph.D.
Lake Forest, IL

Robert M. Guthrie, M.D.
Columbus, OH

Samir A. Hanna, Ph.D.
Lawrenceville, NJ

Stanley L. Hem, Ph.D.
West Lafayette, IN

Joy Hochstadt, Ph.D.
New York, NY

David W. Hughes, Ph.D.
Ottawa, Ontario, Canada

Norman C. Jamieson, Ph.D.
St. Louis, MO

Richard D. Johnson, Pharm.D.,
Ph.D.
Kansas City, MO

Judith K. Jones, M.D., Ph.D.
Arlington, VA

Stanley A. Kaplan, Ph.D.
Menlo Park, CA

Herbert E. Kaufman, M.D.
New Orleans, LA

Donald Kaye, M.D.
Philadelphia, PA

Paul E. Kennedy, Ph.D.
West Conshohocken, PA

Jay S. Keystone, M.D.
Toronto, Ontario, Canada

x

Advisory Panels
For the 1990–1995 Revision Cycle

Members who serve as Chairs are listed first.

The information presented in this text represents an ongoing review of the drugs contained herein and represents a consensus of various viewpoints expressed. The individuals listed below have served on the USP Advisory Panels for the 1990–1995 revision period and have contributed to the development of the 1993 USP DI data base. Such listing does not imply that these individuals have reviewed all of the material in this text or that they individually agree with all statements contained herein.

Anesthesiology
Paul F. White, Ph.D., M.D., *Chair*, Dallas, TX; David R. Bevan, M.B., FFARCS, MRCP, Vancouver, British Columbia; Eugene Y. Cheng, M.D., Milwaukee, WI; Charles J. Coté, M.D., Boston, MA; Roy Cronnelly, M.D., Ph.D., Placerville, CA; Peter Glass, M.D., Durham, NC; Michael B. Howie, M.D., Columbus, OH; Beverly A. Krause, C.R.N.A., M.S., St. Louis, MO; Carl Lynch III, M.D., Ph.D., Charlottesville, VA; Carl Rosow, M.D., Ph.D., Boston, MA; Peter S. Sebel, M.B., Ph.D., Atlanta, GA; Walter L. Way, M.D., San Francisco, CA; Matthew B. Weinger, M.D., San Diego, CA; Richard Weiskopf, M.D., San Francisco, CA; David H. Wong, Pharm.D., M.D., Long Beach, CA

Cardiovascular and Renal Drugs
Burton E. Sobel, M.D., *Chair*, St. Louis, MO; William P. Baker, M.D., Ph.D., Bethesda, MD; Nils U. Bang, M.D., Indianapolis, IN; Emmanuel L. Bravo, M.D., Cleveland, OH; Mary Jo Burgess, M.D., Salt Lake City, UT; James H. Chesebro, M.D., Rochester, MN; Peter Corr, Ph.D., St. Louis, MO; Dwain L. Eckberg, M.D., Richmond, VA; Ruth Eshleman, Ph.D., W. Kingston, RI; William H. Frishman, M.D., Bronx, NY; Edward D. Frohlich, M.D., New Orleans, LA; Martha Hill, Ph.D., R.N., Baltimore, MD; Norman M. Kaplan, M.D., Dallas, TX; Michael Lesch, M.D., Ann Arbor, MI; Manuel Martinez-Maldonado, M.D., Decatur, GA; Patrick A. McKee, M.D., Oklahoma City, OK; Dan M. Roden, M.D., Nashville, TN; Michael R. Rosen, M.D., New York, NY; Jane Schultz, R.N., B.S.N., Rochester, MN; Robert L. Talbert, Pharm.D., San Antonio, TX; Raymond L. Woosley, M.D., Ph.D., Washington, DC

Clinical Immunology/Allergy/Rheumatology
Albert L. Sheffer, M.D., *Chair*, Boston, MA; John A. Anderson, M.D., Detroit, MI; Emil Bardana, Jr., M.D., Portland, OR; John Baum, M.D., Rochester, NY; Debra Danoff, M.D., Montreal, Quebec; Daniel G. de Jesus, M.D., Ph.D., Vanier, Ontario; Elliott F. Ellis, M.D., Jacksonville, FL; Patricia A. Fraser, M.D., Boston, MA; Frederick E. Hargreave,

M.D., Hamilton, Ontario; Evelyn V. Hess, M.D., Cincinnati, OH; Jean M. Jackson, M.D., Boston, MA; Stephen R. Kaplan, M.D., Buffalo, NY; Sandra M. Koehler, Milwaukee, WI; Richard A. Moscicki, M.D., Boston, MA; Shirley Murphy, M.D., Albuquerque, NM; Gary S. Rachelefsky, M.D., Los Angeles, CA; Robert E. Reisman, M.D., Buffalo, NY; Robert L. Rubin, Ph.D., La Jolla, CA; Daniel J. Stechschulte, M.D., Kansas City, KS; Virginia S. Taggert, Bethesda, MD; Joseph A. Tami, Pharm.D., San Antonio, TX; John H. Toogood, M.D., London, Ontario; Martin D. Valentine, M.D., Baltimore, MD; Michael Weinblatt, M.D., Boston, MA; Dennis Michael Williams, Pharm.D., Chapel Hill, NC; Stewart Wong, Ph.D., Brookfield, CT

Clinical Toxicology/Substance Abuse
Theodore G. Tong, Pharm.D., *Chair*, Tucson, AZ; John Ambre, M.D., Ph.D., Chicago, IL; Usoa E. Busto, Pharm.D., Toronto, Ontario; Darryl Inaba, Pharm.D., San Francisco, CA; Edward P. Krenzelok, Pharm.D., Pittsburgh, PA; Michael Montagne, Ph.D., Boston, MA; Sven A. Normann, Pharm.D., Tampa, FL; Gary M. Oderda, Pharm.D., Salt Lake City, UT; Paul Pentel, M.D., Minneapolis, MN; Rose Ann Soloway, R.N., Washington, DC; Daniel A. Spyker, M.D., Ph.D., Rockville, MD; Anthony R. Temple, M.D., Ft. Washington, PA; Anthony Tommasello, Pharm.D., Baltimore, MD; Joseph C. Veltri, Pharm.D., Salt Lake City, UT; William A. Watson, Pharm.D., Kansas City, MO

Consumer Interest/Health Education
Gordon D. Schiff, M.D., *Chair*, Chicago, IL; Michael J. Ackerman, Ph.D., Bethesda, MD; Barbara Aranda-Naranjo, R.N., San Antonio, TX; Frank J. Ascione, Pharm.D., Ph.D., Ann Arbor, MI; Judith I. Brown, Silver Spring, MD; Jose Camacho, Austin, TX; Margaret A. Charters, Ph.D., Syracuse, NY; Jennifer Cross, San Francisco, CA; William G. Harless, Ph.D., Bethesda, MD; Louis H. Kompare, Lake Buena Vista, FL; Margo Kroshus, R.N., B.S.N., Rochester, MN; Marilyn Lister, Wakefield, Quebec; Margaret Lueders, Seattle, WA; Frederick S. Mayer, R.Ph., M.P.H., Sausalito, CA; Nancy Milio, Ph.D., Chapel Hill, NC; Irving Rubin, Port Washington, NY; T. Donald Rucker, Ph.D., River Forest, IL; Stephen B. Soumerai, Sc.D., Boston, MA; Carol A. Vetter, Rockville, MD

Critical Care Medicine
Catherine M. MacLeod, M.D., *Chair*, Chicago, IL; William Banner, Jr., M.D., Salt Lake City, UT; Philip S. Barie, M.D., New York, NY; Thomas P. Bleck, M.D., Charlottesville, VA; Roger C. Bone, M.D., Chicago, IL; Susan S. Fish, Pharm.D., Boston, MA; Edgar R. Gonzalez, Pharm.D., Richmond, VA; Robert Gottesman, Rockville, MD; Michael Halperin, M.D., Denver, CO; John W. Hoyt, M.D., Pittsburgh, PA; Sheldon A. Magder, M.D., Montreal, Quebec; Henry Masur, M.D., Bethesda, MD; Joseph E. Parrillo, M.D., Chicago, IL; Sharon Peters, M.D., St. John's, Newfoundland; Domenic A. Sica, M.D., Richmond, VA; Martin G. Tweeddale, M.B., Ph.D., Vancouver, British Columbia

xiii

toon, Saskatchewan; Richard S. Blum, M.D., East Hills, NY; Amy Cooper-Outlaw, Pharm.D., Atlanta, GA; Joseph W. Cranston, Jr., Ph.D., Chicago, IL; W. Gary Erwin, Pharm.D., Philadelphia, PA; Jere E. Goyan, Ph.D., San Francisco, CA; Duane M. Kirking, Ph.D., Ann Arbor, MI; Karen E. Koch, Pharm.D., Tupelo, MS; Aida A. LeRoy, Pharm.D., Arlington, VA; Jerome Levine, M.D., Baltimore, MD; Richard W. Lindsay, M.D., Charlottesville, VA; Deborah M. Nadzam, R.N., Ph.D., Oak Brook Terrace, IL; William Z. Potter, M.D., Ph.D., Bethesda, MD; Louise R. Rodriquez, M.S., Washington, DC; Stephen P. Spielberg, M.D., Ph.D., Gwynedd Valley, PA; Suzan M. Streichenwein, M.D., Houston, TX; Brian L. Strom, M.D., Philadelphia, PA; Michael Weintraub, M.D., Rockville, MD; Antonio Carlos Zanini, M.D., Ph.D., Sao Paulo, Brazil

Endocrinology
Maria I. New, M.D., *Chair*, New York, NY; Ronald D. Brown, M.D., Oklahoma City, OK; R. Keith Campbell, Pharm.D., Pullman, WA; David S. Cooper, M.D., Baltimore, MD; Betty J. Dong, Pharm.D., San Francisco, CA; Andrea Dunaif, M.D., New York, NY; Anke A. Ehrhardt, Ph.D., New York, NY; Nadir R. Farid, M.D., Riyadh, Saudi Arabia; John G. Haddad, Jr., M.D., Philadelphia, PA; Michael M. Kaplan, M.D., Southfield, MI; Harold E. Lebovitz, M.D., Brooklyn, NY; Marvin E. Levin, M.D., St. Louis, MO; Marvin M. Lipman, M.D., Yonkers, NY; Barbara Lippe, M.D., Los Angeles, CA; Barbara J. Maschak-Carey, R.N., M.S.N., Philadelphia, PA; James C. Melby, M.D., Boston, MA; Walter J. Meyer, III., M.D., Galveston, TX; Rita Nemchik, R.N., M.S., C.D.E., Franklin Lakes, NJ; Daniel A. Notterman, M.D., New York, NY; Ron Gershon Rosenfeld, M.D., Stanford, CA; Paul Saenger, M.D., Bronx, NY; Judson J. Van Wyk, M.D., Chapel Hill, NC; Leonard Wartofsky, M.D., Washington, DC

Family Practice
Robert M. Guthrie, M.D., *Chair*, Columbus, OH; Jack A. Brose, D.O., Athens, OH; Jannet M. Carmichael, Pharm.D., Reno, NV; Jacqueline A. Chadwick, M.D., Phoenix, AZ; Mark E. Clasen, M.D., Ph.D., Houston, TX; Lloyd P. Haskell, M.D., West Borough, MA; Luis A. Izquierdo-Mora, M.D., Rio Piedras, PR; Edward L. Langston, M.D., Indianapolis, IN; Charles D. Ponte, Pharm.D., Morgantown, WV; Jack M. Rosenberg, Pharm.D., Ph.D., Brooklyn, NY; John F. Sangster, M.D., London, Ontario; Theodore L. Yarboro, Sr., M.D., M.P.H., Sharon, PA

Gastroenterology
Gordon L. Klein, M.D., *Chair*, Galveston, TX; Karl E. Anderson, M.D., Galveston, TX; William Balistreri, M.D., Cincinnati, OH; Paul Bass, Ph.D., Madison, WI; Rosemary R. Berardi, Pharm.D., Ann Arbor, MI; Raymond F. Burk, M.D., Nashville, TN; Thomas Q. Garvey, III, M.D., Potomac, MD; Donald J. Glotzer, M.D., Boston, MA; Flavio Habal, M.D., Toronto, Ontario; Paul E. Hyman, M.D., Torrance, CA; Bernard Mehl, D.P.S., New York, NY; William J. Snape, Jr., M.D., Torrance, CA; Ronald D. Soltis, M.D., Minneapolis, MN; C. Noel Williams,

M.S., Washington, DC; Sudesh K. Mahajan, M.D., Allen Park, MI; Craig J. McClain, M.D., Lexington, KY; Jay M. Mirtallo, M.S., Columbus, OH; Sohrab Mobarhan, M.D., Maywood, IL; Robert M. Russell, M.D., Boston, MA; Harold H. Sandstead, M.D., Galveston, TX; William J. Stone, M.D., Nashville, TN; Carlos A. Vaamonde, M.D., Miami, FL; Stanley Wallach, M.D., Jamaica, NY

Obstetrics and Gynecology

Douglas D. Glover, M.D., *Chair*, Morgantown, WV; Rudi Ansbacher, M.D., Ann Arbor, MI; Florence Comite, M.D., New Haven, CT; James W. Daly, M.D., Columbia, MO; Marilynn C. Frederiksen, M.D., Chicago, IL; Charles B. Hammond, M.D., Durham, NC; Barbara A. Hayes, M.A., New Rochelle, NY; Art Jacknowitz, Pharm.D., Morgantown, WV; William J. Ledger, M.D., New York, NY; Andre-Marie Leroux, M.D., Vanier, Ontario; William A. Nahhas, M.D., Dayton, OH; Warren N. Otterson, M.D., Shreveport, LA; Samuel A. Pasquale, M.D., New Brunswick, NJ; Johanna Perlmutter, M.D., Boston, MA; Robert W. Rebar, M.D., Cincinnati, OH; Richard H. Reindollar, M.D., Boston, MA; G. Millard Simmons, M.D., Morgantown, WV; J. Benjamin Younger, M.D., Birmingham, AL

Ophthalmology

Herbert E. Kaufman, M.D., *Chair*, New Orleans, LA; Steven R. Abel, Pharm.D., Indianapolis, IN; Jules Baum, M.D., Boston, MA; Steven M. Drance, M.D., Vancouver, British Columbia; Lee R. Duffner, M.D., Miami, FL; David L. Epstein, M.D., Durham, NC; Allan J. Flach, Pharm.D., M.D., San Francisco, CA; Vincent H. L. Lee, Ph.D., Los Angeles, CA; Steven M. Podos, M.D., New York, NY; Kirk R. Wilhelmus, M.D., Houston, TX; Thom J. Zimmerman, M.D., Ph.D., Louisville, KY

Otorhinolaryngology

Leonard P. Rybak, M.D., *Chair*, Springfield, IL; Robert E. Brummett, Ph.D., Portland, OR; Robert A. Dobie, M.D., San Antonio, TX; Linda J. Gardiner, M.D., New Haven, CT; David Hilding, M.D., Price, UT; David B. Hom, M.D., Minneapolis, MN; Helen F. Krause, M.D., Pittsburgh, PA; Richard L. Mabry, M.D., Dallas, TX; Lawrence J. Marentette, M.D., Minneapolis, MN; Robert A. Mickel, M.D., Ph.D., Los Angeles, CA; Randal A. Otto, M.D., San Antonio, TX; Richard W. Waguespack, M.D., Birmingham, AL; William R. Wilson, M.D., Washington, DC

Parasitic Disease

Jay S. Keystone, M.D., *Chair*, Toronto, Ontario; Michele Barry, M.D., New Haven, CT; Frank J. Bia, M.D., M.P.H., New Haven, CT; David Botero, M.D., Medellin, Colombia; Robert Goldsmith, M.D., Berkeley, CA; Elaine C. Jong, M.D., Seattle, WA; Dennis D. Juranek, M.D., Atlanta, GA; Donald J. Krogstad, M.D., New Orleans, LA; Douglas W. MacPherson, M.D., Hamilton, Ontario; Edward K. Markell, M.D., San Francisco, CA; Theodore Nash, M.D., Bethesda, MD; Murray Wittner, M.D., Bronx, NY

Pulmonary Disease

Harold S. Nelson, M.D., *Chair*, Denver, CO; Richard C. Ahrens, M.D., Iowa City, IA; Eugene R. Bleecker, M.D., Baltimore, MD; William W. Busse, M.D., Madison, WI; Christopher Fanta, M.D., Boston, MA; Mary K. Garcia, R.N., Missouri City, TX; Nicholas Gross, M.D., Hines, IL; Leslie Hendeles, Pharm.D., Gainesville, FL; Elliot Israel, M.D., Boston, MA; Susan Janson-Bjerklie, R.N., Ph.D., San Francisco, CA; John W. Jenne, M.D., Hines, IL; H. William Kelly, Pharm.D., Albuquerque, NM; James P. Kemp, M.D., San Diego, CA; Henry Levison, M.D., Toronto, Ontario; Gail Shapiro, M.D., Seattle, WA; Stanley J. Szefler, M.D., Denver, CO

Radiopharmaceuticals

Carol S. Marcus, Ph.D., M.D., *Chair*, Torrance, CA; Capt. William H. Briner, B.S., Durham, NC; Ronald J. Callahan, Ph.D., Boston, MA; Janet F. Eary, M.D., Seattle, WA; Joanna S. Fowler, Ph.D., Upton, NJ; David L. Gilday, M.D., Toronto, Ontario; David A. Goodwin, M.D., Palo Alto, CA; David L. Laven, N.Ph., C.R.Ph., FASCP, Bay Pines, FL; Andrea H. McGuire, M.D., Des Moines, IA; Peter Paras, Ph.D., Rockville, MD; Barry A. Siegel, M.D., St. Louis, MO; Edward B. Silberstein, M.D., Cincinnati, OH; Dennis P. Swanson, M.S., Pittsburgh, PA; Mathew L. Thakur, Ph.D., Philadelphia, PA; Henry N. Wellman, M.D., Indianapolis, IN

Surgical Drugs and Devices

Lary A. Robinson, M.D., *Chair*, Omaha, NE; Greg Alexander, M.D., Rockville, MD; Norman D. Anderson, M.D., Baltimore, MD; Alan R. Dimick, M.D., Birmingham, AL; Jack Hirsh, M.D., Hamilton, Ontario; Manucher J. Javid, M.D., Madison, WI; Henry J. Mann, Pharm.D., Minneapolis, MN; Kurt M. W. Niemann, M.D., Birmingham, AL; Robert P. Rapp, Pharm.D., Lexington, KY; Ronald Rubin, M.D., Boston, MA

Urology

John A. Belis, M.D., *Chair*, Hershey, PA; Culley C. Carson, M.D., Durham, NC; Richard A. Cohen, M.D., Red Bank, NJ; B. J. Reid Czarapata, R.N., Washington, DC; Jean B. de Kernion, M.D., Los Angeles, CA; Warren Heston, Ph.D., New York, NY; Mark V. Jarowenko, M.D., Hershey, PA; Mary Lee, Pharm.D., Chicago, IL; Marguerite C. Lippert, M.D., Charlottesville, VA; Penelope A. Longhurst, Ph.D., Philadelphia, PA; Tom F. Lue, M.D., San Francisco, CA; Michael G. Mawhinney, Ph.D., Morgantown, WV; Martin G. McLoughlin, M.D., Vancouver, British Columbia; Randall G. Rowland, M.D., Ph.D., Indianapolis, IN; J. Patrick Spirnak, M.D., Cleveland, OH; William F. Tarry, M.D., Morgantown, WV; Keith N. Van Arsdalen, M.D., Philadelphia, PA

Veterinary Medicine

Lloyd E. Davis, D.V.M., Ph.D., *Chair*, Urbana, IL; Arthur L. Aronson, D.V.M., Ph.D., Raleigh, NC; Gordon W. Brumbaugh, D.V.M., Ph.D.,

College Station, TX; Gordon L. Coppoc, D.V.M., Ph.D., West Lafayette, IN; Sidney A. Ewing, D.V.M., Ph.D., Stillwater, OK; Stuart D. Forney, M.S., Fort Collins, CO; Diane K. Gerken, D.V.M., Ph.D., Columbus, OH; William G. Huber, D.V.M., Ph.D., Stillwater, OK; William L. Jenkins, D.V.M., Baton Rouge, LA; V. Corey Langston, D.V.M., Ph.D., Mississippi State, MS; Mark G. Papich, D.V.M., Saskatoon, Saskatchewan; John W. Paul, D.V.M., Somerville, NJ; Thomas E. Powers, D.V.M., Ph.D., Columbus, OH; Charles R. Short, D.V.M., Ph.D., Baton Rouge, LA; Steven L. Sved, Ph.D., Ottawa, Ontario; Richard H. Teske, D.V.M., Ph.D., Rockville, MD; Jeffrey R. Wilcke, D.V.M., M.S., Blacksburg, VA

Headquarters Staff

DRUG INFORMATION DIVISION

Director: Keith W. Johnson

Assistant Director: Georgie M. Cathey

Special Assistant for Patient Counseling and Education Programs: Alice E. Kimball

Administrative Staff: Jaime A. Ramirez *(Administrative Assistant),* Albert Crucillo, Mayra L. Martinez

Senior Drug Information Specialists: Nancy Lee Dashiell, Esther H. Klein, Angela Méndez Mayo *(Spanish Publications Coordinator)*

Drug Information Specialists: Ann Corken, Debra A. Edwards, Jymeann King, Doris Lee, Carol A. Pamer

Computer Applications Specialist: Elizabeth Chew

Publications Development Staff: Diana M. Blais *(Supervisor),* David D. Housley *(Associate),* Anne M. Lawrence *(Assistant),* Dorothy Raymond *(Assistant)*

Library Services: Florence A. Hogan *(Coordinator),* Terri Rikhy *(Assistant)*

Research Assistants: Nancy King, Annamarie J. Sibik

Consultants: Sandra Lee Boyer, Henry Fomundan, Marcelo Vernengo, Gordon K. Wurster

Student Interns/Externs: Arthur Bonner, Howard University; Peter D'Orazio, Howard University; Ellen Frank, University of Pittsburgh; Hyun Kim, University of Texas—Austin; Lucy Kim, Philadelphia College of Pharmacy and Science; Amy O'Donnell, Washington State University

Visiting Scholars: Romaldas Maciulaitis, Kaunas, Lithuania; David Ofori-Adjei, Accra, Ghana; Bose Ogunbunmi, Lagos, Nigeria

USPC ADMINISTRATIVE STAFF

Executive Director: Jerome A. Halperin

Associate Executive Director: Joseph G. Valentino

Assistant Executive Director for Professional and Public Affairs: Jacqueline L. Eng

Director, Operations: J. Robert Strang

Director, Personnel: Arlene Bloom

Controller: Russell L. Williams

Fulfillment/Facilities Manager: Drew J. Lutz

Also Contributing: Barbara Arnold, Kay Kessell, and Marie Kotomori, Proofreaders; Dan Edwards, Typesetter; and Terri A. DeIuliis, Graphics.

PRACTITIONER REPORTING PROGRAMS

Assistant Executive Director for Practitioner Reporting Programs: Diane M. McGinnis

Staff: Robin A. Baldwin, Deirdre Beagan, Shawn C. Becker, Alice C. Curtis, Kay E. McClaine, Ilze Mohseni, Joanne Pease, Susmita Samanta, Anne Paula Thompson, Mary Susan Zmuda

To The Reader

When purchasing a medicine, whether over-the-counter (nonprescription) or with a doctor's prescription, you may have questions about its usefulness to you, the best way to take it, possible side effects, and precautions to take to avoid complications. For instance, some medicines should be taken with meals, others between meals. Some may make you drowsy while others may tend to keep you awake. Alcoholic or other beverages, other medicines, certain foods, or smoking may affect the way your medicine works. As for side effects, some are merely bothersome and may go away while others may require medical attention.

About Your Medicines contains information which may provide general answers to some of your questions as well as suggestions for the correct use of your medicine. *It is important to remember, however, that the human body is very complex and medicines may act differently on different people—and even in the same person at different times. If you want additional information about your medicine or its possible side effects, ask your doctor, nurse, or pharmacist. They are there to help you.*

How To Use This Book

About Your Medicines contains a section of general information about the correct use of any medicine, as well as individual discussions of a wide variety of commonly and not so commonly used medicines. *You should read both the general information and the information specific to the medicine you are taking.*

Each medicine has a generic name that all manufacturers who make that medicine must use. Some manufacturers also create a brand name to put on the label and to use in advertising. *Look in the index* for the generic name or the brand name of the medicine about which you have questions. We have put the generic names and common brand names in the same index, so you do not have to know whether the name you have is a generic name or a brand name. However, it is a good idea for you to learn both the generic and the brand names of the medicines you are using and even to write them down and keep them for future use.

Although the informational entries generally appear in alphabetical order by generic name, there are numerous occasions when closely related medicines are grouped under a family name. Therefore, the surest way to find the page number of the information about each medicine is to *look in the index first.*

The information for each medicine is presented according to the area of the body which is affected. As a general rule, information for one type of use will not be the same as for other types of use. Thus, if you take tetracycline capsules by mouth for their systemic effect in treating an infection, the information will not be the same as for tetracycline ointment, which is applied directly to the skin for its topical effects. And both of these will be different from the information for tetracyclines used in the eye. The common divisions used in this publication are:

- *BUCCAL*—For general effects throughout the body when a medicine is placed in the cheek pocket and slowly absorbed.
- *DENTAL*—For local effects when applied to the teeth or gums.
- *INHALATION*—For local, and in some cases systemic, effects when inhaled into the lungs.
- *INTRA-AMNIOTIC*—For local effects when a medicine is injected into the sac that contains the fetus and amniotic fluid.
- *INTRACAVERNOSAL*—For local effects in the penis when a medicine is given by injection.
- *LINGUAL*—For general effects throughout the body when a medicine is absorbed through the lining of the mouth.
- *MUCOSAL*—For local effects when applied directly to mucous membranes (for example, the inside of the mouth).
- *NASAL*—For local effects when used in the nose.

- *OPHTHALMIC*—For local effects when applied directly to the eyes.
- *ORAL-LOCAL*—For local effects in the gastrointestinal tract when taken by mouth (i.e., not absorbed into the body).
- *OTIC*—For local effects when used in the ear.
- *PARENTERAL-LOCAL*—For local effects in a specific area of the body when given by injection.
- *RECTAL*—For local, and in some cases systemic, effects when used in the rectum.
- *SUBLINGUAL*—For general effects throughout the body when a medicine is placed under the tongue and slowly absorbed.
- *SYSTEMIC*—For general effects throughout the body; applies to most medicines when taken by mouth or given by injection.
- *TOPICAL*—For local effects when applied directly to the skin.
- *VAGINAL*—For local, and in some cases systemic, effects when used in the vagina.

Notice

The information about the drugs contained herein is general in nature and is intended to be used in consultation with your health care providers. It is not intended to replace specific instructions or directions or warnings given to you by your physician or other prescriber or accompanying a particular product. The information is selective and it is not claimed that it includes all known precautions, contraindications, effects, or interactions possibly related to the use of a drug. The information may differ from that contained in the product labeling which is required by law. The information is not sufficient to make an evaluation as to the risks and benefits of taking a particular drug in a particular case and is not medical advice for individual problems and should not alone be relied upon for these purposes. Since the inclusion or exclusion of particular information about a drug is judgmental in nature and since opinion as to drug usage may differ, you may wish to consult additional sources. Should you desire additional information or if you have any questions as to how this information may relate to you in particular, ask your doctor, nurse, pharmacist, or other health care provider.

Because of space constraints, monographs for only the more commonly used medicines have been included in this volume.

Since new drugs are constantly being marketed and since previously unreported side effects, newly recognized precautions, or other new information for any given drug may come to light at any time, continuously updated drug information sources should be consulted as necessary.

There are many brands of drugs on the market. The listing of selected brand names is intended only for ease of reference. The inclusion of a brand name does not mean the USPC has any particular knowledge that the brand listed has properties different from other brands of the same drug, nor should it be interpreted as an endorsement by the USPC. Similarly, the fact that a brand name has not been included does not indicate that that particular brand has been judged to be unsatisfactory or unacceptable.

If any of the information in this book causes you special concern, do not decide against taking any medicine prescribed for you without first checking with your doctor.

About USPC

The information in this volume is prepared by the United States Pharmacopeial Convention, Inc. (USPC), the organization that sets the official standards of strength, quality, purity, packaging, and labeling for medical products used in the United States.

The United States Pharmacopeial Convention is an independent, not-for-profit corporation composed of delegates from the accredited colleges of medicine and pharmacy in the U.S.; state medical and pharmaceutical associations; many national associations concerned with medicines, such as the American Medical Association, the American Nurses Association, the American Dental Association, the National Association of Retail Druggists, and the American Pharmaceutical Association; and various departments of the federal government, including the Food and Drug Administration. In addition, four members of the Convention have been appointed by the Board of Trustees specifically to represent the public. USPC was established 173 years ago, and is the only national body that represents the professions of both pharmacy and medicine.

The first convention came into being on January 1, 1820, and within the year published the first national drug formulary of the United States. The *U.S. Pharmacopeia* of 1820 contained 217 drug names, divided into two groups according to the level of general acceptance and usage.

When Congress passed the first major drug safety law in 1906, the standards recognized by that statute were those set forth in the *United States Pharmacopeia* and in the *National Formulary*. Today, the *USP* and *NF* continue to be the official U.S. compendia for standards for drugs and for the inactive ingredients in drug dosage forms. The *United States Pharmacopeia* is the world's oldest regularly revised national pharmacopeia and is generally accepted as being the most influential.

The work of the USPC is carried out by the Committee of Revision. This committee of experts is elected by the Convention and currently consists of 114 outstanding physicians, pharmacists, dentists, nurses, chemists, microbiologists, and other individuals particularly qualified to judge the merits of drugs and the standards and information that should apply to them. Committee members serve without pay and are assisted by numerous advisory panels, other outside reviewers, and USPC staff.

About *USP DI*

About Your Medicines contains information extracted from *Advice for the Patient* (Volume II of *USP DI*). Volume I contains drug use information in technical language for the physician, dentist, pharmacist, nurse, or other health care provider, and Volume II is its lay language counterpart for use by consumers. Volume III provides information on approved drug products and legal requirements. The monthly *USP DI Update* contains both the practitioner and the patient language information and keeps all volumes up to date. Together, the volumes form the foundation of a coordinated approach to drug-use education. Many health care providers, institutions, and associations in the United States and Canada provide individual drug leaflets based on *Advice for the Patient*. Spanish translations for many medicines are also available.

USP DI was first published in 1980. It is continuously reviewed and revised and is intended for use by prescribers, dispensers, and consumers of medications. The information is developed by the consensus of the USP Committee of Revision and its Advisory Panels and anyone, including users of medicines, may contribute through review and comment on drafts of the monographs.

For further information about *USP DI* or to comment on how the information published in this volume might better meet your information needs, please contact:

USP Drug Information Division
12601 Twinbrook Parkway
Rockville, Maryland 20852
(301) 816-8351

General Information About Use of Medicines

Information about the proper use of medicines is of two types. One type is drug specific and applies to a certain medicine or group of medicines only. The other type is general in nature and applies to the use of any medicine.

The information that follows is general in nature. For your own safety, health, and well-being, however, it is important that you learn about the proper use of your specific medicines as well. You can get this information from your health care provider, or find it in the individual listings of this book.

Before Using Your Medicine

Before you use any medicine, your health care provider should be told:

—if you have ever had an allergic or unusual reaction to any medicine, food, or other substance, such as yellow dye or sulfites.

—if you are on a low-salt, low-sugar, or any other special diet. Most medicines contain more than their active ingredient, and many liquid medicines contain alcohol.

—**if you are pregnant or if you plan to become pregnant.** Certain medicines may cause birth defects or other problems in the unborn child. For other medicines, safe use during pregnancy has not been established. **The use of any medicine during pregnancy must be carefully considered** and should be discussed with a health care professional.

—**if you are breast-feeding.** Some medicines may pass into the breast milk and cause unwanted effects in the baby.

—**if you are now taking or have taken any medicines in the past few weeks.** Don't forget over-the-counter (non-prescription) medicines such as pain relievers, laxatives, and antacids.

—**if you have any medical problems** other than the one(s) for which your medicine was prescribed.

Storage of Your Medicine

It is important to store your medicines properly. Guidelines for proper storage include:

- *Keep out of the reach of children* and in the original container.
- Store away from heat and direct light.
- Do not store capsules or tablets in the bathroom, near the kitchen sink, or in other damp places. Heat or moisture may cause the medicine to break down. Also, do not leave the cotton plug in a medicine container that has been opened since it may draw moisture into the container.

- Keep liquid medicines from freezing.
- Do not store medicines in the refrigerator unless directed to do so.
- Do not leave your medicines in an automobile for long periods of time.
- Do not keep outdated medicine or medicine no longer needed. Be sure that any discarded medicine is out of the reach of children.

Proper Use of Your Medicine

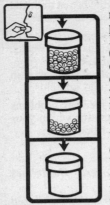

Take medicine only as directed, at the right time, and for the full length of time prescribed by your health care provider. If you are using an over-the-counter (nonprescription) medicine, follow the directions on the label, unless otherwise directed by your health care provider. If you feel that your medicine is not working for you, check with your health care provider.

Unless your pharmacist has packaged different medicines together in a "bubble-pack," different medicines should never be mixed in one container. It is best to keep your medicines tightly capped in their original containers when not in use. Do not remove the label since directions for use and other special information appear on it.

To avoid mistakes, do not take medicine in the dark. Always read the label before taking, noting especially the expiration date, if any, of the contents.

For oral (by mouth) medicines:

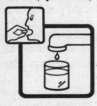

- In general, it is best to take oral medicines with a full glass of water. However, follow your health care provider's directions. Some medicines should be taken with food while others should be taken on an empty stomach.

- When taking most long-acting forms of a medicine, each dose should be swallowed whole. Do not break, crush, or chew before swallowing unless you have been specifically told that it is OK to do so.

- If you are taking liquid medicines, you might consider using a specially marked measuring spoon or other device to measure each dose accurately. Ask your pharmacist about these devices. The average household teaspoon may not hold the right amount of liquid.

- Oral medicine may come in a number of different dosage forms such as tablets, capsules, and liquids. If you have trouble swallowing the dosage form prescribed for you, check with your health care provider. There may be another form that would be better for you.

- Child-resistant caps on medicines for oral use have greatly decreased the number of accidental poisonings and are required by law. However, if you find it hard to open such caps, you may ask your pharmacist for a regular, easier-to-open cap. He or she is authorized by law to furnish you with a regular cap if you request it. You must make this request, however, each time you get a prescription filled.

For skin patches:

- Apply the patch to a clean, dry skin area with little or no hair and free of scars, cuts, or irritation. Remove the previous patch before applying a new one.

- Apply a new patch if the first one becomes loose or falls off.

- Apply each dose to a different area of skin to prevent skin irritation or other problems.

- Do not try to trim or cut the adhesive patch to adjust the dosage. Check with your health care provider if you think the medicine is not working as it should.

For inhalers:

- Medicines that come in inhalers usually come with patient directions. *Read the directions carefully before using the medicine.* If you do not understand the directions, or if you are not sure how to use the inhaler, check with your health care provider.

- Since different types of inhalers may not be used the same way, it is very important to carefully follow the directions given to you.

For ophthalmic (eye) drops:

- To prevent contamination, do not let the eye drop applicator tip touch any surface (including the eye) and keep the container tightly closed.

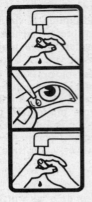

- How to apply: First, wash hands. Tilt head back and, with the index finger, pull lower eyelid away from eye to form a pouch. Drop the medicine into the pouch and gently close eyes. Do not blink. Keep eyes closed for 1 or 2 minutes. In addition, if your medicine is for glaucoma or inflammation of the eye, with middle finger of the same hand, apply pressure to the inside corner of the eye (and continue to apply pressure for 1 or 2 minutes after the medicine has been placed in the eye). This will help prevent the medicine from being absorbed into the body and possibly causing side effects.

  After applying the eye drops, wash hands to remove any medicine that may be on them.

- The bottle may not be full; this is to provide proper drop control.

For ophthalmic (eye) ointments:

- To prevent contamination of the eye ointment, do not let the applicator tip touch any surface (including the eye). After using, wipe the tip of the ointment tube with a clean tissue and keep the tube tightly closed.
- How to apply: First, wash hands. Pull lower eyelid away from eye to form a pouch. Squeeze a thin strip of oint-

ment into the pouch. A 1-cm (approximately ⅓-inch) strip of ointment is usually enough unless otherwise directed. Gently close eyes and keep them closed for 1 or 2 minutes.

- After applying the eye ointment, wash hands to remove any medicine that may be on them.

For nasal (nose) drops:

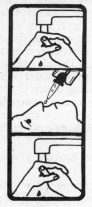

- How to use: Blow nose gently, without squeezing. Tilt head back while standing or sitting up, or lie down on your back on a bed and hang head over the side. Place the drops into each nostril and keep head tilted back for a few minutes to allow medicine to spread throughout the nose.
- Rinse the dropper with hot water and dry with a clean tissue. Replace the cap right after use. To avoid the spread of infection, do not use the container for more than one person.

For nasal (nose) spray:

- How to use: Blow nose gently, without squeezing. With head upright, spray the medicine into each nostril. Sniff briskly while squeezing bottle quickly and firmly.
- Rinse the tip of the spray bottle with hot water, taking care not to suck water into the bottle, and dry with a clean tissue. Replace the cap right after cleaning. To avoid the spread of infection, do not use the container for more than one person.

For otic (ear) drops:

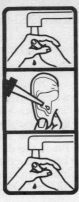

- To prevent contamination of the ear drops, do not touch the applicator tip to any surface (including the ear).
- How to apply: First, wash hands. Lie down or tilt the head so that the ear into which the medicine is to be placed faces up. For adults, gently pull the ear lobe up and back to straighten the ear canal. (For children, gently pull the ear lobe down and back to straighten the ear canal). Drop medicine into the ear canal. Keep ear facing up for several minutes to allow medicine to run to the bottom of the ear canal. A sterile cotton plug may be gently inserted into the ear opening to prevent the medicine from leaking out.
- The bottle may not be full; this is to provide proper drop control.
- Do not rinse dropper after use. Wipe the tip of the dropper with a clean tissue and keep the container tightly closed.

For rectal suppositories:

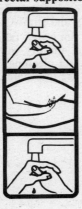

- How to insert suppository: First, wash hands. Remove the foil wrapper and moisten the suppository with water. Lie down on side and push the suppository well up into rectum with finger. If the suppository is too soft to insert because of storage in a warm place, chill the suppository in the refrigerator for 30 minutes or run cold water over it before removing the foil wrapper.
- Wash hands after you have inserted the suppository.

For rectal cream or ointment:

- Bathe and dry the rectal area. Apply a small amount of cream or ointment and rub in gently.
- If your health care provider wants you to insert the medicine into the rectum: First attach the plastic applicator tip onto the opened tube. Insert the applicator tip into the rectum and gently squeeze the tube to deliver the cream. Remove the applicator tip from the tube and wash with hot, soapy water. Replace the cap of the tube after use.
- Wash hands after you have inserted the medicine.

For vaginal medicines:

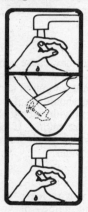

- How to insert the medicine: First, wash hands. Use the special applicator. Follow any special directions that are provided by the manufacturer. However, if you are pregnant, check with your health care provider before using the applicator to insert the medicine.
- Lie on your back with your knees drawn up. Using the applicator, insert the medicine into the vagina as far as you can without using force or causing discomfort. Release the medicine by pushing on the plunger. Wait several minutes before getting up.
- Wash the applicator and your hands with soap and warm water.

Precautions While Using Your Medicine

Never give your medicine to anyone else. It has been prescribed for your personal medical problem and may not be the correct treatment for or may even be harmful to another person.

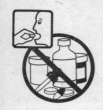

Many medicines should not be taken with other medicines or with alcoholic beverages. Follow your health care provider's directions to help avoid problems.

Before having any kind of surgery (including dental surgery) or emergency treatment, tell the physician or dentist about any medicine you are taking.

If you think you have taken an overdose of any medicine or if a child has taken a medicine by accident: Call your poison control center or your health care provider at once. Keep those telephone numbers handy. Also, keep a bottle of Ipecac Syrup safely stored in your home in case you are told to cause vomiting. Read the directions on the label of Ipecac Syrup before using.

Side Effects of Your Medicine

Along with its intended effects, a medicine may cause some unwanted effects. Some of these side effects may need medical attention, while others may not. It is important for you to know what side effects may occur and what you should do if you notice signs of them. Ask your health care provider about the possible side effects of the medicines you are taking. If you notice any unusual reactions or side effects that you were not told about, check with your health care provider.

Additional Information

It is a good idea for you to learn both the generic and brand names of your medicine and even to write them down and keep them for future use.

Many prescriptions may not be refilled unless your pharmacist has first checked with your health care provider. *To save time, do not wait until you have run out of medicine before requesting a refill*. This is especially important if you must take your medicine every day.

When traveling:

- Carry your medicine with you rather then putting it in your checked luggage. Checked luggage may get lost or misplaced or may be stored in very cold or very hot areas.
- Make sure a source of medicine is available where you are traveling to or take a large enough supply with you to last during your visit. It is a good idea to take a copy of your written prescription with you in case you need it.

If you want more information about your medicines, ask your health care provider. *Do not be embarrassed to ask questions* about any medicine you are taking. To help you remember, it may be helpful to write down any questions and bring them with you on your next visit to your health care provider.

Avoiding Medicine Mishaps

Tips Against Tampering

Over-the-counter (OTC) or nonprescription medicines are now packaged so that signs of tampering can be more easily noticed by the consumer. This may include, for example, packaging where each dose is sealed in its own pouch or where special wrappers, seals, or caps are used on the outer and/or inner containers. Even with this packaging, however, it is important to know that no system is completely safe. You must also do your part by checking for signs of tampering whenever you buy and use a medicine.

The following information may help you detect possible signs of tampering. Some of these can be used only if you already know how the medicine usually looks.

Protecting yourself

General common sense suggestions include the following:

- When buying a drug product, *consider* the dosage form (for example, capsules, syrup), the type of packaging, and whether the tamper-resistant features used, if any, will cause you any problems in opening the container.

- *Look very carefully* at the outer packaging of the drug product before you buy it. After you buy it, also check the inner packaging as soon as possible.

- If the medicine has a protective packaging feature, the package should describe the feature and it should be unbroken. If it does not have the protective packaging as described on its label, *do not buy* the product. If already purchased, return it to the store. Be sure to tell someone in charge about the problem.

- *Don't take* medicines that show even the slightest signs of tampering or don't seem quite right.

- Never take medicines in the dark or in poor lighting. *Look* at the label and each dose of medicine every time you take a dose.

What to look for

Packaging

- Are there bits of paper or glue on the rim of the container that make it seem as if it once had a bottle seal?

- Does the cotton plug or filler in the bottle appear to have been taken out and put back?

- Are there breaks, cracks, or holes in the outer wrapping or protective cover or seal?

- Does the outer covering appear to have been disturbed, unwrapped, or replaced?

- Does the bottle appear to be too full or not full enough?

- Does a plastic or other shrink band (tight-fitting wrap) around the top of the bottle appear distorted or stretched, as though it had been rolled down and then put back into place? Is the seal missing? Has the band been slit and retaped?

- Is the cap on tight?

- Is the bottom of the bottle intact?

- Are the information (including the expiration date) and the lot number on the container the same as those on its outer wrapping or box?

Liquids

- Is it the usual color and thickness?

- Are there particles (small pieces) in the bottom of the bottle or floating in the solution? For some liquids called suspensions, floating particles are normal.

- Is a normally clear liquid cloudy?

- Does it have a strange or different odor (for example, bleach, acid, gasoline-like, or other pungent or sharp odor)?

- Do eye drops have a protective seal? All eye drops must to be sealed when they are made, in order to keep them germ-free. Do not use if there is any sign of a broken or removed seal.

Tablets

- Has their appearance changed? Is the color different? Do they have unusual spots? If they normally are shiny and smooth, are some dull or rough?
- Do the tablets have a strange or different odor or taste?
- Are the tablets all the same size and thickness?
- If there is printing on the tablets, do they all have the same imprint? Is the imprint missing from some?

Capsules

- Are they cracked or dented?
- Do they have their normal shiny appearance or are some dull or have fingerprints on them as though they have been handled?
- If there is printing on the capsules, do they all have the same imprint? Is the imprint missing from some? Do the imprints all line up the same way?
- Are they all the same size and color?
- Are the capsules all the same length?
- Does the filling in all the capsules look the same?
- Do they have an unexpected or unusual odor?

Tubes and jars (ointments, creams, pastes, etc.)

- Is the tube properly sealed? Check the bottom as well as the top of a tube, especially if it is a metal tube crimped up from the bottom like a tube of toothpaste. It should be firmly sealed.
- Are ointments and creams smooth and non-gritty? Have they separated?

Be a wise consumer. Look for signs of tampering before buying a medicine and again each time you take a dose of it. Also, pay attention to the news so you'll know of any tampering that occurs.

It is important to recognize that not every change in the appearance or condition of a product may mean that the package has been tampered with. The manufacturer may have changed the color or the packaging of a medicine or the product may be breaking down with age or may have had rough or unusual handling in shipping. Also, some minor product variations may be normal.

Whenever you suspect anything to be unusual about a medicine or its packaging, have your pharmacist look at it. He or she would know the usual appearance of the packaging and the product.

Accidental Poisoning

Over 1.1 million children 5 years of age and younger were accidentally poisoned in 1991. Of these, over 100,000 required hospital emergency room treatment, according to information provided by the American Association of Poison Control Centers. In 1991, 44 children 5 years of age and younger died as a result of poisoning.

Adults also may be accidentally poisoned, most often through carelessness or lack of information; for example, the sleepy adult who takes a medicine in the dark and winds up getting the wrong one, or the adult who decides to take the medicine prescribed for a friend to treat "the same symptoms."

Drug poisoning, usually from an accidental overdose, is one of the three types of accidental poisoning contributing to these figures. The other two are household chemical poisoning from accidental ingestion or contact, and vapor poisoning—for example, carbon monoxide, usually from a car.

Children are ready victims

The natural curiosity of children makes them ready victims of poisoning. Children explore everywhere and investigate their environment. What they find frequently goes into their mouths. They do not understand danger and possibly cannot read warning labels.

Accidental poisoning from medicine is especially dangerous in small children because the strength of medicines that may be ingested is most often based on their use in adults. Even a small quantity of an adult dose can sometimes poison a child.

Preventing poisoning from medicines

- Store medicines out of the sight and reach of children, preferably in a locked cabinet—not in the medicine cabinet in the bathroom or in a cabinet with foodstuffs.

- Use child-resistant closures on pain relievers and other potentially harmful products whether you have children living with you or only as occasional visitors. Adults who have difficulty opening child-resistant closures may request traditional, easy-to-open packaging for their medicines. Whichever closure you use, store medicines in a secure place.

- Always replace lids and return medicines to their storage place after use, even if you will be using them again soon.

- If you are called to the telephone or to answer the door while you are taking medicine, take the container with you or put the medicine out of the reach of small children. Children act quickly—usually when no one is watching.

- Date medicines when purchased and clean out your medicines periodically. Discard outdated prescription medicines—those past their expiration or "beyond use" date. As medicines grow old, the chemicals in some may change. Many medicines will come with an expiration date on the label. In general, medicines that do not have an expiration date should not be kept for more than one year. Carefully discard any medicines so that children cannot get them. Rinse containers well before discarding in the trash.

• Take only those medicines prescribed for you and give medicines only to those for whom prescribed. A medicine that worked well for one person may harm another.

• It is best to keep all medicines in their original containers with their labels intact. The label contains valuable information for taking the medicine properly. Also, in case of accidental poisoning, it is important to know the ingredients in a drug product and any emergency instructions from the manufacturer. While prescription medicines usually do not list ingredients, information on the label makes it possible for your pharmacist to identify the contents.

• Ask your pharmacist to include on the label the number of tablets or capsules that he or she put in the container. In case of poisoning, it may be important to know roughly how many tablets or capsules were taken.

• Do not trust your memory—read the label before use, every time, and take as directed.

• If a medicine container has no label or the label has been defaced so that you are not absolutely sure what it says, do not use it.

• Turn on a light when taking or giving medicines at night or in a dark room.

• Label medicine containers with poison symbols, especially if you have children, individuals with poor vision, or other persons in your home who cannot read well.

• Teach children that medicine is not candy by calling each medicine by its proper name.

• Do not take medicines in front of children. They may wish to imitate you or, when they play "doctor," may decide to replenish their supply of "pills" with some of those you take.

• Communicate these safety rules to any babysitters you may have and remember them if you babysit or are visiting a house with children. Children are naturally curious and can get into a pocketbook, briefcase, or overnight bag that might contain medicines.

What to do if a poisoning happens

Remember:

• There may be no immediate, significant symptoms or warning signs, particularly in a child.

• Nothing you can give will work equally well in all cases of poisoning. In fact, one "antidote" may counteract the effects of another.

• Many poisons act quickly, leaving little time for treatment.

Therefore:

• Do not wait to see what effect the poison will have or if symptoms of overdose develop. If you think someone has swallowed medicine or a household product, call a Poison Control Center (listed in the white pages of your telephone book under "Poison Control" or inside the front cover with other emergency numbers), health care provider, hospital, or rescue squad, immediately. These numbers should be posted beside every telephone in the house together with those of your pharmacist, the police, fire department, and ambulance services. (Some poison control centers have TTY capability for the deaf. Check with your local center if you or someone in your family requires this service.)

• Have the container with you when you call so you can read the label on the product for ingredients.

• Describe what, when, and how much was taken and the age and condition of the person poisoned—for example, vomiting, choking, drowsy, change in color or temperature of skin, conscious or unconscious, or convulsing.

• *Do not induce vomiting* unless instructed by medical personnel. *Do not induce vomiting or force liquids* into a person who is convulsing, unconscious, or very drowsy.

• Stay calm and in control of the situation.

Keep a bottle of Syrup of Ipecac stored in a secure place in your home for emergency use. It is available at pharmacies in one ounce bottles without prescription. Syrup of Ipecac is often recommended in cases of poisoning to cause vomiting.

Activated Charcoal also is sometimes recommended in certain types of poisoning and you may wish to add a supply to your emergency medicines. It is available without a prescription; however, before using this medicine for poisoning, call for medical advice. There are a number of types of poisoning for which this substance should *not* be used. When you are directed to use it, be aware that Activated Charcoal acts by adsorbing (holding) the poison so that it can be eliminated from the body before it is absorbed into the bloodstream. Therefore, any other medicine taken within two hours of the Activated Charcoal may similarly be tied up and not taken up by the body. Also, if you are told to use both Syrup of Ipecac and Activated Charcoal to treat poisoning, do not take the Activated Charcoal until *after* you have taken the Syrup of Ipecac to cause vomiting and the vomiting has stopped, usually about 30 minutes.

A first aid book that describes emergency treatment of poisoning or a chart of emergency measures to take that can be posted in some central place in your home can be useful if medical help is not readily available in your area. If you must rely on these sources of information, however, familiarize yourself fully with the various procedures listed so that in an emergency you will not waste time trying to match the poison with treatment.

Getting the Most Out of Your Medicines

To get the most out of your medicines, you must make an informed decision as to whether to take the medicine at all, to know about the medicine and its effects, and follow precise directions for use.

Most consumers are concerned with getting best value for money spent. Nevertheless, there are many who ignore this consideration when it comes to medicines. These are the people—up to 50% of all drug consumers in the United States according to some research studies—who do not follow drug use directions accurately.

Communicating With Your Health Care Provider

As the purchaser from your health care provider of his or her knowledge, skills, and office services, you must weigh the advice given and determine whether you accept it and are willing to follow it. To make that decision, you need to have information from your health care provider about the therapy being recommended. How are you going to get it? The same way you get information about any other service or thing you buy. You will have to ask questions—and answer some too. Communication is a two-way street.

Giving information

To make an intelligent diagnosis and prescription for care, your health care provider needs to know about your past and present medical history, including all the illnesses you have ever had; current symptoms; the drugs you are taking; any allergies or sensitivities to foods, medicines, or other things; your smoking, drinking, and exercise habits; vaccinations; operations; accidents requiring hospitalization; illnesses that run in your family; the cause of death of your closest relatives; and other relevant information.

Many health care providers have a standard "medical history" form they will ask you to fill out when they see you initially, or they may ask the questions and write down the answers for you. If you are visiting a health care provider for the first time, prepare yourself before you go by thinking about the questions that might be asked and jotting down the answers—including dates—so that you won't forget an important item. Once your "medical history" is in the health care provider's files, subsequent visits will take less time.

You will, however, have to supply each health care provider you see—every time you see one—with complete information about what happened since your last visit so that your records can be updated and the health care provider can make sound recommendations for your continued treatment, or treatment of your new problem.

It will simplify things if you develop a similar "medical history" file for yourself at home and keep one for each family member for whom you are responsible. Setting up the file will take time, but once established, you have only to keep it up-to-date and remember to take it with you when you see a health care provider. It is better than having to repeat the information time after time and running the risk of confusing or forgetting details.

It is also a good idea to carry a card in your wallet summarizing your chronic medical conditions, the medicines you are taking for each, and your allergies and drug sensitivities—and keep it current. Many pharmacists provide these cards as a service.

"Medical history" checklist

A "medical history" checklist covers the following information:

- All the serious illnesses you have ever had and the approximate dates.

- Your current symptoms, if any.
- All the medicines you are taking now or have taken within the last few weeks, prescription and nonprescription (including pain relievers, antacids, laxatives, and cold medicines). This is especially important if you are seeing more than one health care provider; if you are having surgery, including dental or emergency treatment; or if you obtain your medicines from more than one source.
- Any allergies or sensitivities to medicines, foods, or other substances.
- Your smoking, drinking, and exercise habits.
- Any recent changes in lifestyle or personal habits. New job? Retired? Change of residence? Death in family? Married? Divorced? Other?
- Any special diet you are on—low-sugar, low-sodium, or a diet to lose or gain weight.
- If you are pregnant, plan to become pregnant, or if you are breast-feeding an infant.
- All the vaccinations and vaccination boosters you have had, with dates if possible.
- Any operations you have had, including dental and those performed on an outpatient basis, and any accidents that have required hospitalization.
- Illnesses that run in your family.
- Cause of death of closest relatives.

Remember, be sure to tell your health care provider at each visit if there have been any changes since your last visit.

Getting information

Assuming you have decided to accept the health care provider's advice, you need to understand what you are being directed to do so that you can follow the instructions. A number of medical problems can be handled without the use of drugs. Some of these lend themselves to a standard list of instructions which your health care provider may have had printed up for your use. If the instructions are not written down, you may want to do that yourself or ask the health care provider to write them down for you. When medicines are prescribed, there are certain things you should understand about each.

If you don't have time to jot down everything while you are still with your doctor or nurse, sit down in the waiting room before you leave and finish filling in the information while it is still fresh in your mind and you still have the possibility of requesting answers to questions. If you have been given a prescription, ask for written information about the drug. You can also get answers to your questions from your pharmacist when you have your prescription filled.

For your health care provider to be able to serve you well, you must communicate all that you know about your present health condition at every visit. In order to benefit from the advice for which you have paid—and you have paid not only in dollars, but in terms of time, taxes, insurance, and transportation costs—your health care provider must communicate full instructions for your care. Then it is up to you as the health care provider's partner in the management of your health care to carry out those instructions precisely. If there is a failure in any part of this system, you will pay an even higher price—physically and financially—for your health care.

What you need to know about your medicines

There are a number of things that you should know about each medicine you are taking. These include:

- The medicine's generic and brand name.
- How it will help you and the expected results. How it make you feel. How long it takes to begin working.
- How much to take at one time.

- How often to take the medicine.
- How long it will be necessary to take the medicine.
- When to take it. Before, during, after meals? At bedtime? At any other special times?
- How to take it. With water? With fruit juice? How much?
- What to do about a missed dose.
- Foods, drinks, or other medicines not to be taken while taking a medicine.
- Restrictions on activities while taking a medicine. May I drive a car or operate other motor vehicles?
- Side effects to be expected. What to do if they appear. How to minimize the side effects. How soon will they go away?
- When to seek help if there are problems.
- How long to wait before reporting no change in symptoms.
- How to store the medicine. Should the unused portion be saved for future use?
- The expiration date.
- The cost of the medicine.
- How to have your prescription refilled, if necessary.

Other issues or important information about your medicine that you may want to consider include the following:

- Ask your health care provider about the ingredients in the prescription and over-the-counter (OTC) medicines you are taking and whether there may be a conflict with some other medicine you are taking regularly or occasionally. Your health care provider can help you avoid dangerous combinations or drug products that contain ingredients to which you are allergic or sensitive.

- You may want to ask your health care provider for help in developing a system for taking your medicines properly, particularly if you are taking a number of them on a daily basis. (When you are a patient in a hospital, ask for instruction in managing your medicines on your own before you are discharged.) Do not hesitate or be embarrassed to ask questions or ask for help.

• If you are over 60 years of age, ask your health care provider if the dose of the medicine prescribed is right for you. Some medicines may have to be given in lower doses to certain older individuals.

• If you are taking several different medicines (for example, more than five), ask your health care provider if all of them are necessary for you. You should take only those medicines that you need.

• Medicines should be kept in the container they came in. However, if this is not possible and you must take medicines during working hours, or when you are otherwise away from home, ask your pharmacist to provide or recommend a suitable container or a more convenient package to transport your medicines safely. Tablets can be broken or chipped or can deteriorate in "pill boxes" thereby delivering a dosage somewhat smaller than you were prescribed to take. Medicines that are similar in appearance can be confused if they are in the same container and you could take the wrong medicine in the wrong amount. In rare cases, some medicines can interact with the metal of these boxes causing harmful effects. Medicines like nitroglycerin can evaporate, altering the quantity you may receive in any given tablet.

• Some people have trouble taking tablets or capsules. Your health care provider will know if another dosage form is available or if the tablets can be crushed or the capsule contents dissolved and taken in a liquid. If this is an ongoing problem, ask the person who prescribes your medicines to write the prescription for the dosage form you can take most comfortably.

• Child-resistant caps are required by law on most prescription medicines for oral use to protect children from accidental poisoning. These containers are designed so that children will have difficulty opening them. Since many adults find these containers to also be adult-resistant, the law allows consumers to request traditional, easy-to-open packaging for their drugs. Remember, however, if you do not use child-resistant packaging, make sure that your medicines are stored where small children cannot see or reach them. If you use child-resistant containers, ask your pharmacist to show you how to open them.

Consumer education is one of the most important responsibilities of your health care provider. To supplement what you learn during your visit to your health care provider, ask if there is any written information about your medicines that you can take home with you. Your health care provider may also have available various reference books or computerized drug information which you may consult for details about precautions, side effects, and proper use of your medicines.

Managing Your Medicines

To get the full benefit from your prescribed medicines—and reduce risks from improper use—it is important to take the right medicine at the right time in the right amount for the length of time prescribed. Bad effects can result from taking too much or too little of a medicine, or taking it too often or not often enough.

Whether you are taking one or several medicines, develop a system for taking them. It can be just as difficult to remember whether you took your once-a-day high blood pressure medicine, as it can be to keep track of a number of medicines to be taken several times during the day. Many medicines also have special instructions that further complicate keeping it all straight. Establish a way of knowing whether you took your medicines and took them properly, then make that a part of your daily routine.

Establishing a system

For the person taking only one or two medicines a day, perhaps all you need to do is take them at the same time you perform some other regular task such as brushing your teeth or getting dressed. Others may find a check-off record a handy way of managing multiple medicines.

Keep your medicine record with a pencil or pen in a handy, visible place next to where you take your medicines. Check off each dose as you take it.

Try to take your medicines on time, but a half hour early or late usually isn't going to upset things drastically. If, however, you are more than several hours late, and particularly if you are getting close to your next dose, check with your health care provider if you did not receive instructions for what to do about a missed dose. You may also find this information in the entries included in this book.

If you skip a dose, for whatever reason, make a note on the back of the record or the bottom of the sheet if there is room, about what happened and what you did.

Be sure to also note in the same place, any unwanted effects or anything unusual that happens to you that may be connected with your medicines, or if the medicine does not do what you expect. But remember, some medicines take a while before they start having a noticeable effect.

With such a record—if you keep it faithfully—you will know for sure whether or not you took your medicine, and you have a complete record for your health care providers to review when you visit any one of them again. This information can help them determine if the medicine is working properly or causing unwanted side effects and, when necessary, to make adjustments in your medicines and/or doses being taken.

If your medicines or the instructions for taking them are changed, correct your record or make a new one. Keep the old record until you are sure you or your health care providers no longer need that information.

This sample record will work for most people. However, some may need to adjust it to meet their special needs. You might also want to color code your medicine containers. If you are having trouble reading labels, codes recognized by touch, like rubber bands, a cotton ball, or a piece of emery board, can be attached to the container. If you code your medicines, be sure these identifications are included on any medicine record you use. Ask you pharmacist to type medicine labels in large letters for ease in reading.

A check-off list is not the only method to record medicine use. If this system does not work for you, ask your health care provider to help you develop an alternative. Be sure he or she knows all the medicines prescribed for you and those nonprescription medicines you take regularly, the hours you usually eat your meals, and any special diet you are following.

Informed management

Your medicines have been prescribed for you and your condition. When they are prescribed, ask what benefits to expect, what side effects may occur, and when to report any side effects you notice. If your symptoms go away, don't decide on your own that you are well and can stop your medicine. If you stop too soon, the symptoms may come back. If your health care provider said to finish all of the medicine, then finish it. However, if you develop diarrhea or some other unpleasant side effect, do not continue with the medicine just because you were told to finish it. Call your health care provider and report the bad effects. A change in dose or in the kind of medicine you are taking may be necessary.

When you are given a prescription for a medicine, ask the person who wrote it to explain it to you. For example, does "four times a day" mean one in the morning, one at noon, one in the evening, and one at bedtime, or does it mean every six hours around the clock? When a prescription says "take as needed," ask how close together the doses can be taken and still be safe; what is the maximum number of doses you can take in one day? Does "take with liquids" mean with water, milk, or something else? Are there some liquids that should avoided? What does "take with food" mean? At every meal time (some people must eat six meals a day), or with a snack? Do not trust your memory—have the instructions written down. To follow the instructions for taking your medicines, you must understand exactly what the prescriber wants you to do in order to "take as directed."

When the pharmacist fills the prescription, you have another opportunity to clarify information received or to ask other questions. Before you leave, check the label on your medicine to be sure it matches the prescription and your understanding of what you are to do. If it does not, ask more questions.

The key to getting the most from your prescribed treatments is following instructions accurately—but intelligently. If you have questions or doubts about the prescribed treatment, do not just decide not to take the medicine or otherwise fail to follow the prescribed regimen. Discuss your questions and doubts with your health care provider.

The time and effort put into setting up a system to manage your medicines and establish a routine for taking them will pay off in the end by relieving anxiety and helping you get the most from your prescribed treatment.

Taking Your Medicine

To take medicines safely and get the greatest benefit from them, it is important to establish regular habits so that you are less likely to make mistakes.

Before taking any medicine, read the label and any accompanying information. Consult books to learn the purpose, side effects, and other information you may need about the medicine to take it safely and intelligently. If you have unanswered questions, check with your health care provider.

The label on the container of a prescription medicine should bear your first and last name; the name of the prescriber; the pharmacy address and telephone number; the prescription number so it can be located for refills or in case of emergency; the date of dispensing; and directions for use. Some states or provinces may have additional requirements. If the name of the drug product is not on the label, ask the pharmacist to include the brand (if any) and generic names. An expiration date may also appear. All of this information is important in identifying your medicines and using them properly. In general, the labels on the containers should never be removed and all medicines should be kept in their original containers.

Some tips for taking medicines safely and accurately include the following:

- Read the label of each medicine container three times:
  —before you remove it from its storage place,
  —before you take the lid off the container to remove the dose, and
  —before you replace the container in its storage place.
- Never take medicines in the dark even if you believe you know exactly where to find them.
- Use standard measuring devices to take your medicines (the household teaspoon, cup, and glass vary widely in the amount they hold). Ask your pharmacist for help with measuring.
- Set bottles and boxes of medicines on a clear area, well back from the edge of the surface to prevent containers and/or caps from being knocked to the floor.

lix

- When pouring liquid medicines, pick up the container with the label against the palm of your hand to protect it from being stained by dripping medicine.

- Wipe off the top and neck of bottles of liquid medicines to keep labels from being obscured, and to make it less likely that the lid will stick.

- Shake all liquid suspensions of drug products before pouring so that ingredients are mixed thoroughly.

- If you are to take medicine with water, take a full, 8 oz. glassful, not just enough to get it down. Too little liquid with some medicines can prevent the medicine from working like it should or can cause throat irritation if the medicine does not get completely to the stomach.

- Replace the lid on one container before opening another to avoid accidental confusion of lids, labels, and medicines.

- When you are called to the door or telephone or are otherwise interrupted while taking your medicine, take the container with you or put the medicine up out of the reach of small children. It only takes a second for them to take an overdose. When you return, check the label of the medicine to be sure you have the right one before taking it.

- Do not crush tablets or open capsules to take the powder or granules with food or beverages unless you have checked with your health care provider and know that this will not affect the action of the medicine. If you have difficulty swallowing a tablet or capsule, check with your health care provider about the availability of a different dosage form.

- Follow any diet instructions or other treatment measures prescribed by your health care provider.

- If at any point you realize you have taken the wrong medicine or the wrong amount, call your health care provider immediately. In an emergency, call your local emergency number.

When you have finished taking your medicines, mark it down immediately on your medication calendar to avoid "double dosing." Also, make notes of any unusual changes in your body: change in weight, color or amount of urine, perspiration, sputum; your pulse, temperature, or any other items you may have been instructed to observe for your condition or your medicine.

When your medicines are being managed by someone else, for example, when you are a patient in a hospital or nursing home, question what is happening to you and communicate what you know about your previous drug therapy—or any other treatments. If you know you always take one, not two, of a certain tablet, say so and ask that your record be checked before you agree to take the medicine. If you are there for pain in your back and they are putting drops in your eyes, speak up; if you know you took that medicine an hour ago, tell the nurse. Your concerns may be unfounded—your health care provider may have forgotten to tell you about a change in your therapy, and different brands of the same drug may not look alike. Then again, you might be right.

Many hospitals and nursing homes now offer counseling in medicine management as part of their discharge planning for patients. If you or a family member is getting ready to come home, ask your health care provider if you can be part of such instruction since you will have to manage the medicines at home.

The "Expiration Date" on Medicine Labels

To assure that a drug product meets applicable standards of identity, strength, quality, and purity at the time of use, an "expiration date" is added by the manufacturer to the label of most prescription and nonprescription drug products.

The expiration date on a drug product is valid only as long as the product is stored in the original, unopened container under the storage conditions specified by the manufacturer. Among other things, drugs can be affected by humidity, temperature, light, and even air. A medicine taken after the expiration date may have changed in potency or the medicine may have formed harmful material as it deteriorates (for example, as sometimes happens with tetracyclines). In other instances, for injectables, eye drops, or other sterile products, contamination with germs may have occurred. Therefore, the safest rule is not to use any medicine beyond the expiration date.

Preventing deterioration

A drug begins to deteriorate the minute it is made. This rate of deterioration is factored in by the manufacturer in calculating the expiration date. Keeping the drug product in the container supplied by the pharmacist helps slow down deterioration. Storing the drug in the prescribed manner—for example, in a light-resistant container or in a cool, dry place (not the bathroom medicine cabinet)—also helps. The need for medicines to be kept in their pharmacist-dispensed containers and to be stored properly to minimize deterioration cannot be overstressed.

Patients sometimes ask their health care providers to prescribe a large quantity of a particular medicine they are taking in order to "economize." This may be a false economy; especially if, as a result of the medicine's deterioration, the illness is not properly treated, or the medicine causes an unexpected reaction. Therefore, your health care provider may recommend against this practice.

Sometimes deterioration can be recognized by physical changes in the drug, such as a change in odor, or in appearance; for example, aspirin tablets develop a vinegar odor when they break down. These changes are not true of all drugs, however, and the absence of physical changes should not be assumed to mean no deterioration has occurred.

Some liquid medicines mixed at the pharmacy will have a "beyond use" date put on the label by the pharmacist. This expiration date is calculated from the date of preparation in the pharmacy. This is a definite date, after which you should discard any of the medicine that remains.

If your prescription medicines do not bear an "expiration" or "beyond use" date, your dispensing pharmacist is the best person to advise you concerning how long they can be safely utilized.

About the Medicines You Are Taking

New Drugs—From Idea to Marketplace

To be sold legitimately in the United States, new drugs must pass through a rigorous system of approval specified in the Food, Drug, and Cosmetic Act and supervised by the Food and Drug Administration (FDA). Except for certain drugs subject to other regulatory provisions, no new drug for human use may be marketed in this country unless FDA has approved a "New Drug Application" (NDA) for it.

The idea

The creation of a new drug usually starts with an idea. Most likely that idea results from the study of a disease or group of symptoms, or may come from observations of clinical research. This may involve many years of study, or the idea may occur from an accidental discovery in a research laboratory or may be a coincidental discovery, as happened with penicillin.

Idea development takes place most often in the laboratory of a pharmaceutical company, but may also happen in laboratories at research institutions like the National Institutes of Health, at medical centers and universities, or in the laboratory of a chemical company.

Animal testing

The idea for a new drug is first tested on animals to help determine how toxic the substance may be. Most drugs interfere in some way with normal body functions. These animal studies are designed to discover the degree of that interference and the extent of the toxic effects.

After successful animal testing, perhaps over several years, the sponsors of the new drug apply to the FDA for an Investigational New Drug (IND) application—approval to test in humans. As part of their request, the sponsoring manufacturer must submit the information about the drug that was found as a result of the animal studies plus a detailed outline of the proposed human testing and information about the researchers to be involved in the human trials.

Human testing

Drug testing in humans usually consists of three consecutive phases. "Informed consent" must be secured from all volunteers participating in this testing.

Phase I testing is most often done on young, healthy adults. This testing is done on a relatively small number of subjects, generally between 20 and 80. Its purpose is to learn more about the biochemistry of the drug, how it acts on the body, and how the body reacts to it. The procedure differs for some drugs, however. For example, Phase I testing of drugs used to treat cancer involves actual patients with the disease from the beginning of testing.

During Phase II, small controlled clinical studies designed to test the effectiveness and relative safety of the drug are done on closely monitored patients who have the disease for which the drug is being tested. Their numbers seldom go beyond 100 to 200 patients. Some volunteers for Phase II testing who have severely complicating conditions may be excluded.

A "control" group of people of comparable physical and disease types is used to do double-blind, controlled experiments for most drugs. These are conducted by medical investigators thoroughly familiar with the disease and this type of research. In a double-blind experiment, the patient, the health care provider, and other personnel do not know or are "blind" as to whether the patient is receiving the drug being tested, another active drug, or no medicine at all (a placebo or "sugar pill"). This helps eliminate bias and assures the accuracy of results. The findings of these tests are statistically analyzed to determine whether they are "significant" or due to chance alone.

Phase III consists of larger studies. This testing is performed after effectiveness of the drug has been established initially and is intended to gather additional evidence of effectiveness for specific uses of the drug. These studies also help discover adverse drug reactions that may occur with the drug. Phase III studies involve a few hundred to several thousand patients who have the disease the drug is intended to treat.

Patients with additional diseases or those receiving other therapy may be included in later Phase II and Phase III studies, since they would be expected to be representative of certain segments of the population who will be receiving the drug following approval for marketing.

Final approval

When a sponsor believes the investigational studies on a drug have shown it to be safe and effective in treating specific conditions, a New Drug Application (NDA) is submitted to FDA, accompanied by all the documentation from the company's research. This includes everything they know about the medicine as well as the complete records of all the animal and human testing. This documentation can run to many thousands of pages.

The application, together with its documentation, must then be reviewed by FDA physicians, pharmacologists, chemists, statisticians, and other professionals experienced in evaluating new drugs. Proposed information for the physician and pharmacist that is to be placed on the label of the medicine and in its package insert is screened for accuracy, completeness, and conformity to FDA-approved wording.

The regulations call for the FDA to review an NDA within 180 days. This period may be extended and, in fact, takes an average of 2 to 3 years. When all research phases are considered, the actual time it takes from idea to marketplace may be 8 to 10 years or even longer. However, for drugs representing major therapeutic advances, FDA may "fast-track" the approval process to try to get those drugs to patients who need them as soon as possible.

After approval

After a drug is marketed, the manufacturer must inform the FDA of any unexpected side effects or toxicity that comes to its attention. Consumers and health care professionals have an important role in helping to identify any previously unreported effects. New information may be added to the drug's labeling or the FDA can withdraw approval for marketing at any time if new evidence indicates the drug presents an "imminent hazard."

Generic drugs

After a new drug is approved for marketing, a patent will generally protect the financial interests of the drug's developer for a number of years after approval. The traditional protection period is for 17 years but in reality the period is much less because of the extended period of time needed to gain approval before marketing can begin. Recognizing that a considerable part of a drug's patent life may be tied up in the approval process, Congress in 1984 passed a law providing patent extension for drugs whose commercial sale may have been unduly delayed because of the approval process.

Any manufacturer can apply for permission to produce and market a drug after the patent for the drug has expired. Following a procedure called an Abbreviated New Drug Application (ANDA), the applicant must show that its product is bioequivalent to the originator's product. Although the extensive clinical testing the originator had to complete during the drug's development does not have to be repeated, comparative testing between the products in question must be done to ensure that the products will indeed be therapeutically equivalent.

Drug Names

Every drug must have a nonproprietary name; that is, a name that is available for each manufacturer of it to use. These names are commonly called generic names.

Although FDA requires that the generic name of a drug product be placed on its labeling, manufacturers often coin brand (trade) names to use in promotion of their particular product. In general, brand names are shorter, catchier, and easier to use than the corresponding generic name. The brand name manufacturer will then emphasize its proprietary product name (i.e., one that cannot be used by anyone else) in its advertising and other promotions. In many instances, the consumer may not recognize that a drug being sold under one particular brand name is indeed available under other brand names or by generic name. Ask your pharmacist if you have any questions about the names of your medicines.

Drug Quality

After an NDA or an ANDA has been approved, the manufacturer of that product must then meet all requirements relating to production, including current Good Manufacturing Practice regulations of the Food and Drug Administration (FDA) and any applicable standards relating to strength, quality, purity, packaging, and labeling that are established by the *United States Pharmacopeia* (USP).

It should be obvious that the mere placing of a brand name on the label does not in itself assure the quality of the product inside the container. Rather, the quality of a product depends on the manufacturer's ability to create a good mix of inactive ingredients into which to put the active ingredient to make the final dosage form (for example, tablet, capsule, syrup, or suppository) *and* to do so consistently from batch to batch.

Routine product testing by the manufacturer is required by the Good Manufacturing Practice regulations of the FDA (the FDA itself does not routinely test all products, except in cases where there is a suspicion that something might be wrong). In addition to governmental standards, drug products must meet public standards of strength, quality, and purity that are published in the USP. In order to market their products, all manufacturers in the United States must meet USP-established standards unless they specifically choose not to meet the standards for a particular product, in which case that product's label must state that it is "not USP" (this occurs very rarely).

Differences in Drug Products

Although standards to ensure strength, quality, purity, and bioequivalence exist for drug products, the standards allow for variations in certain factors that may produce other differences from product to product. These product variations may be important or of concern to some patients since not all patients are "equivalent." For example, the size, shape, and coating may vary and, therefore, be harder or easier for some patients to swallow; an oral liquid will taste good to some patients and taste awful to others; one manufacturer may use lactose as an inactive ingredient in its product while a therapeutically equivalent product may use some other inactive ingredient; one product may contain sugar or alcohol while another product may not.

In deciding to use one therapeutically equivalent product over another, consumers should keep the following in mind:

• Consider convenience factors that may be important in relation to the use of a drug product (for example, ease of taking a particular dosage form).

• Don't overlook the convenience of the package. The package must protect the drug in accordance with USP requirements, but packages can be quite different in their ease of carrying, storing, opening, and measuring.

• If you have a known allergy or any type of dietary restriction, you need to be aware of the pharmaceutic or "inactive" ingredients that may be present in medicines you have to take. These inactive ingredients may vary from product to product.

- Price is always a consideration. The selection of the specific product to be dispensed may be the most significant factor in the price of a prescription. Talk to the pharmacist about it. Depending on state laws and regulations, the consumer may need to talk to the physician first about changing brands, as the pharmacist may have no alternative but to dispense the specific product the physician originally prescribed.

Aside from differences in the drug product, there are many other factors that you often cannot control that may influence the effectiveness of a medicine. For example, your diet, body chemistry, medical conditions, or other drugs you are taking may affect how much of a dose of a particular medicine gets into the body.

For a majority of the drugs you might take, slight differences in the amount of drug made available to the body will not make any therapeutic difference. For other drugs, the precise amount that gets into the body is more critical. For example, some heart medicines or medicines for epilepsy may create problems for the patient if the dose delivered to the body varies for some reason.

For those drugs that fall in the critical category, it is probably a good idea to stay on the specific product you started on, with any changes being made only if the prescribing health care provider is aware of the change. Your health care provider can help you with questions about these medicines. Also, if you are on such a medicine and you feel that a certain batch is more potent or does not work as well as previous batches, check with your health care provider.

Drug Monographs

Entries appear alphabetically by generic or "family" names (groupings of closely related medicines). To find the location of brand name entries, refer to the Index at the back of the book.

ACYCLOVIR   Systemic

A commonly used brand name in the U.S. and Canada is Zovirax.
Other commonly used names are aciclovir and acycloguanosine.

Description

Acyclovir (ay-SYE-kloe-veer) belongs to the family of medicines called antivirals, which are used to treat infections
caused by viruses. Usually these medicines work for only
one kind or group of virus infections.

Acyclovir is used to treat the symptoms of herpes virus infections of the genitals (sex organs), the skin, the brain, and
mucous membranes. Although acyclovir will not cure herpes,
it does help relieve the pain and discomfort and helps the
sores (if any) heal faster. Acyclovir is also used to treat
chickenpox.

Acyclovir may also be used for other virus infections as
determined by your doctor. However, it does not work in
treating certain viruses, such as the common cold.

Acyclovir is available only with your doctor's prescription,
in the following dosage forms:

Oral
- Capsules (U.S.)
- Oral suspension (U.S.)
- Tablets (Canada)

Parenteral
- Injection (U.S. and Canada)

*It is very important that you read and understand the fol-
lowing information.* If any of it causes you special concern,
check with your doctor. Also, *if you have any questions* or
if you want more information about this medicine or your
medical problem, *ask your doctor, nurse, or pharmacist.*

Before Using This Medicine

In deciding to use a medicine, the risks of taking the medicine must be weighed against the good it will do. This is a
decision you and your doctor will make. For acyclovir, the
following should be considered:

Allergies—Tell your doctor if you have ever had any unusual or allergic reaction to acyclovir or ganciclovir. Also tell your doctor and pharmacist if you are allergic to any other substances, such as foods, sulfites or other preservatives, or dyes.

Pregnancy—Acyclovir has been used in pregnant women and has not been reported to cause birth defects or other problems. However, studies have not been done in humans. Studies in rabbits have shown that acyclovir given by injection may keep the fetus from becoming attached to the lining of the uterus (womb). However, acyclovir has not been shown to cause birth defects or other problems in mice given many times the usual human dose, or in rats or rabbits given several times the usual human dose.

Breast-feeding—Acyclovir passes into the breast milk. However, it has not been reported to cause problems in nursing babies.

Children—A limited number of studies have been done using oral acyclovir in children, and it has not caused different effects or problems in children than it does in adults.

Older adults—Acyclovir has been used in the elderly and has not been shown to cause different side effects or problems in older people than it does in younger adults.

Other medicines—Although certain medicines should not be used together at all, in many cases two different medicines may be used together even if an interaction might occur. In these cases, changes in dose or other precautions may be necessary. If you are receiving acyclovir by injection it is especially important that your doctor and pharmacist know if you are taking any of the following:

- Carmustine (e.g., BiCNU) or
- Cisplatin (e.g., Platinol) or
- Combination pain medicine containing acetaminophen and aspirin (e.g., Excedrin) or other salicylates or
- Cyclosporine (e.g., Sandimmune) or
- Deferoxamine (e.g., Desferal) (with long-term use) or
- Gold salts (medicine for arthritis) or
- Inflammation or pain medicine, except narcotics, or
- Lithium (e.g., Lithane) or
- Other medicine for infection or

- Penicillamine (e.g., Cuprimine) or
- Plicamycin (e.g., Mithracin) or
- Streptozocin (e.g., Zanosar)—Concurrent use of these medicines with acyclovir by injection may increase the chance for side effects, especially when kidney disease is present

Other medical problems—The presence of other medical problems may affect the use of acyclovir. Make sure you tell your doctor if you are receiving acyclovir by injection and have any of the following medical problems, especially:

- Kidney disease—Kidney disease may increase blood levels of acyclovir, increasing the chance of side effects
- Nerve disease—Acyclovir by injection may increase the chance for nervous system side effects

Before you begin using any new medicine (prescription or nonprescription) or if you develop any new medical problem while you are using this medicine, check with your doctor, nurse, or pharmacist.

Proper Use of This Medicine

Patient information about the treatment of herpes is available with this medicine. Read it carefully before using this medicine.

Acyclovir is best used as soon as possible after the symptoms of herpes infection (for example, pain, burning, blisters) begin to appear.

Acyclovir capsules, tablets, and oral suspension may be taken with meals.

If you are taking acyclovir for the *treatment of chickenpox*, it is best to start taking acyclovir as soon as possible after the first sign of the chickenpox rash, usually within one day.

If you are using *acyclovir oral suspension*, use a specially marked measuring spoon or other device to measure each dose accurately. The average household teaspoon may not hold the right amount of liquid.

Do not use after the expiration date on the label. The medicine may not work properly. Check with your pharmacist if you have any questions about this.

To help clear up your herpes infection, *keep taking acyclovir for the full time of treatment,* even if your symptoms begin to clear up after a few days. *Do not miss any doses.* However, *do not use this medicine more often or for a longer time than your doctor ordered.*

Dosing—The dose of acyclovir will be different for different patients. *Follow your doctor's orders or the directions on the label.* The following information includes only the average doses of acyclovir. Your dose may be different if you have kidney disease. *If your dose is different, do not change it* unless your doctor tells you to do so.

- The number of capsules or tablets or teaspoonful of suspension that you take depends on the strength of the medicine. Also, *the number of doses you take each day, the time allowed between doses, and the length of time you take the medicine depend on the medical problem for which you are taking acyclovir.*

- For *oral* dosage forms (capsules, oral suspension, or tablets):

  —Adults and children 12 years of age and older: 200 to 800 milligrams two to five times a day for up to ten days.

  —Children 2 to 12 years of age: Treatment of chickenpox, up to 800 milligrams per dose (dose is based on body weight) four times a day for five days.

  —Children up to 2 years of age: Dose must be determined by the doctor.

- For *injection* dosage form:

  —Adults and children 12 years of age and older: Dose is based on body weight (5 to 10 milligrams of acyclovir per kilogram [2.3 to 4.6 milligrams per pound] of body weight). It is given slowly into a vein over at least a one-hour period and repeated every eight hours for up to ten days.

  —Children up to 12 years of age: Dose is based on body weight or body size. It is given slowly into a vein over at least a one-hour period and repeated every eight hours for up to ten days.

Missed dose—If you do miss a dose of this medicine, take it as soon as possible. However, if it is almost time for your next dose, skip the missed dose and go back to your regular dosing schedule. Do not double doses.

Storage—To store this medicine:
- Keep out of the reach of children.
- Store away from heat and direct light.
- Do not store the capsule or tablet form of this medicine in the bathroom, near the kitchen sink, or in other damp places. Heat or moisture may cause the medicine to break down.
- Do not keep outdated medicine or medicine no longer needed. Be sure that any discarded medicine is out of the reach of children.

Precautions While Using This Medicine

Women with genital herpes may be more likely to get cancer of the cervix (mouth of the womb). Therefore, it is very important that Pap tests be taken at least once a year to check for cancer. Cervical cancer can be cured if found and treated early.

If your symptoms do not improve within a few days, or if they become worse, check with your doctor.

The areas affected by herpes should be kept as clean and dry as possible. Also, wear loose-fitting clothing to avoid irritating the sores (blisters).

It is important to remember that acyclovir will not keep you from spreading herpes to others.

Herpes infection of the genitals can be caught from or spread to your partner during any sexual activity. Even though you may get herpes if your partner has no symptoms, the infection is more likely to be spread if sores are present. This is true until the sores are completely healed and the scabs have fallen off. *Therefore, it is best to avoid any sexual activity if either you or your sexual partner has any symptoms of herpes.* The use of a latex condom ("rubber") may help prevent the spread of herpes. However, spermicidal (sperm-killing) jelly or a diaphragm will probably not help.

Side Effects of This Medicine

Along with its needed effects, a medicine may cause some unwanted effects. Although not all of these side effects may occur, if they do occur they may need medical attention.

Check with your doctor immediately if any of the following side effects occur:

> *For acyclovir injection only*
> > *More common*
> > > Pain, swelling, or redness at place of injection
> >
> > *Less common (more common with rapid injection)*
> > > Abdominal or stomach pain; decreased frequency of urination or amount of urine; increased thirst; loss of appetite; nausea or vomiting; unusual tiredness or weakness
> >
> > *Rare*
> > > Confusion; convulsions (seizures); hallucinations (seeing, hearing, or feeling things that are not there); trembling

Other side effects may occur that usually do not need medical attention. These side effects may go away during treatment as your body adjusts to the medicine. However, check with your doctor if any of the following side effects continue or are bothersome:

> *For oral acyclovir only*
> > *Less common (especially seen with long-term use or high doses)*
> > > Diarrhea; headache; lightheadedness; nausea or vomiting

Other side effects not listed above may also occur in some patients. If you notice any other effects, check with your doctor.

Additional Information

Once a medicine has been approved for marketing for a certain use, experience may show that it is also useful for other medical problems. Although not specifically included in product labeling, acyclovir by injection is used in certain patients with the following medical conditions:

- Disseminated neonatal herpes simplex (widespread infection in the newborn)
- Herpes simplex (prevention of)

Other than the above information, there is no additional information relating to proper use, precautions, or side effects for these uses.

ALLOPURINOL Systemic

Some commonly used brand names are:

In the U.S.

Lopurin   Zyloprim

Generic name product may also be available.

In Canada

Alloprin   Purinol
Apo-Allopurinol   Zyloprim
Novopurol

Description

Allopurinol (al-oh-PURE-i-nole) is used to treat chronic gout (gouty arthritis). This condition is caused by too much uric acid in the blood.

This medicine works by causing less uric acid to be produced by the body. Allopurinol will not relieve a gout attack that has already started. Also, it does not cure gout, but it will help prevent gout attacks. However, it works only after you have been taking it regularly for a few months. Allopurinol will help prevent gout attacks only as long as you continue to take it.

Allopurinol is also used to prevent or treat other medical problems that may occur if too much uric acid is present in the body. These include certain kinds of kidney stones or other kidney problems.

Allopurinol is available only with your doctor's prescription in the following dosage form:

Oral
  • Tablets (U.S. and Canada)

It is very important that you read and understand the following information. If any of it causes you special concern, check with your doctor. Also, *if you have any questions* or if you want more information about this medicine or your medical problem, *ask your doctor, nurse, or pharmacist.*

Before Using This Medicine

In deciding to use a medicine, the risks of taking the medicine must be weighed against the good it will do. This is a decision you and your doctor will make. For allopurinol, the following should be considered:

Allergies—Tell your doctor if you have ever had any unusual or allergic reaction to allopurinol. Also tell your doctor and pharmacist if you are allergic to any other substances, such as foods, preservatives, or dyes.

Pregnancy—Although studies on birth defects have not been done in humans, allopurinol has not been reported to cause problems in humans. In one study in mice, large amounts of allopurinol caused birth defects and other unwanted effects. However, allopurinol did not cause birth defects or other problems in rats or rabbits given doses up to 20 times the amount usually given to humans.

Breast-feeding—Allopurinol passes into the breast milk. However, this medicine has not been reported to cause problems in nursing babies.

Children—This medicine has been tested in children and, in effective doses, has not been shown to cause different side effects or problems than it does in adults.

Older adults—Many medicines have not been studied specifically in older people. Therefore, it may not be known whether they work exactly the same way they do in younger adults or if they cause different side effects or problems in older people. There is no specific information comparing use of allopurinol in the elderly with use in other age groups.

Other medicines—Although certain medicines should not be used together at all, in other cases two different medicines may be used together even if an interaction might occur. In these cases, your doctor may want to change the dose, or other precautions may be necessary. When you are taking allopurinol, it is especially important that your doctor and pharmacist know if you are taking any of the following:

- Anticoagulants (blood thinners)—Allopurinol may increase the chance of bleeding; changes in the dose of the anticoagulant may be needed, depending on blood test results

- Azathioprine (e.g., Imuran) or
- Mercaptopurine (e.g., Purinethol)—Allopurinol may cause higher blood levels of azathioprine or mercaptopurine, leading to an increased chance of serious side effects

Other medical problems—The presence of other medical problems may affect the use of allopurinol. Make sure you tell your doctor if you have any other medical problems, especially:

- Diabetes mellitus (sugar diabetes) or
- High blood pressure or
- Kidney disease—There is an increased risk of severe allergic reactions or other serious effects; a change in the dose of allopurinol may be needed

Proper Use of This Medicine

If this medicine upsets your stomach, it may be taken after meals. If stomach upset (indigestion, nausea, vomiting, diarrhea, or stomach pain) continues, check with your doctor.

In order for this medicine to help you, it must be taken regularly as ordered by your doctor.

To help prevent kidney stones while taking allopurinol, adults should drink at least 10 to 12 full glasses (8 ounces each) of fluids each day unless otherwise directed by their doctor. Check with the doctor about the amount of fluids that children should drink each day while receiving this medicine. Also, your doctor may want you to take another medicine to make your urine less acid. It is important that you follow your doctor's instructions very carefully.

For patients taking allopurinol for *gout:*

- After you begin to take allopurinol, gout attacks may continue to occur for a while. However, if you take this medicine regularly as directed by your doctor, the attacks will gradually become less frequent and less painful. After you have been taking allopurinol regularly for several months, they may stop completely.

- Allopurinol is used to help prevent gout attacks. It will not relieve an attack that has already started. *Even if you take another medicine for gout attacks, continue to take this medicine also.*

Missed dose—If you miss a dose of this medicine, take it as soon as possible. However, if it is almost time for your next dose, skip the missed dose and go back to your regular dosing schedule. Do not double doses.

Storage—To store this medicine:

- Keep out of the reach of children.
- Store away from heat and direct light.
- Do not store this medicine in the bathroom, near the kitchen sink, or in other damp places. Heat or moisture may cause the medicine to break down.
- Do not keep outdated medicine or medicine no longer needed. Be sure that any discarded medicine is out of the reach of children.

Before you begin using any new medicine (prescription or nonprescription) or if you develop any new medical problem while you are using this medicine, check with your doctor, nurse, or pharmacist.

Precautions While Using This Medicine

Your doctor should check your progress at regular visits. A blood test may be needed to make sure that this medicine is working properly and is not causing unwanted effects.

Drinking too much alcohol may increase the amount of uric acid in the blood and lessen the effects of allopurinol. Therefore, people with gout and other people with too much uric acid in the body should be careful to limit the amount of alcohol they drink.

Taking too much vitamin C may make the urine more acidic and increase the possibility of kidney stones forming while you are taking allopurinol. Therefore, check with your doctor before you take vitamin C while taking this medicine.

Check with your doctor immediately:
- *if you notice a skin rash, hives, or itching while you are taking allopurinol.*
- *if chills, fever, joint pain, muscle aches or pains, sore throat, or nausea or vomiting occur, especially if they occur together with or shortly after a skin rash.*

Very rarely, these effects may be the first signs of a serious reaction to the medicine.

Allopurinol may cause some people to become drowsy or less alert than they are normally. *Make sure you know how you react to this medicine before you drive, use machines, or do anything else that could be dangerous if you are not alert.*

Side Effects of This Medicine

Along with its needed effects, a medicine may cause some unwanted effects. Although not all of these side effects may occur, if they do occur they may need medical attention.

Stop taking this medicine and check with your doctor immediately if any of the following side effects occur:

More common

Skin rash or sores, hives, or itching

Rare

Black, tarry stools; bleeding sores on lips; blood in urine or stools; chills, fever, muscle aches or pains, nausea, or vomiting—especially if occurring with or shortly after a skin rash; difficult or painful urination; pinpoint red spots on skin; redness, tenderness, burning, or peeling of skin; red and/or irritated eyes; red, thickened, or scaly skin; shortness of breath, troubled breathing, tightness in chest, or wheezing; sores, ulcers, or white spots in mouth or on lips; sore throat and fever; sudden decrease in amount of urine; swelling in upper abdominal (stomach) area; swelling of face, fingers, feet, or lower legs; unusual bleeding or bruising; unusual weakness; weight gain (rapid); yellow eyes or skin

Also, check with your doctor as soon as possible if any of the following side effects occur:

Rare

Loosening of fingernails; numbness, tingling, pain, or weakness in hands or feet; pain in lower back or side; unexplained nosebleeds

Other side effects may occur that usually do not need medical attention. These side effects may go away during treatment as your body adjusts to the medicine. However, check with your doctor if any of the following side effects continue or are bothersome:

Less common or rare

Diarrhea; drowsiness; headache occurring without other side effects; indigestion; nausea or vomiting occurring without a skin rash or other side effects; stomach pain occurring without other side effects; unusual hair loss

Other side effects not listed above may also occur in some patients. If you notice any other effects, check with your doctor.

AMANTADINE Systemic

Some commonly used brand names are:

In the U.S.

Symadine

Symmetrel

Generic name product may also be available.

In Canada

Symmetrel

Description

Amantadine (a-MAN-ta-deen) is an antiviral. It is used to prevent or treat certain influenza (flu) infections (type A). It may be given alone or along with flu shots. Amantadine will not work for colds, other types of flu, or other virus infections.

Amantadine also is an antidyskinetic. It is used to treat Parkinson's disease, sometimes called paralysis agitans or shaking palsy. It may be given alone or with other medicines for Parkinson's disease. By improving muscle control and reducing stiffness, this medicine allows more normal movements of the body as the disease symptoms are reduced. Amantadine is also used to treat stiffness and shaking caused by certain medicines used to treat nervous, mental, and emotional conditions.

Amantadine may be used for other conditions as determined by your doctor.

Amantadine is available only with your doctor's prescription, in the following dosage forms:
Oral
- Capsules (U.S. and Canada)
- Syrup (U.S. and Canada)

It is very important that you read and understand the following information. If any of it causes you special concern, check with your doctor. Also, *if you have any questions* or if you want more information about this medicine or your medical problem, *ask your doctor, nurse, or pharmacist.*

Before Using This Medicine

In deciding to use a medicine, the risks of taking the medicine must be weighed against the good it will do. This is a decision you and your doctor will make. For amantadine, the following should be considered:

Allergies—Tell your doctor if you have ever had any unusual or allergic reaction to amantadine. Also tell your doctor and pharmacist if you are allergic to any other substances, such as foods, preservatives, or dyes.

Pregnancy—Studies have not been done in humans. However, studies in some animals have shown that amantadine is harmful to the fetus and causes birth defects.

Breast-feeding—Amantadine passes into breast milk. However, the effects of amantadine in neonates and infants are not known.

Children—This medicine has been tested in children over one year of age and has not been shown to cause different side effects or problems in these children than it does in adults. There is no specific information comparing the use of amantadine in children under one year of age with use in other age groups.

Older adults—Elderly people are especially sensitive to the effects of amantadine. Confusion, difficult urination, blurred vision, constipation, and dry mouth, nose, and throat may be especially likely to occur.

Other medicines—Although certain medicines should not be used together at all, in other cases two different medicines may be used together even if an interaction might occur. In these cases, your doctor may want to change the dose, or other precautions may be necessary. When you are taking amantadine, it is especially important that your doctor and pharmacist know if you are taking any of the following:

- Amphetamines or
- Appetite suppressants (diet pills), except fenfluramine (e.g., Pondimin), or
- Caffeine (e.g., NoDoz) or
- Chlophedianol (e.g., Ulone) or
- Cocaine or
- Medicine for asthma or other breathing problems or
- Medicine for colds, sinus problems, or hay fever or other allergies (including nose drops or sprays) or
- Methylphenidate (e.g., Ritalin) or
- Nabilone (e.g., Cesamet) or
- Pemoline (e.g., Cylert)—The use of amantadine with these medicines may increase the chance of unwanted effects such as nervousness, irritability, trouble in sleeping, and possibly seizures or irregular heartbeat
- Anticholinergics (medicine for abdominal or stomach spasms or cramps)—The use of amantadine with these medicines may increase the chance of unwanted effects such as blurred vision, dryness of the mouth, confusion, hallucinations, and nightmares

Other medical problems—The presence of other medical problems may affect the use of amantadine. Make sure you tell your doctor if you have any other medical problems, especially:

- Eczema (recurring)—Amantadine may cause or worsen eczema
- Epilepsy or other seizures (history of)—Amantadine may increase the frequency of seizures in patients with a seizure disorder
- Heart disease or other circulation problems or
- Swelling of feet and ankles—Amantadine may increase the chance of swelling of the feet and ankles, and may worsen heart disease or circulation problems
- Kidney disease—Amantadine is removed from the body by the kidneys; patients with kidney disease will need to receive a lower dose of amantadine
- Mental or emotional illness—Higher doses of amantadine may cause confusion, hallucinations, and nightmares

Before you begin using any new medicine (prescription or nonprescription) or if you develop any new medical problem while you are using this medicine, check with your doctor, nurse, or pharmacist.

Proper Use of This Medicine

For patients *taking amantadine to prevent or treat flu infections:*

- Talk to your doctor about the possibility of getting a flu shot if you have not had one yet.
- This medicine is *best taken before exposure, or as soon as possible after exposure,* to people who have the flu.
- To help keep you from getting the flu, *keep taking this medicine for the full time of treatment.* Or if you already have the flu, you should still continue taking this medicine for the full time of treatment even if you begin to feel better after a few days. This will help to clear up your infection completely. If you stop taking this medicine too soon, your symptoms may return. This medicine should be taken for at least 2 days after all your flu symptoms have disappeared.
- This medicine works best when there is a constant amount in the blood. *To help keep the amount constant,*

do not miss any doses. Also, it is best to take the doses at evenly spaced times day and night. For example, if you are to take 2 doses a day, the doses should be spaced about 12 hours apart. If this interferes with your sleep or other daily activities, or if you need help in planning the best times to take your medicine, check with your doctor, nurse, or pharmacist.

- **Missed dose**—If you do miss a dose of this medicine, take it as soon as possible. This will help to keep a constant amount of medicine in the blood. However, if it is almost time for your next dose, skip the missed dose and go back to your regular dosing schedule. Do not double doses.

- If you are using the oral liquid form of amantadine, use a specially marked measuring spoon or other device to measure each dose accurately. The average household teaspoon may not hold the right amount of liquid.

For patients *taking amantadine for Parkinson's disease or movement problems* caused by certain medicines used to treat nervous, mental, and emotional conditions:

- *Take this medicine exactly as directed by your doctor.* Do not miss any doses and do not take more medicine than your doctor ordered.

- **Missed dose**—If you do miss a dose of this medicine, take it as soon as possible. However, if it is within 4 hours of your next dose, skip the missed dose and go back to your regular dosing schedule. Do not double doses.

- Improvement in the symptoms of Parkinson's disease usually occurs in about 2 days. However, in some patients this medicine must be taken for up to 2 weeks before full benefit is seen.

Storage—To store this medicine:

- Keep out of the reach of children.
- Store away from heat and direct light.
- Do not store the capsule form of this medicine in the bathroom, near the kitchen sink, or in other damp places. Heat or moisture may cause the medicine to break down.

- Keep the oral liquid form of this medicine from freezing.
- Do not keep outdated medicine or medicine no longer needed. Be sure that any discarded medicine is out of the reach of children.

Precautions While Using This Medicine

Drinking alcoholic beverages while taking this medicine may cause increased side effects such as circulation problems, dizziness, lightheadedness, fainting, or confusion. Therefore, *you should not drink alcoholic beverages while you are taking this medicine.*

This medicine may cause some people to become dizzy, confused, or lightheaded, or to have blurred vision or trouble concentrating. *Make sure you know how you react to this medicine before you drive, use machines, or do anything else that could be dangerous if you are dizzy or are not alert or able to see well.* If these reactions are especially bothersome, check with your doctor.

Getting up suddenly from a lying or sitting position may also be a problem because of the dizziness, lightheadedness, or fainting that may be caused by this medicine. Getting up slowly may help. If this problem continues or gets worse, check with your doctor.

Amantadine may cause dryness of the mouth, nose, and throat. For temporary relief of mouth dryness, use sugarless candy or gum, melt bits of ice in your mouth, or use a saliva substitute. However, if your mouth continues to feel dry for more than 2 weeks, check with your medical doctor or dentist. Continuing dryness of the mouth may increase the chance of dental disease, including tooth decay, gum disease, and fungus infections.

This medicine may cause purplish red, net-like, blotchy spots on the skin. This problem occurs more often in females and usually occurs on the legs and/or feet after taking this medicine regularly for a month or more. Although the blotchy spots may remain as long as you are taking this medicine, they usually go away gradually within 2 to 12 weeks after you stop taking this medicine. If you have any questions about this, check with your doctor.

For patients *taking amantadine to prevent or treat flu infections:*
- If your symptoms do not improve within a few days, or if they become worse, check with your doctor.

For patients *taking amantadine for Parkinson's disease or movement problems* caused by certain medicines used to treat nervous, mental, and emotional conditions:
- *Patients with Parkinson's disease must be careful not to overdo physical activities as their condition improves and body movements become easier* since injuries resulting from falls may occur. Such activities must be gradually increased to give your body time to adjust to changing balance, circulation, and coordination.
- Some patients may notice that this medicine gradually loses its effect while they are taking it regularly for a few months. If you notice this, check with your doctor. Your doctor may want to adjust the dose or stop the medicine for a while and then restart it to restore its effect.
- *Do not suddenly stop taking this medicine without first checking with your doctor* since your Parkinson's disease may get worse very quickly. Your doctor may want you to reduce your dose gradually before stopping the medicine completely.

Side Effects of This Medicine

Along with its needed effects, a medicine may cause some unwanted effects. Although not all of these side effects may occur, if they do occur they may need medical attention.

Check with your doctor immediately if any of the following side effects occur:

Less common
> Blurred vision; confusion (especially in elderly patients); difficult urination (especially in elderly patients); fainting; hallucinations (seeing, hearing, or feeling things that are not there)

Rare

Convulsions (seizures); decreased vision or any change in vision; difficulty in coordination; irritation and swelling of the eye; mental depression; skin rash; swelling of feet or lower legs; unexplained shortness of breath

Other side effects may occur that usually do not need medical attention. These side effects may go away during treatment as your body adjusts to the medicine. However, check with your doctor if any of the following side effects continue or are bothersome:

More common

Difficulty concentrating; dizziness or lightheadedness; headache; irritability; loss of appetite; nausea; nervousness; purplish red, net-like, blotchy spots on skin; trouble in sleeping or nightmares

Less common or rare

Constipation; dryness of the mouth, nose, and throat; vomiting

Other side effects not listed above may also occur in some patients. If you notice any other effects, check with your doctor.

Additional Information

Once a medicine has been approved for marketing for a certain use, experience may show that it is also useful for other medical problems. Although this use is not included in product labeling, amantadine is used in certain patients with the following medical condition:

- Unusual tiredness or weakness associated with multiple sclerosis

Other than the above information, there is no additional information relating to proper use, precautions, or side effects for this use.

ANABOLIC STEROIDS   Systemic

This information applies to the following medicines:

Nandrolone (NAN-droe-lone)
Oxandrolone (ox-AN-droe-lone)

Oxymetholone (ox-i-METH-oh-lone)
Stanozolol (stan-OH-zoe-lole)

Some commonly used brand names are:

For Nandrolone
   In the U.S.

Anabolin	Hybolin Decanoate
Anabolin LA-100	Hybolin-Improved
Androlone	Kabolin
Androlone 50	Nandrobolic
Androlone D	Nandrobolic L.A.
Deca-Durabolin	Neo-Durabolic
Durabolin	

   Generic name product may also be available.

   In Canada

Deca-Durabolin	Durabolin

For Oxandrolone†‡
   In the U.S.
      Anavar

For Oxymetholone
   In the U.S.
      Anadrol
   In Canada
      Anapolon 50

For Stanozolol
   In the U.S.
      Winstrol
   In Canada
      Winstrol

---

†Not commercially available in Canada.
‡Product is no longer being manufactured but may still be in circulation.

Description

This medicine belongs to the group of medicines known as anabolic (an-a-BOL-ik) steroids. They are related to testosterone, a male sex hormone. Anabolic steroids help to rebuild tissues that have become weak because of serious injury or illness. A diet high in proteins and calories is necessary with anabolic steroid treatment.

Anabolic steroids are used for several reasons:
- to help patients gain weight after a severe illness, injury, or continuing infection. They also are used when patients fail to gain or maintain normal weight because of unexplained medical reasons.
- to treat certain types of anemia.
- to treat certain kinds of breast cancer in some women.
- to treat hereditary angioedema, which causes swelling of the face, arms, legs, throat, windpipe, bowels, or sexual organs.

Anabolic steroids may also be used for other conditions as determined by your doctor.

Anabolic steroids are available only with your doctor's prescription, in the following dosage forms:

Oral
　Oxandrolone
　　- Tablets (U.S.)
　Oxymetholone
　　- Tablets (U.S. and Canada)
　Stanozolol
　　- Tablets (U.S. and Canada)

Parenteral
　Nandrolone
　　- Injection (U.S. and Canada)

It is very important that you read and understand the following information. If any of it causes you special concern, check with your doctor. Also, *if you have any questions* or if you want more information about this medicine or your medical problem, *ask your doctor, nurse, or pharmacist.*

Before Using This Medicine

In deciding to use a medicine, the risks of taking the medicine must be weighed against the good it will do. This is a decision you and your doctor will make. For anabolic steroids, the following should be considered:

Allergies—Tell your doctor if you have ever had any unusual or allergic reaction to anabolic steroids or androgens (male sex hormones). Also tell your doctor and pharmacist if you are allergic to any other substances, such as foods, preservatives, or dyes.

Pregnancy—Anabolic steroids are not recommended during pregnancy. They may cause the development of male features in the female fetus and premature growth and development of male features in the male fetus. Be sure you have discussed this with your doctor.

Breast-feeding—It is not known whether anabolic steroids can cause problems in nursing babies. There is very little experience with their use in mothers who are breast-feeding.

Children—Anabolic steroids may cause children to stop growing. In addition, they may make male children develop too fast sexually and may cause male-like changes in female children.

Older adults—When elderly male patients are treated with anabolic steroids, they may have an increased risk of enlarged prostate or cancer of the prostate.

Athletes—Anabolic steroids are banned and tested for by the U.S. Olympic Committee (USOC), International Olympic Committee (IOC), and National Collegiate Athletic Association (NCAA). Anabolic steroid use can lead to disqualification of athletes in most athletic events.

Use of these medicines by athletes to build muscle tissue and improve performance is not recommended. There is no good medical evidence to support the belief that the use of these medicines by athletes will increase muscle strength. When used for this purpose, they may even be dangerous to the health because of unwanted effects such as too much fluid in the body, liver disease, and liver cancer in males and females; reduced fertility and/or swelling of breasts in males; and hoarseness or deepening of voice, unnatural hair growth, or unusual hair loss in females.

Other medicines—Although certain medicines should not be used together at all, in other cases two different medicines may be used together even if an interaction might occur. In these cases, your doctor may want to change the dose, or

other precautions may be necessary. When you are taking anabolic steroids, it is especially important that your doctor and pharmacist know if you are taking any of the following:

- Acetaminophen (e.g., Tylenol) (with long-term, high-dose use) or
- Amiodarone (e.g., Cordarone) or
- Androgens (male hormones) or
- Anti-infectives by mouth or by injection (medicine for infection) or
- Antithyroid agents (medicine for overactive thyroid) or
- Carbamazepine (e.g., Tegretol) or
- Carmustine (e.g., BiCNU) or
- Chloroquine (e.g., Aralen) or
- Dantrolene (e.g., Dantrium) or
- Daunorubicin (e.g., Cerubidine) or
- Disulfiram (e.g., Antabuse) or
- Divalproex (e.g., Depakote) or
- Estrogens (female hormones) or
- Etretinate (e.g., Tegison) or
- Gold salts (medicine for arthritis) or
- Hydroxychloroquine (e.g., Plaquenil) or
- Mercaptopurine (e.g., Purinethol) or
- Methotrexate (e.g., Mexate) or
- Methyldopa (e.g., Aldomet) or
- Naltrexone (e.g., Trexan) (with long-term, high-dose use) or
- Oral contraceptives (birth control pills) containing estrogen or
- Phenothiazines (acetophenazine [e.g., Tindal], chlorpromazine [e.g., Thorazine], fluphenazine [e.g., Prolixin], mesoridazine [e.g., Serentil], perphenazine [e.g., Trilafon], prochlorperazine [e.g., Compazine], promazine [e.g., Sparine], promethazine [e.g., Phenergan], thioridazine [e.g., Mellaril], trifluoperazine [e.g., Stelazine], triflupromazine [e.g., Vesprin], trimeprazine [e.g., Temaril]) or
- Phenytoin (e.g., Dilantin) or
- Plicamycin (e.g., Mithracin) or
- Valproic acid (e.g., Depakene)—Taking anabolic steroids with any of these medicines may increase the chances of liver damage. Your doctor may want you to have extra blood tests to check for this if you must take both medicines
- Anticoagulants, oral (blood thinners you take by mouth)—Anabolic steroids can increase the effect of these medicines and possibly cause excessive bleeding

Other medical problems—The presence of other medical problems may affect the use of anabolic steroids. Make sure you tell your doctor if you have any other medical problems, especially:

- Breast cancer (in males and some females)
- Diabetes mellitus (sugar diabetes)—Anabolic steroids can decrease blood sugar levels
- Enlarged prostate or
- Prostate cancer—Anabolic steroids may make these conditions worse by causing more enlargement of the prostate or more growth of a tumor
- Heart or blood vessel disease—Anabolic steroids can worsen these conditions by increasing blood cholesterol levels
- Kidney disease
- Liver disease
- Too much calcium in the blood (or history of) (in females)—Anabolic steroids may worsen this condition by raising the amount of calcium in the blood even more

Proper Use of This Medicine

Take this medicine only as directed. Do not take more of it and do not take it more often than your doctor ordered. To do so may increase the chance of side effects.

In order for this medicine to work properly, it is important that you follow a diet high in proteins and calories. If you have any questions about this, check with your doctor, nurse, or pharmacist.

Missed dose—If you miss a dose of this medicine and your dosing schedule is:

- One dose a day— Take the missed dose as soon as possible. However, if you do not remember it until the next day, skip the missed dose and go back to your regular dosing schedule. Do not double doses.
- More than one dose a day—Take the missed dose as soon as possible. However, if it is almost time for your next dose, skip the missed dose and go back to your regular dosing schedule. Do not double doses.

If you have any questions about this, check with your doctor.

Storage—To store this medicine:

- Keep out of the reach of children.
- Store away from heat and direct light.

- Do not store the tablet form of this medicine in the bathroom, near the kitchen sink, or in other damp places. Heat or moisture may cause the medicine to break down.
- Keep the liquid form of this medicine from freezing.
- Do not keep outdated medicine or medicine no longer needed. Be sure that any discarded medicine is out of the reach of children.

Precautions While Using This Medicine

Your doctor should check your progress at regular visits to make sure that this medicine does not cause unwanted effects.

For diabetic patients:

- This medicine may affect blood sugar levels. If you notice a change in the results of your blood or urine sugar tests or if you have any questions, check with your doctor.

Side Effects of This Medicine

Tumors of the liver, liver cancer, or peliosis hepatis, a form of liver disease, have occurred during long-term, high-dose therapy with anabolic steroids. Although these effects are rare, they can be very serious and may cause death. Discuss these possible effects with your doctor.

Along with its needed effects, a medicine may cause some unwanted effects. Although not all of these side effects may occur, if they do occur they may need medical attention.

Check with your doctor immediately if any of the following side effects occur:

>*For both females and males*
>>*Less common*
>>>Yellow eyes or skin
>>*Rare (with long-term use)*
>>>Black, tarry, or light-colored stools; dark-colored urine; purple- or red-colored spots on body or inside the mouth or nose; sore throat and/or fever; vomiting of blood

Also, check with your doctor as soon as possible if any of the following side effects occur:

For both females and males
   Less common
      Bone pain; nausea or vomiting; sore tongue; swelling of
      feet or lower legs; unusual bleeding; unusual weight
      gain
Rare (with long-term use)
      Abdominal or stomach pain; feeling of discomfort (con-
      tinuing); headache (continuing); hives; loss of appetite
      (continuing); unexplained weight loss; unpleasant
      breath odor (continuing)
For females only
   More common
      Acne or oily skin; enlarging clitoris; hoarseness or deep-
      ening of voice; irregular menstrual periods; unnatural
      hair growth; unusual hair loss
   Less common
      Mental depression; unusual tiredness
For young males (boys) only
   More common
      Acne; enlarging penis; increased frequency of erections;
      unnatural hair growth
   Less common
      Unexplained darkening of skin
For sexually mature males only
   More common
      Enlargement of breasts or breast soreness; frequent or
      continuing erections; frequent urge to urinate
For elderly males only
   Less common
      Difficult or frequent urination

Other side effects may occur that usually do not need medical attention. These side effects may go away during treatment as your body adjusts to the medicine. However, check
with your doctor if any of the following side effects continue
or are bothersome:
For both females and males
   Less common
      Chills; diarrhea; feeling of abdominal or stomach fullness;
      muscle cramps; trouble in sleeping; unusual decrease
      or increase in sexual desire

For males only
  More common
    Acne
Less common
    Decreased sexual ability

Other side effects not listed above may also occur in some patients. If you notice any other effects, check with your doctor.

Additional Information

Once a medicine has been approved for marketing for a certain use, experience may show that it is also useful for other medical problems. Although these uses are not included in product labeling, anabolic steroids may be used in certain patients with the following medical conditions:

- Certain blood clotting diseases
- Growth failure
- Turner's syndrome

Other than the above information, there is no additional information relating to proper use, precautions, or side effects for these uses.

ANGIOTENSIN-CONVERTING ENZYME (ACE) INHIBITORS   Systemic

This information applies to the following medicines:
  Benazepril (ben-AY-ze-pril)
  Captopril (KAP-toe-pril)
  Enalapril (e-NAL-a-pril)
  Enalaprilat (e-NAL-a-pril-at)
  Fosinopril (foe-SIN-oh-pril)
  Lisinopril (lyse-IN-oh-pril)
  Quinapril (KWIN-a-pril)
  Ramipril (ra-MI-pril)
Some commonly used brand names are:

For Benazepril†
  In the U.S.
    Lotensin

For Captopril
  In the U.S.
    Capoten
  In Canada
    Capoten

For Enalapril
  In the U.S.
    Vasotec
  In Canada
    Vasotec

For Enalaprilat
  In the U.S.
    Vasotec
  In Canada
    Vasotec

For Fosinopril†
  In the U.S.
    Monopril

For Lisinopril
  In the U.S.
    Prinivil
    Zestril
  In Canada
    Prinivil
    Zestril

For Quinapril†
  In the U.S.
    Accupril

For Ramipril†
  In the U.S.
    Altace

†Not commercially available in Canada.

Description

ACE inhibitors belong to the class of medicines called high blood pressure medicines (antihypertensives). They are used to treat high blood pressure (hypertension).

High blood pressure adds to the workload of the heart and arteries. If it continues for a long time, the heart and arteries may not function properly. This can damage the blood vessels of the brain, heart, and kidneys, resulting in a stroke, heart failure, or kidney failure. High blood pressure may also increase the risk of heart attacks. These problems may be less likely to occur if blood pressure is controlled.

Some of these medicines are also used to treat congestive heart failure.

These medicines may also be used for other conditions as determined by your doctor.

The exact way that these medicines work is not known. They block an enzyme in the body that is necessary to produce a substance that causes blood vessels to tighten. As a result, they relax blood vessels. This lowers blood pressure and increases the supply of blood and oxygen to the heart.

These medicines are available only with your doctor's prescription, in the following dosage forms:

  Oral

    Benazepril
      • Tablets (U.S.)
    Captopril
      • Tablets (U.S. and Canada)
    Enalapril
      • Tablets (U.S. and Canada)
    Fosinopril
      • Tablets (U.S.)
    Lisinopril
      • Tablets (U.S. and Canada)
    Quinapril
      • Tablets (U.S.)
    Ramipril
      • Capsules (U.S.)

  Parenteral

    Enalaprilat
      • Injection (U.S. and Canada)

It is very important that you read and understand the following information. If any of it causes you special concern, check with your doctor. Also, *if you have any questions* or if you want more information about this medicine or your medical problem, *ask your doctor, nurse, or pharmacist.*

Before Using This Medicine

In deciding to use a medicine, the risks of taking the medicine must be weighed against the good it will do. This is a decision you and your doctor will make. For the angiotensin-converting enzyme (ACE) inhibitors, the following should be considered:

Allergies—Tell your doctor if you have ever had any unusual or allergic reaction to benazepril, captopril, enalapril, fosinopril, lisinopril, quinapril, or ramipril. Also tell your doctor and pharmacist if you are allergic to any other substances, such as foods, preservatives, or dyes.

Pregnancy—Use of angiotensin-converting enzyme (ACE) inhibitors during pregnancy, especially in the second and third trimesters (after the first three months) can cause low blood pressure, severe kidney failure, too much potassium, or even death in the newborn. *Therefore, it is important that you check with your doctor immediately if you think that you may be pregnant.* Be sure that you have discussed this with your doctor before taking this medicine. In addition, if you are taking:

- *Benazepril*—Benazepril has not been shown to cause birth defects in animals when given in doses more than 3 times the highest recommended human dose.

- *Captopril*—Studies in rabbits and rats at doses up to 400 times the recommended human dose have shown that captopril causes an increase in deaths of the fetus and newborn. Also, captopril has caused deformed skulls in the offspring of rabbits given doses 2 to 70 times the recommended human dose.

- *Enalapril*—Studies in rats at doses many times the recommended human dose have shown that use of enalapril causes the fetus to be smaller than normal. Studies in rabbits have shown that enalapril causes an increase in fetal death. Enalapril has not been shown to cause birth defects in rats or rabbits.

- *Fosinopril*—Studies in rats have shown that fosinopril causes the fetus to be smaller than normal. Studies in rabbits have shown that fosinopril causes fetal death, probably due to extremely low blood pressure. In rats, birth defects such as skeletal and facial deformities were seen. However, it is not clear that the deformities were related to fosinopril. Birth defects were not seen in rabbits.

- *Lisinopril*—Studies in mice and rats at doses many times the recommended human dose have shown that use of lisinopril causes a decrease in successful pregnancies, a decrease in the weight of infants, and an increase in infant deaths. It has also caused a decrease in successful pregnancies and abnormal bone growth in rabbits. Lisinopril has not been shown to cause birth defects in mice, rats, or rabbits.

- *Quinapril*—Studies in rats have shown that quinapril causes lower birth weights and changes in kidney structure of the fetus. However, birth defects were not seen in rabbits given quinapril.

- *Ramipril*—Studies in animals have shown that ramipril causes lower birth weights.

Breast-feeding—

- *Benazepril, captopril, and fosinopril*—These medicines pass into breast milk.

- *Enalapril, lisinopril, quinapril, or ramipril* —It is not known whether these medicines pass into breast milk. However, these medicines have not been reported to cause problems in nursing babies.

Children—Children may be especially sensitive to the blood pressure–lowering effect of ACE inhibitors. This may increase the chance of side effects or other problems during treatment. Therefore, it is especially important that you discuss with the child's doctor the good that this medicine may do as well as the risks of using it.

Older adults—This medicine has been tested in a limited number of patients 65 years of age or older and has not been shown to cause different side effects or problems in older people than it does in younger adults.

Other medicines—Although certain medicines should not be used together at all, in other cases two different medicines

may be used together even if an interaction might occur. In these cases, your doctor may want to change the dose, or other precautions may be necessary. When you are taking or receiving ACE inhibitors it is especially important that your doctor and pharmacist know if you are taking any of the following:

- Diuretics (water pills)—Effects on blood pressure may be increased. In addition, some diuretics make the increase in potassium in the blood caused by ACE inhibitors even greater
- Potassium-containing medicines or supplements or
- Salt substitutes or
- Low-salt milk—Use of these substances with ACE inhibitors may result in an unusually high potassium level in the blood, which can lead to heart rhythm and other problems

Other medical problems—The presence of other medical problems may affect the use of the ACE inhibitors. Make sure you tell your doctor if you have any other medical problems, especially:

- Diabetes mellitus (sugar diabetes)—Increased risk of potassium levels in the body becoming too high
- Heart or blood vessel disease or
- Heart attack or stroke (recent)—Lowering blood pressure may make problems resulting from these conditions worse
- Kidney disease or
- Liver disease—Effects may be increased because of slower removal from the body
- Kidney transplant—Increased risk of kidney disease caused by ACE inhibitors
- Systemic lupus erythematosus (SLE)—Increased risk of blood problems caused by ACE inhibitors
- Previous reaction to any ACE inhibitor involving hoarseness; swelling of face, mouth, hands, or feet; or sudden trouble in breathing—Reaction is more likely to occur again

Before you begin using any new medicine (prescription or nonprescription) or if you develop any new medical problem while you are using this medicine, check with your doctor, nurse, or pharmacist.

Proper Use of This Medicine

To help you remember to take your medicine, try to get into the habit of taking it at the same time each day.

For patients taking *captopril:*

- This medicine is best taken on an empty stomach 1 hour before meals, unless you are otherwise directed by your doctor.

For patients taking this medicine *for high blood pressure:*

- In addition to the use of the medicine your doctor has prescribed, treatment for your high blood pressure may include weight control and care in the types of foods you eat, especially foods high in sodium. Your doctor will tell you which of these are most important for you. You should check with your doctor before changing your diet.

- Many patients who have high blood pressure will not notice any signs of the problem. In fact, many may feel normal. It is very important that you *take your medicine exactly as directed* and that you keep your appointments with your doctor even if you feel well.

- Remember that this medicine will not cure your high blood pressure but it does help control it. Therefore, you must continue to take it as directed if you expect to lower your blood pressure and keep it down. *You may have to take high blood pressure medicine for the rest of your life.* If high blood pressure is not treated, it can cause serious problems such as heart failure, blood vessel disease, stroke, or kidney disease.

Missed dose—If you miss a dose of this medicine, take it as soon as possible. However, if it is almost time for your next dose, skip the missed dose and go back to your regular dosing schedule. Do not double doses.

Storage—To store this medicine:

- Keep out of the reach of children.
- Store away from heat and direct light.

- Do not store in the bathroom, near the kitchen sink, or in other damp places. Heat or moisture may cause the medicine to break down.
- Do not keep outdated medicine or medicine no longer needed. Be sure that any discarded medicine is out of the reach of children.

Precautions While Using This Medicine

It is important that your doctor check your progress at regular visits to make sure that this medicine is working properly and to check for unwanted effects.

For patients taking this medicine *for high blood pressure:*
- *Do not take other medicines unless they have been discussed with your doctor.* This especially includes over-the-counter (nonprescription) medicines for appetite control, asthma, colds, cough, hay fever, or sinus problems, since they may tend to increase your blood pressure.

Dizziness or lightheadedness may occur after the first dose of this medicine, especially if you have been taking a diuretic (water pill). Make sure you know how you react to this medicine before you drive, use machines, or do anything else that could be dangerous if you are dizzy.

Check with your doctor right away if you become sick while taking this medicine, especially with severe or continuing nausea and vomiting or diarrhea. These conditions may cause you to lose too much water and lead to low blood pressure.

Dizziness, lightheadedness, or fainting may also occur if you exercise or if the weather is hot. Heavy sweating can cause loss of too much water and low blood pressure. Use extra care during exercise or hot weather.

Avoid alcoholic beverages until you have discussed their use with your doctor. Alcohol may make the low blood pressure effect worse and/or increase the possibility of dizziness or fainting.

Before having any kind of surgery (including dental surgery) or emergency treatment, tell the medical doctor or dentist in charge that you are taking this medicine.

For patients taking *captopril or fosinopril:*

- Before you have any medical tests, tell the doctor in charge that you are taking this medicine. The results of some tests may be affected by this medicine.

Side Effects of This Medicine

Along with its needed effects, a medicine may cause some unwanted effects. Although not all of these side effects may occur, if they do occur they may need medical attention.

Check with your doctor immediately if any of the following side effects occur:

Rare

Fever and chills; hoarseness; swelling of face, mouth, hands, or feet; trouble in swallowing or breathing (sudden)

Check with your doctor as soon as possible if any of the following side effects occur:

Less common

Dizziness, lightheadedness, or fainting; skin rash, with or without itching, fever, or joint pain

Rare

Abdominal pain, abdominal distention, fever, nausea, or vomiting; chest pain

Signs and symptoms of too much potassium in the body

Confusion; irregular heartbeat; nervousness; numbness or tingling in hands, feet, or lips; shortness of breath or difficulty breathing; weakness or heaviness of legs

Other side effects may occur that usually do not need medical attention. These side effects may go away during treatment as your body adjusts to the medicine. However, check with your doctor if any of the following side effects continue or are bothersome:

More common

Cough (dry, continuing)

Less common
> Diarrhea; headache; loss of taste; nausea; unusual tiredness

Other side effects not listed above may also occur in some patients. If you notice any other effects, check with your doctor.

Additional Information

Once a medicine has been approved for marketing for a certain use, experience may show that it is also useful for other medical problems. Although these uses are not included in product labeling, ACE inhibitors are used in certain patients with the following medical conditions:

- Hypertension in scleroderma (high blood pressure in patients with hardening and thickening of the skin)
- Renal crisis in scleroderma (kidney problems in patients with hardening and thickening of the skin)

Other than the above information, there is no additional information relating to proper use, precautions, or side effects for these uses.

ANTICHOLINERGICS/ ANTISPASMODICS   Systemic

This information applies to the following medicines:
> Anisotropine (an-iss-oh-TROE-peen)
> Atropine (A-troe-peen)
> Belladonna (bell-a-DON-a)
> Clidinium (kli-DI-nee-um)
> Dicyclomine (dye-SYE-kloe-meen)
> Glycopyrrolate (glye-koe-PYE-roe-late)
> Homatropine (hoe-MA-troe-peen)
> Hyoscyamine (hye-oh-SYE-a-meen)
> Isopropamide (eye-soe-PROE-pa-mide)
> Mepenzolate (me-PEN-zoe-late)
> Methantheline (meth-AN-tha-leen)
> Methscopolamine (meth-skoe-POL-a-meen)
> Oxyphencyclimine (ox-i-fen-SYE-kli-meen)
> Pirenzepine (peer-EN-ze-peen)
> Propantheline (proe-PAN-the-leen)

Scopolamine (scoe-POL-a-meen)
Tridihexethyl (trye-dye-hex-ETH-il)

Some commonly used brand names are:

For Anisotropine†
In the U.S.
    Valpin 50
      Generic name product may also be available.
Another commonly used name is octatropine.

For Atropine
In the U.S.
      Generic name product available.
In Canada
      Generic name product available.

For Belladonna†
In the U.S.
      Generic name product available.

For Clidinium†
In the U.S.
    Quarzan

For Dicyclomine
In the U.S.

Antispas	Neoquess
A-Spas	Or-Tyl
Bentyl	Spasmoject
Di-Spaz	

    Generic name product may also be available.

In Canada

Bentylol	Lomine
Formulex	Spasmoban

Another commonly used name is dicycloverine.

For Glycopyrrolate
In the U.S.

Robinul	Robinul Forte

    Generic name product may also be available.

In Canada

Robinul	Robinul Forte

Another commonly used name is glycopyrronium bromide.

For Homatropine†
In the U.S.
    Homapin

For Hyoscyamine
   In the U.S.
      Anaspaz   Levsin
      Cystospaz   Levsinex Timecaps
      Cystospaz-M   Levsin S/L
      Gastrosed   Neoquess

   In Canada
      Levsin

For Isopropamide†
   In the U.S.
      Darbid

For Mepenzolate†
   In the U.S.
      Cantil

For Methantheline†
   In the U.S.
      Banthine

Another commonly used name is methanthelinium.

For Methscopolamine†
   In the U.S.
      Pamine

Another commonly used name for methscopolamine is hyoscine methobromide.

For Oxyphencyclimine†
   In the U.S.
      Daricon

For Pirenzepine*
   In Canada
      Gastrozepin

For Propantheline
   In the U.S.
      Norpanth   Pro-Banthine
      Generic name product may also be available.

   In Canada
      Pro-Banthine   Propanthel

For Scopolamine
   In the U.S.
      Transderm-Scōp
      Generic name product may also be available.

   In Canada
      Buscopan   Transderm-V

Another commonly used name for scopolamine is hyoscine hydrobromide.

For Tridihexethyl†
  In the U.S.
    Pathilon

---

*Not commercially available in the U.S.
†Not commercially available in Canada.

Description

The anticholinergics/antispasmodics are a group of medicines that include the natural belladonna alkaloids (atropine, belladonna, hyoscyamine, and scopolamine) and related products.

The anticholinergics/antispasmodics are used to relieve cramps or spasms of the stomach, intestines, and bladder. Some are used together with antacids or other medicine in the treatment of peptic ulcer. Others are used to prevent nausea, vomiting, and motion sickness.

Anticholinergics/antispasmodics are also used in certain surgical and emergency procedures. In surgery, some are given by injection before anesthesia to help relax you and to decrease secretions, such as saliva. During anesthesia and surgery, atropine, glycopyrrolate, hyoscyamine, and scopolamine are used to help keep the heartbeat normal. Atropine is also given by injection to help relax the stomach and intestines for certain types of examinations. Some anticholinergics are also used to treat poisoning caused by medicines such as neostigmine and physostigmine, certain types of mushrooms, and poisoning by "nerve" gases or organic phosphorous pesticides (for example, demeton [Systox], diazinon, malathion, parathion, and ronnel [Trolene]). Also, anticholinergics can be used for painful menstruation, runny nose, and to prevent urination during sleep.

These medicines may also be used for other conditions as determined by your doctor.

The anticholinergics/antispasmodics are available only with your doctor's prescription in the following dosage forms:

Oral

  Anisotropine
    • Tablets (U.S.)

Atropine
- Tablets (U.S.)
- Soluble tablets (U.S.)

Belladonna
- Tincture (U.S.)

Clidinium
- Capsules (U.S.)

Dicyclomine
- Capsules (U.S. and Canada)
- Syrup (U.S. and Canada)
- Tablets (U.S. and Canada)
- Extended-release Tablets (Canada)

Glycopyrrolate
- Tablets (U.S. and Canada)

Homatropine
- Tablets (U.S.)

Hyoscyamine
- Extended-release capsules (U.S.)
- Elixir (U.S.)
- Oral solution (U.S. and Canada)
- Tablets (U.S.)

Isopropamide
- Tablets (U.S.)

Mepenzolate
- Tablets (U.S.)

Methantheline
- Tablets (U.S.)

Methscopolamine
- Tablets (U.S.)

Oxyphencyclimine
- Tablets (U.S.)

Pirenzepine
- Tablets (Canada)

Propantheline
- Tablets (U.S. and Canada)

Scopolamine
- Tablets (Canada)

Tridihexethyl
- Tablets (U.S.)

Parenteral

Atropine
- Injection (U.S. and Canada)

Dicyclomine
- Injection (U.S. and Canada)

> Glycopyrrolate
> - Injection (U.S. and Canada)
>
> Hyoscyamine
> - Injection (U.S. and Canada)
>
> Scopolamine
> - Injection (U.S. and Canada)
>
> *Rectal*
>
> Scopolamine
> - Suppositories (Canada)
>
> *Transdermal*
>
> Scopolamine
> - Transdermal disk (U.S. and Canada)

It is very important that you read and understand the following information. If any of it causes you special concern, check with your doctor. Also, *if you have any questions* or if you want more information about this medicine or your medical problem, *ask your doctor, nurse, or pharmacist.*

Before Using This Medicine

In deciding to use a medicine, the risks of taking the medicine must be weighed against the good it will do. This is a decision you and your doctor will make. For anticholinergics/antispasmodics the following should be considered:

Allergies—Tell your doctor if you have ever had any unusual or allergic reaction to any of the natural belladonna alkaloids (atropine, belladonna, hyoscyamine, and scopolamine), iodine or iodides, or any related products. Also, tell your doctor and pharmacist if you are allergic to any other substances, such as foods, preservatives, or dyes.

Pregnancy—If you are pregnant or if you may become pregnant, make sure your doctor knows if your medicine contains any of the following:

- *Atropine*—Atropine has not been shown to cause birth defects or other problems in animals. However, when injected into humans during pregnancy, atropine has been reported to increase the heartbeat of the fetus.
- *Belladonna*—Studies on effects in pregnancy have not been done in either humans or animals.

- *Clidinium*—Clidinium has not been studied in pregnant women. However, clidinium has not been shown to cause birth defects or other problems in animal studies.
- *Dicyclomine*—Dicyclomine has been associated with a few cases of human birth defects but dicyclomine has not been confirmed as the cause.
- *Glycopyrrolate*—Glycopyrrolate has not been studied in pregnant women. However, glycopyrrolate did not cause birth defects in animal studies, but did decrease the chance of becoming pregnant and in the newborn's chance of surviving after weaning.
- *Hyoscyamine*—Studies on effects in pregnancy have not been done in either humans or animals. However, when injected into humans during pregnancy, hyoscyamine has been reported to increase the heartbeat of the fetus.
- *Isopropamide*—Studies on effects in pregnancy have not been done in either humans or animals.
- *Mepenzolate*—Mepenzolate has not been studied in pregnant women. However, studies in animals have not shown that mepenzolate causes birth defects or other problems.
- *Propantheline*—Studies on effects in pregnancy have not been done in either humans or animals.
- *Scopolamine*—Studies on effects in pregnancy have not been done in either humans or animals.

Breast-feeding—Although these medicines may pass into the breast milk, they have not been reported to cause problems in nursing babies. However, the flow of breast milk may be reduced in some patients. The use of dicyclomine in nursing mothers has been reported to cause breathing problems in infants.

Children—Unusual excitement, nervousness, restlessness, or irritability and unusual warmth, dryness, and flushing of skin are more likely to occur in children, who are usually more sensitive to the effects of anticholinergics. Also, when anticholinergics are given to children during hot weather, a rapid increase in body temperature may occur. In infants and children, especially those with spastic paralysis or brain damage, this medicine may be more likely to cause severe side effects. Shortness of breath or difficulty in breathing has occurred in children taking dicyclomine.

Older adults—Confusion or memory loss; constipation; difficult urination; drowsiness; dryness of mouth, nose, throat, or skin; and unusual excitement, nervousness, restlessness, or irritability may be more likely to occur in the elderly, who are usually more sensitive than younger adults to the effects of anticholinergics. Also, eye pain may occur, which may be a sign of glaucoma.

Athletes—Scopolamine is banned, and in some cases, tested for in competitors in biathlon and modern pentathlon events by U.S. Olympic Committee (USOC) Use of scopolamine can lead to disqualification of athletes in these events.

Other medicines—Although certain medicines should not be used together at all, in other cases two different medicines may be used together even if an interaction might occur. In these cases, your doctor may want to change the dose, or other precautions may be necessary. When you are taking anticholinergics/antispasmodics, it is especially important that your doctor and pharmacist know if you are taking any of the following:

- Antacids or
- Diarrhea medicine containing kaolin or attapulgite or
- Ketoconazole (e.g., Nizoral)—Using these medicines with an anticholinergic may lessen the effects of the anticholinergic
- Central nervous system (CNS) depressants (medicines that cause drowsiness)—Taking scopolamine with CNS depressants may increase the effects of either medicine
- Other anticholinergics (medicine for abdominal or stomach spasms or cramps) or
- Tricyclic antidepressants (amitriptyline [e.g., Elavil], amoxapine [e.g., Asendin], clomipramine [e.g., Anafranil], desipramine [e.g., Pertofrane], doxepin [e.g., Sinequan], imipramine [e.g., Tofranil], nortriptyline [e.g., Aventyl], protriptyline [e.g., Vivactil], trimipramine [e.g., Surmontil])—Taking anticholinergics with tricyclic antidepressants or other anticholinergics may cause an increase the effects of the anticholinergic

- Potassium chloride (e.g., Kay Ciel)—Using this medicine with an anticholinergic may make gastrointestinal problems caused by potassium worse

Other medical problems—The presence of other medical problems may affect the use of anticholinergics/antispasmodics. Make sure you tell your doctor if you have any other medical problems, especially:

- Bleeding problems (severe)—These medicines may increase heart rate, which would make bleeding problems worse
- Brain damage (in children)—May increase the CNS effects of this medicine
- Colitis (severe) or
- Dryness of mouth (severe and continuing) or
- Enlarged prostate or
- Fever or
- Glaucoma or
- Heart disease or
- Hernia (hiatal) or
- High blood pressure (hypertension) or
- Intestinal blockage or other intestinal problems or
- Lung disease (chronic) or
- Myasthenia gravis or
- Toxemia of pregnancy or
- Urinary tract blockage or difficult urination—These medicines may make these conditions worse
- Down's syndrome (mongolism)—These medicines may cause an increase in pupil dilation and heart rate
- Kidney disease or
- Liver disease—Higher blood levels may occur and cause an increase in side effects
- Overactive thyroid—These medicines may further increase heart rate
- Spastic paralysis (in children)—This condition may increase the effects of the anticholinergic

Before you begin using any new medicine (prescription or nonprescription) or if you develop any new medical problem while you are using this medicine, check with your doctor, nurse, or pharmacist.

Proper Use of This Medicine

Take this medicine only as directed. Do not take more of it, do not take it more often, and do not take it for a longer time than your doctor ordered. To do so may increase the chance of side effects.

Missed dose—If you miss a dose of this medicine, take it as soon as possible. However, if it is almost time for your next dose, skip the missed dose and go back to your regular dosing schedule. Do not double doses.

For patients *taking any of these medicines by mouth:*
- Take this medicine 30 minutes to 1 hour before meals unless otherwise directed by your doctor.

To use the *rectal suppository* form of *scopolamine:*
- If the suppository is too soft to insert, chill it in the refrigerator for 30 minutes or run cold water over it before removing the foil wrapper.
- To insert the suppository: First remove the foil wrapper and moisten the suppository with cold water. Lie down on your side and use your finger to push the suppository well up into the rectum.

To use the *transdermal disk* form of *scopolamine:*
- This medicine usually comes with patient directions. Read them carefully before using this medicine.
- Wash and dry your hands thoroughly before and after handling.
- Apply the disk to the hairless area of skin behind the ear. Do not place over any cuts or irritations.

Storage—To store this medicine:
- Keep out of the reach of children. Overdose is especially dangerous in young children.
- Store away from heat and direct light.
- Do not store the capsule or tablet form of this medicine in the bathroom, near the kitchen sink, or in other damp places. Heat or moisture may cause the medicine to break down.

- Keep the liquid form of this medicine tightly closed and keep it from freezing. Do not refrigerate the syrup form of this medicine.
- Do not keep outdated medicine or medicine no longer needed. Be sure that any discarded medicine is out of the reach of children.

Precautions While Using This Medicine

If you think you or someone else may have taken an over-dose, get emergency help at once. Taking an overdose of any of the belladonna alkaloids or taking scopolamine with alcohol or other CNS depressants may lead to unconsciousness and possibly death. Some signs of overdose are clumsiness or unsteadiness; dizziness; severe drowsiness; fever; hallucinations (seeing, hearing, or feeling things that are not there); confusion; shortness of breath or troubled breathing; slurred speech; unusual excitement, nervousness, restlessness, or ir-ritability; fast heartbeat; and unusual warmth, dryness, and flushing of skin.

These medicines may make you sweat less, causing your body temperature to increase. *Use extra care not to become overheated during exercise or hot weather while you are taking this medicine,* since overheating may result in heat stroke. Also hot baths or saunas may make you dizzy or faint while you are taking this medicine.

Check with your doctor before you stop using this medicine. Your doctor may want you to reduce gradually the amount you are using before stopping completely. Stopping this med-icine may cause withdrawal side effects such as vomiting, sweating, and dizziness.

Anticholinergics may cause some people to have blurred vision. *Make sure your vision is clear before you drive or do anything else that could be dangerous if you are not able to see well.* These medicines may also cause your eyes to become more sensitive to light than they are normally. Wearing sunglasses may help lessen the discomfort from bright light.

These medicines, especially in high doses, may cause some people to become dizzy or drowsy. *Make sure you know how you react to this medicine before you drive, use machines, or do anything else that could be dangerous if you are dizzy or are not alert.*

Dizziness, lightheadedness, or fainting may occur, especially when you get up from a lying or sitting position. Getting up slowly may help lessen this problem.

These medicines may cause dryness of the mouth, nose, and throat. For temporary relief of mouth dryness, use sugarless candy or gum, melt bits of ice in your mouth, or use a saliva substitute. However, if your mouth continues to feel dry for more than 2 weeks, check with your medical doctor or dentist. Continuing dryness of the mouth may increase the chance of dental disease, including tooth decay, gum disease, and fungus infections.

For patients taking *isopropamide:*
- Make sure your doctor knows if you are planning to have any future thyroid tests. The results of the thyroid test may be affected by the iodine in this medicine.

For patients taking *scopolamine:*
- This medicine will add to the effects of alcohol and other CNS depressants (medicines that slow down the nervous system, possibly causing drowsiness). Some examples of CNS depressants are antihistamines or medicine for hay fever, other allergies, or colds; sedatives, tranquilizers, or sleeping medicine; prescription pain medicine or narcotics; barbiturates; medicine for seizures; muscle relaxants; or anesthetics, including some dental anesthetics. *Check with your doctor before taking any of the above while you are using this medicine.*

For patients *taking any of these medicines by mouth:*
- Do not take this medicine within 2 or 3 hours of taking antacids or medicine for diarrhea. Taking antacids or antidiarrhea medicines and this medicine too close together may prevent this medicine from working properly.

Side Effects of This Medicine

Along with its needed effects, a medicine may cause some unwanted effects. Although not all of these side effects may occur, if they do occur they may need medical attention.

Check with your doctor as soon as possible if any of the following side effects occur:

Rare

Confusion (especially in the elderly); dizziness, lightheadedness (continuing), or fainting; eye pain; skin rash or hives

Symptoms of overdose

Blurred vision (continuing) or changes in near vision; clumsiness or unsteadiness; confusion; convulsions (seizures); difficulty in breathing, muscle weakness (severe), or tiredness (severe); dizziness; drowsiness (severe); dryness of mouth, nose, or throat (severe); fast heartbeat; fever; hallucinations (seeing, hearing, or feeling things that are not there); slurred speech; unusual excitement, nervousness, restlessness, or irritability; unusual warmth, dryness, and flushing of skin

Other side effects may occur that usually do not need medical attention. These side effects may go away during treatment as your body adjusts to the medicine. However, check with your doctor if any of the following side effects continue or are bothersome:

More common

Constipation (less common with hyoscyamine); decreased sweating; dryness of mouth, nose, throat, or skin

Less common or rare

Bloated feeling; blurred vision; decreased flow of breast milk; difficult urination; difficulty in swallowing; drowsiness (more common with high doses of any of these medicines and with usual doses of scopolamine when given by mouth or by injection); false sense of well-being (for scopolamine only); headache; increased sensitivity of eyes to light; lightheadedness (with injection); loss of memory; nausea or vomiting; redness or other signs of irritation at place of injection; trouble in sleeping (for scopolamine only); unusual tiredness or weakness

For patients using *scopolamine:*

- After you stop using scopolamine, your body may need time to adjust. The length of time this takes depends on the amount of scopolamine you were using and how long you used it. During this period of time check with your doctor if you notice any of the following side effects:

Anxiety; irritability; nightmares; trouble in sleeping

For patients using the *transdermal disk* of *scopolamine:*

- While using the disk or even after removing it, your eyes may become more sensitive to light than usual. You may also notice the pupil in one eye is larger than the other. Check with your doctor if this side effect continues or is bothersome.

Other side effects not listed above may also occur in some patients. If you notice any other effects, check with your doctor.

Additional Information

Once a medicine has been approved for marketing for a certain use, experience may show that it is also useful for other medical problems. Although these uses are not included in product labeling, anticholinergics/antispasmodics are used in certain patients with the following medical conditions:

- Diarrhea
- Excessive watering of mouth

Other than the above information, there is no additional information relating to proper use, precautions, or side effects for these uses.

ANTICOAGULANTS   Systemic

This information applies to the following medicines:
> Anisindione (an-iss-in-DYE-one)
> Dicumarol (dye-KOO-ma-role)
> Warfarin (WAR-far-in)

This information does *not* apply to heparin.

Some commonly used brand names are:

For Anisindione
> *In the U.S.*
>> Miradon

For Dicumarol
> *In the U.S.*
>> Generic name product available.

Another commonly used name is dicoumarol.

For Warfarin
> *In the U.S.*
>> Coumadin   Sofarin
>> Panwarfin
>> Generic name product may also be available.

> *In Canada*
>> Coumadin   Warfilone

Description

Anticoagulants decrease the clotting ability of the blood and therefore help to prevent harmful clots from forming in the blood vessels. These medicines are sometimes called blood thinners, although they do not actually thin the blood. They also will not dissolve clots that already have formed, but they may prevent the clots from becoming larger and causing more serious problems. They are often used as treatment for certain blood vessel, heart, and lung conditions.

In order for an anticoagulant to help you without causing serious bleeding, it must be used properly and all of the precautions concerning its use must be followed exactly. Be sure that you have discussed the use of this medicine with your doctor. It is very important that you understand all of your doctor's orders and that you are willing and able to follow them exactly.

Anticoagulants are available only with your doctor's prescription, in the following dosage forms:

Oral

Anisindione
- Tablets (U.S.)

Dicumarol
- Tablets (U.S.)

Warfarin
- Tablets (U.S. and Canada)

Parenteral

Warfarin
- Injection (U.S.)

It is very important that you read and understand the following information. If any of it causes you special concern, check with your doctor. Also, *if you have any questions* or if you want more information about this medicine or your medical problem, *ask your doctor, nurse, or pharmacist.*

Before Using This Medicine

In deciding to use a medicine, the risks of taking the medicine must be weighed against the good it will do. This is a decision you and your doctor will make. For anticoagulants, the following should be considered:

Allergies—Tell your doctor if you have ever had any unusual or allergic reaction to an anticoagulant. Also tell your doctor and pharmacist if you are allergic to any other substances, such as foods, preservatives, or dyes.

Pregnancy—Anticoagulants may cause birth defects. They may also cause other problems affecting the physical or mental growth of the fetus or newborn baby. In addition, use of this medicine during the last 6 months of pregnancy may increase the chance of severe, possibly fatal, bleeding in the fetus. If taken during the last few weeks of pregnancy, anticoagulants may cause severe bleeding in both the fetus and the mother before or during delivery and in the newborn infant.

Do not begin taking this medicine during pregnancy, and do not become pregnant while taking it, unless you have first discussed the possible effects of this medicine with your doctor. Also, if you suspect that you may be pregnant and you are already taking an anticoagulant, check with your doctor at once. Your doctor may suggest that you take a different anticoagulant that is less likely to harm the fetus or the newborn infant during all or part of your pregnancy. Anticoagulants may also cause severe bleeding in the mother if taken soon after the baby is born.

Breast-feeding—Warfarin is not likely to cause problems in nursing babies. Other anticoagulants may pass into the breast milk. A blood test can be done to see if unwanted effects are occurring in the nursing baby. If necessary, another medicine that will overcome any unwanted effects of the anticoagulant can be given to the baby.

Children—Very young babies may be especially sensitive to the effects of anticoagulants. This may increase the chance of bleeding during treatment.

Older adults—Elderly people are especially sensitive to the effects of anticoagulants. This may increase the chance of bleeding during treatment.

Other medicines—Although certain medicines should not be used together at all, in other cases two different medicines may be used together even if an interaction might occur. In these cases, your doctor may want to change the dose, or other precautions may be necessary. *Many different medicines can affect the way anticoagulants work in your body.* Therefore, it is very important that your doctor and pharmacist know if you are taking *any* other prescription or nonprescription (over-the-counter [OTC]) medicine, even aspirin, laxatives, vitamins, or antacids.

Other medical problems—The presence of other medical problems may affect the use of anticoagulants. Make sure you tell your doctor if you have *any* other medical problems, or if you are now being treated by any other medical doctor or dentist. Many medical problems and treatments will affect the way your body responds to this medicine.

Also, it is important that you tell your doctor if you have recently had any of the following conditions or medical procedures:

- Childbirth or
- Falls or blows to the body or head or
- Fever lasting more than a couple of days or
- Heavy or unusual menstrual bleeding or
- Insertion of intrauterine device (IUD) or
- Medical or dental surgery or
- Severe or continuing diarrhea or
- Spinal anesthesia or
- X-ray (radiation) treatment—The risk of serious bleeding may be increased

Before you begin using any new medicine (prescription or nonprescription) or if you develop any new medical problem while you are using this medicine, check with your doctor, nurse, or pharmacist.

Proper Use of This Medicine

Take this medicine only as directed by your doctor. Do not take more or less of it, do not take it more often, and do not take it for a longer time than your doctor ordered. This is especially important for elderly patients, who are especially sensitive to the effects of anticoagulants.

Your doctor should check your progress at regular visits. A blood test must be taken regularly to see how fast your blood is clotting. This will help your doctor decide on the proper amount of anticoagulant you should be taking each day.

Missed dose—If you miss a dose of this medicine, take it as soon as possible. Then go back to your regular dosing schedule. If you do not remember until the next day, do not take the missed dose at all and do not double the next one. *Doubling the dose may cause bleeding.* Instead, go back to your regular dosing schedule. It is recommended that you keep a record of each dose as you take it to avoid mistakes. Also, be sure to give your doctor a record of any doses you miss. If you have any questions about this, check with your doctor.

Storage—To store this medicine:
- Keep out of the reach of children.
- Store away from heat and direct light.
- Do not store this medicine in the bathroom, near the kitchen sink, or in other damp places. Heat or moisture may cause the medicine to break down.
- Do not keep outdated medicine or medicine no longer needed. Be sure that any discarded medicine is out of the reach of children.

Precautions While Using This Medicine

Tell all medical doctors, dentists, and pharmacists you go to that you are taking this medicine.

Check with your doctor, nurse, or pharmacist before you start or stop taking any other medicine. This includes any nonprescription (over-the-counter [OTC]) medicine, even aspirin or acetaminophen. Many medicines change the way this medicine affects your body. You may not be able to take the other medicine, or the dose of your anticoagulant may need to be changed.

It is important that you carry identification stating that you are using this medicine. If you have any questions about what kind of identification to carry, check with your doctor, nurse, or pharmacist.

While you are taking this medicine, it is very important that you avoid sports and activities that may cause you to be injured. Report to your doctor any falls, blows to the body or head, or other injuries, since serious internal bleeding may occur without your knowing about it.

Be careful to avoid cutting yourself. This includes taking special care in brushing your teeth and in shaving. Use a soft toothbrush and floss gently. Also, it is best to use an electric shaver rather than a blade.

Drinking too much alcohol may change the way this anticoagulant affects your body. You should not drink regularly on a daily basis or take more than 1 or 2 drinks at any time. If you have any questions about this, check with your doctor.

The foods that you eat may also affect the way this medicine affects your body. Eat a normal, balanced diet while you are taking this medicine. Do not go on a reducing diet, make other changes in your eating habits, start taking vitamins, or begin using other nutrition supplements unless you have first checked with your doctor, nurse, or pharmacist. Also, check with your doctor if you are unable to eat for several days or if you have continuing stomach upset, diarrhea, or fever. These precautions are important because the effects of the anticoagulant depend on the amount of vitamin K in your body. Therefore, it is best to have the same amount of vitamin K in your body every day. Some multiple vitamins and some nutrition supplements contain vitamin K. Vitamin K is also present in meats, dairy products (such as milk, cheese, and yogurt), and green, leafy vegetables (such as broccoli, cabbage, collard greens, kale, lettuce, and spinach). It is especially important that you do not make large changes in the amounts of these foods that you eat every day while you are taking an anticoagulant.

After you stop taking this medicine, your body will need time to recover before your blood clotting ability returns to normal. Your pharmacist or doctor can tell you how long this will take depending on which anticoagulant you were taking. Use the same caution during this period of time as you did while you were taking the anticoagulant.

Side Effects of This Medicine

Along with its needed effects, a medicine may cause some unwanted effects. Although not all of these side effects may occur, if they do occur they may need medical attention.

Check with your doctor immediately if any of the following side effects occur:

Less common or rare

Blue or purple color of toes and pain in toes; cloudy or dark urine; difficult or painful urination; sores, ulcers, or white spots in mouth or throat; sore throat and fever or chills; sudden decrease in amount of urine; swelling of face, feet, or lower legs; unusual tiredness or weakness; unusual weight gain; yellow eyes or skin

Since many things can affect the way your body reacts to this medicine, you should always watch for signs of unusual bleeding. Unusual bleeding may mean that your body is getting more medicine than it needs. *Check with your doctor immediately if any of the following signs of overdose occur:*

Bleeding from gums when brushing teeth; unexplained bruising or purplish areas on skin; unexplained nosebleeds; unusually heavy bleeding or oozing from cuts or wounds; unusually heavy or unexpected menstrual bleeding

Signs and symptoms of bleeding inside the body

Abdominal or stomach pain or swelling; back pain or backaches; blood in urine; bloody or black tarry stools; constipation; coughing up blood; dizziness; headache (severe or continuing); joint pain, stiffness, or swelling; vomiting blood or material that looks like coffee grounds

Also, check with your doctor as soon as possible if any of the following side effects occur:

Less common or rare

Diarrhea (more common with dicumarol); nausea or vomiting; skin rash, hives, or itching; stomach cramps or pain

For patients taking *anisindione* (e.g., Miradon):

• Depending on your diet, this medicine may cause your urine to turn orange. Since it may be hard to tell the difference between blood in the urine and this normal color change, check with your doctor if you notice any color change in your urine.

Other side effects may occur that usually do not need medical attention. These side effects may go away during treatment as your body adjusts to the medicine. However, check with your doctor if any of the following side effects continue or are bothersome:

More common

Bloated feeling or gas (with dicumarol)

Less common

Blurred vision or other vision problems (with anisindione); loss of appetite; unusual hair loss

Other side effects not listed above may also occur in some patients. If you notice any other effects, check with your doctor.

ANTICONVULSANTS, HYDANTOIN Systemic

This information applies to the following medicines:
  Ethotoin (ETH-oh-toyn)
  Mephenytoin (me-FEN-i-toyn)
  Phenytoin (FEN-i-toyn)

Some commonly used brand names are:

For Ethotoin†
  In the U.S.
    Peganone

For Mephenytoin
  In the U.S.
    Mesantoin

  In Canada
    Mesantoin

For Phenytoin
  In the U.S.
    Dilantin   Dilantin-30 Pediatric
    Dilantin-125   Diphenylan
    Dilantin Infatabs   Phenytex
    Dilantin Kapseals

    Generic name product may also be available.

  In Canada
    Dilantin   Dilantin-125
    Dilantin-30   Dilantin Infatabs

Another commonly used name is diphenylhydantoin.

---

†Not commercially available in Canada.

Description

Hydantoin anticonvulsants (hye-DAN-toyn an-tye-kon-VUL-sants) are used most often to control certain convulsions or seizures in the treatment of epilepsy. Phenytoin may also be used for other conditions as determined by your doctor.

In seizure disorders, these medicines act on the central nervous system (CNS) to reduce the number and severity of seizures. Hydantoin anticonvulsants may also produce some unwanted effects. These depend on the patient's individual condition, the amount of medicine taken, and how long it has been taken. It is important that you know what the side effects are and when to call your doctor if they occur.

Hydantoin anticonvulsants are available only with your doctor's prescription, in the following dosage forms:

Oral
Ethotoin
- Tablets (U.S.)
Mephenytoin
- Tablets (U.S. and Canada)
Phenytoin
- Extended capsules (U.S. and Canada)
- Prompt capsules (U.S.)
- Oral suspension (U.S. and Canada)
- Chewable tablets (U.S. and Canada)

Parenteral
Phenytoin
- Injection (U.S. and Canada)

It is very important that you read and understand the following information. If any of it causes you special concern, check with your doctor. Also, *if you have any questions* or if you want more information about this medicine or your medical problem, *ask your doctor, nurse, or pharmacist.*

Before Using This Medicine

In deciding to use a medicine, the risks of taking the medicine must be weighed against the good it will do. This is a decision you and your doctor will make. For hydantoin anticonvulsants, the following should be considered:

Allergies—Tell your doctor if you have ever had any unusual or allergic reaction to any hydantoin anticonvulsant medicine. Also tell your doctor and pharmacist if you are allergic to any other substance, such as foods, preservatives, or dyes.

Pregnancy—Although most mothers who take medicine for seizure control deliver normal babies, there have been reports of increased birth defects when these medicines were used during pregnancy. It is not definitely known if any of these medicines are the cause of such problems.

Also, pregnancy may cause a change in the way hydantoin anticonvulsants are absorbed in your body. You may have more seizures, even though you are taking your medicine regularly. Your doctor may need to increase the anticonvulsant dose during your pregnancy.

In addition, when taken during pregnancy, this medicine may cause a bleeding problem in the mother during delivery and in the newborn. This may be prevented by giving vitamin K to the mother during delivery, and to the baby immediately after birth.

Breast-feeding—Ethotoin and phenytoin pass into the breast milk in small amounts. They have not been reported to cause unwanted effects in nursing babies. However, your doctor may want you to take another medicine or to stop breast-feeding during treatment. It is not known whether mephenytoin passes into breast milk. Be sure you have discussed the risks and benefits of the medicine with your doctor.

Children—Some side effects, especially bleeding, tender, or enlarged gums and enlarged facial features are more likely to occur in children and young adults. Also, unusual and excessive hair growth may occur, which is more noticeable in young girls. In addition, some children may not do as well in school after using high doses of this medicine for a long time.

Older adults—Some medicines may affect older patients differently than they do younger patients. Overdose is more likely to occur in elderly patients and in patients with liver disease.

Athletes—Hydantoin anticonvulsants are banned and, in some cases, tested for in competitors in biathlon and modern pentathlon events by the U.S. Olympic Committee (USOC).

Other medicines—Although certain medicines should not be used together at all, in other cases 2 different medicines may be used together even if an interaction might occur. In these cases, your doctor may want to change the dose, or other precautions may be necessary. When you are taking or receiving hydantoin anticonvulsants, it is especially important that your doctor and pharmacist know if you are taking any of the following:

- Adrenocorticoids (cortisone-like medicines) or
- Estrogens (female hormones) or
- Oral contraceptives (birth-control pills) containing estrogens—Hydantoin anticonvulsants may decrease the effects of these medicines; use of hydantoin anticonvulsants with oral, estrogen-containing contraceptives may result in breakthrough bleeding and contraceptive failure; the amount of estrogen in the oral contraceptive may need to be increased to stop the bleeding and decrease the risk of pregnancy

- Alcohol or
- Central nervous system (CNS) depressants—Long-term use of alcohol may decrease the blood levels of hydantoin anticonvulsants, resulting in decreased effects; use of hydantoin anticonvulsants in cases where a large amount of alcohol is consumed may increase the blood levels of the hydantoin, resulting in an increased risk of side effects

- Aminophylline (e.g., Somophyllin) or
- Caffeine (e.g., NoDoz) or
- Oxtriphylline (e.g., Choledyl) or
- Theophylline (e.g., Somophyllin-T)—Hydantoin anticonvulsants may make these medicines less effective

- Amiodarone (e.g., Cordarone)—Use with phenytoin and possibly with other hydantoin anticonvulsants may increase blood levels of the hydantoin, resulting in an increase in serious side effects

- Antacids or
- Medicine containing calcium—Use of antacids or calcium supplements may decrease the absorption of phenytoin; doses of antacids and phenytoin or calcium supplements and phenytoin should be taken 2 to 3 hours apart

- Anticoagulants (blood thinners) or
- Chloramphenicol (e.g., Chloromycetin) or
- Cimetidine (e.g., Tagamet) or
- Disulfiram (e.g., Antabuse) (medicine for alcoholism) or
- Isoniazid (INH) (e.g., Nydrazid) or
- Phenylbutazone (e.g., Butazolidin) or
- Sulfonamides (sulfa drugs)—Blood levels of hydantoin anticonvulsants may be increased, increasing the risk of serious side effects; hydantoin anticonvulsants may increase the effects of the anticoagulants at first, but with continued use may decrease the effects of these medicines

- Diazoxide (e.g., Proglycem)—Use with hydantoin anticonvulsants may decrease the effects of both medicines; therefore, these medicines should not be taken together
- Fluconazole (e.g., Diflucan)—Blood levels of phenytoin may be increased, increasing the chance of side effects
- Lidocaine—Risk of slow heartbeat may be increased. Other effects of lidocaine may be decreased because hydantoin anticonvulsants may cause it to be removed from the body more quickly
- Methadone (e.g., Dolophine, Methadose)—Long-term use of phenytoin may bring on withdrawal symptoms in patients being treated for drug dependence
- Phenacemide (e.g., Phenurone)—Use with hydantoin anticonvulsants may increase the risk of serious side effects
- Streptozocin (e.g., Zanosar)—Phenytoin may decrease the effects of streptozocin; therefore, these medicines should not be used together
- Valproic acid (e.g., Depakene, Depakote)—Use with phenytoin, and possibly other hydantoin anticonvulsants, may increase seizure frequency and increase the risk of serious liver side effects, especially in infants

Other medical problems—The presence of other medical problems may affect the use of hydantoin anticonvulsants. Make sure you tell your doctor if you have any other medical problems, especially:

- Alcohol abuse—Blood levels of phenytoin may be decreased, decreasing its effects
- Blood disease—Risk of serious infections rarely may be increased by hydantoin anticonvulsants
- Diabetes mellitus (sugar diabetes) or
- Porphyria or
- Systemic lupus erythematosus—Hydantoin anticonvulsants may make the condition worse
- Fever above 101 °F for longer than 24 hours—Blood levels of hydantoin anticonvulsants may be decreased, decreasing the medicine's effects
- Heart disease—Administration of phenytoin by injection may change the rhythm of the heart
- Kidney disease or
- Liver disease—Blood levels of hydantoin anticonvulsants may be increased, leading to an increase in serious side effects

- Thyroid disease—Blood levels of thyroid hormones may be decreased

Before you begin using any new medicine (prescription or nonprescription) or if you develop any new medical problem while you are using this medicine, check with your doctor, nurse, or pharmacist.

Proper Use of This Medicine

For patients taking the *liquid form* of this medicine:

- Shake the bottle well before using.
- Use a specially marked measuring spoon, a plastic syringe, or a small measuring cup to measure each dose accurately. The average household teaspoon may not hold the right amount of liquid.

For patients taking the *chewable tablet form* of this medicine:

- Tablets may be chewed or crushed before they are swallowed, or may be swallowed whole.

For patients taking the *capsule form* of this medicine:

- Swallow the capsule whole.

If this medicine upsets your stomach, take it with food, unless otherwise directed by your doctor. The medicine should always be taken at the same time in relation to meals to make sure that it is absorbed in the same way.

To control your medical problem, *take this medicine every day* exactly as ordered by your doctor. Do not take more or less of it than your doctor ordered. To help you remember to take the medicine at the correct times, try to get into the habit of taking it at the same time each day.

Missed dose—*If you miss a dose of this medicine* and your dosing schedule is:

- One dose a day—Take the missed dose as soon as possible. However, if you do not remember the missed dose until the next day, skip it and go back to your regular dosing schedule. Do not double doses.

- More than one dose a day—Take the missed dose as soon as possible. However, if it is within 4 hours of your next dose, skip the missed dose and go back to your regular dosing schedule. Do not double doses.

If you miss doses for 2 or more days in a row, check with your doctor.

Storage—To store this medicine:
- Keep out of the reach of children.
- Store away from heat and direct light.
- Do not store in the bathroom, near the kitchen sink, or in other damp places. Heat or moisture may cause the medicine to break down.
- Keep the liquid form of this medicine from freezing. Do not refrigerate.
- Do not keep outdated medicine or medicine no longer needed. Be sure any discarded medicine is out of the reach of children.

Precautions While Using This Medicine

Your doctor should check your progress at regular visits, especially during the first few months of treatment with this medicine. During this time the amount of medicine you are taking may have to be changed often to meet your individual needs.

Do not start or stop taking any other medicine without your doctor's advice. Other medicines may affect the way this medicine works.

This medicine will add to the effects of alcohol and other CNS depressants (medicines that slow down the nervous system, possibly causing drowsiness). Some examples of CNS depressants are antihistamines or medicine for hay fever, other allergies, or colds; sedatives, tranquilizers, or sleeping medicine; prescription pain medicine or narcotics; barbiturates; other medicine for seizures; muscle relaxants; or anesthetics, including some dental anesthetics. *Check with your doctor before taking any of the above while you are using this medicine.*

Do not take this medicine within 2 to 3 hours of taking antacids or medicine for diarrhea. Taking these medicines too close to taking hydantoin anticonvulsants may make the hydantoins less effective.

Do not change brands or dosage forms of phenytoin without first checking with your doctor. Different products may not work the same way. If you refill your medicine and it looks different, check with your pharmacist.

If you have been taking this medicine regularly for several weeks or more, do not suddenly stop taking it. Your doctor may want you to reduce gradually the amount you are taking before stopping completely.

Your doctor may want you to carry a medical identification card or bracelet stating that you are taking this medicine.

For diabetic patients:
- This medicine may affect blood sugar levels. If you notice a change in the results of your blood or urine sugar tests or if you have any questions, check with your doctor.

Before you have any medical tests, tell the medical doctor in charge that you are taking this medicine. The results of some tests (including the dexamethasone, metyrapone, or Schilling tests, and certain thyroid function tests) may be affected by this medicine.

Before having any kind of surgery, dental treatment, or emergency treatment, tell the medical doctor or dentist in charge that you are taking this medicine.

This medicine may cause some people to become dizzy, light-headed, drowsy, or less alert than they are normally. After you have taken this medicine for a while, this effect may not be so bothersome. However, *make sure you know how you react to this medicine before you drive, use machines, or do anything else that could be dangerous if you are dizzy or are not alert.*

For patients taking *phenytoin* or *mephenytoin*:
- In some patients (usually younger patients), tenderness, swelling, or bleeding of the gums (gingival hyperplasia)

may appear soon after phenytoin or mephenytoin treatment is started. To help prevent this, brush and floss your teeth carefully and regularly and massage your gums. Also, *see your dentist every 3 months to have your teeth cleaned. If you have any questions about how to take care of your teeth and gums, or if you notice any tenderness, swelling, or bleeding of your gums, check with your medical doctor or dentist.*

Side Effects of This Medicine

Along with its needed effects, a medicine may cause some unwanted effects. Although not all of these side effects may occur, if they do occur they may need medical attention.

Check with your doctor as soon as possible if any of the following side effects or signs of overdose occur:

More common

Bleeding, tender, or enlarged gums (rare with ethotoin); clumsiness or unsteadiness; confusion; continuous, uncontrolled back-and-forth and/or rolling eye movements—may be sign of overdose; enlarged glands in neck or underarms; fever; increase in seizures; mood or mental changes; muscle weakness or pain; skin rash or itching; slurred speech or stuttering—may be sign of overdose; sore throat; trembling—may be sign of overdose; unusual excitement, nervousness, or irritability

Rare

Bone malformations; burning pain at place of injection; chest discomfort; chills and fever; dark urine; dizziness; frequent breaking of bones; headache; joint pain; learning difficulties—in children taking high doses for a long time; light gray–colored stools; loss of appetite; nausea or vomiting; pain of penis on erection; restlessness or agitation; slowed growth; stomach pain (severe); troubled or quick, shallow breathing; uncontrolled jerking or twisting movements of hands, arms, or legs; uncontrolled movements of lips, tongue, or cheeks; unusual bleeding (such as nosebleeds) or bruising; unusual tiredness or weakness; weight loss (unusual); yellow eyes or skin

Rare (with long-term use of phenytoin)

Numbness, tingling, or pain in hands or feet

Symptoms of overdose
> Blurred or double vision; clumsiness or unsteadiness (severe); confusion (severe); dizziness or drowsiness (severe); staggering walk

Other side effects may occur that usually do not need medical attention. These side effects may go away during treatment as your body adjusts to the medicine. However, check with your doctor if any of the following side effects continue or are bothersome:

More common
> Constipation; dizziness (mild); drowsiness (mild)

Less common
> Diarrhea (with ethotoin); enlargement of jaw; muscle twitching; swelling of breasts—in males; thickening of lips; trouble in sleeping; unusual and excessive hair growth on body and face (more common with phenytoin); widening of nose tip

Other side effects not listed above may also occur in some patients. If you notice any other effects, check with your doctor.

Additional Information

Once a medicine has been approved for marketing for a certain use, experience may show that it is also useful for other medical problems. Although these uses are not included in product labeling, phenytoin is used in certain patients with the following medical conditions:

- Cardiac arrythmias caused by digitalis glycosides (changes in your heart rhythm)
- Episodic dyscontrol (certain behavior disorders)
- Myotonia congenita or
- Myotonic muscular dystrophy or
- Neuromyotonia (certain muscle disorders)
- Paroxysmal choreoathetosis (certain movement disorders)
- Recessive dystrophic epidermolysis bullosa (an hereditary skin disorder)
- Tricyclic antidepressant poisoning
- Trigeminal neuralgia (tic douloureux)

Other than the above information, there is no additional information relating to proper use, precautions, or side effects for these uses.

ANTIDEPRESSANTS, MONOAMINE OXIDASE (MAO) INHIBITOR   Systemic

This information applies to the following medicines:

 Isocarboxazid (eye-soe-kar-BOX-a-zid)
 Phenelzine (FEN-el-zeen)
 Tranylcypromine (tran-ill-SIP-roe-meen)

Note: This information does *not* apply to furazolidone, procarbazine, or selegiline.

Some commonly used brand names are:

For Isocarboxazid
 In the U.S.
  Marplan

 In Canada
  Marplan

For Phenelzine
 In the U.S.
  Nardil

 In Canada
  Nardil

For Tranylcypromine
 In the U.S.
  Parnate

 In Canada
  Parnate

Description

Monoamine oxidase (MAO) inhibitors are taken by mouth to relieve certain types of mental depression. They work by blocking the action of a chemical substance known as monoamine oxidase (MAO) in the nervous system.

Although these medicines are very effective for certain patients, they may also cause some unwanted reactions if not taken in the right way. It is very important to avoid certain foods, beverages, and medicines while you are being treated with an MAO inhibitor. Your doctor, nurse, or pharmacist will help you obtain a list to carry in your wallet or purse as a reminder of which products you should avoid.

MAO inhibitors are available only with your doctor's prescription, in the following dosage forms:

Oral
Isocarboxazid
• Tablets (U.S. and Canada)
Phenelzine
• Tablets (U.S. and Canada)
Tranylcypromine
• Tablets (U.S. and Canada)

It is very important that you read and understand the following information. If any of it causes you special concern, check with your doctor. Also, *if you have any questions* or if you want more information about this medicine or your medical problem, *ask your doctor, nurse, or pharmacist*.

Before Using This Medicine

In deciding to use a medicine, the risks of taking the medicine must be weighed against the good it will do. This is a decision you and your doctor will make. For monoamine oxidase (MAO) inhibitors, the following should be considered:

Allergies—Tell your doctor if you have ever had any unusual or allergic reaction to any MAO inhibitor. Also tell your doctor and pharmacist if you are allergic to any other substances, such as foods, preservatives, or dyes.

Diet—Dangerous reactions such as sudden high blood pressure may result when MAO inhibitors are taken with certain foods or drinks. The following foods should be avoided:

• Foods that have a high tyramine content (most common in foods that are aged or fermented to increase their flavor), such as cheeses; fava or broad bean pods; yeast or meat extracts; smoked or pickled meat, poultry or fish; fermented sausage (bologna, pepperoni, salami, summer sausage) or other fermented meat; sauerkraut;

or any overripe fruit. If a list of these foods and beverages is not given to you, ask your doctor, nurse, or pharmacist to provide one.

- Alcoholic beverages or alcohol-free or reduced-alcohol beer and wine.
- Large amounts of caffeine-containing food or beverages such as coffee, tea, cola, or chocolate.

Pregnancy—Tranylcypromine (and probably isocarboxazid and phenelzine) crosses the placenta. A limited study in humans showed an increased risk of birth defects when these medicines were taken during the first trimester. In animal studies, MAO inhibitors caused a slowing of growth and increased excitability in the newborn when very large doses were given to the mother during pregnancy.

Breast-feeding—Tranylcypromine passes into the breast milk; it is not known whether isocarboxazid or phenelzine passes into breast milk. Problems in nursing babies have not been reported.

Children—Studies on these medicines have been done only in adult patients and there is no specific information comparing use of MAO inhibitors in children with use in other age groups. However, animal studies have shown that these medicines may slow growth in the young. Therefore, be sure to discuss with your doctor the use of these medicines in children.

Older adults—Dizziness or lightheadedness may be especially likely to occur in elderly patients, who are usually more sensitive than younger adults to these effects of MAO inhibitors.

Use by athletes—MAO inhibitors are banned and, in some cases, tested for in competitors in biathlon and modern pentathlon events by the United States Olympic Committee (USOC). Use of MAO inhibitors can lead to the disqualification of athletes in these events.

Other medicines—Although certain medicines should not be used together at all, in other cases 2 different medicines may be used together even if an interaction might occur. In these cases, your doctor may want to change the dose, or other precautions may be necessary. When you are taking MAO inhibitors, it is especially important that your doctor and pharmacist know if you are taking any of the following:

- Amphetamines or
- Antihypertensives (high blood pressure medicine) or
- Appetite suppressants (diet pills) or
- Cyclobenzaprine (e.g., Flexeril) or
- Fluoxetine (e.g., Prozac) or
- Levodopa (e.g., Dopar, Larodopa) or
- Maprotiline (e.g., Ludiomil) or
- Medicine for asthma or other breathing problems or
- Medicines for colds, sinus problems, or hay fever or other allergies (including nose drops or sprays) or
- Meperidine (e.g., Demerol) or
- Methylphenidate (e.g., Ritalin) or
- Monoamine oxidase (MAO) inhibitors, other, including furazolidone (e.g., Furoxone), procarbazine (e.g., Matulane), or selegiline (e.g., Eldepryl), or
- Tricyclic antidepressants (amitriptyline [e.g., Elavil], amoxapine [e.g., Asendin], clomipramine [e.g., Anafranil], desipramine [e.g., Pertofrane], doxepin [e.g., Sinequan], imipramine [e.g., Tofranil], nortriptyline [e.g., Aventyl], protriptyline [e.g., Vivactil], trimipramine [e.g., Surmontil])—Using these medicines while you are taking or within 2 weeks of taking MAO inhibitors may cause serious side effects such as sudden highly elevated body temperature, extremely high blood pressure, severe convulsions, and death; however, sometimes certain of these medicines may be used together under close supervision by your doctor
- Antidiabetics, oral (diabetes medicine you take by mouth) or
- Insulin—MAO inhibitors may change the amount of antidiabetic medicine you need to take
- Buspirone (e.g., BuSpar)—Use with MAO inhibitors may cause high blood pressure
- Carbamazepine (e.g., Tegretol)—Use with MAO inhibitors may increase seizures
- Central nervous system (CNS) depressants (medicines that cause drowsiness)—Using these medicines with MAO inhibitors may increase the CNS and other depressant effects
- Cocaine—Cocaine use by persons taking MAO inhibitors, including furazolidone and procarbazine, may cause a severe increase in blood pressure

- Dextromethorphan—Use with MAO inhibitors may cause excitement, high blood pressure, and fever
- Trazodone or
- Tryptophan used as a food supplement or a sleep aid—Use of these medicines by persons taking MAO inhibitors, including furazolidone and procarbazine, may cause mental confusion, excitement, shivering, trouble in breathing, or fever

Other medical problems—The presence of other medical problems may affect the use of MAO inhibitors. Make sure you tell your doctor if you have any other medical problems, especially:

- Alcohol abuse—Drinking alcohol while you are taking an MAO inhibitor may cause serious side effects
- Angina (chest pain) or
- Headaches (severe or frequent)—These conditions may interfere with warning signs of other more serious side effects
- Asthma or bronchitis—Some medicines used to treat these conditions may cause serious side effects when used while you are taking an MAO inhibitor
- Diabetes mellitus (sugar diabetes)—These medicines may change the amount of insulin or oral antidiabetic medication that you need
- Epilepsy—Seizures may occur more often
- Heart or blood vessel disease or
- Liver disease or
- Mental illness (or history of) or
- Parkinson's disease or
- Recent heart attack or stroke—MAO inhibitors may make the condition worse
- High blood pressure—Condition may be affected by these medicines
- Kidney disease—Higher blood levels of MAO inhibitors may occur, which increases the chance of side effects
- Overactive thyroid or
- Pheochromocytoma (PCC)—Serious side effects may occur

Proper Use of This Medicine

Sometimes this medicine must be taken for several weeks before you begin to feel better. Your doctor should check your progress at regular visits, especially during the first few months of treatment, to make sure that this medicine is working properly and to check for unwanted effects.

Take this medicine only as directed by your doctor. Do not take more of it, do not take it more often, and do not take it for a longer time than your doctor ordered.

Missed dose—If you miss a dose of this medicine, take it as soon as possible. However, if it is within 2 hours of your next dose, skip the missed dose and go back to your regular dosing schedule. Do not double doses.

Storage—To store this medicine:

- Keep out of the reach of children.
- Store away from heat and direct light.
- Do not store in the bathroom, near the kitchen sink, or in other damp places. Heat or moisture may cause the medicine to break down.
- Do not keep outdated medicine or medicine no longer needed. Be sure that any discarded medicine is out of the reach of children.

Precautions While Using This Medicine

When taken with certain foods, drinks, or other medicines, MAO inhibitors can cause very dangerous reactions such as sudden high blood pressure (also called hypertensive crisis). To avoid such reactions, *obey the following rules of caution:*

- Do not eat foods that have a high tyramine content (most common in foods that are aged or fermented to increase their flavor), such as cheeses; fava or broad bean pods; yeast or meat extracts; smoked or pickled meat, poultry, or fish; fermented sausage (bologna, pepperoni, salami, and summer sausage) or other fermented meat; sauerkraut; or any overripe fruit. If a list of these foods is not given to you, ask your doctor, nurse, or pharmacist to provide one.
- Do not drink alcoholic beverages or alcohol-free or reduced-alcohol beer and wine.
- Do not eat or drink large amounts of caffeine-containing food or beverages such as coffee, tea, cola, or chocolate.

- Do not take any other medicine unless approved or prescribed by your doctor. This especially includes over-the-counter (OTC) or nonprescription medicine, such as that for colds (including nose drops or sprays), cough, asthma, hay fever, and appetite control; "keep awake" products; or products that make you sleepy.

This medicine will add to the effects of alcohol and other CNS depressants (medicines that slow down the nervous system, possibly causing drowsiness). Some examples of CNS depressants are antihistamines or medicine for hay fever, other allergies, or colds; sedatives, tranquilizers, or sleeping medicine; prescription pain medicine or narcotics; barbiturates; medicine for seizures; muscle relaxants; or anesthetics, including some dental anesthetics. *Check with your doctor before taking any of the above while you are using this medicine.*

Check with your doctor or hospital emergency room immediately if severe headache, stiff neck, chest pains, fast heartbeat, or nausea and vomiting occur while you are taking this medicine. These may be symptoms of a serious side effect that should have a doctor's attention.

Do not stop taking this medicine without first checking with your doctor. Your doctor may want you to reduce gradually the amount you are using before stopping completely.

Dizziness, lightheadedness, or fainting may occur, especially when you get up from a lying or sitting position. *Getting up slowly may help.* When you get up from lying down, sit on the edge of the bed with your feet dangling for 1 or 2 minutes. Then stand up slowly. If the problem continues or gets worse, check with your doctor.

This medicine may cause blurred vision or make some people drowsy or less alert than they are normally. *Make sure you know how you react to this medicine before you drive, use machines, or do anything else that could be dangerous if you are unable to see well or are not alert.*

Before having any kind of surgery, dental treatment, or emergency treatment, tell the medical doctor or dentist in charge that you are using this medicine or have used it within the past 2 weeks.

Your doctor may want you to carry an identification card stating that you are using this medicine.

For patients with *angina* (chest pain):
- This medicine may cause you to have an unusual feeling of good health and energy. However, *do not suddenly increase the amount of exercise you get without discussing it with your doctor.* Too much activity could bring on an attack of angina.

For *diabetic* patients:
- This medicine may affect blood sugar levels. While you are using this medicine, be especially careful in testing for sugar in your blood or urine. If you have any questions about this, check with your doctor.

After you stop using this medicine, you must continue to obey the rules of caution for at least 2 weeks concerning food, drink, and other medicine, since these things may continue to react with MAO inhibitors.

Side Effects of This Medicine

Along with its needed effects, a medicine may cause some unwanted effects. Although not all of these side effects may occur, if they do occur they may need medical attention.

Stop taking this medicine and get emergency help immediately if any of the following side effects occur:

Symptoms of unusually high blood pressure (hypertensive crisis)

   Chest pain (severe); enlarged pupils; fast or slow heartbeat; headache (severe); increased sensitivity of eyes to light; increased sweating (possibly with fever or cold, clammy skin); nausea and vomiting; stiff or sore neck

Check with your doctor as soon as possible if any of the following side effects occur:

More common

   Dizziness or lightheadedness (severe), especially when getting up from a lying or sitting position

Less common

Diarrhea; fast or pounding heartbeat; swelling of feet or lower legs; unusual excitement or nervousness

Rare

Dark urine; fever; skin rash; slurred speech; sore throat; staggering walk; yellow eyes or skin

Symptoms of overdose

Anxiety (severe); confusion; convulsions (seizures); cool, clammy skin; dizziness (severe); drowsiness (severe); fast and irregular pulse; fever; hallucinations (seeing, hearing, or feeling things that are not there); headache (severe); high or low blood pressure; muscle stiffness; sweating; troubled breathing; trouble in sleeping (severe); unusual irritability

Other side effects may occur that usually do not need medical attention. These side effects may go away during treatment as your body adjusts to the medicine. However, check with your doctor if any of the following side effects continue or are bothersome:

More common

Blurred vision; decreased amount of urine; decreased sexual ability; dizziness or lightheadedness (mild), especially when getting up from a lying or sitting position; drowsiness; headache (mild); increased appetite (especially for sweets) or weight gain; increased sweating; muscle twitching during sleep; restlessness; shakiness or trembling; tiredness and weakness; trouble in sleeping; weakness

Less common or rare

Chills; constipation; decreased appetite; dryness of mouth

Other side effects not listed above may also occur in some patients. If you notice any other effects, check with your doctor.

Additional Information

Once a medicine has been approved for marketing for a certain use, experience may show that it is also useful for other medical problems. Although these uses are not included in product labeling, phenelzine and tranylcypromine are used in certain patients with the following medical conditions:

- Headache
- Panic disorder

Other than the above information, there is no additional information relating to proper use, precautions, or side effects for this use.

ANTIDEPRESSANTS, TRICYCLIC Systemic

This information applies to the following medicines:
   Amitriptyline (a-mee-TRIP-ti-leen)
   Amoxapine (a-MOX-a-peen)
   Clomipramine (cloe-MIP-ra-meen)
   Desipramine (dess-IP-ra-meen)
   Doxepin (DOX-e-pin)
   Imipramine (im-IP-ra-meen)
   Nortriptyline (nor-TRIP-ti-leen)
   Protriptyline (proe-TRIP-ti-leen)
   Trimipramine (trye-MIP-ra-meen)

Some commonly used brand names are:

For Amitriptyline
   In the U.S.
   Elavil   Endep
   Emitrip   Enovil

   Generic name product may also be available.

   In Canada
   Apo-Amitriptyline   Novotriptyn
   Elavil   PMS Amitriptyline
   Levate

   Generic name product may also be available.

For Amoxapine
   In the U.S.
   Asendin

   Generic name product may also be available.

   In Canada
   Asendin

For Clomipramine
   In the U.S.
   Anafranil

   In Canada
   Anafranil

For Desipramine
In the U.S.
    Norpramin

    Generic name product may also be available.

In Canada
    Norpramin
    Pertofrane

For Doxepin
In the U.S.
    Sinequan

    Generic name product may also be available.

In Canada
    Novo-Doxepin   Triadapin
    Sinequan

For Imipramine
In the U.S.
    Janimine   Tofranil
    Norfranil   Tofranil-PM
    Tipramine

    Generic name product may also be available.

In Canada
    Apo-Imipramine   PMS Imipramine
    Impril   Tofranil
    Novopramine

    Generic name product may also be available.

For Nortriptyline
In the U.S.
    Aventyl
    Pamelor

In Canada
    Aventyl

For Protriptyline
In the U.S.
    Vivactil

In Canada
    Triptil

For Trimipramine
In the U.S.
    Surmontil

    Generic name product may also be available.

In Canada
    Apo-Trimip   Surmontil
    Rhotrimine

Description

Tricyclic antidepressants ("mood elevators") are used to relieve mental depression.

One form of this medicine (imipramine) is also used to treat enuresis (bedwetting) in children. Another form (clomipramine) is used to treat obsessive-compulsive disorders. Tricyclic antidepressants may be used for other conditions as determined by your doctor.

These medicines are available only with your doctor's prescription, in the following dosage forms:

Oral

Amitriptyline
- Syrup (Canada)
- Tablets (U.S. and Canada)

Amoxapine
- Tablets (U.S. and Canada)

Clomipramine
- Capsules (U.S.)
- Tablets (Canada)

Desipramine
- Tablets (U.S. and Canada)

Doxepin
- Capsules (U.S. and Canada)
- Oral solution (U.S.)

Imipramine
- Capsules (U.S.)
- Tablets (U.S. and Canada)

Nortriptyline
- Capsules (U.S. and Canada)
- Oral solution (U.S.)

Protriptyline
- Tablets (U.S. and Canada)

Trimipramine
- Capsules (U.S. and Canada)
- Tablets (Canada)

Parenteral

Amitriptyline
- Injection (U.S.)

Imipramine
- Injection (U.S.)

It is very important that you read and understand the following information. If any of it causes you special concern, check with your doctor. Also, *if you have any questions* or if you want more information about this medicine or your medical problem, *ask your doctor, nurse, or pharmacist.*

Before Using This Medicine

In deciding to use a medicine, the risks of taking the medicine must be weighed against the good it will do. This is a decision you and your doctor will make. For tricyclic antidepressants, the following should be considered:

Allergies—Tell your doctor if you have ever had any unusual or allergic reaction to any tricyclic antidepressant or to carbamazepine, maprotiline, or trazodone. Also tell your doctor and pharmacist if you are allergic to any other substances, such as foods, preservatives, or dyes.

Pregnancy—Studies have not been done in pregnant women. However, there have been reports of newborns suffering from muscle spasms and heart, breathing, and urinary problems when their mothers had taken tricyclic antidepressants immediately before delivery. Also, studies in animals have shown that some tricyclic antidepressants may cause unwanted effects in the fetus.

Breast-feeding—Tricyclic antidepressants pass into the breast milk. Doxepin has been reported to cause drowsiness in the nursing baby.

Children—Children are especially sensitive to the effects of this medicine. This may increase the chance of side effects during treatment. However, side effects in children taking this medicine for bedwetting usually disappear upon continued use. The most common of these are nervousness, sleeping problems, tiredness, and mild stomach upset. If these side effects continue or are bothersome, check with your doctor.

Older adults—Drowsiness, dizziness, confusion, vision problems, dryness of mouth, constipation, and problems in urinating are more likely to occur in elderly patients, who are usually more sensitive than younger adults to the effects of tricyclic antidepressants.

Athletes—Tricyclic antidepressants are banned and, in some cases, tested for in competitors in biathlon and modern pentathlon events by the U.S. Olympic Committee (USOC).

Other medicines—Although certain medicines should not be used together at all, in other cases 2 different medicines may be used together even if an interaction might occur. In these cases, your doctor may want to change the dose, or other precautions may be necessary. When you are taking a tricyclic antidepressant, it is especially important that your doctor and pharmacist know if you are taking any of the following:

- Antipsychotics (medicine for mental illness) or
- Clonidine (e.g., Catapres)—Using these medicines with tricyclic antidepressants may increase the CNS depressant effects and increase the chance of serious side effects
- Antithyroid agents (medicine for overactive thyroid) or
- Cimetidine (e.g., Tagamet)—Using these medicines with tricyclic antidepressants may increase the chance of serious side effects
- Amphetamines or
- Appetite suppressants (diet pills) or
- Ephedrine or
- Epinephrine (e.g., Adrenalin) or
- Isoproterenol (e.g., Isuprel) or
- Medicine for asthma or other breathing problems or
- Medicine for colds, sinus problems, or hay fever or other allergies or
- Phenylephrine (e.g., Neo-Synephrine)—Using these medicines with tricyclic antidepressants may increase the risk of serious effects on the heart
- Central nervous system (CNS) depressants—Using these medicines with tricyclic antidepressants may increase the CNS depressant effects
- Guanadrel (e.g., Hylorel) or
- Guanethidine (e.g., Ismelin)—Tricyclic antidepressants may keep these medicines from working as well
- Methyldopa (e.g., Aldomet) or
- Metoclopramide (e.g., Reglan) or
- Metyrosine (e.g., Demser) or
- Pemoline (e.g., Cylert) or
- Pimozide (e.g., Orap) or
- Promethazine (e.g., Phenergan) or

- Rauwolfia alkaloids (alseroxylon [e.g., Rauwiloid], deserpidine [e.g., Harmonyl], rauwolfia serpentina [e.g., Raudixin], reserpine [e.g., Serpasil]) or
- Trimeprazine (e.g., Temaril)—Tricyclic antidepressants may cause certain side effects to be more severe and occur more often
- Metrizamide—The risk of seizures may be increased
- Monoamine oxidase (MAO) inhibitors (furazolidone [e.g., Furoxone], isocarboxazid [e.g., Marplan], phenelzine [e.g., Nardil], procarbazine [e.g., Matulane], selegiline [e.g., Eldepryl], tranylcypromine [e.g., Parnate])—Taking tricyclic antidepressants while you are taking or within 2 weeks of taking monoamine oxidase (MAO) inhibitors may cause sudden highly elevated body temperature, extremely high blood pressure, severe convulsions, and death; however, sometimes certain of these medicines may be used together under close supervision by your doctor

Other medical problems—The presence of other medical problems may affect the use of tricyclic antidepressants. Make sure you tell your doctor if you have any other medical problems, especially:

- Alcohol abuse (or history of)—Drinking alcohol may cause increased CNS depressant effects
- Asthma or
- Bipolar disorder (manic-depressive illness) or
- Blood disorders or
- Convulsions (seizures) or
- Difficult urination or
- Enlarged prostate or
- Glaucoma or increased eye pressure or
- Heart disease or
- High blood pressure (hypertension) or
- Schizophrenia—Tricyclic antidepressants may make the condition worse
- Kidney disease or
- Liver disease—Higher blood levels of tricyclic antidepressants may result, increasing the chance of side effects
- Overactive thyroid or
- Stomach or intestinal problems—Tricyclic antidepressants may cause an increased chance of serious side effects

Before you begin using any new medicine (prescription or nonprescription) or if you develop any new medical problem while you are using this medicine, check with your doctor, nurse, or pharmacist.

Proper Use of This Medicine

To lessen stomach upset, take this medicine with food, even for a daily bedtime dose, unless your doctor has told you to take it on an empty stomach.

Take this medicine only as directed by your doctor, to benefit your condition as much as possible. Do not take more of it, do not take it more often, and do not take it for a longer time than your doctor ordered.

Sometimes this medicine must be taken for several weeks before you begin to feel better. Your doctor should check your progress at regular visits.

To use *doxepin oral solution:*

- This medicine is to be taken by mouth even though it comes in a dropper bottle. The amount you should take should be measured with the dropper provided with your prescription and diluted just before you take each dose. Dilute each dose with about one-half glass (4 ounces) of water, milk, citrus fruit juice, tomato juice, or prune juice. Do not mix this medicine with grape juice or carbonated beverages since these may decrease the medicine's effectiveness.

- Doxepin oral solution must be mixed immediately before you take it. Do not prepare it ahead of time.

Missed dose—If you miss a dose of this medicine and your dosing schedule is:

- One dose a day at bedtime—Do not take the missed dose in the morning since it may cause disturbing side effects during waking hours. Instead, check with your doctor.

- More than one dose a day—Take the missed dose as soon as possible. However, if it is almost time for your next dose, skip the missed dose, and go back to your regular dosing schedule. Do not double doses.

If you have any questions about this, check with your doctor.

Storage—To store this medicine:

- Keep out of the reach of children. Overdose of this medicine is very dangerous in young children.
- Store away from heat and direct light.
- Do not store the tablet or capsule form of this medicine in the bathroom, near the kitchen sink, or in other damp places. Heat or moisture may cause the medicine to break down.
- Keep the liquid form of this medicine from freezing.
- Do not keep outdated medicine or medicine no longer needed. Be sure that any discarded medicine is out of the reach of children.

Precautions While Using This Medicine

It is very important that your doctor check your progress at regular visits to allow dosage adjustments and to help reduce side effects.

This medicine will add to the effects of alcohol and other CNS depressants (medicines that slow down the nervous system, possibly causing drowsiness). Some examples of CNS depressants are antihistamines or medicine for hay fever, other allergies, or colds; sedatives, tranquilizers, or sleeping medicine; prescription pain medicine or narcotics; barbiturates; medicine for seizures; muscle relaxants; or anesthetics, including some dental anesthetics. *Check with your medical doctor or dentist before taking any of the above while you are taking this medicine.*

This medicine may cause some people to become drowsy. *If this occurs, do not drive, use machines, or do anything else that could be dangerous if you are not alert.*

Dizziness, lightheadedness, or fainting may occur, especially when you get up from a lying or sitting position. Getting up slowly may help. If this problem continues or gets worse, check with your doctor.

This medicine may cause dryness of the mouth. For temporary relief, use sugarless gum or candy, melt bits of ice in your mouth, or use a saliva substitute. However, if your mouth continues to feel dry for more than 2 weeks, check with your medical doctor or dentist. Continuing dryness of the mouth may increase the chance of dental disease, including tooth decay, gum disease, and fungus infections.

Tricyclic antidepressants may cause your skin to be more sensitive to sunlight than it is normally. Exposure to sunlight, even for brief periods of time, may cause a skin rash, itching, redness or other discoloration of the skin, or a severe sunburn. When you begin taking this medicine:

- Stay out of direct sunlight, especially between the hours of 10:00 a.m. and 3:00 p.m., if possible.
- Wear protective clothing, including a hat. Also, wear sunglasses.
- Apply a sun block product that has a skin protection factor (SPF) of at least 15. Some patients may require a product with a higher SPF number, especially if they have a fair complexion. If you have any questions about this, check with your doctor or pharmacist.
- Apply a sun block lipstick that has an SPF of at least 15 to protect your lips.
- Do not use a sunlamp or tanning bed or booth.

If you have a severe reaction from the sun, check with your doctor.

Before you have any medical tests, tell the medical doctor in charge that you are taking this medicine. The results of the metyrapone test may be affected by this medicine.

Before having any kind of surgery, dental treatment, or emergency treatment, tell the medical doctor or dentist in charge that you are using this medicine.

For diabetic patients:
- This medicine may affect blood sugar levels. If you notice a change in the results of your blood or urine sugar tests or if you have any questions, check with your doctor.

Do not stop taking this medicine without first checking with your doctor. Your doctor may want you to reduce gradually the amount you are using before stopping completely. This may help prevent a possible worsening of your condition and reduce the possibility of withdrawal symptoms such as headache, nausea, and/or an overall feeling of discomfort.

The effects of this medicine may last for 3 to 7 days after you have stopped taking it. Therefore, all the precautions stated here must be observed during this time.

For patients taking protriptyline:
- If taken late in the day, protriptyline may interfere with nighttime sleep.

Side Effects of This Medicine

Along with its needed effects, a medicine may cause some unwanted effects. Although not all of these side effects may occur, if they do occur they may need medical attention.

Stop taking this medicine and get emergency help immediately if any of the following side effects occur:

Reported for amoxapine only—rare

Convulsions (seizures); difficult or fast breathing; fever with increased sweating; high or low (irregular) blood pressure; loss of bladder control; muscle stiffness (severe); pale skin; unusual tiredness or weakness

Check with your doctor as soon as possible if any of the following side effects occur:

Less common

Blurred vision; confusion or delirium; constipation (especially in the elderly); decreased sexual ability (more common with amoxapine and clomipramine); difficulty in speaking or swallowing; eye pain; fainting; fast or irregular heartbeat (pounding, racing, skipping); hallucinations; loss of balance control; mask-like face; nervousness or restlessness; problems in urinating; shakiness or trembling; shuffling walk; slowed movements; stiffness of arms and legs

Reported for amoxapine only (in addition to the above)— less common

Lip smacking or puckering; puffing of cheeks; rapid or worm-like movements of tongue; uncontrolled chewing movements; uncontrolled movements of hands, arms, or legs

Rare

Anxiety; breast enlargement in both males and females; hair loss; inappropriate secretion of milk—in females; increased sensitivity to sunlight; irritability; muscle twitching; red or brownish spots on skin; ringing, buzzing, or other unexplained sounds in the ears; seizures (more common with clomipramine); skin rash and itching; sore throat and fever; swelling of face and tongue; swelling of testicles (more common with amoxapine); trouble with teeth or gums (more common with clomipramine); weakness; yellow eyes or skin

Symptoms of acute overdose

Confusion; convulsions (seizures); disturbed concentration; drowsiness (severe); enlarged pupils; fast, slow, or irregular heartbeat; fever; hallucinations (seeing, hearing, or feeling things that are not there); restlessness and agitation; shortness of breath or troubled breathing; unusual tiredness or weakness (severe); vomiting

Other side effects may occur that usually do not need medical attention. These side effects may go away during treatment as your body adjusts to the medicine. However, check with your doctor if any of the following side effects continue or are bothersome:

More common

Dizziness; drowsiness; dryness of mouth; headache; increased appetite (may include craving for sweets); nausea; tiredness or weakness (mild); unpleasant taste; weight gain

Less common

Diarrhea; heartburn; increased sweating; trouble in sleeping (more common with protriptyline, especially when taken late in the day); vomiting

Certain side effects of this medicine may occur after you have stopped taking it. Check with your doctor if you notice any of the following effects:

Headache; irritability; nausea, vomiting, or diarrhea; restlessness; trouble in sleeping, with vivid dreams; unusual excitement

Reported for amoxapine only (in addition to the above)

Lip smacking or puckering; puffing of cheeks; rapid or worm-like movements of the tongue; uncontrolled chewing movements; uncontrolled movements of arms or legs

Other side effects not listed above also may occur in some patients. If you notice any other effects, check with your doctor.

Additional Information

Once a medicine has been approved for marketing for a certain use, experience may show that it is also useful for other medical problems. Although these uses are not included in product labeling, tricyclic antidepressants are used in certain patients with the following medical conditions:

- Attention deficit hyperactivity disorder (hyperactivity in children) (desipramine, imipramine, and protriptyline)
- Bulimia (uncontrolled eating, followed by vomiting) (amitriptyline, clomipramine, desipramine, and imipramine)
- Cocaine withdrawal (desipramine and imipramine)
- Headache prevention (for certain types of frequent or continuing headaches) (most tricyclic antidepressants)
- Itching with hives due to cold temperature exposure (doxepin)
- Narcolepsy (extreme tendency to fall asleep suddenly) (clomipramine, desipramine, imipramine, and protriptyline)
- Neurogenic pain (a type of continuing pain) (amitriptyline, clomipramine, desipramine, doxepin, imipramine, nortriptyline, and trimipramine)
- Panic disorder (clomipramine, desipramine, doxepin, nortriptyline, and trimipramine)
- Stomach ulcer (amitriptyline, doxepin, and trimipramine)
- Urinary incontinence (imipramine)

Other than the above information, there is no additional information relating to proper use, precautions, or side effects for these uses.

ANTIDIABETICS, ORAL   Systemic

This information applies to the following medicines:

Acetohexamide (a-set-oh-HEX-a-mide)
Chlorpropamide (klor-PROE-pa-mide)
Glipizide (GLIP-i-zide)
Glyburide (GLYE-byoo-ride)
Tolazamide (tole-AZ-a-mide)
Tolbutamide (tole-BYOO-ta-mide)

Some commonly used brand names are:

For Acetohexamide
In the U.S.
   Dymelor
   Generic name product may also be available.

In Canada
   Dimelor
   Generic name product may also be available.

For Chlorpropamide
In the U.S.
   Diabinese   Glucamide
   Generic name product may also be available.

In Canada
   Apo-Chlorpropamide   Novopropamide
   Diabinese
   Generic name product may also be available.

For Glipizide
In the U.S.
   Glucotrol

For Glyburide
In the U.S.
   DiaBeta   Micronase
In Canada
   DiaBeta   Euglucon
   Another commonly used name is glibenclamide.

For Tolazamide
In the U.S.
   Tolamide   Tolinase
   Generic name product may also be available.

For Tolbutamide
In the U.S.
   Oramide   Orinase
   Generic name product may also be available.

In Canada
   Apo-Tolbutamide   Novobutamide
   Mobenol   Orinase
   Generic name product may also be available.

Description

Oral antidiabetics (diabetes medicine you take by mouth)
may help reduce the amount of sugar in the blood by causing
your pancreas gland to make more insulin. They are used
to treat certain types of diabetes mellitus (sugar diabetes).

Oral antidiabetics can usually be used only by adults who develop diabetes after 30 years of age and who do not require insulin shots (or who usually do not require more than 20 Units of insulin a day) to control their condition. This type of diabetic patient is said to have non–insulin-dependent diabetes mellitus (or NIDDM), sometimes known as maturity-onset or Type II diabetes. Oral antidiabetics do not help diabetic patients who have insulin-dependent diabetes mellitus (or IDDM), sometimes known as juvenile-onset or Type I diabetes.

Chlorpropamide may also be used for other conditions as determined by your doctor.

Oral antidiabetic medicines do not help diabetic patients who are insulin-dependent (type I). However, non–insulin-dependent (type II) diabetic patients who are taking oral antidiabetics may have to temporarily switch to insulin if they:

- develop diabetic coma or ketoacidosis.
- have a severe injury or burn.
- develop a severe infection.
- are to have major surgery.
- are pregnant.

Before you begin treatment with this medicine, you and your doctor should talk about the good the medicine will do as well as the risks of using it. You should also find out about other possible ways to treat your diabetes such as by diet alone or by diet plus insulin.

Oral antidiabetics are available only with your doctor's prescription, in the following dosage forms:

Oral

Acetohexamide
- Tablets (U.S. and Canada)

Chlorpropamide
- Tablets (U.S. and Canada)

Glipizide
- Tablets (U.S.)

Glyburide
- Tablets (U.S. and Canada)

Tolazamide
  • Tablets (U.S.)
Tolbutamide
  • Tablets (U.S. and Canada)

It is very important that you read and understand the following information. If any of it causes you special concern, check with your doctor. Also, *if you have any questions* or if you want more information about this medicine or your medical problem, *ask your doctor, nurse, or pharmacist.*

Before Using This Medicine

In deciding to use a medicine, the risks of taking the medicine must be weighed against the good it will do. This is a decision you and your doctor will make. For oral antidiabetic medicines, the following should be considered:

Allergies—Tell your doctor if you have ever had any unusual or allergic reaction to oral antidiabetic medicines, or to sulfonamide-type (sulfa) medications, including thiazide diuretics (a certain type of water pill). Also tell your doctor and pharmacist if you are allergic to any other substances, such as foods, preservatives, or dyes.

Diet—If you have non–insulin-dependent (type II) diabetes, your doctor may try to control your condition by prescribing a personal meal plan for you before prescribing medicine. Such a diet is low in refined carbohydrates (foods such as sugar and candy used for quick energy) and fat. The daily number of calories in this meal plan should be adjusted by a dietitian to help you reach and maintain a proper body weight. Oral antidiabetics are less effective if you are greatly overweight. It may be very important for you to follow a planned weight reduction diet. In addition, meals and snacks are arranged to meet the energy needs of your body at different times of the day.

Many people with type II diabetes are able to control their diabetes by carefully following their prescribed meal and exercise plan. Oral antidiabetics are prescribed only when additional help is needed.

Pregnancy—Oral antidiabetics should not be used during pregnancy. Insulin may be needed to keep blood sugar levels as close to normal as possible. Poor control of blood sugar levels may cause birth defects or death of the fetus. In addition, use of oral antidiabetics during pregnancy may cause the newborn baby to have low blood sugar levels. This may last for several days following birth.

Breast-feeding—Chlorpropamide passes into the breast milk and its use is not recommended because it could cause low blood sugar in the baby. Although it is not known if the other oral antidiabetics pass into breast milk and these medicines have not been shown to cause problems in humans, the chance always exists.

Children—There is little information about the use of oral antidiabetic agents in children. Type II diabetes is unusual in this age group.

Older adults—The elderly may be more sensitive than younger adults to the effects of oral antidiabetics. Also, elderly patients who take chlorpropamide are more likely to retain (keep) too much body water.

Other medicines—Although certain medicines should not be used together at all, in other cases two different medicines may be used together even if an interaction might occur. In these cases, your doctor may want to change the dose, or other precautions may be necessary. *Do not take any other medicine, unless prescribed or approved by your doctor.* When you are taking oral antidiabetic drugs, it is especially important that your doctor and pharmacist know if you are taking any of the following:

- Anticoagulants (blood thinners)—The effect of either the blood thinner or the antidiabetic medicine may be increased or decreased if the 2 medicines are used together
- Appetite control medicines or
- Asthma medicines or
- Cough or cold medicines or
- Hay fever or allergy medicines—Many medicines (including nonprescription [over-the-counter]) products can affect the control of your blood glucose (sugar)

- Aspirin or other salicylates or
- Chloramphenicol (e.g., Chloromycetin) or
- Guanethidine (e.g., Ismelin) or
- Sulfonamides (sulfa medicine)—These medicines may increase the chances of low blood sugar

- Beta-blockers (acebutolol [e.g., Sectral], atenolol [e.g., Tenormin], carteolol [e.g., Cartrol], labetalol [e.g., Normodyne], metoprolol [e.g., Lopressor], nadolol [e.g., Corgard], oxprenolol [e.g., Trasicor], penbutolol [e.g., Levatol], pindolol [e.g., Visken], propranolol [e.g., Inderal], sotalol [e.g., Sotacor], timolol [e.g., Blocadren])—Beta-blockers may increase the risk of high or low blood sugar occurring. They can also block symptoms of low blood sugar (such as fast heartbeat or high blood pressure). Because of this, a diabetic patient might not know that he or she had low blood sugar and might not immediately take the proper steps to raise the blood sugar level. Beta-blockers can also cause low blood sugar to last longer

- Monoamine oxidase (MAO) inhibitors (furazolidone [e.g., Furoxone], isocarboxazid [e.g., Marplan], pargyline [e.g., Eutonyl], phenelzine [e.g., Nardil], procarbazine [e.g., Matulane], or tranylcypromine [e.g., Parnate])—Taking oral antidiabetic medicines while you are taking (or within 2 weeks of taking) monoamine oxidase (MAO) inhibitors may increase the chances of low blood sugar occurring

Other medical problems—The presence of other medical problems may affect the use of the oral antidiabetic medicines. Make sure you tell your doctor if you have any other medical problems, especially:

- Heart disease—Chlorpropamide causes some patients to retain (keep) more body water than usual. Heart disease may worsened by this extra body water
- Infection (severe)—Insulin may be needed temporarily to control diabetes in patients with severe infection because changes in blood sugar may occur rapidly and without much warning
- Kidney disease or
- Liver disease—Low blood sugar may be more likely to occur because the kidney or liver is not able to get the medicine out of the blood stream as it normally would. Also, people with kidney disease who take chlorpropamide are more likely to retain (keep) too much body water
- Thyroid disease

- Underactive adrenal glands (untreated) or
- Underactive pituitary gland (untreated)—Patients with these conditions may be more likely to develop low blood sugar (hypoglycemia) while taking oral antidiabetic medicines

Before you begin using any new medicine (prescription or nonprescription) or if you develop any new medical problem while you are using this medicine, check with your doctor, nurse, or pharmacist.

Proper Use of This Medicine

Follow carefully your special meal plan, since this is the most important part of controlling your diabetes and is necessary if the medicine is to work properly.

Take your oral antidiabetics only as directed by your doctor. Do not take more or less of it than your doctor ordered, and take it at the same time each day. This will help to control your blood sugar levels.

Missed dose—If you miss a dose of this medicine, take it as soon as possible. However, if it is almost time for your next dose, skip the missed dose and go back to your regular dosing schedule. Do not double doses.

Storage—To store this medicine:
- Keep out of the reach of children.
- Store away from heat and direct light.
- Do not store in the bathroom, near the kitchen sink, or in other damp places. Heat or moisture may cause the medicine to break down.
- Do not keep outdated medicine or medicine no longer needed. Be sure that any discarded medicine is out of the reach of children.

Precautions While Using This Medicine

Your doctor will want to check your progress at regular visits, especially during the first few weeks that you take this medicine.

Test for sugar in your blood or urine as directed by your doctor. This is important in making sure your diabetes is being controlled and provides an early warning when it is not.

Do not take any other medicine, unless prescribed or approved by your doctor. This especially includes nonprescription (over-the-counter [OTC]) medicine such as that for colds, cough, asthma, hay fever, or appetite control.

Avoid drinking alcoholic beverages until you have discussed their use with your doctor. Some patients who drink alcohol while taking this medicine may suffer stomach pain, nausea, vomiting, dizziness, pounding headache, sweating, or flushing (redness of face and skin). In addition, alcohol may produce hypoglycemia (low blood sugar).

Oral antidiabetic medicines may cause your skin to be more sensitive to sunlight than it is normally. Exposure to sunlight, even for brief periods of time, may cause a skin rash, itching, redness or other discoloration of the skin, or a severe sunburn.

When you begin taking this medicine:
- Stay out of direct sunlight, especially between the hours of 10:00 a.m. and 3:00 p.m., if possible.
- Wear protective clothing, including a hat. Also, wear sunglasses.
- Apply a sun block product that has a skin protection factor (SPF) of at least 15. Some patients may require a product with a higher SPF number, especially if they have a fair complexion. If you have any questions about this, check with your doctor or pharmacist.
- Apply a sun block lipstick that has an SPF of at least 15 to protect your lips.
- Do not use a sunlamp or tanning bed or booth.

If you have a severe reaction from the sun, check with your doctor.

Eat or drink something containing sugar and check with your doctor right away if mild symptoms of low blood sugar (hypoglycemia) appear. Good sources of sugar are glucose tablets or gel or fruit juice, corn syrup, honey, non-diet soft drinks, or sugar cubes or table sugar (dissolved in water). It is a good idea also to check your blood sugar to confirm that it is low.

- *If severe symptoms such as convulsions (seizures) or unconsciousness occur, diabetics should not eat or drink anything.* There is a chance that they could choke from not swallowing correctly. Emergency medical help should be obtained immediately.

- *Symptoms of low blood sugar (hypoglycemia) are:*
  Abdominal or stomach pain (mild)
  Anxious feeling
  Chills (continuing)
  Cold sweats
  Confusion
  Convulsions (seizures)
  Cool pale skin
  Difficulty in concentration
  Drowsiness
  Excessive hunger
  Fast heartbeat
  Headache (continuing)
  Nausea or vomiting (continuing)
  Nervousness
  Shakiness
  Unconsciousness
  Unsteady walk
  Unusual tiredness or weakness
  Vision changes

- Different people may have different symptoms of hypoglycemia. It is important that you learn your own signs of low blood sugar so that you can treat it quickly.

- *These symptoms may occur if you:*
  —delay or miss a scheduled meal or snack.
  —exercise much more than usual.
  —cannot eat because of nausea and vomiting.
  —drink a significant amount of alcohol.

- *Tell someone to take you to your doctor or to a hospital right away if the symptoms do not improve after eating or drinking a sweet food.*

- Even if you correct these symptoms by eating sugar, it is very important to call your doctor or hospital emergency service right away, since the blood sugar–lowering effects of this medicine may last for days and the symptoms may return often during this time.

Before having any kind of surgery, dental treatment, or emergency treatment, tell the medical doctor or dentist in charge that you are taking this medicine.

You should wear a medical I.D. bracelet or chain at all times. In addition, you should carry an identification card that says you have diabetes and that lists your medications.

Side Effects of This Medicine

The use of oral antidiabetics has been reported to increase the risk of death from heart and blood vessel disease. A report based on a study by the University Group Diabetes Program (UGDP) compared the use of one of the oral medicines (tolbutamide) to the use of diet alone or diet plus insulin. Although only tolbutamide was studied, other oral antidiabetics may cause a similar effect since all these medicines are related chemically and in the way they work.

Along with their needed effects, oral antidiabetics may cause some unwanted effects. Although not all of these side effects may occur, if they do occur they may need medical attention.

Check with your doctor as soon as possible if any of the following side effects occur:

Rare

Chest pain; chills; coughing up blood; dark urine; fever; general feeling of illness; increased sweating; itching of the skin; light-colored stools; increased amounts of sputum (phlegm); shortness of breath; sore throat; unusual bleeding or bruising; unusual tiredness or weakness (continuing and unexplained); yellow eyes or skin

Symptoms of overdose (hypoglycemia)

Abdominal or stomach pain (mild); anxious feeling; chills (continuing); cold sweats; confusion; convulsions (seizures); cool, pale skin; difficulty in concentration; drowsiness; excessive hunger; fast heartbeat; headache (continuing); nausea or vomiting (continuing); nervousness; shakiness; unconsciousness; unsteady walk; unusual tiredness or weakness; vision changes

Other side effects may occur that usually do not need medical attention. These side effects may go away during treatment as your body adjusts to the medicine. However, check with your doctor if any of the following side effects continue or are bothersome:

More common

Changes in taste (for tolbutamide); constipation; diarrhea; dizziness; drowsiness (mild); headache; heartburn; increased or decreased appetite; nausea; vomiting; stomach pain, fullness, or discomfort

Less common or rare

Hives; increased sensitivity of skin to sun; skin redness, itching, or rash

For patients taking chlorpropamide:

- Some patients who take chlorpropamide may retain (keep) more body water than usual. Check with your doctor as soon as possible if any of the following signs occur:

Breathing difficulty; shortness of breath

Other side effects not listed above may also occur in some patients. If you notice any other effects, check with your doctor.

Additional Information

Once a medicine has been approved for marketing for a certain use, experience may show that it is also useful for other medical problems. Although this use is not included in product labeling, chlorpropamide is used in certain patients with the following medical condition:

- Diabetes insipidus (water diabetes)

If you are taking this medicine for water diabetes, the advice listed above that relates to diet and urine testing for patients with *sugar* diabetes *does not apply to you*. However, the advice about hypoglycemia (low blood sugar) does apply to you. Call your doctor right away if you feel any of the symptoms described.

ANTIDYSKINETICS Systemic

This information applies to the following medicines:

    Benztropine (BENZ-troe-peen)
    Biperiden (bye-PER-i-den)
    Ethopropazine (eth-oh-PROE-pa-zeen)
    Procyclidine (proe-SYE-kli-deen)
    Trihexyphenidyl (trye-hex-ee-FEN-i-dill)

Note: This information does *not* apply to Amantadine, Carbidopa and Levodopa, Diphenhydramine, Haloperidol, and Levodopa.

Some commonly used brand names are:

For Benztropine
    In the U.S.
        Cogentin
        Generic name product may also be available.

    In Canada

Apo-Benztropine	Cogentin
Bensylate	PMS Benztropine

        Generic name product may also be available.

Another commonly used name is benzatropine.

For Biperiden
    In the U.S. and Canada
        Akineton

For Ethopropazine
In the U.S.
Parsidol
In Canada
Parsitan

Another commonly used name is profenamine.

For Procyclidine
In the U.S.
Kemadrin
In Canada
Kemadrin   Procyclid
PMS Procyclidine

For Trihexyphenidyl
In the U.S.
Artane   Trihexane
Artane Sequels   Trihexy
Generic name product may also be available.
In Canada
Aparkane   Artane Sequels
Apo-Trihex   Novohexidyl
Artane   PMS Trihexyphenidyl

Description

Antidyskinetics are used to treat Parkinson's disease, sometimes referred to as "shaking palsy." By improving muscle control and reducing stiffness, this medicine allows more normal movements of the body as the disease symptoms are reduced. It is also used to control severe reactions to certain medicines such as reserpine (e.g., Serpasil) (medicine to control high blood pressure) or phenothiazines, chlorprothixene (e.g., Taractan), thiothixene (e.g., Navane), loxapine (e.g., Loxitane), and haloperidol (e.g., Haldol) (medicines for nervous, mental, and emotional conditions).

Antidyskinetics may also be used for other conditions as determined by your doctor.

These medicines are available only with your doctor's prescription in the following dosage forms:

Oral
Benztropine
• Tablets (U.S. and Canada)

Biperiden
  • Tablets (U.S. and Canada)
Ethopropazine
  • Tablets (U.S. and Canada)
Procyclidine
  • Elixir (Canada)
  • Tablets (U.S. and Canada)
Trihexyphenidyl
  • Extended-release capsules (U.S. and Canada)
  • Elixir (U.S. and Canada)
  • Tablets (U.S. and Canada)

Parenteral
Benztropine
  • Injection (U.S. and Canada)
Biperiden
  • Injection (U.S.)

It is very important that you read and understand the following information. If any of it causes you special concern, do not decide against using this medicine without first checking with your doctor. Also, *if you have any questions* or if you want more information about this medicine or your medical problem, *ask your doctor, nurse, or pharmacist.*

Before Using This Medicine

In deciding to use a medicine, the risks of taking the medicine must be weighed against the good it will do. This is a decision you and your doctor will make. For antidyskinetics, the following should be considered:

Allergies—Tell your doctor if you have ever had any unusual or allergic reaction to antidyskinetics. Also tell your doctor and pharmacist if you are allergic to any other substances, such as foods, preservatives, or dyes.

Pregnancy—Studies on effects in pregnancy have not been done in either humans or animals. However, antidyskinetics have not been shown to cause problems in humans.

Breast-feeding—Antidyskinetics have not been reported to cause problems in nursing babies. However, since these medicines tend to decrease the secretions of the body, it is possible that the flow of breast milk may be reduced in some patients.

Children—Children may be especially sensitive to the effects of antidyskinetics. This may increase the chance of side effects during treatment.

Older adults—Agitation, confusion, disorientation, hallucinations, memory loss, and mental changes are more likely to occur in elderly patients, who are usually more sensitive to the effects of antidyskinetics.

Other medicines—Although certain medicines should not be used together at all, in other cases 2 different medicines may be used together even if an interaction might occur. In these cases, your doctor may want to change the dose, or other precautions may be necessary. When you are taking an antidyskinetic, it is especially important that your doctor and pharmacist know if you are taking any of the following:

- Antacids—May interfere with the effects of the antidyskinetics; allow at least 1 hour between doses of the different medicines
- Anticholinergics (medicine for abdominal or stomach spasms or cramps) or
- Central nervous system (CNS) depressants—Using these medicines together with antidyskinetics may result in additive effects, increasing the chance of unwanted effects

Other medical problems—The presence of other medical problems may affect the use of antidyskinetics. Make sure you tell your doctor if you have any other medical problems, especially:

- Difficult urination or
- Enlarged prostate or
- Glaucoma or
- Heart or blood vessel disease or
- High blood pressure or
- Intestinal blockage or
- Myasthenia gravis or
- Uncontrolled movements of hands, mouth, or tongue—Antidyskinetics may make the condition worse
- Kidney disease or
- Liver disease—Higher blood levels of the antidyskinetics may result, increasing the chance of side effects

Before you begin using any new medicine (prescription or nonprescription) or if you develop any new medical problem while you are using this medicine, check with your doctor, nurse, or pharmacist.

Proper Use of This Medicine

Take this medicine only as directed by your doctor. Do not take more of it, do not take it more often, and do not take it for a longer period of time than your doctor ordered. To do so may increase the chance of side effects.

To lessen stomach upset, take this medicine with meals or immediately after meals, unless otherwise directed by your doctor.

Missed dose—If you miss a dose of this medicine, take it as soon as possible. However, if it is within 2 hours of your next dose, skip the missed dose and go back to your regular dosing schedule. Do not double doses.

Storage—To store this medicine:
- Keep out of the reach of children.
- Store away from heat and direct light.
- Do not store the capsule or tablet form of this medicine in the bathroom, near the kitchen sink, or in other damp places. Heat or moisture may cause the medicine to break down.
- Keep the liquid form of this medicine from freezing.
- Do not keep outdated medicine or medicine no longer needed. Be sure that any discarded medicine is out of the reach of children.

Precautions While Using This Medicine

Your doctor should check your progress at regular visits, especially for the first few months you take this medicine. This will allow your dosage to be changed as necessary to meet your needs.

Your doctor may want you to have your eyes examined by an ophthalmologist (eye doctor) before and also sometime later during treatment.

Do not stop taking this medicine without first checking with your doctor. Your doctor may want you to reduce gradually the amount you are taking before stopping completely, to prevent side effects or the worsening of your condition.

This medicine will add to the effects of alcohol and other CNS depressants (medicines that slow down the nervous system, possibly causing drowsiness). Some examples of CNS depressants are antihistamines or medicine for hay fever, other allergies, or colds; sedatives, tranquilizers, or sleeping medicine; prescription pain medicine or narcotics; barbiturates; medicine for seizures; muscle relaxants; or anesthetics, including some dental anesthetics. *Check with your doctor before taking any of the above while you are using this medicine.*

Do not take this medicine within 1 hour of taking antacids or medicine for diarrhea. Taking these medicines too close together will make this medicine less effective.

If you think you or anyone else has taken an overdose of this medicine, get emergency help at once. Taking an overdose of this medicine may lead to unconsciousness. Some signs of an overdose are clumsiness or unsteadiness; seizures; severe drowsiness; fast heartbeat; hallucinations (seeing, hearing, or feeling things that are not there); mood or mental changes; shortness of breath or troubled breathing; trouble in sleeping; and unusual warmth, dryness, and flushing of skin.

This medicine may cause your eyes to become more sensitive to light than they are normally. Wearing sunglasses and avoiding too much exposure to bright light may help lessen the discomfort.

This medicine may cause some people to have blurred vision or to become drowsy, dizzy, or less alert than they are normally. *Make sure you know how you react to this medicine before you drive, use machines, or do anything else that could be dangerous if you are dizzy or are not alert or able to see well.*

Dizziness, lightheadedness, or fainting may occur, especially when you get up from lying or sitting. Getting up slowly may help. If the problem continues or gets worse, check with your doctor.

This medicine may make you sweat less, causing your body temperature to increase. *Use extra care to avoid becoming overheated during exercise or hot weather while you are taking this medicine, since overheating may result in heat stroke.* Also, hot baths or saunas may make you feel dizzy or faint while you are taking this medicine.

This medicine may cause dryness of the mouth. For temporary relief, use sugarless candy or gum, melt bits of ice in your mouth, or use a saliva substitute. However, if your mouth continues to feel dry for more than 2 weeks, check with your medical doctor or dentist. Continuing dryness of the mouth may increase the chance of dental disease, including tooth decay, gum disease, and fungus infections.

Side Effects of This Medicine

Along with its needed effects, a medicine may cause some unwanted effects. Although not all of these side effects may occur, if they do occur they may need medical attention.

Check with your doctor as soon as possible if any of the following side effects occur:

Rare

Confusion (more common in the elderly or with high doses); eye pain; skin rash

Symptoms of overdose

Clumsiness or unsteadiness; drowsiness (severe); dryness of mouth, nose, or throat (severe); fast heartbeat; hallucinations (seeing, hearing, or feeling things that are not there); mood or mental changes; seizures; shortness of breath or troubled breathing; trouble in sleeping; warmth, dryness, and flushing of skin

Other side effects may occur that usually do not need medical attention. These side effects may go away during treatment as your body adjusts to the medicine. However, check with your doctor if any of the following side effects continue or are bothersome:

More common

Blurred vision; constipation; decreased sweating; difficult or painful urination (especially in older men); drowsiness; dryness of mouth, nose, or throat; increased sensitivity of eyes to light; nausea or vomiting

Less common or rare

Dizziness or lightheadedness when getting up from a lying or sitting position; false sense of well-being (especially in the elderly or with high doses); headache; loss of memory (especially in the elderly); muscle cramps; nervousness; numbness or weakness in hands or feet; soreness of mouth and tongue; stomach upset or pain; unusual excitement (more common with large doses of trihexyphenidyl)

After you stop using this medicine, your body may need time to adjust. The length of time this takes depends on the amount of medicine you were using and how long you used it. During this period of time check with your doctor if you notice any of the following side effects:

Anxiety; difficulty in speaking or swallowing; dizziness or light-headedness when getting up from a lying or sitting position; fast heartbeat; loss of balance control; mask-like face; muscle spasms, especially of face, neck, and back; restlessness or desire to keep moving; shuffling walk; stiffness of arms or legs; trembling and shaking of hands and fingers; trouble in sleeping; twisting movements of body

Other side effects not listed above may also occur in some patients. If you notice any other effects, check with your doctor.

ANTIHISTAMINES Systemic

This information applies to the following medicines:

Astemizole (a-STEM-mi-zole)
Azatadine (a-ZA-ta-deen)
Bromodiphenhydramine (broe-moe-dye-fen-HYE-dra-meen)
Brompheniramine (brome-fen-EER-a-meen)
Carbinoxamine (kar-bi-NOX-a-meen)
Cetirizine (se-TI-ra-zeen)
Chlorpheniramine (klor-fen-EER-a-meen)
Clemastine (KLEM-as-teen)

Cyproheptadine (si-proe-HEP-ta-deen)
Dexchlorpheniramine (dex-klor-fen-EER-a-meen)
Dimenhydrinate (dye-men-HYE-dri-nate)
Diphenhydramine (dye-fen-HYE-dra-meen)
Diphenylpyraline (dye-fen-il-PEER-a-leen)
Doxylamine (dox-ILL-a-meen)
Hydroxyzine (hye-DROX-i-zeen)
Loratadine (lor-AT-a-deen)
Phenindamine (fen-IN-da-meen)
Pyrilamine (peer-ILL-a-meen)
Terfenadine (ter-FEN-a-deen)
Tripelennamine (tri-pel-ENN-a-meen)
Triprolidine (trye-PROE-li-deen)

Some commonly used brand names are:

For Astemizole
In the U.S.
    Hismanal

In Canada
    Hismanal

For Azatadine
In the U.S.
    Optimine

In Canada
    Optimine

For Bromodiphenhydramine

Another commonly used name for bromodiphenhydramine is bromazine.
Bromodiphenhydramine is not available by itself in the U.S. and Canada.
However, it is available in cough/cold combination products.

For Brompheniramine
In the U.S.

Bromphen	Dimetane
Chlorphed	Dimetane Extentabs
Codimal-A	Histaject Modified
Conjec-B	Nasahist B
Cophene-B	ND-Stat Revised
Dehist	Oraminic II
Diamine T.D.	Veltane

Generic name product may also be available.

In Canada
Dimetane   Dimetane Extentabs

For Carbinoxamine

Carbinoxamine is not available by itself in the U.S. and Canada. However, it is available in cough/cold combination products.

For Cetirizine*
In Canada
    Reactine

For Chlorpheniramine
In the U.S.

Aller-Chlor
Chlo-Amine
Chlor-100
Chlorate
Chlor-Niramine
Chlor-Pro
Chlor-Pro 10
Chlorspan-12
Chlortab-4
Chlortab-8
Chlor-Trimeton

Chlor-Trimeton Repetabs
Genallerate
PediaCare Allergy
 Formula
Pfeiffer's Allergy
Phenetron
Phenetron Lanacaps
Telachlor
Teldrin
Trymegen

Generic name product may also be available.

In Canada
Chlor-Tripolon   Novopheniram

Another commonly used name is chlorphenamine.

For Clemastine
In the U.S.
Tavist   Tavist-1
In Canada
Tavist

For Cyproheptadine
In the U.S.
Periactin

Generic name product may also be available.

In Canada
Periactin

For Dexchlorpheniramine
In the U.S.
Dexchlor   Polaramine
Poladex T.D.   Polaramine Repetabs

Generic name product may also be available.

In Canada
Polaramine   Polaramine Repetabs

For Dimenhydrinate
In the U.S.

Calm X
Dimetabs
Dinate
Dommanate
Dramamine
Dramamine Chewable
Dramamine Liquid
Dramanate
Dramocen

Dramoject
Dymenate
Hydrate
Marmine
Nico-Vert
Tega-Vert
Triptone Caplets
Vertab

Generic name product may also be available.

In Canada
Apo-Dimenhydrinate   Novodimenate
Gravol   PMS-Dimenhydrinate
Gravol L/A   Travamine
Nauseatol

Generic name product may also be available.

For Diphenhydramine
In the U.S.

AllerMax Caplets   Fynex
Aller-med   Genahist
Banophen   Gen-D-phen
Banophen Caplets   Hydramine
Beldin   Hydramine Cough
Belix   Hydramyn
Bena-D 10   Hydril
Bena-D 50   Hyrexin-50
Benadryl   Nervine Nighttime Sleep-Aid
Benadryl 25   Nidryl
Benadryl Kapseals   Noradryl
Benahist 10   Nordryl
Benahist 50   Nordryl Cough
Ben-Allergin-50   Nytol Maximum Strength
Benoject-10   Nytol with DPH
Benoject-50   Phendry
Benylin Cough   Phendry Children's
Bydramine Cough   Allergy Medicine
Compoz   Sleep-Eze 3
Diphenacen-50   Sominex Formula 2
Diphenadryl   Tusstat
Diphen Cough   Twilite Caplets
Diphenhist   Uni-Bent Cough
Diphenhist Captabs   Wehdryl-10
Dormarex 2   Wehdryl-50

Generic name product may also be available.

In Canada
Allerdryl   Insomnal
Benadryl

Generic name product may also be available.

For Diphenylpyraline
Diphenylpyraline is not available by itself in the U.S. and Canada. However, it is available in cough/cold combination products.

For Doxylamine
In the U.S.
Unisom Nighttime Sleep Aid

In Canada
Doxylamine is not available by itself in Canada. However, it is available in cough/cold combination products.

For Hydroxyzine
In the U.S.

Anxanil	Quiess
Atarax	Vistaject-25
E-Vista	Vistaject-50
Hydroxacen	Vistaril
Hyzine-50	Vistazine 50

Generic name product may also be available.

In Canada

Apo-Hydroxyzine	Multipax
Atarax	Novohydroxyzin

Generic name product may also be available.

For Loratadine*
In Canada
Claritin

For Phenindamine†
In the U.S.
Nolahist

For Pyrilamine†
In the U.S.
Nisaval

Generic name product may also be available.
Another commonly used name is mepyramine.

For Terfenadine
In the U.S.
Seldane
In Canada
Seldane   Seldane Caplets

For Tripelennamine
In the U.S.

PBZ	Pelamine
PBZ-SR	

Generic name product may also be available.

In Canada
Pyribenzamine

For Triprolidine
In the U.S.

Actidil	Myidil
Alleract	

Generic name product may also be available.
In Canada

Triprolidine is not available by itself in Canada. However, it is available in cough/cold combination products.

---

*Not commercially available in the U.S.
†Not commercially available in Canada.

Description

Antihistamines are used to relieve or prevent the symptoms of hay fever and other types of allergy. They work by preventing the effects of a substance called histamine, which is produced by the body.

Some of the antihistamines are also used to prevent motion sickness, nausea, vomiting, and dizziness. In patients with Parkinson's disease, diphenhydramine may be used to decrease stiffness and tremors. Also, the syrup form of diphenhydramine is used to relieve the cough due to colds or hay fever. In addition, since antihistamines may cause drowsiness as a side effect, some of them may be used to help people go to sleep.

Hydroxyzine is used in the treatment of nervous and emotional conditions to help control anxiety. It can also be used to help control anxiety and produce sleep before surgery.

Antihistamines may also be used for other conditions as determined by your doctor.

Some antihistamine preparations are available only with your doctor's prescription. Others are available without a prescription. However, your doctor may have special instructions on the proper dose of the medicine for your medical condition.

These medicines are available in the following dosage forms:

Oral

Astemizole
- Oral suspension (Canada)
- Tablets (U.S. and Canada)

Azatadine
- Tablets (U.S. and Canada)

Brompheniramine
- Elixir (U.S. and Canada)
- Tablets (U.S. and Canada)
- Extended-release tablets (U.S. and Canada)

Cetirizine
- Tablets (Canada)

Chlorpheniramine
- Extended-release capsules (U.S.)
- Syrup (U.S. and Canada)
- Tablets (U.S. and Canada)
- Chewable tablets (U.S.)
- Extended-release tablets (U.S. and Canada)

Clemastine
- Syrup (U.S. and Canada)
- Tablets (U.S. and Canada)

Cyproheptadine
- Syrup (U.S. and Canada)
- Tablets (U.S. and Canada)

Dexchlorpheniramine
- Syrup (U.S. and Canada)
- Tablets (U.S. and Canada)
- Extended-release tablets (U.S. and Canada)

Dimenhydrinate
- Capsules (U.S.)
- Extended-release capsules (Canada)
- Elixir (Canada)
- Syrup (U.S.)
- Tablets (U.S. and Canada)
- Chewable tablets (U.S.)

Diphenhydramine
- Capsules (U.S. and Canada)
- Elixir (U.S. and Canada)
- Syrup (U.S.)
- Tablets (U.S.)

Doxylamine
- Tablets (U.S.)

Hydroxyzine
- Capsules (U.S. and Canada)
- Oral suspension (U.S.)
- Syrup (U.S. and Canada)
- Tablets (U.S.)

Loratadine
- Tablets (Canada)

Phenindamine
- Tablets (U.S.)

Pyrilamine
- Tablets (U.S.)

Terfenadine
- Oral suspension (Canada)
- Tablets (U.S. and Canada)

Tripelennamine
  • Elixir (U.S.)
  • Tablets (U.S. and Canada)
  • Extended-release tablets (U.S.)
Triprolidine
  • Syrup (U.S.)
  • Tablets (U.S.)

Parenteral
Brompheniramine
  • Injection (U.S.)
Chlorpheniramine
  • Injection (U.S. and Canada)
Dimenhydrinate
  • Injection (U.S. and Canada)
Diphenhydramine
  • Injection (U.S. and Canada)
Hydroxyzine
  • Injection (U.S. and Canada)

Rectal
Dimenhydrinate
  • Suppositories (Canada)

It is very important that you read and understand the following information. If any of it causes you special concern, check with your doctor or pharmacist. Also, *if you have any questions* or if you want more information about this medicine or your medical problem, *ask your doctor, nurse, or pharmacist.*

Before Using This Medicine

In deciding to use a medicine, the risks of taking the medicine must be weighed against the good it will do. This is a decision you and your doctor will make. For antihistamines, the following should be considered:

Allergies—Tell your doctor if you have ever had any unusual or allergic reaction to antihistamines. Also tell your doctor and pharmacist if you are allergic to any other substances, such as foods, preservatives, or dyes.

Diet—Make certain your doctor and pharmacist know if you are on a low-sodium, low-sugar, or any other special diet.

Most medicines contain more than their active ingredient, and many liquid medicines contain alcohol.

Pregnancy—Most antihistamines have not been studied in pregnant women. Although these antihistamines have not been shown to cause problems in humans, studies in animals have shown that some other antihistamines, such as meclizine (e.g., Antivert) and cyclizine (e.g., Marezine), may cause birth defects.

Also, studies in animals have shown that terfenadine, when given in doses several times the human dose, lowers the birth weight and increases the risk of death of the offspring.

Hydroxyzine is not recommended for use in the first months of pregnancy since it has been shown to cause birth defects in animal studies when given in doses up to many times the usual human dose. Be sure you have discussed this with your doctor.

Breast-feeding—Small amounts of antihistamines pass into the breast milk. Use is not recommended since babies are more susceptible to the side effects of antihistamines, such as unusual excitement or irritability. Also, since these medicines tend to decrease the secretions of the body, it is possible that the flow of breast milk may be reduced in some patients. It is not known yet whether astemizole, loratadine, and terfenadine cause these same side effects.

Children—Serious side effects, such as convulsions (seizures), are more likely to occur in younger patients and would be of greater risk to infants than to older children or adults. In general, children are more sensitive to the effects of antihistamines. Also, nightmares or unusual excitement, nervousness, restlessness, or irritability may be more likely to occur in children.

Older adults—Elderly patients are usually more sensitive to the effects of antihistamines. Confusion; difficult or painful urination; dizziness; drowsiness; feeling faint; or dryness of mouth, nose, or throat may be more likely to occur in elderly patients. Also, nightmares or unusual excitement, nervousness, restlessness, or irritability may be more likely to occur in elderly patients.

Other medicines—Although certain medicines should not be used together at all, in other cases different medicines may be used together even if an interaction might occur. In these cases, your doctor may want to change the dose, or other precautions may be necessary. When you are taking antihistamines it is especially important that your doctor and pharmacist know if you are taking any of the following:

- Anticholinergics (medicine for abdominal or stomach spasms or cramps)—Side effects, such as dryness of mouth, of antihistamines or anticholinergics may be more likely to occur
- Central nervous system (CNS) depressants—Effects, such as drowsiness, of CNS depressants or antihistamines may be worsened; also, taking maprotiline or tricyclic antidepressants may cause some side effects of either of these medicines, such as dryness of mouth, to become more severe
- Erythromycin (e.g., E-Mycin) or
- Ketoconazole (e.g., Nizoral)—Use of these medicines with terfenadine may cause heart problems, such as an irregular heartbeat; these medicines should not be used together
- Monoamine oxidase (MAO) inhibitors (furazolidone [e.g., Furoxone], isocarboxazid [e.g., Marplan], phenelzine [e.g., Nardil], procarbazine [e.g., Matulane], tranylcypromine [e.g., Parnate])—If you are now taking, or have taken within the past 2 weeks, any of the MAO inhibitors, the side effects of the antihistamines may become more severe; these medicines should not be used together

Other medical problems—The presence of other medical problems may affect the use of antihistamines. Make sure you tell your doctor if you have any other medical problems, especially:

- Enlarged prostate or
- Urinary tract blockage or difficult urination—Antihistamines may make urinary problems worse
- Glaucoma—These medicines may cause a slight increase in inner eye pressure that may make the condition worse
- Liver disease—Higher blood levels of astemizole or terfenadine may result, which may increase the chance of heart problems

Before you begin using any new medicine (prescription or nonprescription) or if you develop any new medical problem while you are using this medicine, check with your doctor, nurse, or pharmacist.

Proper Use of This Medicine

Antihistamines are used to relieve or prevent the symptoms of your medical problem. Take them only as directed. Do not take more of them and do not take them more often than recommended on the label, unless otherwise directed by your doctor. To do so may increase the chance of side effects.

Missed dose—If you are taking this medicine regularly and you miss a dose, take it as soon as possible. However, if it is almost time for your next dose, skip the missed dose and go back to your regular dosing schedule. Do not double doses.

For patients *taking this medicine by mouth:*

- Antihistamines can be taken with food or a glass of water or milk to lessen stomach irritation if necessary.
- If you are taking the extended-release tablet form of this medicine, swallow the tablets whole. Do not break, crush, or chew before swallowing.

For patients taking *dimenhydrinate or diphenhydramine for motion sickness:*

- Take this medicine at least 30 minutes or, even better, 1 to 2 hours before you begin to travel.

For patients using the *suppository form of this medicine:*

- To insert suppository: First remove the foil wrapper and moisten the suppository with cold water. Lie down on side and use your finger to push the suppository well up into the rectum. If the suppository is too soft to insert, chill the suppository in the refrigerator for 30 minutes or run cold water over it, before removing the foil wrapper.

For patients using the *injection form of this medicine:*

- If you will be giving yourself the injections, make sure you understand exactly how to give them. If you have any questions about this, check with your doctor, nurse, or pharmacist.

Storage—To store this medicine:

- Keep out of the reach of children, since overdose may be very dangerous in children.
- Store away from heat and direct light.
- Do not store the capsule or tablet form of this medicine in the bathroom medicine cabinet, near the kitchen sink, or in other damp places. Heat or moisture may cause the medicine to break down.
- Keep the liquid form of this medicine from freezing.
- Do not keep outdated medicine or medicine no longer needed. Be sure that any discarded medicine is out of the reach of children.

Precautions While Using This Medicine

Before you have any skin tests for allergies, tell the doctor in charge that you are taking this medicine. The results of the test may be affected by this medicine.

When taking antihistamines on a regular basis, make sure your doctor knows if you are taking large amounts of aspirin at the same time (as in arthritis or rheumatism). Effects of too much aspirin, such as ringing in the ears, may be covered up by the antihistamine.

Antihistamines will add to the effects of alcohol and other CNS depressants (medicines that slow down the nervous system, possibly causing drowsiness). Some examples of CNS depressants are sedatives, tranquilizers, or sleeping medicine; prescription pain medicine or narcotics; barbiturates; medicine for seizures; muscle relaxants; or anesthetics, including some dental anesthetics. *Check with your doctor before taking any of the above while you are using this medicine.*

This medicine may cause some people to become drowsy or less alert than they are normally. Even if taken at bedtime, it may cause some people to feel drowsy or less alert on arising. Some antihistamines are more likely to cause drowsiness than others (astemizole, loratadine, and terfenadine, for example, rarely produce this effect). *Make sure you know how you react to the antihistamine you are taking before you drive, use machines, or do anything else that could be dangerous if you are not alert.*

Antihistamines may cause dryness of the mouth, nose, and throat. Some antihistamines are more likely to cause dryness of the mouth than others (astemizole, loratadine, and terfenadine, for example, rarely produce this effect). For temporary relief of mouth dryness, use sugarless candy or gum, melt bits of ice in your mouth, or use a saliva substitute. However, if your mouth continues to feel dry for more than 2 weeks, check with your medical doctor or dentist. Continuing dryness of the mouth may increase the chance of dental disease, including tooth decay, gum disease, and fungus infections.

For patients using *dimenhydrinate, diphenhydramine, or hydroxyzine:*

- This medicine controls nausea and vomiting. For this reason, it may cover up the signs of overdose caused by other medicines or the symptoms of appendicitis. This will make it difficult for your doctor to diagnose these conditions. Make sure your doctor knows that you are taking this medicine if you have other symptoms of appendicitis such as stomach or lower abdominal pain, cramping, or soreness. Also, if you think you may have taken an overdose of any medicine, tell your doctor that you are taking this medicine.

For patients using *diphenhydramine or doxylamine as a sleeping aid:*

- If you are already taking a sedative or tranquilizer, do not take this medicine without consulting your doctor first.

Side Effects of This Medicine

Along with its needed effects, a medicine may cause some unwanted effects. Although not all of these side effects may occur, if they do occur they may need medical attention.

Check with your doctor immediately if the following side effect occurs:

Less common or rare—with high doses of astemizole or terfenadine only

Fast or irregular heartbeat

Also, check with your doctor as soon as possible if any of the following side effects occur:

Less common or rare

Sore throat and fever; unusual bleeding or bruising; unusual tiredness or weakness

Symptoms of overdose

Clumsiness or unsteadiness; convulsions (seizures); drowsiness (severe); dryness of mouth, nose, or throat (severe); feeling faint; flushing or redness of face; hallucinations (seeing, hearing, or feeling things that are not there); shortness of breath or troubled breathing; trouble in sleeping

Other side effects may occur that usually do not need medical attention. These side effects may go away during treatment as your body adjusts to the medicine. However, check with your doctor or pharmacist if any of the following side effects continue or are bothersome:

More common—rare with astemizole, loratadine, and terfenadine; less common with cetirizine

Drowsiness; thickening of mucus

Less common or rare

Blurred vision or any change in vision; confusion; difficult or painful urination; dizziness; dryness of mouth, nose, or throat; fast heartbeat; increased sensitivity of skin to sun; increased sweating; loss of appetite (increased appetite with astemizole and cyproheptadine); nightmares; ringing or buzzing in ears; skin rash; stomach upset or stomach pain (more common with pyrilamine and tripelennamine); unusual excitement, nervousness, restlessness, or irritability; weight gain (with astemizole and cyproheptadine only)

Other side effects not listed above may also occur in some patients. If you notice any other effects, check with your doctor or pharmacist.

Additional Information

Once a medicine has been approved for marketing for a certain use, experience may show that it is also useful for other medical problems. Although this use is not included in product labeling, astemizole, cetirizine, loratadine, and terfenadine are used in certain patients with asthma.

Other than the above information, there is no additional information relating to proper use, precautions, or side effects for this use.

ANTIHISTAMINES AND DECONGESTANTS   Systemic

Some commonly used brand names are:

In the U.S.—

Actacin[25]
Actagen[25]
Actifed[25]
Actifed 12-Hour[25]
Alamine[11]
Alersule[9]
Allent[6]
Allerest[11]
Allerest 12 Hour[11]
Allerest 12 Hour
   Caplets[11]
Allerfrin[25]
Allergy Formula Sinutab [18]
Allergy Relief Medicine[11]
Allerphed[25]
Amaril D[13]
Amaril D Spantab[13]
Anamine[14]
Anamine T.D.[14]
Aprodrine[25]

A.R.M. Maximum
   Strength Caplets[11]
Atrohist Sprinkle[5]
Benadryl Decongestant[19]
Benylin Decongestant[19]
Brexin L.A.[14]
Bromatap[4]
Bromatapp[4]
Bromfed[6]
Bromfed-PD[6]
Bromophen T.D.[3]
Brompheril[18]
Carbiset[7]
Carbodec[7]
Carbodec TR[7]
Cardec-S[7]
Cenafed Plus[25]
Chlorafed[14]
Chlorafed H.S. Timecelles[14]
Chlorafed Timecelles[14]

Chlor-Rest[11]
Chlor-Trimeton Decongestant[14]
Chlor-Trimeton Decongestant Repetabs[14]
Codimal-L.A.[14]
Coltab Children's[9]
Comhist[12]
Comhist LA[12]
Condrin-LA[11]
Conex D.A.[11]
Contac 12-Hour[11]
Contac Maximum Strength 12-Hour Caplets[11]
Cophene No.2[14]
Co-Pyronil 2[14]
Dallergy-D[9][14]
Dallergy Jr.[6]
Decohist[9]
Deconamine[14]
Deconamine SR[14]
Decongestabs[13]
Dehist[11]
Demazin[11]
Demazin Repetabs[11]
Dexaphen SA[18]
Dexophed[18]
Dihistine[9]
Dimaphen S.A.[3]
Dimetane Decongestant[2]
Dimetane Decongestant Caplets[2]
Dimetapp[4]
Dimetapp Extentabs[4]
Disobrom[18]
Disophrol[18]
Disophrol Chronotabs[18]
Dorcol Children's Cold Formula[14]

Drixoral[6][18]
Drize[11]
Duralex[14]
Dura-Tap PD[14]
Dura-Vent/A[11]
Endafed[6]
Fedahist[14]
Fedahist Decongestant[14]
Fedahist Gyrocaps[14]
Fedahist Timecaps[14]
Genac[25]
Genamin[11]
Genatap[4]
Gencold[11]
Histabid Duracaps[11]
Histalet[14]
Histalet Forte[16]
Histamic[13]
Histatab Plus[9]
Histatan[15]
Hista-Vadrin[10]
Histor-D[9]
12-Hour Cold[11]
Isoclor[14]
Isoclor Timesules[14]
Klerist-D[14]
Kronofed-A Jr. Kronocaps[14]
Kronofed-A Kronocaps[14]
Myfed[25]
Myfedrine Plus[14]
Myhistine[9]
Myminic[11]
Myphetapp[4]
Naldecon[13]
Naldecon Pediatric Drops[13]
Naldecon Pediatric Syrup[13]
Naldelate[13]
Naldelate Pediatric Syrup[13]
Nalgest[13]

Napril[14]
Nasahist[10]
ND Clear T.D.[14]
New-Decongest[13]
New-Decongest
    Pediatric Syrup[13]
Nolamine[8]
Norafed[25]
Noraminic[11]
Normatane[3]
Novafed A[14]
Novahistine[9]
Oragest S.R.[11]
Oraminic Spancaps[11]
Ornade Spansules[11]
Panadyl[23]
PediaCare Cold Formula[14]
Phenergan-D[23]
Phenergan VC[22]
Phentox Compound[13]
Pherazine VC[22]
Poly-Histine-D[20]
Poly-Histine-D Ped[20]
Prometh VC Plain[22]
Promethazine VC[22]
Pseudo-Chlor[14]
Pseudo-gest Plus[14]
Resaid S.R.[11]
Resporal TR[18]
Rhinolar-EX[11]
Rhinolar-EX 12[11]
Rinade B.I.D.[14]
Rondec[7]
Rondec Drops[7]
Rondec-TR[7]
R-Tannate[15]

Ru-Tuss[9]
Ru-Tuss II[11]
Ryna[14]
Rynatan[15]
Seldane-D[24]
Sinucon Pediatric
    Drops[13]
Snaplets-D[11]
Sudafed Plus[14]
Tamine S.R.[3]
Tavist-D[17]
T-Dry[14]
T-Dry Junior[14]
Triaminic-12[11]
Triaminic Allergy[11]
Triaminic Chewables[11]
Triaminic Cold[11]
Triaminic Oral
    Infant Drops[21]
Triaminic TR[21]
Trifed[25]
Trinalin Repetabs[1]
Trind[11]
Tri-Nefrin
    Extra Strength[11]
Triofed[25]
Triotann[15]
Tri-Phen-Chlor[13]
Tri-Phen-Chlor T.D.[13]
Triphenyl[11]
Triphenyl T.D.[21]
Tripodrine[25]
Triposed[25]
Tussanil Plain[9]
Vasominic T.D.[13]
Veltap[3]

In Canada—

Actifed[25]
Benylin Cold[14]
Chlor-Tripolon
  Decongestant[11] [14]
Chlor-Tripolon
  Decongestant Extra
  Strength[14]
Chlor-Tripolon
  Decongestant Repetabs[14]
Corsym[11]
Dimetapp[3]
Dimetapp Extentabs[3]

Dimetapp Oral
  Infant Drops[3]
Drixoral[18]
Drixtab[18]
Novahistex[14]
Ornade[11]
Ornade-A.F.[11]
Ornade Spansules[11]
Triaminic[11] [21]
Triaminic Oral
  Infant Drops[21]
Trinalin Repetabs[1]

Note: For quick reference the following antihistamine and decongestant combinations are numbered to match the corresponding brand names.

This information applies to the following medicines:

1. Azatadine (a-ZA-ta-deen) and Pseudoephedrine (soo-doe-e-FED-rin)
2. Brompheniramine (brome-fen-EER-a-meen) and Phenylephrine (fen-ill-EF-rin)
3. Brompheniramine, Phenylephrine, and Phenylpropanolamine (fen-ill-proe-pa-NOLE-a-meen)*†
4. Brompheniramine and Phenylpropanolamine
5. Brompheniramine, Phenyltoloxamine (fen-ill-toe-LOX-a-meen), and Phenylephrine
6. Brompheniramine and Pseudoephedrine
7. Carbinoxamine (kar-bi-NOX-a-meen) and Pseudoephedrine
8. Chlorpheniramine (klor-fen-EER-a-meen), Phenindamine (fen-IN-da-meen), and Phenylpropanolamine
9. Chlorpheniramine and Phenylephrine
10. Chlorpheniramine, Phenylephrine, and Phenylpropanolamine
11. Chlorpheniramine and Phenylpropanolamine*
12. Chlorpheniramine, Phenyltoloxamine, and Phenylephrine
13. Chlorpheniramine, Phenyltoloxamine, Phenylephrine, and Phenylpropanolamine
14. Chlorpheniramine and Pseudoephedrine
15. Chlorpheniramine, Pyrilamine (peer-ILL-a-meen), and Phenylephrine
16. Chlorpheniramine, Pyrilamine, Phenylephrine, and Phenylpropanolamine
17. Clemastine (KLEM-as-teen) and Phenylpropanolamine
18. Dexbrompheniramine (dex-brom-fen-EER-a-meen) and Pseudoephedrine*
19. Diphenhydramine (dye-fen-HYE-dra-meen) and Pseudoephedrine
20. Pheniramine (fen-EER-a-meen), Phenyltoloxamine, Pyrilamine, and Phenylpropanolamine
21. Pheniramine, Pyrilamine, and Phenylpropanolamine
22. Promethazine (proe-METH-a-zeen) and Phenylephrine
23. Promethazine and Pseudoephedrine

24. Terfenadine (ter-FEN-a-deen) and Pseudoephedrine
25. Triprolidine (trye-PROE-li-deen) and Pseudoephedrine*

---

*Generic name product may also be available in the U.S.
†Generic name product may also be available in Canada.

Description

Antihistamine and decongestant combinations are used to treat the nasal congestion (stuffy nose), sneezing, and runny nose caused by colds and hay fever.

Antihistamines work by preventing the effects of a substance called histamine, which is produced by the body. Antihistamines contained in these combinations are: brompheniramine, chlorpheniramine, dexbrompheniramine, diphenhydramine, pheniramine, phenyltoloxamine, pyrilamine, terfenadine, and triprolidine.

The decongestants, such as phenylephrine, phenylpropanolamine (also known as PPA), and pseudoephedrine produce a narrowing of blood vessels. This leads to clearing of nasal congestion, but it may also cause an increase in blood pressure in patients who have high blood pressure.

Some of these combinations are available only with your doctor's prescription. Others are available without a prescription; however, your doctor may have special instructions on the proper dose of the medicine for your medical condition. They are available in the following dosage forms:

Oral

Azatadine and Pseudoephedrine
- Extended-release tablets (U.S. and Canada)

Brompheniramine and Phenylephrine
- Elixir (U.S.)
- Tablets (U.S.)

Brompheniramine, Phenylephrine, and Phenylpropanolamine
- Elixir (U.S. and Canada)
- Oral solution (Canada)
- Tablets (Canada)
- Extended-release tablets (U.S. and Canada)

Brompheniramine and Phenylpropanolamine
- Elixir (U.S.)
- Tablets (U.S.)
- Extended-release tablets (U.S.)

Brompheniramine, Phenyltoloxamine, and Phenylephrine
- Extended-release capsules (U.S.)

Brompheniramine and Pseudoephedrine
- Extended-release capsules (U.S.)
- Syrup (U.S.)
- Tablets (U.S.)

Carbinoxamine and Pseudoephedrine
- Oral solution (U.S.)
- Syrup (U.S.)
- Tablets (U.S.)
- Extended-release tablets (U.S.)

Chlorpheniramine, Phenindamine, and Phenylpropanolamine
- Extended-release tablets (U.S.)

Chlorpheniramine and Phenylephrine
- Extended-release capsules (U.S.)
- Elixir (U.S.)
- Syrup (U.S.)
- Tablets (U.S.)
- Chewable tablets (U.S.)

Chlorpheniramine, Phenylephrine, and Phenylpropanolamine
- Extended-release capsules (U.S.)
- Tablets (U.S.)

Chlorpheniramine and Phenylpropanolamine
- Extended-release capsules (U.S. and Canada)
- Granules (U.S.)
- Oral solution (U.S. and Canada)
- Extended-release oral suspension (Canada)
- Syrup (U.S. and Canada)
- Tablets (U.S.)
- Chewable tablets (U.S.)
- Extended-release tablets (U.S.)

Chlorpheniramine, Phenyltoloxamine, and Phenylephrine
- Extended-release capsules (U.S.)
- Tablets (U.S.)

Chlorpheniramine, Phenyltoloxamine, Phenylephrine, and Phenylpropanolamine
- Extended-release capsules (U.S.)
- Oral solution (U.S.)
- Syrup (U.S.)
- Extended-release tablets (U.S.)

Chlorpheniramine and Pseudoephedrine
- Capsules (U.S. and Canada)
- Extended-release capsules (U.S. and Canada)
- Oral solution (U.S.)
- Syrup (U.S.)
- Tablets (U.S. and Canada)
- Extended-release tablets (U.S. and Canada)

Chlorpheniramine, Pyrilamine, and Phenylephrine
- Oral suspension (U.S.)
- Tablets (U.S.)
- Extended-release tablets (U.S.)

Chlorpheniramine, Pyrilamine, Phenylephrine, and Phenylpropanolamine
- Tablets (U.S.)

Clemastine and Phenylpropanolamine
- Extended-release tablets (U.S.)

Dexbrompheniramine and Pseudoephedrine
- Extended-release capsules (Canada)
- Syrup (Canada)
- Tablets (U.S. and Canada)
- Extended-release tablets (U.S. and Canada)

Diphenhydramine and Pseudoephedrine
- Capsules (U.S.)
- Oral solution (U.S.)
- Tablets (U.S.)

Pheniramine, Phenyltoloxamine, Pyrilamine, and Phenylpropanolamine
- Extended-release capsules (U.S.)
- Elixir (U.S.)

Pheniramine, Pyrilamine, and Phenylpropanolamine
- Oral solution (U.S. and Canada)
- Extended-release tablets (U.S. and Canada)

Promethazine and Phenylephrine
- Syrup (U.S.)

Promethazine and Pseudoephedrine
- Tablets (U.S.)

Terfenadine and Pseudoephedrine
- Extended-release tablets (U.S.)

Triprolidine and Pseudoephedrine
- Capsules (U.S.)
- Extended-release capsules (U.S.)
- Syrup (U.S. and Canada)
- Tablets (U.S. and Canada)

It is very important that you read and understand the following information. If any of it causes you special concern,

check with your doctor or pharmacist. Also, *if you have any questions* or if you want more information about this medicine or your medical problem, *ask your doctor, nurse, or pharmacist.*

Before Using This Medicine

If you are taking this medicine without a prescription, carefully read and follow any precautions on the label. For antihistamine and decongestant combinations, the following should be considered:

Allergies—Tell your doctor if you have ever had any unusual or allergic reaction to antihistamines or to amphetamine, dextroamphetamine (e.g., Dexedrine), ephedrine (e.g., Ephed II), epinephrine (e.g., Adrenalin), isoproterenol (e.g., Isuprel), metaproterenol (e.g., Alupent), methamphetamine (e.g., Desoxyn), norepinephrine (e.g., Levophed), phenylephrine (e.g., Neo-Synephrine), pseudoephedrine (e.g., Sudafed), PPA (e.g., Dexatrim), or terbutaline (e.g., Brethine).

Pregnancy—The occasional use of antihistamine and decongestant combinations is not likely to cause problems in the fetus or in the newborn baby. However, when these medicines are used at higher doses and/or for a long time, the chance that problems might occur may increase. For the individual ingredients of these combinations, the following apply:

- *Alcohol*—Some of these combination medicines contain alcohol. Too much use of alcohol during pregnancy may cause birth defects.
- *Antihistamines*—Antihistamines have not been shown to cause problems in humans.
- *Phenylephrine*—Studies on birth defects have not been done in either humans or animals with phenylephrine.
- *Phenylpropanolamine*—Studies on birth defects have not been done in either humans or animals with phenylpropanolamine. However, it seems that women who take phenylpropanolamine in the weeks following delivery are more likely to suffer mental or mood changes.
- *Pseudoephedrine*—Studies on birth defects with pseudoephedrine have not been done in humans. In animal

studies pseudoephedrine did not cause birth defects but did cause a decrease in average weight, length, and rate of bone formation in the animal fetus when administered in high doses.

- *Promethazine*—Phenothiazines, such as promethazine (contained in some of these combination medicines [e.g., Phenergan-D]), have been shown to cause jaundice and muscle tremors in a few newborn infants whose mothers received phenothiazines during pregnancy. Also, the newborn baby may have blood clotting problems if promethazine is taken by the mother within 2 weeks before delivery.

Breast-feeding—Small amounts of antihistamines and decongestants pass into the breast milk. Use is not recommended since the chances are greater for this medicine to cause side effects, such as unusual excitement or irritability, in the nursing baby. Also, since antihistamines tend to decrease the secretions of the body, it is possible that the flow of breast milk may be reduced in some patients. It is not known yet whether terfenadine causes these same side effects.

Children—Very young children are usually more sensitive to the effects of this medicine. Increases in blood pressure, nightmares or unusual excitement, nervousness, restlessness, or irritability may be more likely to occur in children. Also, mental changes may be more likely to occur in young children taking combination medicines that contain phenylpropanolamine. *Before giving any of these combination medicines to a child, check the package label very carefully. Some of these medicines are too strong for use in children.* If you are not certain whether a specific product can be given to a child, or if you have any questions about the amount to give, check with your doctor, nurse, or pharmacist.

Older adults—Confusion, difficult and painful urination, dizziness, drowsiness, dryness of mouth, or convulsions (seizures) may be more likely to occur in the elderly, who are usually more sensitive to the effects of this medicine. Also, nightmares or unusual excitement, nervousness, restlessness, or irritability may be more likely to occur in elderly patients.

Athletes—Stimulants, such as decongestants (e.g., phenylephrine, phenylpropanolamine, pseudoephedrine), are tested for by the U.S. Olympic Committee (USOC) and the National Collegiate Athletic Association (NCAA). These two groups have set limits on the amount of stimulants in the urine they consider to be acceptable. An athlete will be disqualified for competition if the amount of these substances in the urine is above those limits.

Other medicines—Although certain medicines should not be used together at all, in other cases different medicines may be used together even if an interaction might occur. In these cases, your doctor may want to change the dose, or other precautions may be necessary. When you are taking antihistamines it is especially important that your doctor and pharmacist know if you are taking any of the following:

- Anticholinergics (medicine for abdominal or stomach spasms or cramps)—Side effects, such as dryness of mouth, of antihistamines or anticholinergics may be more likely to occur

- Central nervous system (CNS) depressants—Effects, such as drowsiness, of CNS depressants or antihistamines may be worsened

- Erythromycin (e.g., E-Mycin) or
- Ketoconazole (e.g., Nizoral)—Use of these medicines with the terfenadine-containing combination may cause heart problems, such as an irregular heartbeat; these medicines should not be used together

- Monoamine oxidase (MAO) inhibitors (furazolidone [e.g., Furoxone], isocarboxazid [e.g., Marplan], phenelzine [e.g., Nardil], procarbazine [e.g., Matulane], selegiline [e.g., Eldepryl], tranylcypromine [e.g., Parnate])—If you are now taking, or have taken within the past 2 weeks, any of the MAO inhibitors, the side effects of the antihistamines may become more severe; these medicines should not be used together

- Rauwolfia alkaloids (alseroxylon [e.g., Rauwiloid], deserpidine [e.g., Harmonyl], rauwolfia serpentina [e.g., Raudixin], reserpine [e.g., Serpasil])—These medicines may increase or decrease the effect of the decongestant

- Tricyclic antidepressants (amitriptyline [e.g., Elavil], amoxapine [e.g., Asendin], clomipramine [e.g., Anafranil], desipramine [e.g., Pertofrane], doxepin [e.g., Sinequan], imipramine [e.g., Tofranil], maprotiline [e.g., Ludiomil], nortriptyline [e.g., Aventyl], protriptyline [e.g., Vivactil], trimipramine [e.g., Surmontil])—Effects, such as drowsiness, of CNS depressants or antihistamines may be worsened; also, taking these medicines together may cause some of their side effects, such as dryness of mouth, to become more severe

Also, if you are taking one of the combinations containing phenylpropanolamine or pseudoephedrine and are also taking:

- Amantadine (e.g., Symmetrel) or
- Amphetamines or
- Appetite suppressants (diet pills), except fenfluramine (e.g., Pondimin) or
- Beta-blockers (acebutolol [e.g., Sectral], atenolol [e.g., Tenormin], carteolol [e.g., Cartrol], labetalol [e.g., Normodyne], metoprolol [e.g., Lopressor], nadolol [e.g., Corgard], oxprenolol [e.g., Trasicor], penbutolol [e.g., Levatol], pindolol [e.g., Visken], propanolol [e.g., Inderal], sotalol [e.g., Sotacor], timolol [e.g., Blocadren]) or
- Caffeine (e.g., NoDoz) or
- Chlophedianol (e.g., Ulo) or
- Medicine for asthma or other breathing problems or
- Medicine for colds, sinus problems, or hay fever or other allergies (including nose drops or sprays) or
- Methylphenidate (e.g., Ritalin) or
- Pemoline (e.g., Cylert)—Using any of these medicines together with an antihistamine and decongestant combination may cause excessive stimulant side effects, such as difficulty in sleeping, heart rate problems, nervousness, and irritability

Other medical problems—The presence of other medical problems may affect the use of antihistamine and decongestant combinations. Make sure you tell your doctor if you have any other medical problems, especially:

- Diabetes mellitus (sugar diabetes)—The decongestant in this medicine may put diabetic patients at a greater risk of having heart or blood vessel disease
- Enlarged prostate or
- Urinary tract blockage or difficult urination—Some of the effects of antihistamines may make urinary problems worse
- Glaucoma—A slight increase in inner eye pressure may occur

- Heart or blood vessel disease or
- High blood pressure—The decongestant in this medicine may cause the blood pressure to increase and may also speed up the heart rate
- Liver disease—Higher blood levels of terfenadine may result, which may increase the chance of heart problems (for terfenadine-containing combination only)
- Overactive thyroid—If the overactive thyroid has caused a fast heart rate, the decongestant in this medicine may cause the heart rate to speed up further

Before you begin using any new medicine (prescription or nonprescription) or if you develop any new medical problem while you are using this medicine, check with your doctor, nurse, or pharmacist.

Proper Use of This Medicine

Take this medicine only as directed. Do not take more of it and do not take it more often than recommended on the label, unless otherwise directed by your doctor. To do so may increase the chance of side effects.

If this medicine irritates your stomach, you may take it with food or a glass of water or milk, to lessen the irritation.

For patients *taking the extended-release capsule or tablet form of this medicine:*
- Swallow it whole.
- Do not crush, break, or chew before swallowing.
- If the capsule is too large to swallow, you may mix the contents of the capsule with applesauce, jelly, honey, or syrup and swallow without chewing.

Missed dose—If you are taking this medicine regularly and you miss a dose, take it as soon as possible. However, if it is almost time for your next dose, skip the missed dose and go back to your regular dosing schedule. Do not double doses.

Storage—To store this medicine:
- Keep out of the reach of children.
- Store away from heat and direct light.

- Do not store in the bathroom, near the kitchen sink, or in other damp places. Heat or moisture may cause the medicine to break down.
- Keep the liquid form of this medicine from freezing.
- Do not keep outdated medicine or medicine no longer needed. Be sure that any discarded medicine is out of the reach of children.

Precautions While Using This Medicine

Before you have any skin tests for allergies, tell the doctor in charge that you are taking this medicine. The results of the test may be affected by the antihistamine in this medicine.

When taking antihistamines (contained in this combination medicine) on a regular basis, make sure your doctor knows if you are taking large amounts of aspirin at the same time (as in arthritis or rheumatism). Effects of too much aspirin, such as ringing in the ears, may be covered up by the antihistamine.

The antihistamine in this medicine will add to the effects of alcohol and other CNS depressants (medicines that slow down the nervous system, possibly causing drowsiness). Some examples of CNS depressants are other antihistamines or medicine for hay fever, other allergies, or colds; sedatives, tranquilizers, or sleeping medicine; prescription pain medicine or narcotics; barbiturates; medicine for seizures; muscle relaxants; or anesthetics, including some dental anesthetics. *Check with your doctor before taking any of the above while you are taking this medicine.*

The antihistamine in this medicine may cause some people to become drowsy, dizzy, or less alert than they are normally. *Some antihistamines are more likely to cause drowsiness than others (terfenadine, for example, rarely produces this effect). Make sure you know how you react before you drive, use machines, or do anything else that could be dangerous if you are dizzy or are not alert.*

The decongestant in this medicine may add to the central nervous system (CNS) stimulant and other effects of phenylpropanolamine (PPA)-containing diet aids. *Do not use medicines for diet or appetite control while taking this medicine unless you have checked with your doctor.*

The decongestant in this medicine may cause some people to be nervous or restless or to have trouble in sleeping. If you have trouble in sleeping, *take the last dose of this medicine for each day a few hours before bedtime.* If you have any questions about this, check with your doctor.

Antihistamines may cause dryness of the mouth, nose, and throat. Some antihistamines are more likely to cause dryness of the mouth than others (terfenadine, for example, rarely produces this effect). For temporary relief, use sugarless candy or gum, melt bits of ice in your mouth, or use a saliva substitute. However, if your mouth continues to feel dry for more than 2 weeks, check with your dentist. Continuing dryness of the mouth may increase the chance of dental disease, including tooth decay, gum disease, and fungus infections.

For patients *using promethazine-containing medicine:*
- This medicine controls nausea and vomiting. For this reason, it may cover up the signs of overdose caused by other medicines or the symptoms of intestinal blockage. This will make it difficult for your doctor to diagnose these conditions. Make sure your doctor knows that you are taking this medicine if you have other symptoms such as stomach or lower abdominal pain, cramping, or soreness. Also, if you think you may have taken an overdose of any medicine, tell your doctor that you are taking this medicine.

Side Effects of This Medicine

Along with its needed effects, a medicine may cause some unwanted effects. Although serious side effects occur rarely when this medicine is taken as recommended, they may be more likely to occur if:
- too much medicine is taken.
- it is taken in large doses.
- it is taken for a long period of time.

Get emergency help immediately if any of the following symptoms of overdose occur:

Clumsiness or unsteadiness; convulsions (seizures); drowsiness (severe); dryness of mouth, nose, or throat (severe); flushing or redness of face; hallucinations (seeing, hearing, or feeling things that are not there); headache (continuing); shortness of breath or troubled breathing; slow, fast, or irregular heartbeat; trouble in sleeping

For promethazine only

Muscle spasms (especially of neck and back); restlessness; shuffling walk; tic-like (jerky) movements of head and face; trembling and shaking of hands

Also, check with your doctor as soon as possible if any of the following side effects occur:

Rare

Mood or mental changes; sore throat and fever; tightness in chest; unusual bleeding or bruising; unusual tiredness or weakness

Other side effects may occur that usually do not need medical attention. These side effects may go away during treatment as your body adjusts to the medicine. However, check with your doctor or pharmacist if any of the following side effects continue or are bothersome:

More common—rare with terfenadine-containing combination

Drowsiness; thickening of the bronchial secretions

Less common—more common with high doses

Blurred vision; confusion; difficult or painful urination; dizziness; dryness of mouth, nose, or throat; headache; loss of appetite; nightmares; pounding heartbeat; ringing or buzzing in ears; skin rash; stomach upset or pain (more common with pyrilamine and tripelennamine); unusual excitement, nervousness, restlessness, or irritability

Other side effects not listed above may also occur in some patients. If you notice any other effects, check with your doctor.

ANTIHISTAMINES, PHENOTHIAZINE-DERIVATIVE Systemic

This information applies to the following medicines:

    Methdilazine (meth-DILL-a-zeen)
    Promethazine (proe-METH-a-zeen)
    Trimeprazine (trye-MEP-ra-zeen)

Some commonly used brand names are:

For Methdilazine†
    In the U.S.
        Tacaryl

For Promethazine
    In the U.S.

Anergan 25	Pro-50
Anergan 50	Prometh-25
Pentazine	Prometh-50
Phenameth	Promethegan
Phenazine 25	Prorex-25
Phenazine 50	Prorex-50
Phencen-50	Prothazine
Phenergan	Prothazine Plain
Phenergan Fortis	V-Gan-25
Phenergan Plain	V-Gan-50
Phenoject-50	

        Generic name product may also be available.

    In Canada

Histantil	PMS Promethazine
Phenergan	

        Generic name product may also be available.

For Trimeprazine
    In the U.S.
        Temaril

        Generic name product may also be available.

    Another commonly used name for trimeprazine is alimemazine.

    In Canada
        Panectyl

---

†Not commercially available in Canada.

Description

Phenothiazine (FEE-noe-THYE-a-zeen)-derivative antihistamines are used to relieve or prevent the symptoms of hay fever and other types of allergy. They work by preventing the effects of a substance called histamine, which is produced by the body.

Some of these antihistamines are also used to prevent motion sickness, nausea, vomiting, and dizziness. In addition, some of them may be used to help people go to sleep and control their anxiety before or after surgery.

Phenothiazine-derivative antihistamines may also be used for other conditions as determined by your doctor.

In the U.S. these antihistamines are available only with your doctor's prescription. In Canada some are available without a prescription. However, your doctor may have special instructions on the proper dose of the medicine for your medical condition.

These medicines are available in the following dosage forms:

Oral

Methdilazine
- Syrup (U.S.)
- Tablets (U.S.)
- Chewable tablets (U.S.)

Promethazine
- Syrup (U.S. and Canada)
- Tablets (U.S. and Canada)

Trimeprazine
- Extended-release capsules (U.S.)
- Syrup (U.S. and Canada)
- Tablets (U.S. and Canada)

Parenteral

Promethazine
- Injection (U.S. and Canada)

Rectal

Promethazine
- Suppositories (U.S.)

It is very important that you read and understand the following information. If any of it causes you special concern, check with your doctor. Also, *if you have any questions* or if you want more information about this medicine or your medical problem, *ask your doctor, nurse, or pharmacist.*

Before Using This Medicine

In deciding to use a medicine, the risks of taking the medicine must be weighed against the good it will do. This is a decision you and your doctor will make. For phenothiazine-derivative antihistamines, the following should be considered:

Allergies—Tell your doctor if you have ever had any unusual or allergic reaction to these medicines or to phenothiazines. Also tell your doctor and pharmacist if you are allergic to any other substances, such as foods, preservatives, or dyes.

Pregnancy—Methdilazine, promethazine, and trimeprazine have not been studied in pregnant women. In animal studies, promethazine has not been shown to cause birth defects. However, other phenothiazine medicines have been shown to cause jaundice and muscle tremors in a few newborn babies whose mothers received them during pregnancy. Also, the newborn baby may have blood clotting problems if promethazine is taken by the mother within 2 weeks before delivery.

Breast-feeding—Small amounts of antihistamines pass into the breast milk. Use is not recommended since babies are more sensitive to the side effects of antihistamines, such as unusual excitement or irritability. Also, with the use of phenothiazine-derivative antihistamines there is the chance that the nursing baby may be more at risk of having difficulty in breathing while sleeping or of the sudden infant death syndrome (SIDS). However, more studies are needed to confirm this.

In addition, since these medicines tend to decrease the secretions of the body, it is possible that the flow of breast milk may be reduced in some patients.

Children—Serious side effects, such as convulsions (seizures), are more likely to occur in younger patients and would be of greater risk to infants than to older children or adults. In general, children are more sensitive to the effects of antihistamines. Also, nightmares or unusual excitement, nervousness, restlessness, or irritability may be more likely to occur in children. *The use of phenothiazine-derivative* *antihistamines is not recommended in children who have a history of difficulty in breathing while sleeping, or a family history of sudden infant death syndrome (SIDS).*

Children who show signs of Reye's syndrome should not be given phenothiazine-derivative antihistamines, especially by injection. Seizures or uncontrolled movements that may occur with phenothiazine-derivative antihistamines may be thought to be symptoms of Reye's syndrome.

Adolescents—Adolescents who show signs of Reye's syndrome should not be given phenothiazine-derivative antihistamines, especially by injection. Seizures or uncontrolled movements that may occur with phenothiazine-derivative antihistamines may be thought to be symptoms of Reye's syndrome.

Older adults—Elderly patients are especially sensitive to the effects of antihistamines. Confusion; difficult or painful urination; dizziness; drowsiness; feeling faint; or dryness of mouth, nose, or throat may be more likely to occur in elderly patients. Also, nightmares or unusual excitement, nervousness, restlessness, or irritability may be more likely to occur in elderly patients. In addition, uncontrolled movements may be more likely to occur in elderly patients taking phenothiazine-derivative antihistamines.

Other medicines—Although certain medicines should not be used together at all, in other cases two different medicines may be used together even if an interaction might occur. In these cases, your doctor may want to change the dose, or other precautions may be necessary. When taking phenothiazine-derivative antihistamines, it is especially important that your doctor and pharmacist know if you are taking/receiving any of the following:

- Amoxapine (e.g., Asendin) or
- Antipsychotics (medicine for mental illness) or
- Methyldopa (e.g., Aldomet) or
- Metoclopramide (e.g., Reglan) or
- Metyrosine (e.g., Demser) or
- Pemoline (e.g., Cylert) or
- Pimozide (e.g., Orap) or

- Rauwolfia alkaloids (alseroxylon [e.g., Rauwiloid], deserpidine [e.g., Harmonyl], rauwolfia serpentina [e.g., Raudixin], reserpine [e.g., Serpasil])—Side effects, such as uncontrolled body movements, of these medicines may become more severe and frequent if they are used together with phenothiazine-derivative antihistamines
- Anticholinergics (medicine for abdominal or stomach spasms or cramps)—Side effects of phenothiazine-derivative antihistamines or anticholinergics, such as dryness of mouth, may be more likely to occur
- Antithyroid agents (medicine for overactive thyroid)—Serious side effects may be more likely to occur when antithyroid agents are taken together with phenothiazine-derivative antihistamines
- Central nervous system (CNS) depressants—Effects of CNS depressants or antihistamines, such as drowsiness, may be made more severe; also, taking maprotiline or tricyclic antidepressants may cause some side effects of antihistamines, such as dryness of mouth, to become more severe
- Contrast agent, injected into spinal canal—If you are having an x-ray test of the head, spinal canal, or nervous system for which you are going to receive an injection into the spinal canal, phenothiazine-derivative antihistamines may increase the chance of seizures; stop taking any phenothiazine-derivative antihistamine 48 hours before the test and do not start taking it until 24 hours after the test
- Levodopa—When used together with phenothiazine-derivative antihistamines, the levodopa may not work as it should
- Monoamine oxidase (MAO) inhibitors (furazolidone [e.g., Furoxone], isocarboxazid [e.g., Marplan], phenelzine [e.g., Nardil], procarbazine [e.g., Matulane], tranylcypromine [e.g., Parnate])—If you are now taking or have taken within the past 2 weeks any of the MAO inhibitors, the side effects of the phenothiazine-derivative antihistamines may become more severe; these medicines should not be used together

Other medical problems—The presence of other medical problems may affect the use of antihistamines. Make sure you tell your doctor if you have any other medical problems, especially:

- Asthma attacks—Although antihistamines open bronchial passages that are narrowed due to allergies, they may also cause secretions to become thick so that during an asthma attack it might be difficult to cough them up

- Blood disease or
- Heart or blood vessel disease—These medicines may cause more serious conditions to develop
- Enlarged prostate or
- Urinary tract blockage or difficult urination—Phenothiazine-derivative antihistamines may cause urinary problems to become worse
- Epilepsy or
- Reye's syndrome—Phenothiazine-derivative antihistamines, especially promethazine given by injection, may increase the chance of seizures or uncontrolled movements
- Glaucoma—These medicines may cause a slight increase in inner eye pressure that may worsen the condition
- Jaundice—Phenothiazine-derivative antihistamines may make the condition worse
- Liver disease—Phenothiazine-derivative antihistamines may build up in the body, which may increase the chance of side effects such as muscle spasms

Before you begin using any new medicine (prescription or nonprescription) or if you develop any new medical problem while you are using this medicine, check with your doctor, nurse, or pharmacist.

Proper Use of This Medicine

Antihistamines are used to relieve or prevent the symptoms of your medical problem. Take them only as directed. Do not take more of them and do not take them more often than recommended on the label, unless otherwise directed by your doctor. To do so may increase the chance of side effects.

For patients *taking this medicine by mouth:*

- Antihistamines can be taken with food or a glass of water or milk to lessen stomach irritation if necessary.
- If you are taking the *extended-release capsule* form of this medicine, swallow it whole. Do not break, crush, or chew before swallowing.

For patients taking *promethazine for motion sickness:*

- Take this medicine 30 minutes to 1 hour before you begin to travel.

For patients using the *suppository form of this medicine:*

- To insert suppository: First remove the foil wrapper and moisten the suppository with cold water. Lie down on side and use your finger to push the suppository well up into the rectum. If the suppository is too soft to insert, chill the suppository in the refrigerator for 30 minutes or run cold water over it, before removing the foil wrapper.

For patients using the *injection form of this medicine:*

- If you will be giving yourself the injections, make sure you understand exactly how to give them. If you have any questions about this, check with your doctor, nurse, or pharmacist.

Missed dose—If you are taking this medicine regularly and you miss a dose, take it as soon as possible. However, if it is almost time for your next dose, skip the missed dose and go back to your regular dosing schedule. Do not double doses.

Storage—To store this medicine:

- Keep out of the reach of children, since overdose may be very dangerous in children.
- Store away from heat and direct light.
- Do not store the capsule or tablet form of this medicine in the bathroom medicine cabinet, near the kitchen sink, or in other damp places. Heat or moisture may cause the medicine to break down.
- Keep the liquid form of this medicine from freezing.
- Do not keep outdated medicine or medicine no longer needed. Be sure that any discarded medicine is out of the reach of children.

Precautions While Using This Medicine

Tell the doctor in charge that you are taking this medicine before you have any skin tests for allergies. The results of the test may be affected by this medicine.

When taking phenothiazine-derivative antihistamines on a regular basis, make sure your doctor knows if you are taking large amounts of aspirin at the same time (as in arthritis or rheumatism). Effects of too much aspirin, such as ringing in the ears, may be covered up by the antihistamine.

Phenothiazine-derivative antihistamines will add to the effects of alcohol and other CNS depressants (medicines that slow down the nervous system, possibly causing drowsiness). Some examples of CNS depressants are sedatives, tranquilizers, or sleeping medicine; prescription pain medicine or narcotics; barbiturates; medicine for seizures; muscle relaxants; or anesthetics, including some dental anesthetics. *Check with your doctor before taking any of the above while you are using this medicine.*

This medicine may cause some people to become drowsy or less alert than they are normally. Even if taken at bedtime, it may cause some people to feel drowsy or less alert on arising. *Make sure you know how you react to the phenothiazine-derivative antihistamine you are taking before you drive, use machines, or do anything else that could be dangerous if you are not alert.*

Phenothiazine-derivative antihistamines may cause dryness of the mouth, nose, and throat. For temporary relief of mouth dryness, use sugarless candy or gum, melt bits of ice in your mouth, or use a saliva substitute. However, if your mouth continues to feel dry for more than 2 weeks, check with your medical doctor or dentist. Continuing dryness of the mouth may increase the chance of dental disease, including tooth decay, gum disease, and fungus infections.

This medicine controls nausea and vomiting. For this reason, it may cover up the signs of overdose caused by other medicines or the symptoms of appendicitis. This will make it difficult for your doctor to diagnose these conditions. Make sure your doctor knows that you are taking this medicine if you have other symptoms of appendicitis such as stomach or lower abdominal pain, cramping, or soreness. Also, if you think you may have taken an overdose of any medicine, tell your doctor that you are taking this medicine.

Side Effects of This Medicine

Along with its needed effects, a medicine may cause some unwanted effects. Although not all of these side effects may occur, if they do occur they may need medical attention.

Check with your doctor as soon as possible if any of the following side effects occur:

Less common or rare

Sore throat and fever; unusual bleeding or bruising; unusual tiredness or weakness

Symptoms of overdose

Clumsiness or unsteadiness; convulsions (seizures); drowsiness (severe); dryness of mouth, nose, or throat (severe); feeling faint; flushing or redness of face; hallucinations (seeing, hearing, or feeling things that are not there); muscle spasms (especially of neck and back); restlessness; shortness of breath or troubled breathing; shuffling walk; tic-like (jerky) movements of head and face; trembling and shaking of hands; trouble in sleeping

Other side effects may occur that usually do not need medical attention. These side effects may go away during treatment as your body adjusts to the medicine. However, check with your doctor or pharmacist if any of the following side effects continue or are bothersome:

More common

Drowsiness (less common with methdilazine); thickening of mucus

Less common or rare

Blurred vision or any change in vision; burning or stinging of rectum (with rectal suppository); confusion; difficult or painful urination; dizziness; dryness of mouth, nose, or throat; fast heartbeat; feeling faint; increased sensitivity of skin to sun; increased sweating; loss of appetite; nightmares; ringing or buzzing in ears; skin rash; unusual excitement, nervousness, restlessness, or irritability

Other side effects not listed above may also occur in some patients. If you notice any other effects, check with your doctor or pharmacist.

ANTI-INFLAMMATORY ANALGESICS Systemic

This information applies to the following medicines:
  Diclofenac (dye-KLOE-fen-ak)
  Diflunisal (dye-FLOO-ni-sal)
  Fenoprofen (fen-oh-PROE-fen)
  Floctafenine (flok-ta-FEN-een)
  Flurbiprofen (flure-BI-proe-fen)
  Ibuprofen (eye-byoo-PROE-fen)
  Indomethacin (in-doe-METH-a-sin)
  Ketoprofen (kee-toe-PROE-fen)
  Meclofenamate (me-kloe-FEN-am-ate)
  Mefenamic (me-fe-NAM-ik) Acid
  Naproxen (na-PROX-en)
  Phenylbutazone (fen-ill-BYOO-ta-zone)
  Piroxicam (peer-OX-i-kam)
  Sulindac (sul-IN-dak)
  Tiaprofenic (tie-a-pro-FEN-ik) Acid
  Tolmetin (TOLE-met-in)

This information does *not* apply to aspirin or other salicylates or to etodolac (e.g., Lodine) or ketorolac (e.g., Toradol).

Some commonly used brand names are:

For Diclofenac
  In the U.S.
    Voltaren
  In Canada
    Voltaren
    Voltaren SR

For Diflunisal
  In the U.S.
    Dolobid
  In Canada
    Dolobid

For Fenoprofen
  In the U.S.
    Nalfon
    Nalfon 200
    Generic name product may also be available.
  In Canada
    Nalfon

For Floctafenine*
  In Canada
    Idarac

For Flurbiprofen
In the U.S.
    Ansaid

In Canada
    Ansaid
    Froben

    Generic name product may also be available.

For Ibuprofen
In the U.S.

Aches-N-Pain	Ifen
Advil	Medipren
Advil Caplets	Medipren Caplets
Children's Advil	Midol 200 Caplets
Dolgesic	Motrin
Genpril	Motrin-IB
Genpril Caplets	Motrin-IB Caplets
Haltran	Nuprin
Ibren	Nuprin Caplets
Ibumed	Pamprin-IB
Ibuprin	PediaProfen
Ibupro-600	Profen
Ibuprohm	Ro-Profen
Ibuprohm Caplets	Rufen
Ibu-Tab	Trendar
Ibutex	

    Generic name product may also be available.

In Canada

Actiprofen Caplets	Medipren Caplets
Advil	Motrin
Advil Caplets	Motrin-IB Caplets
Amersol	Novoprofen
Apo-Ibuprofen	Nuprin
Medipren	

    Generic name product may also be available.

For Indomethacin
In the U.S.

Indameth	Indocin SR
Indocin	

    Generic name product may also be available.

In Canada

Apo-Indomethacin	Indocid SR
Indocid	Novomethacin

Another commonly used name is indometacin.

For Ketoprofen
In the U.S.
    Orudis

In Canada
Orudis   Rhodis
Orudis-E   Rhodis-E
Orudis-SR

For Meclofenamate†
In the U.S.
Meclofen
Meclomen
Generic name product may also be available.

For Mefenamic Acid
In the U.S.
Ponstel
Generic name product may also be available.
In Canada
Ponstan

For Naproxen
In the U.S.
Anaprox   Naprosyn
Anaprox DS
In Canada
Anaprox   Naxen
Apo-Napro-Na   Novonaprox
Apo-Naproxen   Novonaprox Sodium
Naprosyn   Synflex
Naprosyn-SR

For Phenylbutazone
In the U.S.
Butatab   Butazone
Butazolidin
Generic name product may also be available.
In Canada
Alka-Butazolidin   Butazolidin
Alkabutazone   Intrabutazone
Alka-Phenylbutazone   Novobutazone
Apo-Phenylbutazone   Phenylone Plus
Generic name product may also be available.

For Piroxicam
In the U.S.
Feldene
In Canada
Apo-Piroxicam   Novopirocam
Feldene

For Sulindac
In the U.S.
Clinoril
Generic name product may also be available.

In Canada
   Apo-Sulin   Novo-Sundac
   Clinoril

For Tiaprofenic Acid*
In Canada
   Surgam

For Tolmetin
In the U.S.
   Tolectin 200   Tolectin DS
   Tolectin 600

In Canada
   Tolectin 200   Tolectin 600
   Tolectin 400

---

*Not commercially available in the U.S.
†Not commercially available in Canada.

Description

Anti-inflammatory analgesics (also called nonsteroidal anti-inflammatory drugs [NSAIDs]) are used to relieve some symptoms caused by arthritis (rheumatism), such as inflammation, swelling, stiffness, and joint pain. However, this medicine does not cure arthritis and will help you only as long as you continue to take it.

Some of these medicines are also used to relieve other kinds of pain or to treat other painful conditions, such as:

- gout attacks;
- bursitis;
- tendinitis;
- sprains, strains, or other injuries; or
- menstrual cramps.

Ibuprofen is also used to reduce fever.

Anti-inflammatory analgesics may also be used to treat other conditions as determined by your doctor.

Any anti-inflammatory analgesic can cause side effects, especially when it is used for a long time or in large doses. Some of the side effects are painful or uncomfortable. Others can be more serious, resulting in the need for medical care and sometimes even death. If you will be taking this medicine for more than one or two months or in large amounts, you should discuss with your doctor the good that it can do as well as the risks of taking it. Also, it is a good idea to ask your doctor about other forms of treatment that might help to reduce the amount of this medicine that you take and/or the length of treatment.

One of the anti-inflammatory analgesics, phenylbutazone, is especially likely to cause very serious side effects. These serious side effects are more likely to occur in patients 40 years of age or older than in younger adults, and the risk becomes greater as the patient's age increases. Before you take phenylbutazone, be sure that you have discussed its use with your doctor. *Also, do not use phenylbutazone to treat any painful condition other than the one for which it was prescribed by your doctor.*

Although ibuprofen may be used instead of aspirin to treat many of the same medical problems, it must not be used by people who are allergic to aspirin.

The 200-mg strength of ibuprofen is available without a prescription. However, your medical doctor or dentist may have special instructions on the proper dose of ibuprofen for your medical condition.

Other anti-inflammatory analgesics and other strengths of ibuprofen are available only with your medical doctor's or dentist's prescription. These medicines are available in the following dosage forms:

> *Oral*
>> Diclofenac
>>> • Delayed-release tablets (U.S. and Canada)
>>> • Extended-release tablets (Canada)
>> Diflunisal
>>> • Tablets (U.S. and Canada)
>> Fenoprofen
>>> • Capsules (U.S. and Canada)
>>> • Tablets (U.S. and Canada)
>> Floctafenine
>>> • Tablets (Canada)
>> Flurbiprofen
>>> • Tablets (U.S. and Canada)

Ibuprofen
- Capsules (Canada)
- Oral suspension (U.S.)
- Tablets (U.S. and Canada)

Indomethacin
- Capsules (U.S. and Canada)
- Extended-release capsules (U.S. and Canada)
- Oral suspension (U.S.)

Ketoprofen
- Capsules (U.S. and Canada)
- Delayed-release tablets (Canada)
- Extended-release tablets (Canada)

Meclofenamate
- Capsules (U.S.)

Mefenamic Acid
- Capsules (U.S. and Canada)

Naproxen
- Oral suspension (U.S. and Canada)
- Tablets (U.S. and Canada)
- Extended-release tablets (Canada)

Phenylbutazone
- Capsules (U.S.)
- Tablets (U.S. and Canada)
- Buffered tablets (Canada)
- Delayed-release tablets (Canada)

Piroxicam
- Capsules (U.S. and Canada)

Sulindac
- Tablets (U.S. and Canada)

Tiaprofenic Acid
- Tablets (Canada)

Tolmetin
- Capsules (U.S. and Canada)
- Tablets (U.S. and Canada)

Rectal

Diclofenac
- Suppositories (Canada)

Indomethacin
- Suppositories (U.S. and Canada)

Ketoprofen
- Suppositories (Canada)

Naproxen
- Suppositories (Canada)

Piroxicam
- Suppositories (Canada)

It is very important that you read and understand the following information. If any of it causes you special concern, check with your doctor. Also, *if you have any questions* or if you want more information about this medicine or your medical problem, *ask your doctor, nurse, or pharmacist.*

Before Using This Medicine

In deciding to use a medicine, the risks of taking the medicine must be weighed against the good it will do. This is a decision you and your doctor will make. For the anti-inflammatory analgesics, the following should be considered:

Allergies—Tell your doctor if you have ever had any unusual or allergic reaction to any of the anti-inflammatory analgesics, or to any of the following medicines:

- Aspirin or other salicylates
- Ketorolac (e.g., Toradol)
- Oxyphenbutazone (e.g., Oxalid, Tandearil)
- Suprofen (e.g., Suprol)
- Zomepirac (e.g., Zomax)

Also tell your doctor and pharmacist if you are allergic to any other substances, such as foods, preservatives, or dyes.

Diet—Make certain your doctor and pharmacist know if you are on any special diet, such as a low-sodium or low-sugar diet. Some of these medicines contain sodium or sugar.

Pregnancy—Studies on birth defects with these medicines have not been done in humans. However, there is a chance that these medicines may cause unwanted effects on the heart or blood flow of the fetus or newborn baby if they are taken regularly during the last few months of pregnancy. Also, studies in animals have shown that these medicines, if taken late in pregnancy, may increase the length of pregnancy, prolong labor, or cause other problems during delivery.

Studies in animals have not shown that fenoprofen, floctafenine, flurbiprofen, ibuprofen, ketoprofen, naproxen, phenylbutazone, piroxicam, tiaprofenic acid, or tolmetin causes birth defects. Diflunisal caused birth defects of the spine and ribs in rabbits, but not in mice or rats. Diclofenac and meclofenamate caused unwanted effects on the formation of bones in animals. Indomethacin caused slower development of bones and damage to nerves in animals. In some animal studies, sulindac caused unwanted effects on the development of bones and organs. Studies on birth defects with mefenamic acid have not been done in animals.

Even though most of these medicines did not cause birth defects in animals, many of them did cause other harmful or toxic effects on the fetus, usually when they were given in such large amounts that the pregnant animals became sick.

Breast-feeding—
- *For indomethacin:* Indomethacin passes into the breast milk and has been reported to cause unwanted effects in nursing babies.
- *For phenylbutazone:* Phenylbutazone passes into the breast milk and may cause unwanted effects, such as blood problems, in nursing babies.
- *For meclofenamate:* Use of meclofenamate by nursing mothers is not recommended because in animal studies it caused unwanted effects on the newborn's development.
- *For piroxicam:* Studies in animals have shown that piroxicam may decrease the amount of milk.

Although other anti-inflammatory analgesics have not been reported to cause problems in nursing babies, diclofenac, diflunisal, fenoprofen, mefenamic acid, flurbiprofen, naproxen, piroxicam, and tolmetin pass into the breast milk. It is not known whether floctafenine, ibuprofen, ketoprofen, meclofenamate, sulindac, or tiaprofenic acid passes into human breast milk.

Children—
- *For ibuprofen:* Ibuprofen has been tested in children 6 months of age and older with fevers and in children 12 months of age and older with arthritis. It has not been shown to cause different side effects or problems than it does in adults.

- *For indomethacin and for tolmetin:* Indomethacin and tolmetin have been tested in children 2 years of age and older and have not been shown to cause different side effects or problems than they do in adults.
- *For naproxen:* Studies with naproxen in children 2 years of age and older have shown that skin rash may be more likely to occur.
- *For other anti-inflammatory analgesics:* There is no specific information on the use of other anti-inflammatory analgesics in children.

Most of these medicines, especially indomethacin and phenylbutazone, can cause serious side effects in any patient. Therefore, it is especially important that you discuss with the child's doctor the good that this medicine may do as well as the risks of using it.

Older adults—Certain side effects, such as confusion, swelling of the face, feet, or lower legs, or sudden decrease in the amount of urine, may be especially likely to occur in elderly patients, who are usually more sensitive than younger adults to the effects of anti-inflammatory analgesics. Also, elderly people are more likely than younger adults to get very sick if these medicines cause stomach problems. With phenylbutazone, blood problems may also be more likely to occur in the elderly.

Other medicines—Although certain medicines should not be used together at all, in other cases two different medicines may be used together even if an interaction might occur. In these cases, your doctor may want to change the dose, or other precautions may be necessary. When you are taking an anti-inflammatory analgesic, it is especially important that your doctor and pharmacist know if you are taking any of the following:

- Amphotericin B by injection (e.g., Fungizone) or
- Antineoplastics (cancer medicine) or
- Antithyroid agents (medicine for overactive thyroid) or
- Azathioprine (e.g., Imuran) or
- Chloramphenicol (e.g., Chloromycetin) or
- Colchicine or
- Cyclophosphamide (e.g., Cytoxan) or

- Flucytosine (e.g., Ancobon) or
- Interferon (e.g., Intron A, Roferon-A) or
- Mercaptopurine (e.g., Purinethol) or
- Penicillamine (e.g., Cuprimine)—The chance of serious side effects may be increased, especially with phenylbutazone

- Anticoagulants (blood thinners) or
- Cefamandole (e.g., Mandol) or
- Cefoperazone (e.g., Cefobid) or
- Cefotetan (e.g., Cefotan) or
- Heparin or
- Moxalactam (e.g., Moxam) or
- Plicamycin (e.g., Mithracin)—The chance of bleeding may be increased

- Aspirin—The chance of serious side effects may be increased if aspirin is used together with an anti-inflammatory analgesic on a regular basis

- Digitalis glycosides (heart medicine) or
- Lithium (e.g., Lithane) or
- Methotrexate (e.g., Mexate) or
- Phenytoin (e.g., Dilantin)—Higher blood levels of these medicines and an increased chance of side effects may occur

- Probenecid (e.g., Benemid)—Higher blood levels of the anti-inflammatory analgesic and an increased chance of side effects may occur

- Triamterene (e.g., Dyrenium)—The chance of kidney problems may be increased, especially with indomethacin

- Zidovudine (e.g., AZT, Retrovir)—The chance of serious side effects may be increased, especially with indomethacin or phenylbutazone

Other medical problems—The presence of other medical problems may affect the use of anti-inflammatory analgesics. Make sure you tell your doctor if you have any other medical problems, especially:

- Alcohol abuse or
- Bleeding problems or
- Colitis, stomach ulcer, or other stomach problems or
- Diabetes mellitus (sugar diabetes) or
- Hepatitis or other liver disease or
- Kidney disease or history of or
- Rectal irritation or bleeding, recent, or
- Systemic lupus erythematosus (SLE) or
- Tobacco use (or recent history of)—The chance of side effects may be increased

- Anemia or
- Asthma or
- Epilepsy or
- Fluid retention (swelling of feet or lower legs) or
- Heart disease or
- High blood pressure or
- Mental illness or
- Parkinson's disease or
- Polymyalgia rheumatica or
- Temporal arteritis—Some anti-inflammatory analgesics may make these conditions worse
- Ulcers, sores, or white spots in mouth—Ulcers, sores, or white spots in the mouth sometimes mean that the medicine is causing serious side effects; if these sores or spots are already present before you start taking the medicine, it will be harder for you and your doctor to recognize that these side effects might be occurring

Before you begin using any new medicine (prescription or nonprescription) or if you develop any new medical problem while you are using this medicine, check with your doctor, nurse, or pharmacist.

Proper Use of This Medicine

For patients taking *a capsule, tablet (including caplet), or liquid form* of this medicine:

- To lessen stomach upset, these medicines should be taken with food or an antacid. This is especially important when you are taking indomethacin, mefenamic acid, phenylbutazone, or piroxicam, which should always be taken with food or an antacid. Your doctor may want you to take the first few doses of other anti-inflammatory analgesics 30 minutes before meals or 2 hours after meals. This helps the medicine to work a little faster when you first begin to take it. However, after the first few doses, take the medicine with food or an antacid.
- It is not necessary to take delayed-release (enteric-coated) tablets with food or an antacid, because the enteric coating helps protect your stomach from the irritating effects of the medicine.

- If you will be taking your medicine together with an antacid, one that contains magnesium and aluminum hydroxides (e.g., Maalox) may be the best kind of antacid to use, unless your doctor has directed you to use another antacid. However, do not mix the liquid form of ibuprofen, indomethacin, or naproxen together with an antacid, or any other liquid, before taking it. To do so may cause the medicine to break down. If stomach upset (indigestion, nausea, vomiting, stomach pain, or diarrhea) continues or if you have any questions about how you should be taking this medicine, check with your doctor, nurse, or pharmacist.

- *Take tablet or capsule forms of these medicines with a full glass (8 ounces) of water.* Also, do not lie down for about 15 to 30 minutes after taking the medicine. This helps to prevent irritation that may lead to trouble in swallowing.

- Some anti-inflammatory analgesic tablets must be swallowed whole, not crushed or broken. These include diclofenac tablets (e.g., Voltaren), diflunisal tablets (e.g., Dolobid), ketoprofen delayed-release (enteric-coated) tablets (e.g., Orudis-E), ketoprofen extended-release tablets (e.g., Orudis-SR), naproxen extended-release tablets (e.g., Naprosyn-SR), phenylbutazone tablets (e.g., Butazolidin), and phenylbutazone delayed-release (enteric-coated) tablets (e.g., Intrabutazone).

For patients using *a suppository form* of this medicine:

- If the suppository is too soft to insert, chill it in the refrigerator for 30 minutes or run cold water over it before removing the foil wrapper.

- To insert the suppository: First remove the foil wrapper and moisten the suppository with cold water. Lie down on your side and use your finger to push the suppository well up into the rectum.

- Indomethacin suppositories should be kept inside the rectum for at least one hour so that all of the medicine can be absorbed by your body. This helps the medicine work better.

For patients taking *200-mg (nonprescription) strength ibu-profen:*

- This medicine comes with a patient information sheet. Read it carefully. If you have any questions about this information, check with your doctor or pharmacist.

For safe and effective use of this medicine, do not take more of it, do not take it more often, and do not take it for a longer time than ordered by your medical doctor or dentist or directed on the 200-mg (nonprescription) strength ibu-profen package label. Taking too much of any of these medicines may increase the chance of unwanted effects, especially in elderly patients.

When used for severe or continuing arthritis, this medicine must be taken regularly as ordered by your doctor in order for it to help you. These medicines usually begin to work within one week, but in severe cases up to two weeks or even longer may pass before you begin to feel better. Also, several weeks may pass before you feel the full effects of the medicine.

For patients taking *mefenamic acid:*

- *Always take mefenamic acid with food or antacids.*
- *Do not take mefenamic acid for more than 7 days at a time* unless otherwise directed by your doctor. To do so may increase the chance of side effects, especially in elderly patients.

For patients taking *phenylbutazone:*

- Phenylbutazone is intended to treat your current medical problem only. *Do not take it for any other aches or pains.* Also, phenylbutazone should be used for the shortest time possible because of the chance of serious side effects, especially in patients who are 40 years of age or older.

Missed dose—If your medical doctor or dentist has ordered you to take this medicine according to a regular schedule, and you miss a dose, take it as soon as you remember. However, if it is almost time for your next dose, skip the missed dose and go back to your regular dosing schedule. (For long-acting medicines or extended-release dosage forms that are only taken once or twice a day, take the missed dose only if you remember within an hour or two after the dose should have been taken. If you do not remember until later, skip the missed dose and go back to your regular dosing schedule.) Do not double doses.

Storage—To store this medicine:
- Keep out of the reach of children.
- Store away from heat and direct light.
- Do not store tablets or capsules in the bathroom, near the kitchen sink, or in other damp places. Heat or moisture may cause the medicine to break down.
- Keep liquid and suppository forms of this medicine from freezing.
- Do not keep outdated medicine or medicine no longer needed. Be sure that any discarded medicine is out of the reach of children.

Precautions While Using This Medicine

If you will be taking this medicine for a long time, as for arthritis (rheumatism), your doctor should check your progress at regular visits. Your doctor may want to do certain tests to find out if unwanted effects are occurring, especially if you are taking phenylbutazone. The tests are very important because serious side effects, including ulcers, bleeding, or blood problems, can occur without any warning.

Stomach problems may be more likely to occur if you drink alcoholic beverages while being treated with this medicine. Also, alcohol may add to the depressant side effects of phenylbutazone. Therefore, *do not regularly drink alcoholic beverages while taking this medicine,* unless otherwise directed by your doctor.

Taking acetaminophen or aspirin or other salicylates together with an anti-inflammatory analgesic may increase the chance of unwanted effects. The risk will depend on how much of each medicine you take every day, and on how long you take the medicines together. If your medical doctor or dentist directs you to take these medicines together on a regular basis, follow his or her directions carefully. However, *do not take acetaminophen or aspirin or other salicylates together with this medicine for more than a few days, unless your doctor has directed you to do so and is following your progress.*

For patients taking *the buffered form of phenylbutazone (e.g., Alka-Butazolidin):*

- If you are also taking a tetracycline antibiotic, *do not take buffered phenylbutazone within 1 to 3 hours of taking the antibiotic.* Buffered phenylbutazone contains antacids that may make the tetracycline less effective in treating your infection by causing less of it to be absorbed into your body.

Before having any kind of surgery (including dental surgery), tell the medical doctor or dentist in charge that you are taking this medicine.

This medicine may cause some people to become confused, drowsy, dizzy, lightheaded, or less alert than they are normally. They may also cause blurred vision or other vision problems in some people. *Make sure you know how you react to this medicine before you drive, use machines, or do anything else that could be dangerous if you are dizzy or are not alert and able to see well.* If these reactions are especially bothersome, check with your doctor.

For patients taking *mefenamic acid:*

- If diarrhea occurs while you are using this medicine, *stop taking it and check with your doctor immediately. Do not take it again without first checking with your doctor,* because severe diarrhea may occur each time you take it.

Some people who take anti-inflammatory analgesics may become more sensitive to sunlight than they are normally. Exposure to sunlight, even for brief periods of time, may cause severe sunburn; skin rash, redness, itching, or discoloration; or vision changes. When you begin taking this medicine:

- Stay out of direct sunlight, especially between the hours of 10:00 a.m. and 3:00 p.m., if possible.

- Wear protective clothing, including a hat and sunglasses.
- Apply a sun block product that has a skin protection factor (SPF) of at least 15. Some patients may require a product with a higher SPF number, especially if they have a fair complexion. If you have any questions about this, check with your doctor or pharmacist.
- Do not use a sunlamp or tanning bed or booth.

If you have a severe reaction from the sun, check with your doctor.

Serious side effects, including ulcers or bleeding, can occur during treatment with this medicine. Sometimes serious side effects can occur without any warning. However, possible warning signs often occur, including severe abdominal or stomach cramps, pain, or burning; black, tarry stools; severe, continuing nausea, heartburn, or indigestion; and/or vomiting of blood or material that looks like coffee grounds. *Stop taking this medicine and check with your doctor immediately if you notice any of these warning signs.*

Check with your doctor immediately if chills, fever, muscle aches or pains, or other influenza-like symptoms occur, especially if they occur shortly before, or together with, a skin rash. Very rarely, these effects may be the first signs of a serious reaction to this medicine.

Anti-inflammatory analgesics may cause a serious type of allergic reaction called anaphylaxis. Although this is rare, it may occur more often in patients who are allergic to aspirin or to any other anti-inflammatory analgesic. *Anaphylaxis requires immediate medical attention.* The most serious signs of this reaction are very fast or irregular breathing, gasping for breath, wheezing, or fainting. Other signs may include changes in color of the skin of the face; very fast but irregular heartbeat or pulse; hive-like swellings on the skin; and puffiness or swellings of the eyelids or around the eyes. If these effects occur, get emergency help at once. Ask someone to drive you to the nearest hospital emergency room. If this is not possible, do not try to drive yourself. Call an ambulance, lie down, cover yourself to keep warm, and prop your feet higher than your head. Stay in that position until help arrives.

For patients taking *ibuprofen* without a prescription:
* Check with your medical doctor or dentist:
  —if your symptoms do not improve or if they get worse.
  —if you are using this medicine to bring down a fever and the fever lasts more than 3 days or returns.
  —if the painful area becomes red or swollen.

Side Effects of This Medicine

Along with its needed effects, a medicine may cause some unwanted effects. Although not all of these side effects may occur, if they do occur they may need medical attention.

Stop taking this medicine and check with your doctor immediately if any of the following side effects occur:

More common—for mefenamic acid only
Diarrhea

More common—for phenylbutazone only
Swelling of face, hands, feet, or lower legs; weight gain (rapid)

Symptoms of phenylbutazone overdose
Bluish color of fingernails, lips, or skin; headache (severe and continuing)

Rare—for all anti-inflammatory analgesics
Abdominal or stomach pain, cramping, or burning (severe); bloody or black tarry stools; chest pain; convulsions (seizures); fainting; hive-like swellings (large) on face, eyelids, mouth, lips, or tongue; nausea, heartburn, and/or indigestion (severe and continuing); shortness of breath, troubled breathing, wheezing, or tightness in chest or fast or irregular breathing; sore throat, fever, and chills; sudden decrease in amount of urine; unusual bleeding or bruising; vomiting of blood or material that looks like coffee grounds

Also, check with your doctor as soon as possible if any of the following side effects occur:

More common
Bleeding from rectum (with suppositories); headache (severe), especially in the morning (for indomethacin only); skin rash

Less common or rare

Bleeding or crusting sores on lips; bloody or cloudy urine or any problem with urination, such as difficult, burning, or painful urination; frequent urge to urinate; sudden, large increase in the amount of urine; or loss of bladder control; blurred vision or any change in vision; burning feeling in throat, chest, or stomach; confusion, forgetfulness, mental depression, or other mood or mental changes; cough or hoarseness; decreased hearing, any other change in hearing, or ringing or buzzing in ears; eye pain, irritation, dryness, redness, and/or swelling; fever with or without chills; hallucinations (seeing, hearing, or feeling things that are not there); headache (severe), throbbing, or with fever and stiff neck; hives, itching of skin, or any other skin problem, such as redness, tenderness, burning, peeling, thickening, or scaliness; increased blood pressure; irregular heartbeat; loosening or splitting of fingernails; muscle cramps, pain, or weakness; numbness, tingling, pain, or weakness in hands or feet; pain in lower back and/or side (severe); pinpoint red spots on skin; sores, ulcers, or white spots on lips or in mouth; spitting blood; swelling and/or tenderness in upper abdominal or stomach area; swelling of face, feet, or lower legs (if taking phenylbutazone, stop taking it and check with your doctor immediately); swollen and/or painful glands (especially in the neck or throat area); thirst (continuing); unexplained nosebleeds; unexplained runny nose or sneezing; unexplained, unexpected, or unusually heavy vaginal bleeding; unusual tiredness or weakness; weight gain (rapid) (if taking phenylbutazone, stop taking it and check with your doctor immediately); yellow eyes or skin

Other side effects may occur that usually do not need medical attention. These side effects may go away during treatment as your body adjusts to the medicine. However, check with your doctor if any of the following side effects continue or are bothersome:

More common

Abdominal or stomach cramps, pain, or discomfort (mild to moderate); diarrhea (if taking mefenamic acid, stop taking it and check with your doctor immediately); dizziness, drowsiness, or lightheadedness; headache (mild to moderate); heartburn, indigestion, nausea, or vomiting

Less common or rare

Bitter taste or other taste change; bloated feeling, gas, or constipation; decreased appetite or loss of appetite; fast or pounding heartbeat; flushing or hot flushes; general feeling of discomfort or illness; increased sensitivity of skin to sunlight; increased sweating; irritation, dryness, or soreness of mouth; nervousness, irritability, or trembling; rectal irritation (with suppositories); trouble in sleeping; unexplained weight loss; unusual tiredness or weakness without any other symptoms

Although not all of the side effects listed above have been reported for all of these medicines, they have been reported for at least one of them. However, since all anti-inflammatory analgesics are very similar, it is possible that any of the above side effects may occur with any of these medicines.

Some side effects may occur many days or weeks after you have stopped using phenylbutazone. During this time *check with your doctor immediately* if you notice any of the following side effects:

Sore throat and fever; ulcers, sores, or white spots in mouth; unusual bleeding or bruising; unusual tiredness or weakness

Other side effects not listed above may also occur in some patients. If you notice any other effects, check with your doctor.

BENZODIAZEPINES Systemic

This information applies to the following medicines:

Alprazolam (al-PRAZ-oh-lam)
Bromazepam (broe-MA-ze-pam)
Chlordiazepoxide (klor-dye-az-e-POX-ide)
Clonazepam (kloe-NA-ze-pam)
Clorazepate (klor-AZ-e-pate)
Diazepam (dye-AZ-e-pam)
Estazolam (ess-TA-zoe-lam)
Flurazepam (flure-AZ-e-pam)
Halazepam (hal-AZ-e-pam)
Ketazolam (kee-TAY–zoe-lam)
Lorazepam (lor-AZ-e-pam)
Nitrazepam (nye-TRA-ze-pam)

Oxazepam (ox-AZ-e-pam)
Prazepam (PRAZ-e-pam)
Quazepam (KWA-ze-pam)
Temazepam (tem-AZ-e-pam)
Triazolam (trye-AY-zoe-lam)

Some commonly used brand names are:

For Alprazolam
In the U.S.
Xanax

In Canada
Apo-Alpraz   Nu-Alpraz
Novo-Alprazol   Xanax

For Bromazepam*
In Canada
Lectopam

For Chlordiazepoxide
In the U.S.
Libritabs   Lipoxide
Librium

Generic name product may also be available.

In Canada
Apo-Chlordiazepoxide   Novopoxide
Librium   Solium

For Clonazepam
In the U.S.
Klonopin

In Canada
Rivotril

For Clorazepate
In the U.S.
Gen-XENE   Tranxene T-Tab
Tranxene-SD

Generic name product may also be available.

In Canada
Apo-Clorazepate   Tranxene
Novoclopate

For Diazepam
In the U.S.
Diazepam Intensol   Valrelease
T-Quil   Vazepam
Valium   Zetran

Generic name product may also be available.

In Canada

Apo-Diazepam	PMS Diazepam
Diazemuls	Valium
Novodipam	Vivol

Generic name product may also be available.

For Estazolam†
In the U.S.
ProSom

For Flurazepam
In the U.S.
Dalmane
Durapam

Generic name product may also be available.

In Canada

Apo-Flurazepam	Novoflupam
Dalmane	Somnol

For Halazepam†
In the U.S.
Paxipam

For Ketazolam*
In Canada
Loftran

For Lorazepam
In the U.S.

Alzapam	Lorazepam Intensol
Ativan	

Generic name product may also be available.

In Canada

Apo-Lorazepam	Novolorazem
Ativan	Nu-Loraz

For Nitrazepam*
In Canada
Mogadon

For Oxazepam
In the U.S.
Serax

Generic name product may also be available.

In Canada

Apo-Oxazepam	Serax
Novoxapam	Zapex

For Prazepam†
In the U.S.
Centrax

Generic name product may also be available.

For Quazepam†
> *In the U.S.*
>> Doral

For Temazepam
> *In the U.S.*
>> Razepam   Restoril
>>
>> Generic name product may also be available.
>
> *In Canada*
>> Restoril

For Triazolam
> *In the U.S.*
>> Halcion
>
> *In Canada*
>> Apo-Triazo   Novotriolam
>> Halcion   Nu-Triazo
>>
>> Generic name product may also be available.

---

*Not commercially available in the U.S.
†Not commercially available in Canada.

Description

Benzodiazepines (ben-zoe-dye-AZ-e-peens) belong to the group of medicines called central nervous system (CNS) depressants (medicines that slow down the nervous system).

Some benzodiazepines are used to relieve nervousness or tension. Others are used in the treatment of insomnia (trouble in sleeping). However, if used regularly (for example, every day) for insomnia, they are usually not effective for more than a few weeks.

One of the benzodiazepines, diazepam, is also used to help relax muscles or relieve muscle spasm. Another benzodiazepine, alprazolam, is also used in the treatment of panic disorder. Clonazepam, clorazepate, and diazepam are also used to treat certain convulsive (seizure) disorders, such as epilepsy. The benzodiazepines may also be used for other conditions as determined by your doctor.

Benzodiazepines should not be used for nervousness or tension caused by the stress of everyday life.

These medicines are available only with your doctor's prescription, in the following dosage forms:

Oral

Alprazolam
- Tablets (U.S. and Canada)

Bromazepam
- Tablets (Canada)

Chlordiazepoxide
- Capsules (U.S. and Canada)
- Tablets (U.S.)

Clonazepam
- Tablets (U.S. and Canada)

Clorazepate
- Capsules (U.S. and Canada)
- Tablets (U.S.)

Diazepam
- Extended-release capsules (U.S.)
- Oral solution (U.S.)
- Tablets (U.S. and Canada)

Estazolam
- Tablets (U.S.)

Flurazepam
- Capsules (U.S. and Canada)
- Tablets (Canada)

Halazepam
- Tablets (U.S.)

Ketazolam
- Capsules (Canada)

Lorazepam
- Oral solution (U.S.)
- Tablets (U.S. and Canada)
- Sublingual tablets (Canada)

Nitrazepam
- Tablets (Canada)

Oxazepam
- Capsules (U.S.)
- Tablets (U.S. and Canada)

Prazepam
- Capsules (U.S.)
- Tablets (U.S.)

Quazepam
- Tablets (U.S.)

Temazepam
- Capsules (U.S. and Canada)
- Tablets (U.S.)

Triazolam
- Tablets (U.S. and Canada)

Parenteral
    Chlordiazepoxide
        • Injection (U.S. and Canada)
    Diazepam
        • Injection (U.S. and Canada)
    Lorazepam
        • Injection (U.S. and Canada)

Rectal
    Diazepam
        • Rectal solution (U.S. and Canada)

It is very important that you read and understand the following information. If any of it causes you special concern, check with your doctor. Also, *if you have any questions* or if you want more information about this medicine or your medical problem, *ask your doctor, nurse, or pharmacist.*

Before Using This Medicine

In deciding to use a medicine, the risks of taking the medicine must be weighed against the good it will do. This is a decision you and your doctor will make. For benzodiazepines, the following should be considered:

Allergies—Tell your doctor if you have ever had any unusual or allergic reaction to benzodiazepines. Also tell your doctor and pharmacist if you are allergic to any other substances, such as foods, preservatives, or dyes.

Pregnancy—Chlordiazepoxide and diazepam have been reported to increase the chance of birth defects when used during the first 3 months of pregnancy. Although similar problems have not been reported with the other benzodiazepines, the chance always exists since all of the benzodiazepines are related.

Studies in animals have shown that clonazepam, lorazepam, and temazepam cause birth defects or other problems, including death of the animal fetus.

Too much use of benzodiazepines during pregnancy may cause the baby to become dependent on the medicine. This may lead to withdrawal side effects after birth. Also, use of benzodiazepines during pregnancy, especially during the last weeks, may cause drowsiness, slow heartbeat, shortness of breath, or troubled breathing in the newborn infant.

Benzodiazepines given just before or during labor may cause weakness in the newborn infant. When diazepam is given in high doses (especially by injection) within 15 hours before delivery, it may cause breathing problems, muscle weakness, difficulty in feeding, and body temperature problems in the newborn infant.

Breast-feeding—Benzodiazepines may pass into the breast milk and cause drowsiness, slow heartbeat, shortness of breath, or troubled breathing in nursing babies of mothers taking this medicine.

Children—Most of the side effects of these medicines are more likely to occur in children, especially the very young. These patients are usually more sensitive than adults to the effects of benzodiazepines.

When clonazepam is used for long periods of time in children, it may cause unwanted effects on physical and mental growth. These effects may not be noticed until many years later. Before this medicine is given to children for long periods of time, you should discuss its use with your child's doctor.

Older adults—Most of the side effects of these medicines are more likely to occur in the elderly, who are usually more sensitive to the effects of benzodiazepines.

Taking benzodiazepines for trouble in sleeping may cause more daytime drowsiness in elderly patients than in younger adults. In addition, falls and related injuries may be more likely to occur in elderly patients taking benzodiazepines.

Athletes—Benzodiazepines are banned and, in some cases, tested for in competitors in biathlon and modern pentathlon events by the U.S. Olympic Committee (USOC).

Other medicines—Although certain medicines should not be used together at all, in other cases 2 different medicines may be used together even if an interaction might occur. In these cases, your doctor may want to change the dose, or other

precautions may be necessary. When you are taking or receiving benzodiazepines it is especially important that your doctor and pharmacist know if you are taking any of the following:

- Central nervous system (CNS) depressants (medicine that causes drowsiness)—The CNS depressant effects of either these medicines or benzodiazepines may be increased; your doctor may want to change the dose of either or both medicines

Other medical problems—The presence of other medical problems may affect the use of benzodiazepines. Make sure you tell your doctor if you have any other medical problems, especially:

- Alcohol abuse (or history of) or
- Drug abuse or dependence (or history of)—Dependence on benzodiazepines may develop
- Brain disease—CNS depression and other side effects of benzodiazepines may be more likely to occur
- Difficulty in swallowing (in children) or
- Emphysema, asthma, bronchitis, or other chronic lung disease or
- Glaucoma or
- Hyperactivity or
- Mental depression or
- Mental illness (severe) or
- Myasthenia gravis or
- Porphyria or
- Sleep apnea (temporarily stopping of breathing during sleep)—Benzodiazepines may make the condition worse
- Epilepsy or history of seizures—Although clonazepam and diazepam are used in treating epilepsy, starting or suddenly stopping treatment with these medicines may increase seizures
- Kidney or liver disease—Higher blood levels of benzodiazepines may result, increasing the chance of side effects

Before you begin using any new medicine (prescription or nonprescription) or if you develop any new medical problem while you are using this medicine, check with your doctor, nurse, or pharmacist.

Proper Use of This Medicine

For patients taking *diazepam extended-release capsules:*
- Swallow capsules whole.
- Do not crush, break, or chew the capsules before swallowing.

For patients taking *lorazepam oral solution:*
- Each dose may be diluted with water, soda or soda-like beverages, or semisolid food, such as applesauce or pudding.

For patients taking *lorazepam sublingual tablets:*
- Do not chew or swallow the tablet. This medicine is meant to be absorbed through the lining of the mouth. Place the tablet under your tongue (sublingual) and let it slowly dissolve there. Do not swallow for at least 2 minutes.

Take this medicine only as directed by your doctor. Do not take more of it, do not take it more often, and do not take it for a longer time than your doctor ordered. If too much is taken, it may become habit-forming (causing mental or physical dependence).

If you think this medicine is not working properly after you have taken it for a few weeks, *do not increase the dose.* Instead, check with your doctor.

For patients taking this medicine *for epilepsy or other seizure disorder:*
- *In order for this medicine to control your seizures, it must be taken every day in regularly spaced doses as ordered by your doctor.* This is necessary to keep a constant amount of the medicine in the blood. To help keep the amount constant, do not miss any doses.

For patients taking this medicine *for insomnia:*
- *Do not take this medicine when your schedule does not permit you to get a full night's sleep (7 to 8 hours).* If you must wake up before this, you may continue to feel drowsy and may experience memory problems, because

the effects of the medicine have not had time to wear off.

For patients taking *flurazepam:*
- *When you begin to take this medicine, your sleeping problem will improve somewhat the first night. However, 2 or 3 nights may pass before you receive the full effects of this medicine.*

Missed dose—If you are taking this medicine regularly (for example, every day as for epilepsy) and you miss a dose, take it right away if you remember within an hour or so of the missed dose. However, if you do not remember until later, skip the missed dose and go back to your regular dosing schedule. Do not double doses.

Storage—To store this medicine:
- Keep out of the reach of children. Overdose of benzodiazepines may be especially dangerous in children.
- Store away from heat and direct light.
- Do not store the capsule or tablet form of this medicine in the bathroom, near the kitchen sink, or in other damp places. Heat or moisture may cause the medicine to break down.
- Keep the liquid form of this medicine from freezing.
- Do not keep outdated medicine or medicine no longer needed. Be sure that any discarded medicine is out of the reach of children.

Precautions While Using This Medicine

If you will be *taking this medicine regularly for a long time:*
- Your doctor should check your progress at regular visits to make sure that this medicine does not cause unwanted effects. If you are taking clonazepam, this is also important during the first few months of treatment.
- If you are taking this medicine for nervousness or tension or for panic disorder, check with your doctor at least every 4 months to make sure you need to continue taking this medicine.

- If you are taking estazolam, flurazepam, quazepam, temazepam, or triazolam for insomnia (trouble in sleeping), and you think you need this medicine for more than 7 to 10 days, be sure to discuss it with your doctor. Insomnia that lasts longer than this may be a sign of another medical problem.

If you will be taking this medicine in large doses or for a long time, do not stop taking it without first checking with your doctor. Your doctor may want you to reduce gradually the amount you are taking before stopping completely. Stopping this medicine suddenly may cause withdrawal side effects. Also, if you are taking this medicine for epilepsy or another seizure disorder, stopping this medicine suddenly may cause seizures.

For patients taking this medicine *for epilepsy or another seizure disorder:*

- Your doctor may want you to carry a medical identification card or bracelet stating that you are taking this medicine.

This medicine will add to the effects of alcohol and other CNS depressants (medicines that slow down the nervous system, possibly causing drowsiness). Some examples of CNS depressants are antihistamines or medicine for hay fever, other allergies, or colds; sedatives, tranquilizers, or sleeping medicine; prescription pain medicine or narcotics; barbiturates; medicine for seizures; muscle relaxants; or anesthetics, including some dental anesthetics. This effect may last for a few days after you stop taking this medicine. *Check with your doctor before taking any of the above while you are taking this medicine.*

If you think you or someone else may have taken an overdose of this medicine, get emergency help at once. Taking an overdose of a benzodiazepine or taking alcohol or other CNS depressants with the benzodiazepine may lead to unconsciousness and possibly death. Some signs of an overdose are continuing slurred speech or confusion, severe drowsiness, severe weakness, and staggering.

Before you have any medical tests, tell the medical doctor in charge that you are taking this medicine. The results of the metyrapone test may be affected by chlordiazepoxide.

If you develop any unusual and strange thoughts or behavior while you are taking this medicine, be sure to discuss it with your doctor. Some changes that have occurred in people taking this medicine are like those seen in people who drink alcohol and then act in a manner that is not normal. Other changes may be more unusual and extreme, such as confusion, agitation, and hallucinations (seeing, hearing, or feeling things that are not there).

This medicine may cause some people, especially older persons, to become drowsy, dizzy, lightheaded, clumsy or unsteady, or less alert than they are normally. Even if taken at bedtime, it may cause some people to feel drowsy or less alert on arising. *Make sure you know how you react to this medicine before you drive, use machines, or do anything else that could be dangerous if you are dizzy or are not alert.*

If you have been taking this medicine for insomnia, you may have difficulty sleeping (rebound insomnia) for the first few nights after you stop taking the medicine.

Side Effects of This Medicine

Along with its needed effects, a medicine may cause some unwanted effects. Although not all of these side effects may occur, if they do occur they may need medical attention.

Check with your doctor as soon as possible if any of the following side effects occur:

Less common or rare

Behavior problems, including difficulty in concentrating and outbursts of anger; confusion or mental depression; convulsions (seizures); hallucinations (seeing, hearing, or feeling things that are not there); hypotension (low blood pressure); impaired memory—may be more common with triazolam; muscle weakness; skin rash or itching; sore throat, fever, and chills; trouble in sleeping; ulcers or sores in mouth or throat (continuing); uncontrolled movements of body, including the eyes; unusual bleeding or bruising; unusual excitement, nervousness, or irritability; unusual tiredness or weakness (severe); yellow eyes or skin

Symptoms of overdose

Confusion (continuing); drowsiness (severe); shakiness; slow heartbeat, shortness of breath, or troubled breathing; slow reflexes; slurred speech (continuing); staggering; weakness (severe)

Other side effects may occur that usually do not need medical attention. These side effects may go away during treatment as your body adjusts to the medicine. However, check with your doctor if any of the following side effects continue or are bothersome:

More common

Clumsiness or unsteadiness; dizziness or lightheadedness; drowsiness; slurred speech

Less common or rare

Abdominal or stomach cramps or pain; blurred vision or other changes in vision; changes in sexual drive or performance; constipation; diarrhea; dryness of mouth or increased thirst; false sense of well-being; fast or pounding heartbeat; headache; increased bronchial secretions or watering of mouth; muscle spasm; nausea or vomiting; problems with urination; trembling; unusual tiredness or weakness

Not all of the side effects listed above have been reported for each of these medicines, but they have been reported for at least one of them. All of the benzodiazepines are similar, so any of the above side effects may occur with any of these medicines.

For patients having *chlordiazepoxide, diazepam, or lorazepam injected:*

- Check with your doctor if there is redness, swelling, or pain at the place of injection.

After you stop using this medicine, your body may need time to adjust. If you took this medicine in high doses or for a long time, this may take up to 3 weeks. During this period of time check with your doctor if you notice any of the following side effects:

More common
Irritability; nervousness; trouble in sleeping

Less common
Abdominal or stomach cramps; confusion; fast or pounding heartbeat; increased sense of hearing; increased sensitivity to touch and pain; increased sweating; loss of sense of reality; mental depression; muscle cramps; nausea or vomiting; sensitivity of eyes to light; tingling, burning, or prickly sensations; trembling

Rare
Confusion as to time, place, or person; convulsions (seizures); feelings of suspicion or distrust; hallucinations (seeing, hearing, or feeling things that are not there)

Other side effects not listed above may also occur in some patients. If you notice any other effects, check with your doctor.

Additional Information

Once a medicine has been approved for marketing for a certain use, experience may show that it is also useful for other medical problems. Although these uses are not included in product labeling, some of the benzodiazepines are used in certain patients with the following medical conditions:

- Nausea and vomiting caused by cancer chemotherapy
- Tension headache
- Tremors

Other than the above information, there is no additional information relating to proper use, precautions, or side effects for these uses.

BETA-ADRENERGIC BLOCKING AGENTS   Systemic

This information applies to the following medicines:
Acebutolol (a-se-BYOO-toe-lole)
Atenolol (a-TEN-oh-lole)

    Betaxolol (be-TAX-oh-lol)
    Carteolol (KAR-tee-oh-lole)
    Labetalol (la-BET-a-lole)
    Metoprolol (me-TOE-proe-lole)
    Nadolol (NAY-doe-lole)
    Oxprenolol (ox-PREN-oh-lole)
    Penbutolol (pen-BYOO-toe-lole)
    Pindolol (PIN-doe-lole)
    Propranolol (proe-PRAN-oh-lole)
    Sotalol (SOE-ta-lole)
    Timolol (TIM-oh-lole)

Some commonly used brand names are:

For Acebutolol
    In the U.S.
        Sectral
    In Canada
        Monitan
        Sectral

For Atenolol
    In the U.S. and Canada
        Tenormin

For Betaxolol†
    In the U.S.
        Kerlone

For Carteolol†
    In the U.S.
        Cartrol

For Labetalol
    In the U.S.
        Normodyne
        Trandate
    In Canada
        Trandate

For Metoprolol
    In the U.S.
        Lopressor
    In Canada

Apo-Metoprolol	Lopresor
Apo-Metoprolol (Type L)	Lopresor SR
Betaloc	Novometoprol
Betaloc Durules	

    Generic name product may also be available.

For Nadolol
    In the U.S.
        Corgard

   In Canada
      Corgard
      Syn-Nadolol
      Generic name product may also be available.

For Oxprenolol*
   In Canada
      Slow-Trasicor
      Trasicor

For Penbutolol†
   In the U.S.
      Levatol

For Pindolol
   In the U.S.
      Visken
   In Canada
      Syn-Pindolol
      Visken

For Propranolol
   In the U.S.
      Inderal
      Inderal LA
      Generic name product may also be available.
   In Canada
      Apo-Propranolol   Inderal LA
      Detensol   Novopranol
      Inderal   pms Propranolol
      Generic name product may also be available.

For Sotalol*
   In Canada
      Sotacor

For Timolol
   In the U.S.
      Blocadren
   In Canada
      Apo-Timol
      Blocadren

---

  *Not commercially available in the U.S.
  †Not commercially available in Canada.

Description

These medicines belong to a group of medicines known as beta-adrenergic blocking agents, beta-blocking agents, or more commonly, beta-blockers. Beta-blockers are used in the treatment of high blood pressure (hypertension). Some beta-blockers are also used to relieve angina (chest pain) and in heart attack patients to help prevent additional heart attacks. Beta-blockers have also been found useful in a number of other conditions such as correcting irregular heartbeats, preventing migraine headaches, and treating tremors. They may also be used for other conditions as determined by your doctor.

Beta-blockers work by affecting the response to some nerve impulses in certain parts of the body. As a result, they decrease the need for blood and oxygen by the heart by reducing its workload. They also help the heart to beat more regularly.

Beta-adrenergic blocking agents are available only with your doctor's prescription, in the following dosage forms:

Oral

Acebutolol
- Capsules (U.S.)
- Tablets (Canada)

Atenolol
- Tablets (U.S. and Canada)

Betaxolol
- Tablets (U.S.)

Carteolol
- Tablets (U.S.)

Labetalol
- Tablets (U.S. and Canada)

Metoprolol
- Tablets (U.S. and Canada)
- Extended-release tablets (Canada)

Nadolol
- Tablets (U.S. and Canada)

Oxprenolol
- Tablets (Canada)
- Extended-release tablets (Canada)

Penbutolol
- Tablets (U.S.)

Pindolol
- Tablets (U.S. and Canada)

Propranolol
- Extended-release capsules (U.S. and Canada)
- Oral solution (U.S.)
- Tablets (U.S. and Canada)

Sotalol
- Tablets (Canada)

Timolol
- Tablets (U.S. and Canada)

Parenteral

Atenolol
- Injection (U.S.)

Labetalol
- Injection (U.S. and Canada)

Metoprolol
- Injection (U.S. and Canada)

Propranolol
- Injection (U.S. and Canada)

It is very important that you read and understand the following information. If any of it causes you special concern, check with your doctor. Also, *if you have any questions* or if you want more information about this medicine or your medical problem, *ask your doctor, nurse, or pharmacist.*

Before Using This Medicine

In deciding to use a medicine, the risks of taking the medicine must be weighed against the good it will do. This is a decision you and your doctor will make. For the beta-adrenergic blocking agents (also known as beta-blocking agents or, more commonly, beta-blockers), the following should be considered:

Allergies—Tell your doctor if you have ever had any unusual or allergic reaction to the beta-blocker medicine prescribed. Also tell your doctor and pharmacist if you are allergic to any other substances, such as foods, preservatives, or dyes.

Pregnancy—Adequate studies have not been done in pregnant women. However, use of some beta-blockers during pregnancy has been associated with low blood sugar, breathing problems, a lower heart rate, and low blood pressure in the newborn infant. Other reports have shown no unwanted effects on the newborn infant. Animal studies have shown some beta-blockers to cause problems in pregnancy when used in doses many times the usual human dose.

Breast-feeding—Although some beta-blockers pass into the breast milk, these medicines have not been reported to cause problems in nursing babies. However, enough betaxolol passes into breast milk that it could cause effects such as low heart rate or low blood pressure in the infant.

Children—Although there is no specific information about the use of this medicine in children, it is not expected to cause different side effects or problems in children than it does in adults.

Older adults—Some side effects are more likely to occur in the elderly, who are usually more sensitive to the effects of beta-blockers. Also, beta-blockers may reduce tolerance to cold temperatures in elderly patients.

Athletes—Beta-blockers are banned and tested for by the U.S. Olympic Committee (USOC) and National Collegiate Athletic Association (NCAA). Beta-blocker use can lead to disqualification of athletes in most athletic events.

Other medicines—Although certain medicines should not be used together at all, in other cases 2 different medicines may be used together even if an interaction might occur. In these cases, your doctor may want to change the dose, or other precautions may be necessary. When taking or receiving beta-blockers it is especially important that your doctor and pharmacist know if you are taking any of the following:

- Aminophylline (e.g., Somophyllin) or
- Caffeine (e.g., NoDoz) or
- Dyphylline (e.g., Lufyllin) or
- Oxtriphylline (e.g., Choledyl) or
- Theophylline (e.g., Somophyllin-T)—The effects of both these medicines and beta-blockers may be blocked; in addition, theophylline levels in the body may be increased, especially in patients who smoke

- Antidiabetics, oral (diabetes medicine you take by mouth) or
- Insulin—There is an increased risk of hypoglycemia (low blood sugar) or hyperglycemia (high blood sugar); beta-blockers may cover up certain symptoms of hypoglycemia such as

increases in pulse rate and blood pressure, and may make the hypoglycemia last longer

- Clonidine (e.g., Catapres) or
- Diltiazem (e.g., Cardizem) or
- Guanabenz (e.g., Wytensin) or
- Nicardipine (e.g, Cardene) or
- Nifedipine (e.g., Procardia) or
- Nimodipine (e.g., Nimotop) or
- Verapamil (e.g., Calan)—Effects on blood pressure may be increased. In addition, unwanted effects may occur if clonidine, guanabenz, or a beta-blocker is stopped suddenly after use together
- If you use cocaine—Cocaine may block the effects of beta-blockers; in addition, there is an increased risk of high blood pressure, fast heartbeat, and possibly heart problems
- Monoamine oxidase (MAO) inhibitors (furazolidone [e.g., Furoxone], isocarboxazid [e.g., Marplan], pargyline [e.g., Eutonyl], phenelzine [e.g., Nardil], procarbazine [e.g., Matulane], tranylcypromine [e.g., Parnate])—Taking beta-blockers while you are taking or within 2 weeks of taking monoamine oxidase (MAO) inhibitors may cause severe high blood pressure

Other medical problems—The presence of other medical problems may affect the use of the beta blockers. Make sure you tell your doctor if you have any other medical problems, especially:

- Allergy, history of (asthma, eczema, hay fever, hives), or
- Bronchitis or
- Emphysema—Severity and duration of allergic reactions to other substances may be increased; in addition, beta-blockers can increase trouble in breathing
- Bradycardia (unusually slow heartbeat) or
- Heart or blood vessel disease—There is a risk of further decreased heart function; also, if treatment is stopped suddenly, unwanted effects may occur
- Diabetes mellitus (sugar diabetes)—All beta-blockers may cover up fast heartbeat associated with hypoglycemia (low blood sugar), but not dizziness and sweating; in addition, beta-blockers may cause hypoglycemia and circulation problems
- Kidney disease or
- Liver disease—Effects of beta-blockers may be increased

- Mental depression (or history of)—May be increased by beta-blockers
- Overactive thyroid—Sudden withdrawal of beta-blockers may increase symptoms; beta-blockers may cover up fast heartbeat

Before you begin using any new medicine (prescription or nonprescription) or if you develop any new medical problem while you are using this medicine, check with your doctor, nurse, or pharmacist.

Proper Use of This Medicine

For patients taking the *extended-release capsule or tablet* form of this medicine:

- Swallow the capsule or tablet whole.
- Do not crush, break, or chew before swallowing.

For patients taking the *concentrated oral solution* form of *propranolol:*

- This medicine is to be taken by mouth even though it comes in a dropper bottle. The amount you should take is to be measured only with the specially marked dropper.
- Mix the medicine with some water, juice, or carbonated drink. After drinking all the liquid containing the medicine, rinse the glass with a little more liquid and drink that also, to make sure you get all the medicine.

    If you prefer, you may mix this medicine with applesauce or pudding instead.
- This medicine must be freshly mixed just before it is used. Do not keep any that you have not taken after it has been mixed.

Ask your doctor about checking your pulse rate before and after taking beta-blocking agents. Then, while you are taking this medicine, check your pulse regularly. If it is much slower than your usual rate (or less than 50 beats per minute), check with your doctor. A pulse rate that is too slow may cause circulation problems.

To help you remember to take your medicine, try to get into the habit of taking it at the same time each day.

For patients taking this medicine *for high blood pressure:*

- Importance of diet—When prescribing medicine for your condition, your doctor may also prescribe a personal diet for you. Such a diet may be low in sodium (salt). Most people eat much more sodium than they need. Too much sodium in the diet may increase blood pressure. Some foods that contain large amounts of sodium are canned soup, pickles, ketchup, green and ripe olives, relish, frankfurters, soy sauce, and carbonated beverages. Your doctor may want you to limit the amounts of these and other high-sodium foods in your diet. High blood pressure medicine is usually more effective when such a diet is properly followed.

  Also, it may be very important for you to go on a reducing diet. However, check with your doctor before changing your diet.

- Many patients who have high blood pressure will not notice any signs of the problem. In fact, many may feel normal. It is very important that you *take your medicine exactly as directed.* Also, keep your appointments with your doctor even if you feel well.

- Remember that this medicine will not cure your high blood pressure but it does help control it. Therefore, you must continue to take it as directed if you expect to lower your blood pressure and keep it down. *You may have to take high blood pressure medicine for the rest of your life.* If high blood pressure is not treated, it can cause serious problems such as heart failure, blood vessel disease, stroke, or kidney disease.

Missed dose—Do not miss any doses. This is especially important when you are taking only one dose per day. Some conditions may become worse when this medicine is not taken regularly.

If you do miss a dose of this medicine, take it as soon as possible. However, if it is within 4 hours of your next dose (8 hours when using atenolol, betaxolol, carteolol, labetalol, nadolol, penbutolol, sotalol, or extended-release oxprenolol or propranolol), skip the missed dose and go back to your regular dosing schedule. Do not double doses.

Storage—To store this medicine:
- Keep out of the reach of children.
- Store away from heat and direct light.
- Do not store in the bathroom, near the kitchen sink, or in other damp places. Heat or moisture may cause the medicine to break down.
- Do not keep outdated medicine or medicine no longer needed. Be sure that any discarded medicine is out of the reach of children.

Precautions While Using This Medicine

It is important that your doctor check your progress at regular visits. This is to make sure the medicine is working for you and to allow the dosage to be changed if needed.

Do not stop taking this medicine without first checking with your doctor. Your doctor may want you to reduce gradually the amount you are taking before stopping completely. Some conditions may become worse when the medicine is stopped suddenly, and danger of heart attack is increased in some patients.

Make sure that you have enough medicine on hand to last through weekends, holidays, or vacations. You may want to carry an extra written prescription in your billfold or purse in case of an emergency. You can then have it filled if you run out of medicine while you are away from home.

Your doctor may want you to carry a medical identification card stating that you are taking this medicine.

Before having any kind of surgery (including dental surgery) or emergency treatment, tell the medical doctor or dentist in charge that you are taking this medicine.

For *diabetic patients:*
- *This medicine may cause your blood sugar levels to fall.* Also, *this medicine may cover up signs of hypoglycemia (low blood sugar),* such as change in pulse rate.

This medicine may cause some people to become dizzy, drowsy, or lightheaded. *Make sure you know how you react to this medicine before you drive, use machines, or do anything else that could be dangerous if you are dizzy or are not alert.* If the problem continues or gets worse, check with your doctor.

Beta-blockers may make you more sensitive to cold temperatures, especially if you have blood circulation problems. They tend to decrease blood circulation in the skin, fingers, and toes. Dress warmly during cold weather and be careful during prolonged exposure to cold, such as in winter sports.

Chest pain resulting from exercise or physical exertion is usually reduced or prevented by this medicine. This may tempt a patient to be overly active. *Make sure you discuss with your doctor a safe amount of exercise for your medical problem.*

Before you have any medical tests, tell the doctor in charge that you are taking this medicine. The results of some tests may be affected by this medicine.

For patients with *allergies to foods, medicines, or insect stings:*
- There is a chance that this medicine will cause allergic reactions to be worse and harder to treat. If you have a severe allergic reaction while you are being treated with this medicine, check with a doctor right away so that it can be treated.

For patients taking this medicine *for high blood pressure:*
- *Do not take other medicines unless they have been discussed with your doctor.* This especially includes over-the-counter (nonprescription) medicines for appetite control, asthma, colds, cough, hay fever, or sinus problems since they may tend to increase your blood pressure.

For patients taking *labetalol by mouth:*
- *Dizziness, lightheadedness, or fainting may occur, especially when you get up from a lying or sitting position.* This is more likely to occur when you first start

taking labetalol or when the dose is increased. *Getting up slowly may help.* When you get up from lying down, sit on the edge of the bed with your feet dangling for 1 to 2 minutes. Then stand up slowly. If the problem continues or gets worse, check with your doctor.

• The dizziness, lightheadedness, or fainting is also more likely to occur if you drink alcohol, stand for long periods of time, exercise, or if the weather is hot. *While you are taking this medicine, be careful in the amount of alcohol you drink. Also, use extra care during exercise or hot weather or if you must stand for long periods of time.*

For patients receiving *labetalol by injection:*

• It is very important that you lie down flat while receiving labetalol and for up to 3 hours afterward. If you try to get up too soon, you may become dizzy or faint. *Do not try to sit or stand until your doctor tells you to do so.*

Side Effects of This Medicine

Along with its needed effects, a medicine may cause some unwanted effects. Although not all of these side effects may occur, if they do occur they may need medical attention.

Check with your doctor as soon as possible if any of the following side effects occur:

Less common

Breathing difficulty and/or wheezing; cold hands and feet; confusion (especially in elderly); hallucinations (seeing, hearing, or feeling things that are not there); irregular heartbeat; mental depression; nightmares and vivid dreams; skin rash; slow heartbeat (especially less than 50 beats per minute)—more common with nadolol, propranolol, and sotalol; rare with carteolol, labetalol, penbutolol, and pindolol; swelling of ankles, feet, and/or lower legs

Rare

Back pain or joint pain—more common with pindolol; chest pain; dark urine—for acebutolol or labetalol; fever and sore throat; red, scaling, or crusted skin; unusual bleeding and bruising; yellow eyes or skin—for acebutolol or labetalol

Signs and symptoms of overdose (in the order in which they may occur)

> Slow heartbeat; dizziness (severe) or fainting; fast or irregular heartbeat; difficulty in breathing; bluish-colored fingernails or palms of hands; convulsions (seizures)

Other side effects may occur that usually do not need medical attention. These side effects may go away during treatment as your body adjusts to the medicine. However, check with your doctor if any of the following side effects continue or are bothersome:

More common

> Decreased sexual ability; dizziness or lightheadedness; drowsiness (slight); trouble in sleeping; unusual tiredness or weakness

Less common or rare

> Anxiety and/or nervousness; changes in taste—for labetalol only; constipation; diarrhea; dry, sore eyes; frequent urination—for acebutolol and carteolol only; itching of skin; nausea or vomiting; numbness and/or tingling of fingers and/or toes; numbness and/or tingling of skin, especially on scalp—for labetalol only; stomach discomfort; stuffy nose

Although not all of the side effects listed above have been reported for all of these medicines, they have been reported for at least one of them. Since all of the beta-adrenergic blocking agents are very similar, any of the above side effects may occur with any of these medicines. However, they may be more or less common with some agents than with others.

After you have been taking a beta-blocker for a while, it may cause unpleasant or even harmful effects if you stop taking it too suddenly. After you stop taking this medicine or while you are gradually reducing the amount you are taking, check with your doctor right away if any of the following occur:

> Chest pain; fast or irregular heartbeat; general feeling of discomfort or illness or weakness; shortness of breath (sudden); sweating; trembling

For patients taking *labetalol:*

- You may notice a tingling feeling on your scalp when you first begin to take labetalol. This is to be expected and usually goes away after you have been taking labetalol for a while.

Other side effects not listed above may also occur in some patients. If you notice any other effects, check with your doctor.

BRONCHODILATORS, ADRENERGIC Inhalation

This information applies to the following medicines:

Albuterol (al-BYOO-ter-ole)
Bitolterol (bye-TOLE-ter-ole)
Epinephrine (ep-i-NEF-rin)
Fenoterol (fen-OH-ter-ole)
Isoetharine (eye-soe-ETH-a-reen)
Isoproterenol (eye-soe-proe-TER-e-nole)
Metaproterenol (met-a-proe-TER-e-nole)
Pirbuterol (peer-BYOO-ter-ole)
Procaterol (proe-KAY-ter-ole)
Racepinephrine (race-ep-i-NEF-rin)
Terbutaline (ter-BYOO-ta-leen)

Some commonly used brand names are:

For Albuterol
In the U.S.
    Proventil   Ventolin Rotacaps
    Ventolin

    Generic name product may also be available.

In Canada
    Ventolin   Ventolin Rotacaps

Another commonly used name is salbutamol.

For Bitolterol
In the U.S.
    Tornalate

For Epinephrine
In the U.S.
    Adrenalin   Bronkaid Mist Suspension
    AsthmaHaler   Medihaler-Epi
    Bronitin Mist   Primatene Mist
    Bronkaid Mist   Primatene Mist Suspension

    Generic name product may also be available.

In Canada
    Bronkaid Mistometer   Medihaler-Epi

For Fenoterol*
In Canada
    Berotec

For Isoetharine
In the U.S.
    Arm-a-Med Isoetharine   Dey-Dose Isoetharine S/F
    Bronkometer   Dey-Lute Isoetharine
    Bronkosol   Dey-Lute Isoetharine S/F
    Dey-Dose Isoetharine   Dispos-a-Med Isoetharine
    Generic name product may also be available.

For Isoproterenol
In the U.S.
    Aerolone   Isuprel Mistometer
    Dey-Dose Isoproterenol   Medihaler-Iso
    Dispos-a-Med Isoproterenol   Norisodrine Aerotrol
    Isuprel   Vapo-Iso
    Generic name product may also be available.

In Canada
    Isuprel   Medihaler-Iso
    Isuprel Mistometer

For Metaproterenol
In the U.S.
    Alupent   Dey-Lute Metaproterenol
    Arm-a-Med Metaproterenol   Metaprel
    Dey-Dose Metaproterenol
    Generic name product may also be available.

In Canada
    Alupent

For Pirbuterol
In the U.S.
    Maxair

For Procaterol*
In Canada
    Pro-Air

For Racepinephrine
In the U.S.
    AsthmaNefrin   Vaponefrin
    Dey-Dose Racepinephrine

In Canada
    Vaponefrin

For Terbutaline
In the U.S.
Brethaire
In Canada
Bricanyl

*Not commercially available in the U.S.

Description

Adrenergic bronchodilators are medicines that open up the bronchial tubes (air passages) of the lungs. They are taken by oral inhalation to treat the symptoms of bronchial asthma, chronic bronchitis, emphysema, and other lung diseases. They relieve cough, wheezing, shortness of breath, and troubled breathing by increasing the flow of air through the bronchial tubes.

Some of these medicines are also taken by oral inhalation to prevent bronchospasm (wheezing or difficulty in breathing) caused by exercise. In addition, some of these medicines are taken by oral inhalation to prevent attacks of bronchial asthma and bronchospasm. Also, racepinephrine may be used in the treatment of croup.

All of these medicines, except some epinephrine preparations, are available only with your doctor's prescription. Although some of the epinephrine preparations are available without a prescription, your doctor may have special instructions on the proper dose of epinephrine for your medical condition.

These medicines are available in the following dosage forms:
Inhalation
Albuterol
• Capsules for inhalation (U.S. and Canada)
• Inhalation aerosol (U.S. and Canada)
• Inhalation solution (U.S. and Canada)
Bitolterol
• Inhalation aerosol (U.S.)
Epinephrine
• Inhalation aerosol (U.S. and Canada)
• Inhalation solution (U.S.)

Fenoterol
- Inhalation aerosol (Canada)
- Inhalation solution (Canada)

Isoetharine
- Inhalation aerosol (U.S.)
- Inhalation solution (U.S.)

Isoproterenol
- Inhalation aerosol (U.S. and Canada)
- Inhalation solution (U.S. and Canada)

Metaproterenol
- Inhalation aerosol (U.S. and Canada)
- Inhalation solution (U.S. and Canada)

Pirbuterol
- Inhalation aerosol (U.S.)

Procaterol
- Inhalation aerosol (Canada)

Racepinephrine
- Inhalation solution (U.S. and Canada)

Terbutaline
- Inhalation aerosol (U.S. and Canada)

It is very important that you read and understand the following information. If any of it causes you special concern, check with your doctor. Also, *if you have any questions* or if you want more information about this medicine or your medical problem, *ask your doctor, nurse, or pharmacist.*

Before Using This Medicine

In deciding to use a medicine, the risks of taking the medicine must be weighed against the good it will do. This is a decision you and your doctor will make. For inhalation adrenergic bronchodilators, the following should be considered:

Allergies—Tell your doctor if you have ever had any unusual or allergic reaction to albuterol, bitolterol, epinephrine, fenoterol, isoetharine, isoproterenol, metaproterenol, pirbuterol, procaterol racepinephrine, terbutaline, or other inhalation medicines. Also tell your doctor and pharmacist if you are allergic to any other substances, such as foods, preservatives, or dyes.

Pregnancy—
- *For albuterol, bitolterol, and metaproterenol*: Albuterol, bitolterol, and metaproterenol have not been stud-

ied in pregnant women. However, studies in animals have shown that albuterol, bitolterol, and metaproterenol cause birth defects when given in doses many times the usual human inhalation dose.

- *For epinephrine and racepinephrine*: Epinephrine and racepinephrine have not been studied in pregnant women. However, studies in animals have shown that epinephrine causes birth defects when given in doses many times the usual human inhalation dose. Use of epinephrine or racepinephrine during pregnancy may decrease the supply of oxygen to the fetus.

- *For fenoterol*: Fenoterol has not been shown to cause birth defects or other problems in humans.

- *For isoetharine and isoproterenol*: Studies on birth defects with isoetharine or isoproterenol have not been done in either humans or animals.

- *For pirbuterol*: Pirbuterol has not been studied in pregnant women. However, in some animal studies, pirbuterol has been shown to cause miscarriage and death of the animal fetus when given in doses many times the usual human inhalation dose.

- *For procaterol*: Procaterol has not been studied in pregnant women.

- *For terbutaline*: Terbutaline has not been studied in pregnant women. It has not been shown to cause birth defects in animal studies when given in doses many times the human inhalation dose. However, terbutaline may delay labor.

Breast-feeding—

- *For albuterol, bitolterol, fenoterol, isoetharine, isoproterenol, metaproterenol, pirbuterol, and procaterol*: Although it is not known whether albuterol, bitolterol, fenoterol, isoetharine, isoproterenol, metaproterenol, pirbuterol, or procaterol passes into the breast milk, these medicines have not been reported to cause problems in nursing babies.

- *For epinephrine and racepinephrine*: Epinephrine passes into the breast milk. Epinephrine and racepinephrine may cause unwanted side effects in babies of mothers using epinephrine or racepinephrine.

- *For terbutaline*: Although terbutaline passes into the breast milk, it has not been reported to cause problems in nursing babies.

Children—Although there is no specific information about the use of albuterol, bitolterol, fenoterol, isoetharine, isoproterenol, metaproterenol, pirbuterol, procaterol, racepinephrine, or terbutaline in children, these medicines are not expected to cause different side effects or problems in children than they do in adults.

Infants and children may be especially sensitive to the effects of epinephrine. Fainting has occurred after epinephrine was given to children with asthma.

Older adults—Many medicines have not been tested in older people. Therefore, it may not be known whether they work exactly the same way they do in younger adults or if they cause different side effects or problems in older people. There is no specific information about the use of inhalation adrenergic bronchodilators in the elderly.

Athletes—Stimulants, including isoetharine, isoproterenol, and related substances, are banned and tested for in athletes by the U.S. Olympic Committee (USOC). However, the USOC permits the use of albuterol, bitolterol, metaproterenol, pirbuterol, procaterol, and terbutaline in aerosol or inhalation form.

Other medicines—Although certain medicines should not be used together at all, in other cases two different medicines may be used together even if an interaction might occur. In these cases, your doctor may want to change the dose, or other precautions may be necessary. When you are using inhalation adrenergic bronchodilators, it is especially important that your doctor and pharmacist know if you are taking any of the following:

- Beta-blockers (acebutolol [e.g., Sectral], atenolol [e.g., Tenormin], betaxolol [e.g., Betoptic, Kerlone], carteolol [e.g., Cartrol], labetalol [e.g., Normodyne], levobunolol [e.g., Betagan], metoprolol [e.g., Lopressor], nadolol [e.g., Corgard], oxprenolol [e.g., Trasicor], penbutolol [e.g., Levatol], pindolol [e.g., Visken], propranolol [e.g., Inderal], sotalol [e.g., Sotacor], timolol [e.g., Blocadren, Timoptic])—These medicines may prevent the adrenergic bronchodilators from working properly

- Cocaine or
- Ergoloid mesylates (e.g., Hydergine) or
- Ergotamine (e.g., Gynergen) or
- Maprotiline (e.g., Ludiomil) or
- Tricyclic antidepressants (medicine for depression)—The effects of these medicines on the heart and blood vessels may be increased
- Digitalis glycosides (heart medicine)—The chance of irregular heartbeat may be increased
- Monoamine oxidase (MAO) inhibitors (furazolidone [e.g., Furoxone], isocarboxazid [e.g., Marplan], pargyline [e.g., Eutonyl], phenelzine [e.g., Nardil], procarbazine [e.g., Matulane], tranylcypromine [e.g., Parnate])—Using adrenergic bronchodilators while you are taking or within 2 weeks of taking monoamine oxidase (MAO) inhibitors may increase the effects of MAO inhibitors

Other medical problems—The presence of other medical problems may affect the use of inhalation adrenergic bronchodilators. Make sure you tell your doctor if you have any other medical problems, especially:

- Brain damage
- Convulsions (seizures) (or history of)
- Diabetes mellitus (sugar diabetes)—Adrenergic bronchodilators may make the condition worse; your doctor may need to change the dose of your diabetes medicine
- Heart or blood vessel disease or
- High blood pressure—Adrenergic bronchodilators may make the condition worse
- Mental disease—Epinephrine may make the condition worse
- Overactive thyroid—The chance of side effects may be increased
- Parkinson's disease—Epinephrine may temporarily increase certain symptoms of Parkinson's disease, such as rigidity and tremor

Before you begin using any new medicine (prescription or nonprescription) or if you develop any new medical problem while you are using this medicine, check with your doctor, nurse, or pharmacist.

Proper Use of This Medicine

For patients using *epinephrine, isoetharine, isoproterenol, or racepinephrine*:

- Do not use if the solution turns pinkish to brownish in color or if it becomes cloudy.

Some epinephrine preparations are available without a doctor's prescription. However, *do not use this medicine without a doctor's prescription, unless your medical problem has been diagnosed as asthma by a doctor.*

Some of these preparations may come with patient directions. Read them carefully before using this medicine.

If you are using this medicine in a nebulizer or in a combination nebulizer and respirator, make sure you understand exactly how to use it. If you have any questions about this, check with your doctor or pharmacist.

For patients using the *inhalation aerosol* form of this medicine:

- *Keep spray away from the eyes because it may cause irritation.*
- *Do not take more than 2 inhalations of this medicine at any one time,* unless otherwise directed by your doctor. Allow 1 to 2 minutes after the first inhalation to make certain that a second inhalation is necessary.
- Save your applicator. Refill units of this medicine may be available.

Use this medicine only as directed. Do not use more of it and do not use it more often than recommended on the label, unless otherwise directed by your doctor. To do so may increase the chance of serious side effects. Inhalation aerosol medicines have been reported to cause death when too much of the medicine was used.

Missed dose—If you are using this medicine regularly and you miss a dose, use it as soon as possible. Then use any remaining doses for that day at regularly spaced intervals. Do not double doses.

Storage—To store this medicine:

- Keep out of the reach of children.
- Store away from heat.
- Store the solution form of this medicine away from direct light. Store the inhalation aerosol form of this medicine away from direct sunlight.
- Keep the medicine from freezing.
- Do not puncture, break, or burn the inhalation aerosol container, even if it is empty.
- Do not keep outdated medicine or medicine no longer needed. Be sure that any discarded medicine is out of the reach of children.

Precautions While Using This Medicine

If you still have trouble breathing after using this medicine, or if your condition becomes worse, check with your doctor at once.

For *diabetic patients* using *epinephrine*:

- This medicine may cause your blood sugar levels to rise. If you notice a change in the results of your blood or urine sugar tests or if you have any questions, check with your doctor.

For patients using the aerosol form of this medicine:

- If you are also using the inhalation aerosol form of an adrenocorticoid (cortisone-like medicine, such as beclomethasone, dexamethasone, flunisolide, or triamcinolone) or ipratropium, *use the adrenergic bronchodilator inhalation aerosol first and then wait about 5 minutes before using the adrenocorticoid or ipratropium inhalation aerosol,* unless otherwise directed by your doctor. This will allow the adrenocorticoid or ipratropium inhalation aerosol to better reach the passages

of the lungs (bronchioles) after the adrenergic bronchodilator inhalation aerosol opens them.

For patients using *albuterol inhalation aerosol*:
- If you use all of the medicine in one canister (container)
  in less than 2 weeks, check with your doctor. You may
  be using too much of the medicine.

Dryness of the mouth and throat may occur after use of this
medicine. Rinsing the mouth with water after each dose may
help prevent the dryness.

Some of these preparations may contain sulfites as a preservative. Sulfites may cause an allergic reaction in some
people. *If you know that you are allergic to sulfites, do not
use this medicine until you have carefully read the label or
checked with your doctor or pharmacist to make sure the
medicine does not contain sulfites.* Signs of an allergic reaction to sulfites include bluish coloration of skin; severe
dizziness or feeling faint; continuing flushing or redness of
face or skin; increased wheezing or difficulty in breathing;
skin rash, hives, or itching; or swelling of face, lips, or eyelids.
*If any of these signs occur, check with your doctor imme-
diately*.

Side Effects of This Medicine

In some animal studies, albuterol and terbutaline were shown
to increase the chance of benign (not cancerous) tumors.
Terbutaline was also shown to increase the chance of ovarian
cysts. The doses given were many times the inhalation dose
of albuterol and the oral dose of terbutaline given to humans.
It is not known if albuterol or terbutaline increases the chance
of tumors in humans, or if terbutaline increases the chance
of ovarian cysts in humans.

Along with its needed effects, a medicine may cause some
unwanted effects. Although not all of these side effects may
occur, if they do occur they may need medical attention.

*Check with your doctor immediately if any of the following
side effects occur:*
   Bluish coloration of skin; dizziness (severe) or feeling faint;
      flushing or redness of face or skin (continuing); increased

wheezing or difficulty in breathing; skin rash, hives, or itching; swelling of face, lips, or eyelids

Check with your doctor as soon as possible if any of the following side effects occur:

Rare

Chest discomfort or pain; irregular heartbeat; numbness in hands or feet; unusual bruising

With high doses

Hallucinations (seeing, hearing, or feeling things that are not there)

Symptoms of overdose

Chest discomfort or pain (continuing or severe); chills or fever; convulsions (seizures); dizziness or lightheadedness (continuing or severe); fast or slow heartbeat (continuing); headache (continuing or severe); increase or decrease in blood pressure (severe); irregular or pounding heartbeat (continuing or severe); muscle cramps (severe); nausea or vomiting (continuing or severe); shortness of breath or troubled breathing (severe); trembling (severe); unusual anxiety, nervousness, or restlessness; unusually large pupils or blurred vision; unusual paleness and coldness of skin; weakness (severe)

Other side effects may occur that usually do not need medical attention. These side effects may go away during treatment as your body adjusts to the medicine. However, check with your doctor if any of the following side effects continue or are bothersome:

More common

Nervousness or restlessness; trembling

Less common

Coughing or other bronchial irritation; dizziness or lightheadedness; drowsiness; dryness or irritation of mouth or throat; fast or pounding heartbeat; flushing or redness of face or skin; headache; increased sweating; increase in blood pressure; muscle cramps or twitching; nausea or vomiting; trouble in sleeping; unusual paleness; weakness

Not all of the side effects listed above have been reported for each of these medicines, but they have been reported for at least one of them. All of the adrenergic bronchodilators are similar, so any of the above side effects may occur with any of these medicines.

While you are using albuterol, bitolterol, fenoterol, metaproterenol, or terbutaline, you may notice an unusual or unpleasant taste. Also, pirbuterol may cause changes in smell or taste. These effects may be expected and will go away when you stop using the medicine.

Isoproterenol may cause the saliva to turn pinkish to red. This is to be expected while you are using this medicine.

Other side effects not listed above may also occur in some patients. If you notice any other effects, check with your doctor.

BRONCHODILATORS, ADRENERGIC
Oral/Injection

This information applies to the following medicines:
  Albuterol (al-BYOO-ter-ole)
  Ephedrine (e-FED-rin)
  Epinephrine (ep-i-NEF-rin)
  Ethylnorepinephrine (ETH-il-nor-ep-i-NEF-rin)
  Fenoterol (fen-OH-ter-ole)
  Isoproterenol (eye-soe-proe-TER-e-nole)
  Metaproterenol (met-a-proe-TER-e-nole)
  Terbutaline (ter-BYOO-ta-leen)

Some commonly used brand names are:

For Albuterol
  In the U.S.
      Proventil   Ventolin
      Proventil Repetabs
      Generic name product may also be available.

  In Canada
      Novosalmol   Ventolin
Another commonly used name is salbutamol.

For Ephedrine
  In the U.S.
      Ephed II
      Generic name product may also be available.

In Canada
> Generic name product may be available.

For Epinephrine
In the U.S.
Adrenalin	EpiPen Jr. Auto-Injector
EpiPen Auto-Injector	Sus-Phrine

Generic name product may also be available.

In Canada
Adrenalin	EpiPen Jr. Auto-Injector
EpiPen Auto-Injector	

Generic name product may also be available.

For Ethylnorepinephrine
In the U.S.
> Bronkephrine

Fenoterol*
In Canada
> Berotec

For Isoproterenol
In the U.S.
Isuprel	Isuprel Glossets

Generic name product may also be available.

In Canada
> Isuprel

Generic name product may also be available.

For Metaproterenol
In the U.S.
Alupent	Metaprel

Generic name product may also be available.

In Canada
> Alupent

For Terbutaline
In the U.S.
Brethine	Bricanyl

In Canada
> Bricanyl

---

*Not commercially available in the U.S.

Description

Adrenergic bronchodilators are medicines that open up the bronchial tubes (air passages) of the lungs. They are used to treat the symptoms of bronchial asthma, chronic bronchitis, emphysema, and other lung diseases. They relieve cough, wheezing, shortness of breath, and troubled breathing by increasing the flow of air through the bronchial tubes.

Ephedrine may also be used for the relief of nasal congestion in hay fever or other allergies. Ephedrine injection may be used to treat low blood pressure. In addition, ephedrine may be used in the treatment of narcolepsy (uncontrolled desire for sleep or sudden attacks of sleep) and certain types of mental depression.

Epinephrine injection (not including the auto-injector or the sterile suspension) may also be used in certain heart conditions. In addition, epinephrine injection may be used in eye surgery to stop bleeding, reduce congestion, and dilate the pupil. It may also be applied topically to the skin or mucous membranes to stop bleeding.

Epinephrine injection (including the auto-injector but not the sterile suspension) is used in the emergency treatment of allergic reactions to insect stings, medicines, foods, or other substances. It relieves skin rash, hives, and itching; wheezing; and swelling of the lips, eyelids, tongue, and inside of nose.

Isoproterenol injection and tablets may also be used in the treatment of certain heart disorders.

Adrenergic bronchodilators may be used for other conditions as determined by your doctor.

Ephedrine capsules and syrup are available without a prescription. However, your doctor may have special instructions on the proper dose of ephedrine for your medical condition.

All of the other adrenergic bronchodilators are available only with your doctor's prescription.

These medicines are available in the following dosage forms:
Oral
   Albuterol
   • Oral solution (Canada)
   • Syrup (U.S.)
   • Tablets (U.S. and Canada)
   • Extended-release tablets (U.S.)

Ephedrine
- Capsules (U.S.)
- Syrup (U.S.)

Fenoterol
- Tablets (Canada)

Isoproterenol
- Tablets (U.S. and Canada)

Metaproterenol
- Syrup (U.S. and Canada)
- Tablets (U.S. and Canada)

Terbutaline
- Tablets (U.S. and Canada)

Parenteral

Albuterol
- Injection (Canada)

Ephedrine
- Injection (U.S. and Canada)

Epinephrine
- Injection (U.S. and Canada)

Ethylnorepinephrine
- Injection (U.S.)

Isoproterenol
- Injection (U.S. and Canada)

Terbutaline
- Injection (U.S.)

It is very important that you read and understand the following information. If any of it causes you special concern, check with your doctor. Also, *if you have any questions* or if you want more information about this medicine or your medical problem, *ask your doctor, nurse, or pharmacist.*

Before Using This Medicine

In deciding to use a medicine, the risks of taking the medicine must be weighed against the good it will do. This is a decision you and your doctor will make. For adrenergic bronchodilators taken by mouth or given by injection, the following should be considered:

Allergies—Tell your doctor if you have ever had any unusual or allergic reaction to albuterol, ephedrine, epinephrine, ethylnorepinephrine, fenoterol, isoproterenol, metaproterenol, or terbutaline. Also tell your doctor and pharmacist if you are allergic to any other substances, such as foods, preservatives, or dyes.

Pregnancy—

- *For albuterol*: Albuterol has not been studied in pregnant women. However, studies in animals have shown that albuterol causes birth defects when given in doses many times the usual human dose. In addition, although albuterol has been reported to delay preterm labor when taken by mouth, it has not been shown to stop preterm labor or prevent labor at term.

- *For ephedrine*: Studies on birth defects with ephedrine have not been done in either humans or animals. When ephedrine is used just before or during labor, its effects on the newborn infant or on the growth and development of the child are not known.

- *For epinephrine*: Epinephrine has not been studied in pregnant women. However, studies in animals have shown that epinephrine causes birth defects when given in doses many times the usual human dose. Also, use of epinephrine during pregnancy may decrease the supply of oxygen to the fetus. Epinephrine is not recommended for use during labor since it may delay the second stage of labor. In addition, high doses of epinephrine that decrease contractions of the uterus may result in excessive bleeding when used during labor and delivery.

- *For ethylnorepinephrine and isoproterenol*: Studies on birth defects with ethylnorepinephrine or isoproterenol have not been done in either humans or animals.

- *For fenoterol*: Fenoterol has not been shown to cause birth defects or other problems in humans.

- *For metaproterenol*: Metaproterenol has not been studied in pregnant women. However, studies in animals have shown that metaproterenol causes birth defects when given in doses many times the usual human dose. Also, studies in animals have shown that metaproterenol causes death of the animal fetus when given in doses many times the usual human dose.

- *For terbutaline*: Terbutaline has not been studied in pregnant women. It has not been shown to cause birth defects in animal studies when given in doses many times the usual human dose. However, terbutaline given by injection during pregnancy has been reported to cause an unusually fast heartbeat in the fetus. Although terbutaline is used to delay preterm labor, it may also delay labor at term.

Breast-feeding—

- *For albuterol, fenoterol, isoproterenol, and metaproterenol*: It is not known whether albuterol, fenoterol, isoproterenol, or metaproterenol passes into the breast milk. However, these medicines have not been reported to cause problems in nursing babies.
- *For ephedrine and epinephrine*: Ephedrine and epinephrine pass into the breast milk and may cause unwanted side effects in babies of mothers using ephedrine or epinephrine.
- *For terbutaline*: Although terbutaline passes into the breast milk, it has not been reported to cause problems in nursing babies.

Children—Although there is no specific information about the use of albuterol, ethylnorepinephrine, fenoterol, isoproterenol, metaproterenol, or terbutaline in children, these medicines are not expected to cause different side effects or problems in children than they do in adults.

Infants may be especially sensitive to the effects of ephedrine.

Infants and children may be especially sensitive to the effects of epinephrine. Fainting has occurred after epinephrine was given to children with asthma.

Older adults—Many medicines have not been tested in older people. Therefore, it may not be known whether they work exactly the same way they do in younger adults or if they cause different side effects or problems in older people. There is no specific information about the use of adrenergic bronchodilators in the elderly.

Athletes—Stimulants, including isoproterenol and related substances, are banned and tested for in athletes by the U.S. Olympic Committee (USOC). However, the USOC permits the use of albuterol, bitolterol, metaproterenol, pirbuterol, procaterol, and terbutaline in aerosol or inhalation form.

Other medicines—Although certain medicines should not be used together at all, in other cases two different medicines may be used together even if an interaction might occur. In these cases, your doctor may want to change the dose, or other precautions may be necessary. When you are taking adrenergic bronchodilators, it is especially important that your doctor and pharmacist know if you are taking any of the following:

- Beta-blockers (acebutolol [e.g., Sectral], atenolol [e.g., Tenormin], betaxolol [e.g., Betoptic, Kerlone], carteolol [e.g., Cartrol], labetalol [e.g., Normodyne], levobunolol [e.g., Betagan], metoprolol [e.g., Lopressor], nadolol [e.g., Corgard], oxprenolol [e.g., Trasicor], penbutolol [e.g., Levatol], pindolol [e.g., Visken], propranolol [e.g., Inderal], sotalol [e.g., Sotacor], timolol [e.g., Blocadren, Timoptic])—These medicines may prevent the adrenergic bronchodilators from working properly
- Cocaine or
- Ergoloid mesylates (e.g., Hydergine) or
- Ergotamine (e.g., Gynergen) or
- Maprotiline (e.g., Ludiomil) or
- Tricyclic antidepressants (medicine for depression)—The effects of these medicines on the heart and blood vessels may be increased
- Digitalis glycosides (heart medicine)—The chance of irregular heartbeat may be increased
- Monoamine oxidase (MAO) inhibitors (furazolidone [e.g., Furoxone], isocarboxazid [e.g., Marplan], pargyline [e.g., Eutonyl], phenelzine [e.g., Nardil], procarbazine [e.g., Matulane], tranylcypromine [e.g., Parnate])—Taking adrenergic bronchodilators while you are taking or within 2 weeks of taking monoamine oxidase (MAO) inhibitors may increase the effects of MAO inhibitors

Other medical problems—The presence of other medical problems may affect the use of adrenergic bronchodilators. Make sure you tell your doctor if you have any other medical problems, especially:

- Brain damage
- Convulsions (seizures) (history of)
- Diabetes mellitus (sugar diabetes)—Adrenergic bronchodilators may make the condition worse; your doctor may need to change the dose of your diabetes medicine
- Enlarged prostate—Ephedrine may make the condition worse
- Heart or blood vessel disease or
- High blood pressure—Adrenergic bronchodilators may make the condition worse
- Mental disease—Epinephrine may make the condition worse
- Overactive thyroid—The chance of side effects may be increased
- Parkinson's disease—Epinephrine may temporarily increase certain symptoms of Parkinson's disease, such as rigidity and tremor

Before you begin using any new medicine (prescription or nonprescription) or if you develop any new medical problem while you are using this medicine, check with your doctor, nurse, or pharmacist.

Proper Use of This Medicine

For patients taking *albuterol extended-release tablets:*
- Swallow the tablet whole.
- Do not crush, break, or chew before swallowing.

For patients taking *ephedrine:*
- Ephedrine may cause trouble in sleeping. To help prevent this, *take the last dose of ephedrine for each day a few hours before bedtime.* If you have any questions about this, check with your doctor.

For patients taking *isoproterenol sublingual tablets*:
- Do not chew or swallow the tablet. This medicine is meant to be absorbed through the lining of the mouth. Place the tablet under your tongue (sublingual) and let it slowly dissolve there. Do not swallow until the tablet has dissolved completely.

For patients using the *injection* form of this medicine:
- Do not use the epinephrine solution or suspension if it turns pinkish to brownish in color or if the solution becomes cloudy.

- *Use this medicine only for the conditions for which it was prescribed by your doctor.*
- Keep this medicine ready for use at all times. Also, keep the telephone numbers for your doctor and the nearest hospital emergency room readily available.
- Check the expiration date on the injection regularly. Replace the medicine before that date.
- This medicine is for injection only. If you will be giving yourself the injections, make sure you understand exactly how to give them. If you have any questions about this, check with your doctor.

For patients using *epinephrine injection* for an *allergic reaction emergency*:

- If an allergic reaction as described by your doctor occurs, *use the epinephrine injection immediately*.
- Notify your doctor immediately or go to the nearest hospital emergency room. If you have used the epinephrine injection, be sure to tell your doctor.
- If you have been stung by an insect, remove the insect's stinger with your fingernails, if possible. Be careful not to squeeze, pinch, or push it deeper into the skin. Ice packs or sodium bicarbonate (baking soda) soaks, if available, may then be applied to the area stung.
- If you are using the epinephrine auto-injector (automatic injection device):

  —It is important that you do not remove the safety cap on the auto-injector until you are ready to use it. This prevents accidental activation of the device during storage and handling.

  —Epinephrine auto-injector comes with patient directions. Read them carefully before you actually need to use this medicine. Then, when an emergency arises, you will know how to inject the epinephrine.

  —To use the epinephrine auto-injector:

  - Remove the gray safety cap.
  - Place the black tip on the thigh, at a right angle to the leg.

- Press hard into the thigh until the auto-injector functions. Hold in place for several seconds. Then remove the auto-injector and discard.
- Massage the injection area for 10 seconds.

Use this medicine only as directed. Do not use more of it and do not use it more often than your doctor ordered, or more than recommended on the label unless otherwise directed by your doctor. To do so may increase the chance of side effects.

Missed dose—If you are using this medicine regularly and you miss a dose, use it as soon as possible. Then use any remaining doses for that day at regularly spaced intervals. Do not double doses.

Storage—To store this medicine:
- Keep out of the reach of children.
- Store away from heat and direct light.
- Do not store the capsule or tablet form of this medicine in the bathroom, near the kitchen sink, or in other damp places. Heat or moisture may cause the medicine to break down.
- Keep the injection or syrup form of this medicine from freezing.
- Store the suspension form of epinephrine injection in the refrigerator.
- Do not keep outdated medicine or medicine no longer needed. Be sure that any discarded medicine is out of the reach of children.

Precautions While Using This Medicine

If after using this medicine for asthma or other breathing problems you still have trouble breathing, or if your condition becomes worse, check with your doctor at once.

For *diabetic patients* using *epinephrine*:
- This medicine may cause your blood sugar levels to rise. If you notice a change in the results of your blood or urine sugar tests or if you have any questions, check with your doctor.

For patients using *epinephrine injection* (including the auto-injector but not the sterile suspension) or *ethylnorepinephrine injection*:

- Some of the injection preparations may contain sulfites as a preservative. Sulfites may cause an allergic reaction in some people. If you know that you are allergic to sulfites, carefully read the label on the injection or check with your doctor or pharmacist to find out if the injection contains sulfites.
- Although epinephrine injection may contain sulfites, it is still used to treat serious allergic reactions or other emergency conditions because other medicines may not work properly in a life-threatening situation.
- If you have any questions about when or whether you should use an epinephrine injection that contains sulfites, check with your doctor.
- Signs of an allergic reaction to sulfites include bluish coloration of skin; severe dizziness or feeling faint; continuing flushing or redness of face or skin; increased wheezing or difficulty in breathing; skin rash, hives, or itching; or swelling of face, lips, or eyelids. *If any of these signs occur, check with your doctor immediately.*

Side Effects of This Medicine

In some animal studies, albuterol and terbutaline were shown to increase the chance of benign (not cancerous) tumors. Terbutaline was also shown to increase the chance of ovarian cysts. The doses given were many times the oral dose of albuterol or terbutaline given to humans. It is not known if albuterol or terbutaline increases the chance of tumors in humans, or if terbutaline increases the chance of ovarian cysts in humans.

Along with its needed effects, a medicine may cause some unwanted effects. Although not all of these side effects may occur, if they do occur they may need medical attention.

Check with your doctor immediately if any of the following side effects occur:

Bluish coloration of skin; dizziness (severe) or feeling faint; flushing or redness of face or skin (continuing); increased wheezing or difficulty in breathing; skin rash, hives, or itching; swelling of face, lips, or eyelids

Check with your doctor as soon as possible if any of the following side effects occur:

Rare

Chest discomfort or pain; irregular heartbeat

With high doses

Hallucinations (seeing, hearing, or feeling things that are not there); mood or mental changes (reported for ephedrine only)

Symptoms of overdose

Bluish coloration of skin; chest discomfort or pain (continuing or severe); chills or fever; convulsions (seizures); dizziness or lightheadedness (continuing or severe); fast or slow heartbeat (continuing); headache (continuing or severe); increase or decrease in blood pressure (severe); irregular or pounding heartbeat (continuing or severe); muscle cramps (severe); nausea or vomiting (continuing or severe); shortness of breath or troubled breathing (severe); trembling (severe); unusual anxiety, nervousness, or restlessness; unusually large pupils or blurred vision; unusual paleness and coldness of skin; weakness (severe)

Other side effects may occur that usually do not need medical attention. These side effects may go away during treatment as your body adjusts to the medicine. However, check with your doctor if any of the following side effects continue or are bothersome:

More common

Nervousness or restlessness; trembling

Less common

Difficult or painful urination; dizziness or lightheadedness; drowsiness; fast or pounding heartbeat; flushing or redness of face or skin; headache; heartburn; increased sweating; increase in blood pressure; loss of appetite; muscle cramps or twitching; nausea or vomiting; trouble in sleeping; unusual paleness; weakness

Not all of the side effects listed above have been reported for each of these medicines, but they have been reported for at least one of them. All of the adrenergic bronchodilators are similar, so any of the above side effects may occur with any of these medicines.

While you are using albuterol, fenoterol, metaproterenol, or terbutaline, you may notice an unusual or unpleasant taste. This may be expected and will go away when you stop using the medicine.

Isoproterenol sublingual (under-the-tongue) tablets may cause the saliva to turn pinkish to red. This is to be expected while you are using this medicine.

Other side effects not listed above may also occur in some patients. If you notice any other effects, check with your doctor.

Additional Information

Once a medicine has been approved for marketing for a certain use, experience may show that it is also useful for other medical problems. Although these uses are not included in product labeling, some of the adrenergic bronchodilators are used in certain patients with the following medical conditions:

- Premature labor (terbutaline)
- Urticaria (hives) (ephedrine)
- Hemorrhage (bleeding) of gums and teeth (epinephrine)
- Priapism (prolonged abnormal erection of penis) (epinephrine)

Other than the above information, there is no additional information relating to proper use, precautions, or side effects for these uses.

BRONCHODILATORS, XANTHINE-DERIVATIVE Systemic

This information applies to the following medicines:
Aminophylline (am-in-OFF-i-lin)
Dyphylline (DYE-fi-lin)
Oxtriphylline (ox-TRYE-fi-lin)
Theophylline (thee-OFF-i-lin)

Some commonly used brand names are:

For Aminophylline
In the U.S.

Aminophyllin	Somophyllin-DF
Phyllocontin	Truphylline
Somophyllin	

Generic name product may also be available.

In Canada

Corophyllin	Phyllocontin
Palaron	Phyllocontin-350

Generic name product may also be available.

For Dyphylline
In the U.S.

Dilor	Lufyllin
Dilor-400	Lufyllin-400
Dyflex	Neothylline
Dyflex 400	Thylline

Generic name product may also be available.

In Canada
Protophylline

For Oxtriphylline
In the U.S.

Choledyl	Choledyl SA
Choledyl Delayed-release	

Generic name product may also be available.

In Canada

Apo-Oxtriphylline	Choledyl SA
Choledyl	Novotriphyl

For Theophylline
In the U.S.

Accurbron	Sustaire
Aerolate	Theo-24
Aerolate III	Theo 250
Aerolate Jr.	Theobid Duracaps
Aerolate Sr.	Theobid Jr. Duracaps
Aquaphyllin	Theochron
Asmalix	Theoclear-80
Bronkodyl	Theoclear L.A.-130 Cenules
Constant-T	Theoclear L.A.-260 Cenules
Duraphyl	Theocot
Elixicon	Theo-Dur
Elixomin	Theo-Dur Sprinkle
Elixophyllin	Theolair
Elixophyllin SR	Theolair-SR
Lanophyllin	Theomar
Lixolin	Theon
Quibron-T Dividose	Theophylline SR
Quibron-T/SR Dividose	Theospan-SR
Respbid	Theostat 80
Slo-bid Gyrocaps	Theo-Time
Slo-Phyllin	Theovent Long-Acting
Slo-Phyllin Gyrocaps	T-Phyl
Solu-Phyllin	Truxophyllin
Somophyllin-CRT	Uniphyl
Somophyllin-T	

Generic name product may also be available.

In Canada

Elixophyllin	Somophyllin-T
PMS Theophylline	Theochron
Pulmophylline	Theo-Dur
Quibron-T	Theolair
Quibron-T/SR	Theolair-SR
Slo-Bid	Theo-SR
Somophyllin-12	Uniphyl

For Theophylline Sodium Glycinate
In the U.S.
Synophylate

Description

Xanthine-derivative bronchodilators are used to treat and/
or prevent the symptoms of bronchial asthma, chronic bronchitis, and emphysema. These medicines relieve cough,
wheezing, shortness of breath, and troubled breathing. They
work by opening up the bronchial tubes (air passages of the
lungs) and increasing the flow of air through them.

Aminophylline and theophylline may also be used for other conditions as determined by your doctor.

The oral liquid, uncoated or chewable tablet, capsule, and rectal enema dosage forms of xanthine-derivative bronchodilators may be used for treatment of the acute attack and for chronic (long-term) treatment. If rectal enemas are used, they should not be used for longer than 48 hours because they may cause rectal irritation. The enteric-coated tablet and extended-release dosage forms are usually used only for chronic treatment. Sometimes, aminophylline rectal suppositories may be used but they generally are not recommended because of possible poor absorption.

These medicines are available only with your doctor's prescription, in the following dosage forms:

Oral
Aminophylline
- Oral solution (U.S. and Canada)
- Tablets (U.S. and Canada)
- Enteric-coated tablets (U.S.)
- Extended-release tablets (U.S. and Canada)
Dyphylline
- Elixir (U.S. and Canada)
- Oral solution (Canada)
- Tablets (U.S. and Canada)
Oxtriphylline
- Oral solution (U.S. and Canada)
- Syrup (U.S. and Canada)
- Tablets (U.S. and Canada)
- Delayed-release tablets (U.S.)
- Extended-release tablets (U.S. and Canada)
Theophylline
- Capsules (U.S. and Canada)
- Extended-release capsules (U.S. and Canada)
- Elixir (U.S. and Canada)
- Oral solution (U.S. and Canada)
- Oral suspension (U.S.)
- Syrup (U.S.)
- Tablets (U.S. and Canada)
- Extended-release tablets (U.S. and Canada)
Theophylline Sodium Glycinate
- Elixir (U.S.)

Parenteral
  Aminophylline
   • Injection (U.S. and Canada)
  Aminophylline and Sodium Chloride
   • Injection (U.S.)
  Dyphylline
   • Injection (U.S.)
  Theophylline in Dextrose
   • Injection (U.S. and Canada)

Rectal
  Aminophylline
   • Enema (U.S.)
   • Suppositories (U.S. and Canada)

It is very important that you read and understand the following information. If any of it causes you special concern, check with your doctor. Also, *if you have any questions* or if you want more information about this medicine or your medical problem, *ask your doctor, nurse, or pharmacist.*

Before Using This Medicine

In deciding to use a medicine, the risks of taking the medicine must be weighed against the good it will do. This is a decision you and your doctor will make. For xanthine-derivative bronchodilators, the following should be considered:

Allergies—Tell your doctor if you have ever had any unusual or allergic reaction to aminophylline, caffeine, dyphylline, ethylenediamine (contained in aminophylline), oxtriphylline, theobromine, or theophylline. Also tell your doctor and pharmacist if you are allergic to any other substances, such as foods, preservatives, or dyes.

Diet—Make certain your doctor and pharmacist know if you are on any special diet, such as a low-sodium or low-sugar diet or a high-protein, low-carbohydrate or low-protein, high-carbohydrate diet.

Avoid eating or drinking large amounts of caffeine-containing foods or beverages, such as chocolate, cocoa, tea, coffee, and cola drinks, because they may increase the central nervous system (CNS) stimulant effects of the xanthine-derivative bronchodilators.

Also, eating charcoal broiled foods every day while taking aminophylline, oxtriphylline, or theophylline may keep these medicines from working properly.

Pregnancy—Studies on birth defects have not been done in humans. However, some studies in animals have shown that theophylline (including aminophylline and oxtriphylline) causes birth defects when given in doses many times the human dose. Also, use of aminophylline, oxtriphylline, or theophylline during pregnancy may cause unwanted effects such as fast heartbeat, jitteriness, irritability, gagging, vomiting, and breathing problems in the newborn infant. Studies on birth defects with dyphylline have not been done in either humans or animals.

Breast-feeding—Theophylline passes into the breast milk and may cause irritability, fretfulness, or trouble in sleeping in nursing babies of mothers taking aminophylline, oxtriphylline, or theophylline. Although dyphylline passes into the breast milk, it has not been reported to cause problems in nursing babies.

Children—The side effects of xanthine-derivative bronchodilators are more likely to occur in newborn infants, who are usually more sensitive to the effects of these medicines.

Older adults—The side effects of xanthine-derivative bronchodilators are more likely to occur in elderly patients, who are usually more sensitive than younger adults to the effects of these medicines.

Other medicines—Although certain medicines should not be used together at all, in other cases two different medicines may be used together even if an interaction might occur. In these cases, your doctor may want to change the dose, or other precautions may be necessary. When you are taking xanthine-derivative bronchodilators, it is especially important that your doctor and pharmacist know if you are taking any of the following:

- Adrenocorticoids (cortisone-like medicine)—Use of these medicines with aminophylline and sodium chloride injection may result in too much sodium in the blood

- Beta-blockers (acebutolol [e.g., Sectral], atenolol [e.g., Tenormin], betaxolol [e.g., Kerlone], carteolol [e.g., Cartrol], labetalol [e.g., Normodyne], metoprolol [e.g., Lopressor], nadolol [e.g., Corgard], oxprenolol [e.g., Trasicor], penbutolol [e.g., Levatol], pindolol [e.g., Visken], propranolol [e.g., Inderal], sotalol [e.g., Sotacor], timolol [e.g., Blocadren])—Use of these medicines with xanthine-derivative bronchodilators may prevent either the beta-blocker or the bronchodilator from working properly
- Cimetidine (e.g., Tagamet) or
- Ciprofloxacin or
- Erythromycin (e.g., E-Mycin) or
- Nicotine chewing gum (e.g., Nicorette) or
- Norfloxacin or
- Ranitidine (e.g., Zantac) or
- Troleandomycin (e.g., TAO)—These medicines may increase the effects of aminophylline, oxtriphylline, or theophylline
- Phenytoin (e.g., Dilantin)—The effects of phenytoin may be decreased by aminophylline, oxtriphylline, or theophylline
- Smoking tobacco or marijuana—If you smoke or have smoked tobacco or marijuana regularly within the last 2 years, the amount of medicine you need may vary, depending on how much and how recently you have smoked

Other medical problems—The presence of other medical problems may affect the use of xanthine-derivative bronchodilators. Make sure you tell your doctor if you have any other medical problems, especially:

- Alcohol abuse (or history of) or
- Fever or
- Liver disease or
- Respiratory infections, such as influenza (flu)—The effects of aminophylline, oxtriphylline, or theophylline may be increased
- Diarrhea—The absorption of xanthine-derivative bronchodilators, especially the extended-release dosage forms, may be decreased; therefore, the effects of these medicines may be decreased
- Enlarged prostate or
- Heart disease or
- High blood pressure or
- Stomach ulcer (or history of) or other stomach problems—Xanthine-derivative bronchodilators may make the condition worse

- Fibrocystic breast disease—Symptoms of this disease may be increased by xanthine-derivative bronchodilators
- Irritation or infection of the rectum or lower colon—Aminophylline rectal enema may make the condition worse, since rectal use of this medicine may be irritating
- Kidney disease—The effects of dyphylline may be increased
- Overactive thyroid—The effects of aminophylline, oxtriphylline, or theophylline may be decreased

Before you begin using any new medicine (prescription or nonprescription) or if you develop any new medical problem while you are using this medicine, check with your doctor, nurse, or pharmacist.

Proper Use of This Medicine

For patients *taking this medicine by mouth:*

- If you are taking the *capsule, tablet, liquid, or extended-release (not including the once-a-day capsule or tablet) form* of this medicine, *it works best when taken with a glass of water on an empty stomach* (either 30 minutes to 1 hour before meals or 2 hours after meals). That way the medicine will get into the blood sooner. However, in some cases your doctor may want you to take this medicine with meals or right after meals to lessen stomach upset. If you have any questions about how you should be taking this medicine, check with your doctor.

- If you are taking the *once-a-day capsule or tablet form* of this medicine, *some products are to be taken each morning after fasting overnight and at least 1 hour before eating. However, other products are to be taken in the morning or evening with or without food. Be sure you understand exactly how to take the medicine prescribed for you.* Try to take the medicine about the same time each day.

- There are several different forms of xanthine-derivative bronchodilator capsules and tablets. If you are taking:
  —enteric-coated or delayed-release tablets, swallow the tablets whole. Do not crush, break, or chew before swallowing.

—extended-release capsules, swallow the capsule whole. Do not crush, break, or chew before swallowing.

—extended-release tablets, swallow the tablets whole. Do not break (unless tablet is scored for breaking), crush, or chew before swallowing.

For patients using the *aminophylline enema:*

- This medicine usually comes with patient directions. Read them carefully before using this medicine.
- If crystals form in the solution, dissolve them by placing the closed container of solution in warm water. If the crystals do not dissolve, do not use the medicine.

Use this medicine only as directed by your doctor. Do not use more of it, do not use it more often, and do not use it for a longer time than your doctor ordered. To do so may increase the chance of serious side effects.

In order for this medicine to help your medical problem, it must be taken every day in regularly spaced doses as ordered by your doctor. This is necessary to keep a constant amount of this medicine in the blood. To help keep the amount constant, do not miss any doses.

Missed dose—If you do miss a dose of this medicine, take it as soon as possible. However, if it is almost time for your next dose, skip the missed dose and go back to your regular dosing schedule. Do not double doses.

Storage—To store this medicine:

- Keep out of the reach of children.
- Store away from heat and direct light.
- Do not store the capsule or tablet form of this medicine in the bathroom, near the kitchen sink, or in other damp places. Heat or moisture may cause the medicine to break down.
- Keep the liquid form of this medicine from freezing.
- Do not keep outdated medicine or medicine no longer needed. Be sure that any discarded medicine is out of the reach of children.

Precautions While Using This Medicine

Your doctor should check your progress at regular visits, especially for the first few weeks after you begin using this medicine. A blood test may be taken to help your doctor decide whether the dose of this medicine should be changed.

Do not change brands or dosage forms of this medicine without first checking with your doctor. Different products may not work the same way. If you refill your medicine and it looks different, check with your pharmacist.

This medicine may add to the central nervous system (CNS) stimulant effects of caffeine-containing foods or beverages such as chocolate, cocoa, tea, coffee, and cola drinks. *Avoid eating or drinking large amounts of these foods or beverages while using this medicine.* If you have any questions about this, check with your doctor.

For patients using *aminophylline, oxtriphylline, or theophylline*:

- Do not eat charcoal-broiled foods every day while using this medicine since these foods may keep the medicine from working properly.

- *Check with your doctor at once if you develop symptoms of influenza (flu) or a fever* since either of these may increase the chance of side effects with this medicine.

- Also, *check with your doctor if diarrhea occurs* because the dose of this medicine may need to be changed.

For patients using the *aminophylline enema*:

- If burning or other irritation of the rectal area occurs after you use this medicine and if it continues or becomes worse, check with your doctor.

Side Effects of This Medicine

Along with its needed effects, a medicine may cause some unwanted effects. Although not all of these side effects may occur, if they do occur they may need medical attention.

Check with your doctor as soon as possible if any of the following side effects occur:

Less common

Heartburn and/or vomiting

Rare

Skin rash or hives (with aminophylline only)

Symptoms of overdose

Bloody or black, tarry stools; confusion or change in behavior; convulsions (seizures); diarrhea; dizziness or lightheadedness; fast breathing; fast, pounding, or irregular heartbeat; flushing or redness of face; headache; increased urination; irritability; loss of appetite; muscle twitching; nausea (continuing or severe) or vomiting; stomach cramps or pain; trembling; trouble in sleeping; unusual tiredness or weakness; vomiting blood or material that looks like coffee grounds

Other side effects may occur that usually do not need medical attention. These side effects may go away during treatment as your body adjusts to the medicine. However, check with your doctor if any of the following side effects continue or are bothersome:

More common

Nausea; nervousness or restlessness

Less common

Burning or irritation of rectum (for rectal enema only)

Other side effects not listed above may also occur in some patients. If you notice any other effects, check with your doctor.

Additional Information

Once a medicine has been approved for marketing for a certain use, experience may show that it is also useful for other medical problems. Although this use is not included in product labeling, aminophylline and theophylline are used in certain patients with the following medical condition:

- Apnea (breathing problem) in newborns

Other than the above information, there is no additional information relating to proper use, precautions, or side effects for this use.

BUPROPION Systemic†

A commonly used brand name in the U.S. is Wellbutrin.
Another commonly used name is amfebutamone.

---

†Not commercially available in Canada.

Description

Bupropion (byoo-PROE-pee-on) is an antidepressant or "mood elevator." It works in the central nervous system (CNS) to relieve mental depression.

This medicine is available only with your doctor's prescription, in the following dosage form:

Oral
- Tablets (U.S.)

It is very important that you read and understand the following information. If any of it causes you special concern, check with your doctor. Also, *if you have any questions* or if you want more information about this medicine or your medical problem, *ask your doctor, nurse, or pharmacist.*

Before Using This Medicine

In deciding to use a medicine, the risks of taking the medicine must be weighed against the good it will do. This is a decision you and your doctor will make. For bupropion, the following should be considered:

Allergies—Tell your doctor if you have ever had any unusual or allergic reaction to bupropion. Also tell your doctor and pharmacist if you are allergic to any other substances, such as foods, preservatives, or dyes.

Pregnancy—Studies have not been done in pregnant women. However, bupropion has not been reported to cause birth defects or other problems in animal studies.

Breast-feeding—Bupropion passes into breast milk. Because it may cause unwanted effects in nursing babies, use of bupropion is not recommended during breast-feeding.

Children—Studies on this medicine have been done only in adult patients, and there is no specific information comparing use of bupropion in children with use in other age groups.

Older adults—This medicine has been tested in a limited number of patients 60 years of age and older and has not been shown to cause different side effects or problems in older people than it does in younger adults.

Athletes—Bupropion is banned and, in some cases, tested for in competitors in biathlon and modern pentathlon events by the U.S. Olympic Committee (USOC).

Other medicines—Although certain medicines should not be used together at all, in other cases 2 different medicines may be used together even if an interaction might occur. In these cases, your doctor may want to change the dose, or other precautions may be necessary. When you are taking bupropion, it is especially important that your doctor and pharmacist know if you are taking any of the following:

- Alcohol or
- Antipsychotics (medicine for mental illness) or
- Fluoxetine (e.g., Prozac) or
- Lithium (e.g., Lithane) or
- Maprotiline (e.g., Ludiomil) or
- Trazodone (e.g., Desyrel) or
- Tricyclic antidepressants (amitriptyline [e.g., Elavil], amoxapine [e.g., Asendin], clomipramine [e.g., Anafranil], desipramine [e.g., Pertofrane], doxepin [e.g., Sinequan], imipramine [e.g., Tofranil], nortriptyline [e.g., Aventyl], protriptyline [e.g., Vivactil], trimipramine [e.g., Surmontil])—Using these medicines with bupropion may increase the risk of seizures

- Monoamine oxidase (MAO) inhibitors (furazolidone [e.g., Furoxone], isocarboxazid [e.g., Marplan], phenelzine [e.g., Nardil], procarbazine [e.g., Matulane], selegiline [e.g., Eldepryl], tranylcypromine [e.g., Parnate])—Taking bupropion while you are taking or within 2 weeks of taking monoamine oxidase (MAO) inhibitors may increase the chance of side effects; at least 14 days should be allowed between stopping treatment with one medicine and starting treatment with the other

Other medical problems—The presence of other medical problems may affect the use of bupropion. Make sure you tell your doctor if you have any other medical problems, especially:

- Anorexia nervosa or
- Brain tumor or
- Bulimia or
- Head injury, history of, or
- Seizure disorder—The risk of seizures may be increased when bupropion is taken by patients with these conditions
- Bipolar disorder (manic-depressive illness) or
- Other nervous, mental, or emotional conditions—Bupropion may make the condition worse
- Heart attack (recent) or heart disease—Bupropion may cause unwanted effects on the heart
- Kidney disease or
- Liver disease—Higher blood levels of bupropion may result, increasing the chance of side effects

Proper Use of This Medicine

Use bupropion only as directed by your doctor. Do not use more of it, do not use it more often, and do not use it for a longer time than your doctor ordered. To do so may increase the chance of side effects.

To lessen stomach upset, this medicine may be taken with food, unless your doctor has told you to take it on an empty stomach.

Usually this medicine must be taken for several weeks before you feel better. Your doctor should check your progress at regular visits.

Missed dose—If you miss a dose of this medicine, take it as soon as possible. However, if it is within 4 hours of your next dose, skip the missed dose and go back to your regular dosing schedule. Do not double doses.

Storage—To store this medicine:
- Keep out of the reach of children.
- Store away from heat and direct light.
- Do not store in the bathroom, near the kitchen sink, or in other damp places. Heat or moisture may cause the medicine to break down.
- Do not keep outdated medicine or medicine no longer needed. Be sure that any discarded medicine is out of the reach of children.

Precautions While Using This Medicine

Your doctor should check your progress at regular visits, especially during the first few months of treatment with this medicine. The amount of bupropion you take may have to be changed often to meet the needs of your condition and to help avoid unwanted effects.

If you have been taking this medicine regularly, do not stop taking it without first checking with your doctor. Your doctor may want you to reduce gradually the amount you are taking before stopping completely. This will help reduce the possibility of side effects.

Drinking of alcoholic beverages should be limited or avoided, if possible, while taking bupropion. This will help prevent unwanted effects.

This medicine may cause some people to feel a false sense of well-being, or to become drowsy, dizzy, or less alert than they are normally. *Make sure you know how you react to this medicine before you drive, use machines, or do anything else that could be dangerous if you are dizzy or are not alert and clearheaded.*

Side Effects of This Medicine

Along with its needed effects, a medicine may cause some unwanted effects. Although not all of these side effects may occur, if they do occur they may need medical attention.

Check with your doctor as soon as possible if any of the following side effects occur:

More common

Agitation or excitement; anxiety; confusion; fast or irregular heartbeat; headache (severe); restlessness; trouble in sleeping

Less common

Hallucinations; skin rash

Rare

Fainting; convulsions (seizures), especially with higher doses

Other side effects may occur that usually do not need medical attention. These side effects may go away during treatment as your body adjusts to the medicine. However, check with your doctor if any of the following side effects continue or are bothersome:

More common

Constipation; decrease in appetite; dizziness; dryness of mouth; increased sweating; nausea or vomiting; tremor; weight loss (unusual)

Less common

Blurred vision; difficulty concentrating; drowsiness; fever or chills; hostility or anger; tiredness; unusual feeling of well-being

Other side effects not listed above may also occur in some patients. If you notice any other effects, check with your doctor.

BUSPIRONE   Systemic

A commonly used brand name in the U.S. and Canada is BuSpar.

Description

Buspirone (byoo-SPYE-rone) is used to treat certain anxiety disorders or to relieve the symptoms of anxiety. However, buspirone is usually not used for anxiety or tension caused by the stress of everyday life.

It is not known exactly how buspirone works to relieve the symptoms of anxiety.

Buspirone is available only with your doctor's prescription, in the following dosage form:

  Oral
    • Tablets (U.S. and Canada)

It is very important that you read and understand the following information. If any of it causes you special concern, check with your doctor. Also, *if you have any questions* or if you want more information about this medicine or your medical problem, *ask your doctor, nurse, or pharmacist.*

Before Using This Medicine

In deciding to use a medicine, the risks of taking the medicine must be weighed against the good it will do. This is a decision you and your doctor will make. For buspirone, the following should be considered:

Allergies—Tell your doctor if you have ever had any unusual or allergic reaction to buspirone. Also tell your doctor and pharmacist if you are allergic to any other substances, such as foods, preservatives, or dyes.

Pregnancy—Buspirone has not been studied in pregnant women. However, buspirone has not been shown to cause birth defects or other problems in animal studies.

Breast-feeding—It is not known whether buspirone passes into the breast milk of humans. However, this medicine has not been reported to cause problems in nursing babies.

Children—There is no specific information about the use of buspirone in children up to 18 years of age.

Older adults—This medicine has been tested and has not been shown to cause different side effects or problems in older people than it does in younger adults.

Athletes—Buspirone is banned and, in some cases, tested for in competitors in certain events by the U.S. Olympic Committee (USOC) and the National Collegiate Athletic Association (NCAA).

Other medicines—Although certain medicines should not be used together at all, in other cases 2 different medicines may be used together even if an interaction might occur. In these cases, your doctor may want to change the dose, or other precautions may be necessary. When taking buspirone it is especially important that your doctor and pharmacist know if you are taking any of the following:

- Monoamine oxidase (MAO) inhibitors (furazolidone [e.g., Furoxone], isocarboxazid [e.g., Marplan], pargyline [e.g., Eutonyl], phenelzine [e.g., Nardil], procarbazine [e.g., Matulane], tranylcypromine [e.g., Parnate])—Taking buspirone while you are taking or within 2 weeks of taking monoamine oxidase (MAO) inhibitors may cause high blood pressure

Other medical problems—The presence of other medical problems may affect the use of buspirone. Make sure you tell your doctor if you have any other medical problems, especially:

- Drug abuse or dependence (history of)—There is a possibility that buspirone could become habit-forming, causing mental or physical dependence
- Kidney disease or
- Liver disease—The effects of buspirone may be increased, which may increase the chance of side effects

Before you begin using any new medicine (prescription or nonprescription) or if you develop any new medical problem while you are using this medicine, check with your doctor, nurse, or pharmacist.

Proper Use of This Medicine

Take buspirone only as directed by your doctor. Do not take more of it, do not take it more often, and do not take it for a longer time than your doctor ordered. To do so may increase the chance of unwanted effects.

After you begin taking buspirone, 1 to 2 weeks may pass before you feel the full effects of this medicine.

Missed dose—If you are taking this medicine regularly and you miss a dose, take it as soon as possible. However, if it is almost time for your next dose, skip the missed dose and go back to your regular dosing schedule. Do not double doses.

Storage—To store this medicine:
- Keep out of the reach of children.
- Store away from heat and direct light.
- Do not store in the bathroom, near the kitchen sink, or in other damp places. Heat or moisture may cause the medicine to break down.
- Do not keep outdated medicine or medicine no longer needed. Be sure that any discarded medicine is out of the reach of children.

Precautions While Using This Medicine

If you will be using buspirone regularly for a long time, your doctor should check your progress at regular visits to make ysure the medicine does not cause unwanted effects.

Buspirone when taken with alcohol or other CNS depressants (medicines that slow down the nervous system, possibly causing drowsiness) may increase the chance of drowsiness. Some examples of CNS depressants are antihistamines or medicine for hay fever, other allergies, or colds; sedatives, tranquilizers, or sleeping medicine; prescription pain medicine or narcotics; barbiturates; medicine for seizures; muscle relaxants; or anesthetics, including some dental anesthetics. Check with your doctor before taking any of the above while you are taking this medicine.

Buspirone may cause some people to become dizzy, light-headed, drowsy, or less alert than they are normally. *Make sure you know how you react to this medicine before you drive, use machines, or do anything else that could be dangerous if you are dizzy or are not alert.*

If you think you or someone else may have taken an overdose of buspirone, get emergency help at once. Some symptoms of an overdose are severe dizziness or drowsiness; severe stomach upset, including nausea or vomiting; or unusually small pupils.

Side Effects of This Medicine

Along with its needed effects, a medicine may cause some unwanted effects. Although not all of these side effects may occur, if they do occur they may need medical attention.

Check with your doctor as soon as possible if any of the following side effects occur:

Rare

>Chest pain; confusion or mental depression; fast or pounding heartbeat; muscle weakness; numbness, tingling, pain, or weakness in hands or feet; sore throat or fever; uncontrolled movements of the body

Symptoms of overdose

>Dizziness (severe); drowsiness (severe); stomach upset, including nausea or vomiting (severe); unusually small pupils

Other side effects may occur that usually do not need medical attention. These side effects may go away during treatment as your body adjusts to the medicine. However, check with your doctor if any of the following side effects continue or are bothersome:

More common

>Dizziness or lightheadedness; headache; nausea; restlessness, nervousness, or unusual excitement

Less common or rare

>Blurred vision; decreased concentration; drowsiness (more common with doses of more than 20 mg per day); dryness of mouth; muscle pain, spasms, cramps, or stiffness; ring-

ing in the ears; stomach upset; trouble in sleeping, nightmares, or vivid dreams; unusual tiredness or weakness

Other side effects not listed above may also occur in some
patients. If you notice any other effects, check with your
doctor.

BUTALBITAL AND ASPIRIN   Systemic

Some commonly used brand names are:

For Butalbital and Aspirin†
In the U.S.
　　Axotal

For Butalbital, Aspirin‡, and Caffeine
In the U.S.

Butalgen	Isolin
Fiorgen	Isollyl
Fiorinal	Laniroif
Fiormor	Lanorinal
Fortabs	Marnal
Isobutal	Vibutal
Isobutyl	

　　Generic name product may also be available.

In Canada
　　Fiorinal   Tecnal

Other commonly used names for this combination medicine are butalbital-
　　AC and butalbital compound.

---

†Not commercially available in Canada.

‡In Canada, *Aspirin* is a brand name. Acetylsalicylic acid is the generic
name in Canada. ASA, a synonym for acetylsalicylic acid, is the term that
commonly appears on Canadian product labels.

Description

Butalbital (byoo-TAL-bi-tal) and aspirin (AS-pir-in) combination is a pain reliever and relaxant. It is used to treat
tension headaches. Butalbital belongs to the group of medicines called barbiturates (bar-BI-tyoo-rates). Barbiturates
act in the central nervous system (CNS) to produce their
effects.

When you use butalbital for a long time, your body may get used to it so that larger amounts are needed to produce the same effects. This is called tolerance to the medicine. Also, butalbital may become habit-forming (causing mental or physical dependence) when it is used for a long time or in large doses. Physical dependence may lead to withdrawal side effects when you stop taking the medicine. In patients who get headaches, the first symptom of withdrawal may be new (rebound) headaches.

Some of these medicines also contain caffeine (kaf-EEN). Caffeine may help to relieve headaches. However, caffeine can also cause physical dependence when it is used for a long time. This may lead to withdrawal (rebound) headaches when you stop taking it.

Butalbital and aspirin combination is sometimes also used for other kinds of headaches or other kinds of pain, as determined by your doctor.

Butalbital and aspirin combination is available only with your doctor's prescription, in the following dosage forms:

Oral

Butalbital and Aspirin
- Tablets (U.S.)
Butalbital, Aspirin, and Caffeine
- Capsules (U.S. and Canada)
- Tablets (U.S. and Canada)

It is very important that you read and understand the following information. If any of it causes you special concern, check with your doctor. Also, *if you have any questions* or if you want more information about this medicine or your medical problem, *ask your doctor, nurse, or pharmacist.*

Before Using This Medicine

In deciding to use a medicine, the risks of taking the medicine must be weighed against the good it will do. This is a decision you and your doctor will make. For butalbital and aspirin combinations, the following should be considered:

Allergies—Tell your doctor if you have ever had any unusual or allergic reaction to butalbital or other barbiturates; aspirin or other salicylates, including methyl salicylate (oil of wintergreen); caffeine; or any of the following medicines:

Diclofenac (e.g., Voltaren)
Diflunisal (e.g., Dolobid)
Etodolac (e.g., Lodine)
Fenoprofen (e.g., Nalfon)
Floctafenine (e.g., Idarac)
Flurbiprofen, oral (e.g., Ansaid)
Ibuprofen (e.g., Motrin)
Indomethacin (e.g., Indocin)
Ketoprofen (e.g., Orudis)
Ketorolac (e.g., Toradol)
Meclofenamate (e.g., Meclomen)
Mefenamic acid (e.g., Ponstel)
Nabumetone (e.g., Relafen)
Naproxen (e.g., Naprosyn)
Oxyphenbutazone (e.g., Tandearil)
Phenylbutazone (e.g., Butazolidin)
Piroxicam (e.g., Feldene)
Sulindac (e.g., Clinoril)
Suprofen (e.g., Suprol)
Tenoxicam (e.g., Mobiflex)
Tiaprofenic acid (e.g., Surgam)
Tolmetin (e.g., Tolectin)
Zomepirac (e.g., Zomax)

Also tell your doctor and pharmacist if you are allergic to any other substances, such as foods, preservatives, or dyes.

Pregnancy—

- *For butalbital:* Barbiturates such as butalbital have been shown to increase the chance of birth defects in humans. Also, one study in humans has suggested that barbiturates taken during pregnancy may increase the chance of brain tumors in the baby. Butalbital may cause breathing problems in the newborn baby if taken just before or during delivery.

- *For aspirin:* Although studies in humans have not shown that aspirin causes birth defects, it has caused birth defects in animal studies.

  Do not take aspirin during the last 3 months of pregnancy unless it has been ordered by your doctor. Some reports have suggested that use of aspirin late in pregnancy may cause a decrease in the newborn's weight and possible death of the fetus or newborn baby. However, the mothers in these reports had been taking much larger amounts of aspirin than are usually recommended. Studies of mothers taking aspirin in the doses that are usually recommended did not show these unwanted effects.

There is a chance that regular use of aspirin late in pregnancy may cause unwanted effects on the heart or blood flow in the fetus or in the newborn baby. Also, use of aspirin during the last 2 weeks of pregnancy may cause bleeding problems in the fetus before or during delivery or in the newborn baby. In addition, too much use of aspirin during the last 3 months of pregnancy may increase the length of pregnancy, prolong labor, cause other problems during delivery, or cause severe bleeding in the mother before, during, or after delivery.

- *For caffeine:* Studies in humans have not shown that caffeine causes birth defects. However, use of large amounts of caffeine during pregnancy may cause problems with the heart rhythm and the growth of the fetus. Also, studies in animals have shown that caffeine causes birth defects when given in very large doses (amounts equal to the amount in 12 to 24 cups of coffee a day).

Breast-feeding—Although this combination medicine has not been reported to cause problems, the chance always exists, especially if the medicine is taken for a long time or in large amounts.

- *For butalbital:* Barbiturates such as butalbital pass into the breast milk and may cause drowsiness, unusually slow heartbeat, shortness of breath, or troubled breathing in nursing babies.

- *For aspirin:* Aspirin passes into the breast milk. However, taking aspirin in the amounts present in these combination medicines has not been reported to cause problems in nursing babies.

- *For caffeine:* The caffeine in some of these combination medicines passes into the breast milk in small amounts. Taking caffeine in the amounts present in these medicines has not been reported to cause problems in nursing babies. However, studies have shown that nursing babies may appear jittery and have trouble in sleeping when their mothers drink large amounts of caffeine-containing beverages. Therefore, breast-feeding mothers who use caffeine-containing medicines should probably limit the amount of caffeine they take in from other medicines or from beverages.

Children—

- *For butalbital:* Although barbiturates such as butalbital often cause drowsiness, some children become excited after taking them.

- *For aspirin: Do not give a medicine containing aspirin to a child with fever or other symptoms of a virus infection, especially flu or chickenpox, without first discussing its use with your child's doctor.* This is very important because aspirin may cause a serious illness called Reye's syndrome in children with fever caused by a virus infection, especially flu or chickenpox. Children who do not have a virus infection may also be more sensitive to the effects of aspirin, especially if they have a fever or have lost large amounts of body fluid because of vomiting, diarrhea, or sweating. This may increase the chance of side effects during treatment.

- *For caffeine:* There is no specific information comparing use of caffeine in children up to 12 years of age with use in other age groups. However, caffeine is not expected to cause different side effects or problems in children than it does in adults.

Teenagers—*Teenagers with fever or other symptoms of a virus infection, especially flu or chickenpox, should check with a doctor before taking this medicine.* The aspirin in this combination medicine may cause a serious illness called Reye's syndrome in teenagers with fever caused by a virus infection, especially flu or chickenpox.

Older adults—

- *For butalbital:* Confusion, depression, or excitement may be especially likely to occur in elderly patients, who are usually more sensitive than younger adults to the effects of butalbital.

- *For aspirin:* Elderly patients are more sensitive than younger adults to the effects of aspirin. This may increase the chance of side effects during treatment.

- *For caffeine:* Many medicines have not been studied specifically in older people. Therefore, it may not be known whether they work exactly the same way they do in younger adults or if they cause different side effects or problems in older people. There is no specific information comparing use of caffeine in the elderly with use in other age groups.

Athletes—

- *For butalbital:* Butalbital is banned by the U.S. Olympic Committee (USOC) for use in competitors in biathlon and modern pentathlon events. Butalbital use can lead to disqualification of competitors in these events.

- *For caffeine:* Caffeine (present in some butalbital and aspirin combinations) is tested for by the International Olympic Committee (IOC), the USOC, and the National Collegiate Athletic Association (NCAA). These groups have set limits on the amount of caffeine in the urine they consider to be acceptable. An athlete will be disqualified for competition if the amount of caffeine in the urine is above these limits.

Other medicines—Although certain medicines should not be used together at all, in other cases two different medicines may be used together even if an interaction might occur. In these cases, your doctor may want to change the dose, or other precautions may be necessary. When you are taking a butalbital and aspirin combination, it is especially important that your doctor and pharmacist know if you are taking any of the following:

- Adrenocorticoids (cortisone-like medicines) or
- Carbamazepine (e.g., Tegretol) or
- Contraceptives, oral (birth control pills), containing estrogen or
- Corticotropin (e.g., ACTH)—Butalbital may make these medicines less effective

- Antacids, large amounts taken regularly, especially calcium-
  and/or magnesium-containing antacids or sodium bicarbonate (baking soda), or
- Urinary alkalizers (medicine that makes the urine less acid,
  such as acetazolamide [e.g., Diamox], dichlorphenamide [e.g.,
  Daranide], methazolamide [e.g., Neptazane], potassium or
  sodium citrate and/or citric acid)—These medicines may
  cause aspirin to be removed from the body faster than usual,
  which may shorten the time that aspirin is effective; acetazolamide, dichlorphenamide, and methazolamide may also
  increase the chance of side effects when taken together with
  aspirin
- Anticoagulants (blood thinners) or
- Heparin—Use of these medicines together with aspirin may
  increase the chance of bleeding; also, butalbital may cause
  anticoagulants to be less effective
- Antidepressants, tricyclic (amitriptyline [e.g., Elavil], amoxapine [e.g., Asendin], clomipramine [e.g., Anafranil], desipramine [e.g., Pertofrane], doxepin [e.g., Sinequan], imipramine [e.g., Tofranil], nortriptyline [e.g., Aventyl],
  protriptyline [e.g., Vivactil], trimipramine [e.g., Surmontil])
  or
- Central nervous system (CNS) depressants (medicines that
  often cause drowsiness)—These medicines may add to the
  effects of butalbital and increase the chance of drowsiness
  or other side effects
- Divalproex (e.g., Depakote) or
- Methotrexate (e.g., Folex, Mexate) or
- Valproic acid (e.g., Depakene) or
- Vancomycin (e.g., Vancocin)—The chance of serious side effects may be increased
- Probenecid (e.g., Benemid) or
- Sulfinpyrazone (e.g., Anturane)—Aspirin can keep these med-
  icines from working properly for treating gout

Other medical problems—The presence of other medical
problems may affect the use of butalbital and aspirin combinations. Make sure you tell your doctor if you have any
other medical problems, especially:

- Alcohol abuse (or history of) or
- Drug abuse or dependence (or history of)—Dependence on
  butalbital may develop

- Asthma, especially if occurring together with other allergies and nasal polyps (or history of), or
- Emphysema or other chronic lung disease or
- Hyperactivity (in children) or
- Kidney disease or
- Liver disease—The chance of serious side effects may be increased
- Diabetes mellitus (sugar diabetes) or
- Mental depression or
- Overactive thyroid or
- Porphyria (or history of)—Butalbital may make these conditions worse
- Gout—Aspirin can make this condition worse and can also lessen the effects of some medicines used to treat gout
- Heart disease (severe)—The caffeine in some of these combination medicines can make some kinds of heart disease worse
- Hemophilia or other bleeding problems or
- Vitamin K deficiency—Aspirin increases the chance of serious bleeding
- Stomach ulcer, especially with a history of bleeding, or other stomach problems—Aspirin can make your condition worse

Before you begin using any new medicine (prescription or nonprescription) or if you develop any new medical problem while you are using this medicine, check with your doctor, nurse, or pharmacist.

Proper Use of This Medicine

Take this medicine with food or a full glass (8 ounces) of water to lessen stomach irritation.

Do not take this medicine if it has a strong vinegar-like odor. This odor means the aspirin in it is breaking down. If you have any questions about this, check with your doctor or pharmacist.

Take this medicine only as directed by your doctor. Do not take more of it, do not take it more often, and do not take it for a longer time than your doctor ordered. If butalbital and aspirin combination is taken regularly (for example, every day), it may become habit-forming (causing mental or physical dependence). The caffeine in some butalbital and aspirin combinations can also increase the chance of dependence. Dependence is especially likely to occur in patients who take this medicine to relieve frequent headaches. Taking too much of this combination medicine can also lead to stomach problems or to other medical problems.

This medicine will relieve a headache best if you *take it as soon as the headache begins*. If you get warning signs of a migraine, take this medicine as soon as you are sure that the migraine is coming. This may even stop the headache pain from occurring. *Lying down in a quiet, dark room for a while after taking the medicine also helps to relieve headaches.*

People who get a lot of headaches may need to take a different medicine to help prevent headaches. *It is important that you follow your doctor's directions about taking the other medicine, even if your headaches continue to occur.* Headache-preventing medicines may take several weeks to start working. Even after they do start working, your headaches may not go away completely. However, your headaches should occur less often, and they should be less severe and easier to relieve than before. This will reduce the amount of headache relievers that you need. If you do not notice any improvement after several weeks of headache-preventing treatment, check with your doctor.

Missed dose—If your doctor has ordered you to take this medicine according to a regular schedule and you miss a dose, take it as soon as you remember. However, if it is almost time for your next dose, skip the missed dose and go back to your regular dosing schedule. Do not double doses.

Storage—To store this medicine:
- Keep out of the reach of children. Overdose is especially dangerous in young children.
- Store away from heat and direct light.
- Do not store this medicine in the bathroom, near the kitchen sink, or in other damp places. Heat or moisture may cause the medicine to break down.

- Do not keep outdated medicine or medicine no longer needed. Be sure that any discarded medicine is out of the reach of children.

Precautions While Using This Medicine

Check with your doctor:

- If the medicine stops working as well as it did when you first started using it. This may mean that you are in danger of becoming dependent on the medicine. *Do not try to get better pain relief by increasing the dose.*

- *If you are having headaches more often than you did before you started using this medicine.* This is especially important if a new headache occurs within 1 day after you took your last dose of headache medicine, headaches begin to occur every day, or a headache continues for several days in a row. This may mean that you are dependent on the headache medicine. *Continuing to take this medicine will cause even more headaches later on.* Your doctor can give you advice on how to relieve the headaches.

Check the labels of all nonprescription (over-the-counter [OTC]) and prescription medicines you now take. If any contain a barbiturate, aspirin, or other salicylates, including diflunisal, be especially careful, since taking them while taking this medicine may lead to overdose. If you have any questions about this, check with your doctor or pharmacist.

The butalbital in this medicine will add to the effects of alcohol and other CNS depressants (medicines that slow down the nervous system, possibly causing drowsiness). Some examples of CNS depressants are antihistamines or medicine for hay fever, other allergies, or colds; sedatives, tranquilizers, or sleeping medicine; other prescription pain medicine or narcotics; other barbiturates; medicine for seizures; muscle relaxants; or anesthetics, including some dental anesthetics. Also, stomach problems may be more likely to occur if you drink alcoholic beverages while you are taking aspirin. Therefore, *do not drink alcoholic beverages, and check with your doctor before taking any of the medicines listed above, while you are using this medicine.*

This medicine may cause some people to become drowsy, dizzy, or lightheaded. *Make sure you know how you react to this medicine before you drive, use machines, or do anything else that could be dangerous if you are dizzy or are not alert and clearheaded.*

Before having any kind of surgery (including dental surgery) or emergency treatment, tell the medical doctor or dentist in charge that you are taking this medicine. Serious side effects may occur if your medical doctor or dentist gives you certain other medicines without knowing that you have taken butalbital.

Do not take this medicine for 5 days before any planned surgery, including dental surgery, unless otherwise directed by your medical doctor or dentist. Taking aspirin during this time may cause bleeding problems.

Before you have any medical tests, tell the person in charge that you are taking this medicine. Caffeine (present in some butalbital and aspirin combinations) interferes with the results of certain tests that use dipyridamole (e.g., Persantine) to help show how well blood is flowing to your heart. Caffeine should not be taken for 8 to 12 hours before the test. The results of some other tests may also be affected by butalbital and aspirin combinations.

If you have been taking large amounts of this medicine, or if you have been taking it regularly for several weeks or more, *do not suddenly stop using it without first checking with your doctor*. Your doctor may want you to reduce gradually the amount you are taking before stopping completely, to lessen the chance of withdrawal side effects.

If you think you or anyone else may have taken an overdose of this medicine, get emergency help at once. Taking an overdose of this medicine or taking alcohol or CNS depressants with this medicine may lead to unconsciousness or death. Symptoms of overdose of this medicine include convulsions (seizures); hearing loss; confusion; ringing or buzzing in the ears; severe excitement, nervousness, or restlessness; severe dizziness; severe drowsiness; shortness of breath or troubled breathing; and severe weakness.

Side Effects of This Medicine

Along with its needed effects, a medicine may cause some unwanted effects. Although not all of these side effects may occur, if they do occur they may need medical attention.

The following side effects may mean that a serious allergic reaction is occurring. Check with your doctor or get emergency help immediately if they occur, especially if several of them occur at the same time.

Less common or rare

Bluish discoloration or flushing or redness of skin (occurring together with other effects listed in this section); coughing, shortness of breath, troubled breathing, tightness in chest, or wheezing; difficulty in swallowing; dizziness or feeling faint (severe); hive-like swellings (large) on eyelids, face, lips, or tongue; skin rash, itching, or hives; stuffy nose (occurring together with other effects listed in this section)

Also check with your doctor immediately if any of the following side effects occur, especially if several of them occur together:

Rare

Bleeding or crusting sores on lips; chest pain; fever with or without chills; red, thickened, or scaly skin; sores, ulcers, or white spots in mouth (painful); sore throat (unexplained); tenderness, burning, or peeling of skin

Symptoms of overdose

Anxiety, confusion, excitement, irritability, nervousness, restlessness, or trouble in sleeping (severe, especially with products containing caffeine); convulsions (seizures, with products containing caffeine); diarrhea (severe or continuing); dizziness, lightheadedness, drowsiness, or weakness (severe); frequent urination (for products containing caffeine); hallucinations (seeing, hearing, or feeling things that are not there); increased sensitivity to touch or pain (for products containing caffeine); increased thirst; muscle trembling or twitching (for products containing caffeine); nausea or vomiting (severe or continuing), sometimes with blood; ringing or buzzing in ears (continuing) or hearing loss; seeing flashes of "zig-zag" lights (for products containing caffeine); slow, fast, or irregular heartbeat; slow, fast, irregular, or troubled breathing;

slurred speech; staggering; stomach pain (severe); uncontrollable flapping movements of the hands, especially in elderly patients; unusual movements of the eyes; vision problems

Also, check with your doctor as soon as possible if any of the following side effects occur:

Less common or rare
Bloody or black, tarry stools; bloody urine; confusion or mental depression; muscle cramps or pain; pinpoint red spots on skin; swollen or painful glands; unusual bleeding or bruising; unusual excitement (mild)

Other side effects may occur that usually do not need medical attention. These side effects may go away during treatment as your body adjusts to the medicine. However, check with your doctor if any of the following side effects continue or are bothersome:

More common
Bloated or "gassy" feeling; dizziness or lightheadedness (mild); drowsiness (mild); heartburn or indigestion; nausea, vomiting, or stomach pain (occurring without other symptoms of overdose)

Other side effects not listed above may also occur in some patients. If you notice any other effects, check with your doctor.

CALCIUM CHANNEL BLOCKING AGENTS   Systemic

This information applies to the following medicines:

Bepridil (BE-pri-dil)
Diltiazem (dil-TYE-a-zem)
Felodipine (fe-LOE-di-peen)
Flunarizine (floo-NAR-i-zeen)
Isradipine (is-RA-di-peen)
Nicardipine (nye-KAR-de-peen)
Nifedipine (nye-FED-i-peen)
Nimodipine (nye-MOE-di-peen)
Verapamil (ver-AP-a-mil)

Some commonly used brand names are:

For Bepridil†
In the U.S.
Bepadin
Vascor

For Diltiazem
In the U.S.
Cardizem   Cardizem SR
Cardizem CD

In Canada
Apo-Diltiaz   Novo-Diltazem
Cardizem   Nu-Diltiaz
Cardizem SR   Syn-Diltiazem

Generic name product may also be available.

For Felodipine
In the U.S.
Plendil

In Canada
Plendil
Renedil

For Flunarizine*
In Canada
Sibelium

For Isradipine†
In the U.S.
DynaCirc

For Nicardipine
In the U.S.
Cardene
In Canada
Cardene

For Nifedipine
In the U.S.
Adalat   Procardia XL
Procardia

Generic name product may also be available.

In Canada
Adalat   Apo-Nifed
Adalat FT   Novo-Nifedin
Adalat P.A.   Nu-Nifed

For Nimodipine
In the U.S.
Nimotop
In Canada
Nimotop

For Verapamil
  In the U.S.
    Calan   Isoptin SR
    Calan SR   Verelan
    Isoptin

    Generic name product may also be available.

  In Canada
    Apo-Verap   Novo-Veramil
    Isoptin   Nu-Verap
    Isoptin SR

    Generic name product may also be available.

---

*Not commercially available in the U.S.
†Not commercially available in Canada.

Description

Bepridil, diltiazem, felodipine, flunarizine, isradipine, nicardipine, nifedipine, nimodipine, and verapamil belong to the group of medicines called calcium channel blockers.

Calcium channel blocking agents affect the movement of calcium into the cells of the heart and blood vessels. As a result, they relax blood vessels and increase the supply of blood and oxygen to the heart while reducing its workload.

Some of the calcium channel blocking agents are used to relieve and control angina pectoris (chest pain).

Some are also used to treat high blood pressure (hypertension). High blood pressure adds to the workload of the heart and arteries. If it continues for a long time, the heart and arteries may not function properly. This can damage the blood vessels of the brain, heart, and kidneys, resulting in a stroke, heart failure, or kidney failure. High blood pressure may also increase the risk of heart attacks. These problems may be less likely to occur if blood pressure is controlled.

Flunarizine is used to prevent migraine headaches.

Nimodipine is used to prevent and treat problems caused by a burst blood vessel in the head (also known as a ruptured aneurysm or subarachnoid hemorrhage).

Other calcium channel blocking agents may also be used for these and other conditions as determined by your doctor.

These medicines are available only with your doctor's prescription, in the following dosage forms:

Oral

Bepridil
  • Tablets (U.S.)
Diltiazem
  • Extended-release capsules (U.S. and Canada)
  • Tablets (U.S. and Canada)
Felodipine
  • Extended-release tablets (U.S. and Canada)
Flunarizine
  • Capsules (Canada)
Isradipine
  • Capsules (U.S.)
Nicardipine
  • Capsules (U.S. and Canada)
Nifedipine
  • Capsules (U.S. and Canada)
  • Tablets (Canada)
  • Extended-release tablets (U.S. and Canada)
Nimodipine
  • Capsules (U.S. and Canada)
Verapamil
  • Extended-release capsules (U.S.)
  • Tablets (U.S. and Canada)
  • Extended-release tablets (U.S. and Canada)

Parenteral

Diltiazem
  • Injection (U.S.)
Verapamil
  • Injection (U.S. and Canada)

It is very important that you read and understand the following information. If any of it causes you special concern, check with your doctor. Also, *if you have any questions* or if you want more information about this medicine or your medical problem, *ask your doctor, nurse, or pharmacist.*

Before Using This Medicine

In deciding to use a medicine, the risks of taking the medicine must be weighed against the good it will do. This is a decision you and your doctor will make. For the calcium channel blocking agents, the following should be considered:

Allergies—Tell your doctor if you have ever had any unusual or allergic reaction to bepridil, diltiazem, felodipine, flunarizine, isradipine, nicardipine, nifedipine, nimodipine, or verapamil. Also tell your doctor and pharmacist if you are allergic to any other substances, such as foods, preservatives, or dyes.

Pregnancy—Calcium channel blockers have not been studied in pregnant women. However, studies in animals have shown that large doses of calcium channel blockers cause birth defects, prolonged pregnancy, poor bone development, and stillbirth.

Breast-feeding—Although bepridil, diltiazem, nifedipine, verapamil, and possibly other calcium channel blockers, pass into breast milk, they have not been reported to cause problems in nursing babies.

Children—Although there is no specific information comparing use of this medicine in children with use in other age groups, it is not expected to cause different side effects or problems in children than it does in adults.

Older adults—Elderly people may be especially sensitive to the effects of calcium channel blockers. This may increase the chance of side effects during treatment.

Other medicines—Although certain medicines should not be used together at all, in other cases two different medicines may be used together even if an interaction might occur. In these cases, your doctor may want to change the dose, or other precautions may be necessary. When taking calcium channel blockers it is especially important that your doctor and pharmacist know if you are taking any of the following:

- Amphotericin B by injection (e.g., Fungizone) or
- Acetazolamide (e.g., Diamox) or
- Corticosteroids (cortisone-like medicine) or

- Dichlorphenamide (e.g., Daranide) or
- Diuretics (water pills) or
- Methazolamide (e.g., Naptazane)—These medicines can cause hypokalemia (low levels of potassium in the body), which can increase the unwanted effects of bepridil
- Beta-blockers (acebutolol [e.g., Sectral], atenolol [e.g., Tenormin], betaxolol [e.g., Kerlone], carteolol [e.g., Cartrol], labetalol [e.g., Normodyne], metoprolol [e.g., Lopressor], nadolol [e.g., Corgard], oxprenolol [e.g., Trasicor], penbutolol [e.g., Levatol], pindolol [e.g., Visken], propranolol [e.g., Inderal], sotalol [e.g., Sotacor], timolol [e.g., Blocadren])—Effects of both may be increased. In addition, unwanted effects may occur if a calcium channel blocker or a betablocker is stopped suddenly after use together
- Carbamazepine (e.g., Tegretol) or
- Cyclosporine (e.g., Sandimmune) or
- Procainamide (e.g., Pronestyl) or
- Quinidine (e.g., Quinidex)—Effects of these medicines may be increased if they are used with some calcium channel blockers
- Digitalis glycosides (heart medicine)—Effects of these medicines may be increased if they are used with some calcium channel blockers
- Disopyramide (e.g., Norpace)—Effects of some calcium channel blockers on the heart may be increased

Also, tell your doctor or pharmacist if you are using any of the following medicines in the eye:

- Betaxolol (e.g., Betoptic) or
- Levobunolol (e.g., Betagan) or
- Metipranolol (e.g., OptiPranolol) or
- Timolol (e.g., Timoptic)—Effects on the heart and blood pressure may be increased

Other medical problems—The presence of other medical problems may affect the use of the calcium channel blockers. Make sure you tell your doctor if you have any other medical problems, especially:

- Heart rhythm problems (history of)—Bepridil can cause serious heart rhythm problems
- Kidney disease or
- Liver disease—Effects of the calcium channel blocker may be increased

- Mental depression (history of)—Flunarizine may cause mental depression
- Parkinson's disease or similar problems—Flunarizine can cause parkinsonian-like effects
- Other heart or blood vessel disorders—Calcium channel blockers may make some heart conditions worse

Before you begin using any new medicine (prescription or nonprescription) or if you develop any new medical problem while you are using this medicine, check with your doctor, nurse, or pharmacist.

Proper Use of This Medicine

Take this medicine exactly as directed even if you feel well and do not notice any signs of chest pain. Do not take more of this medicine and do not take it more often than your doctor ordered. Do not miss any doses.

For patients taking *bepridil:*
- If this medicine causes upset stomach, it can be taken with meals or at bedtime.

For patients taking *diltiazem extended-release capsules:*
- Swallow the capsule whole, without crushing or chewing it.
- *Do not change to another brand without checking with your physician.* Different brands have different doses. If you refill your medicine and it looks different, check with your pharmacist.

For patients taking *nifedipine or verapamil extended-release capsules:*
- Swallow the capsule whole, without crushing or chewing it.

For patients taking *regular nifedipine or extended-release felodipine or nifedipine tablets:*
- Swallow the tablet whole, without breaking, crushing, or chewing it.
- If you are taking *Procardia XL*, you may sometimes notice what looks like a tablet in your stool. That is just

the empty shell that is left after the medicine has been absorbed into your body.

For patients taking *verapamil extended-release tablets:*
- Swallow the tablet whole, without crushing or chewing it. However, if your doctor tells you to, you may break the tablet in half.
- Take the medicine with food or milk.

For patients taking this medicine *for high blood pressure:*
- In addition to the use of the medicine your doctor has prescribed, appropriate treatment for your high blood pressure may include weight control and care in the types of food you eat, especially foods high in sodium (salt). Your doctor will tell you which factors are most important for you. You should check with your doctor before changing your diet.
- Many patients who have high blood pressure will not notice any signs of the problem. In fact, many may feel normal. It is very important that you *take your medicine exactly as directed* and that you keep your appointments with your doctor even if you feel well.
- Remember that this medicine will not cure your high blood pressure but it does help control it. Therefore, you must continue to take it as directed if you expect to lower your blood pressure and keep it down. *You may have to take high blood pressure medicine for the rest of your life.* If high blood pressure is not treated, it can cause serious problems such as heart failure, blood vessel disease, stroke, or kidney disease.

Missed dose—If you do miss a dose of this medicine, take it as soon as possible. However, if it is almost time for your next dose, skip the missed dose and go back to your regular dosing schedule. Do not double doses.

Storage—To store this medicine:
- Keep out of the reach of children.
- Store away from heat and direct light.

- Do not store in the bathroom, near the kitchen sink, or in other damp places. Heat or moisture may cause the medicine to break down.
- Do not keep outdated medicine or medicine no longer needed. Be sure that any discarded medicine is out of the reach of children.

Precautions While Using This Medicine

It is important that your doctor check your progress at regular visits. This will allow your doctor to make sure the medicine is working properly and to change the dosage if needed.

If you have been using this medicine regularly for several weeks, do not suddenly stop using it. Stopping suddenly may bring on your previous problem. Check with your doctor for the best way to reduce gradually the amount you are taking before stopping completely.

Chest pain resulting from exercise or physical exertion is usually reduced or prevented by this medicine. This may tempt you to be overly active. *Make sure you discuss with your doctor a safe amount of exercise for your medical problem.*

After taking a dose of this medicine you may get a headache that lasts for a short time. This effect is more common if you are taking felodipine, isradipine, or nifedipine. This should become less noticeable after you have taken this medicine for a while. If this effect continues or if the headaches are severe, check with your doctor.

In some patients, tenderness, swelling, or bleeding of the gums may appear soon after treatment with this medicine is started. Brushing and flossing your teeth carefully and regularly and massaging your gums may help prevent this. *See your dentist regularly to have your teeth cleaned. Check with your medical doctor or dentist if you have any questions about how to take care of your teeth and gums, or if you notice any tenderness, swelling, or bleeding of your gums.*

For patients taking *bepridil, diltiazem,* or *verapamil*:

* *Ask your doctor how to count your pulse rate. Then, while you are taking this medicine, check your pulse regularly.* If it is much slower than your usual rate, or less than 50 beats per minute, check with your doctor. A pulse rate that is too slow may cause circulation problems.

For patients taking *flunarizine:*

* This medicine may cause some people to become drowsy or less alert than they are normally. This is more likely to happen when you begin to take it or when you increase the amount of medicine you are taking. *Make sure you know how you react to this medicine before you drive, use machines, or do anything else that could be dangerous if you are not alert.*

For patients taking this medicine *for high blood pressure:*

* *Do not take other medicines unless they have been discussed with your doctor.* This especially includes over-the-counter (nonprescription) medicines for appetite control, asthma, colds, cough, hay fever, or sinus problems, since they may tend to increase your blood pressure.

Side Effects of This Medicine

Along with its needed effects, a medicine may cause some unwanted effects. Although not all of these side effects may occur, if they do occur they may need medical attention.

Not all of the side effects listed below have been reported for each of these medicines, but they have been reported for at least one of them. Since many of the effects of calcium channel blockers are similar, some of these side effects may occur with any of these medicines. However, they may be more common with some of these medicines than with others.

Check with your doctor as soon as possible if any of the following side effects occur:

Less common

Breathing difficulty, coughing, or wheezing; irregular or fast, pounding heartbeat; skin rash; slow heartbeat (less than 50 beats per minute—bepridil, diltiazem, and verapamil only); swelling of ankles, feet, or lower legs (more common with felodipine and nifedipine)

For flunarizine only—less common

Loss of balance control; mask-like face; mental depression; shuffling walk; stiffness of arms or legs; trembling and shaking of hands and fingers; trouble in speaking or swallowing

Rare

Bleeding, tender, or swollen gums; chest pain (may appear about 30 minutes after medicine is taken); fainting; painful, swollen joints (for nifedipine only); trouble in seeing (for nifedipine only)

For flunarizine and verapamil only—rare

Unusual secretion of milk

Other side effects may occur that usually do not need medical attention. These side effects may go away during treatment as your body adjusts to the medicine. However, check with your doctor if any of the following side effects continue or are bothersome:

More common

Drowsiness (for flunarizine only); increased appetite and/or weight gain (for flunarizine only)

Less common

Constipation; diarrhea; dizziness or lightheadedness (more common with bepridil and nifedipine); dryness of mouth (for flunarizine only); flushing and feeling of warmth (more common with nicardipine and nifedipine); headache (more common with felodipine, isradipine, and nifedipine); nausea (more common with bepridil and nifedipine); unusual tiredness or weakness

Other side effects not listed above may also occur in some patients. If you notice any other effects, check with your doctor.

Additional Information

Once a medicine has been approved for marketing for a certain use, experience may show that it is also useful for other medical problems. Although these uses are not included in product labeling, calcium channel blockers are used in certain patients with the following medical conditions:

- Hypertrophic cardiomyopathy (a heart condition) (verapamil)
- Raynaud's phenomenon (circulation problems) (nicardipine and nifedipine)

Other than the above information, there is no additional information relating to proper use, precautions, or side effects for these uses.

CARBAMAZEPINE Systemic

Some commonly used brand names are:

In the U.S.
Epitol
Tegretol
Generic name product may also be available.

In Canada

Apo-Carbamazepine	Tegretol
Mazepine	Tegetrol Chewtabs
Novocarbamaz	Tegetrol CR
PMS Carbamazepine	

Description

Carbamazepine (kar-ba-MAZ-e-peen) is used to control some types of seizures in the treatment of epilepsy. It is also used to relieve pain due to trigeminal neuralgia (tic douloureux). It should not be used for other more common aches or pains.

Carbamazepine may also be used for other conditions as determined by your doctor.

This medicine is available only with your doctor's prescription, in the following dosage forms:

Oral

- Suspension (U.S.)
- Tablets (U.S. and Canada)
- Chewable tablets (U.S. and Canada)
- Extended-release tablets (Canada)

It is very important that you read and understand the following information. If any of it causes you special concern, check with your doctor. Also, *if you have any questions* or if you want more information about this medicine or your medical problem, *ask your doctor, nurse, or pharmacist.*

Before Using This Medicine

In deciding to use a medicine, the risks of taking the medicine must be weighed against the good it will do. This is a decision you and your doctor will make. For carbamazepine, the following should be considered:

Allergies—Tell your doctor if you have ever had any unusual or allergic reaction to carbamazepine or to any of the tricyclic antidepressants, such as amitriptyline, amoxapine, clomipramine, desipramine, doxepin, imipramine, nortriptyline, protriptyline, or trimipramine. Also tell your doctor and pharmacist if you are allergic to any other substances, such as foods, preservatives, or dyes.

Pregnancy—Carbamazepine has not been studied in pregnant women. However, there have been reports of babies having low birth weight, small head size, skull and facial defects, underdeveloped fingernails, and delays in growth when their mothers had taken carbamazepine in high doses during pregnancy. In addition, birth defects have been reported in some babies when the mothers took other medicines for epilepsy during pregnancy. Also, studies in animals have shown that carbamazepine causes birth defects when given in large doses. Therefore, the use of carbamazepine during pregnancy should be discussed with your doctor.

Breast-feeding—Carbamazepine passes into the breast milk, and in some cases the baby may receive enough of it to cause unwanted effects. In animal studies, carbamazepine has affected the growth and appearance of the nursing babies.

Children—Behavior changes are more likely to occur in children.

Older adults—Confusion; restlessness and nervousness; irregular, pounding, or unusually slow heartbeat; and chest pain may be especially likely to occur in elderly patients, who are usually more sensitive than younger adults to the effects of carbamazepine.

Athletes—Carbamazepine is banned and tested for in competitors in biathlon and modern pentathlon events by the U.S. Olympic Committee (USOC).

Other medicines—Although certain medicines should not be used together at all, in other cases two different medicines may be used together even if an interaction might occur. In these cases, your doctor may want to change the dose, or other precautions may be necessary. When you are taking carbamazepine, it is especially important that your doctor and pharmacist know if you are taking any of the following:

- Adrenocorticoids (cortisone-like medicine)—The effects of adrenocorticoids may be decreased
- Anticoagulants (blood thinners)—The effects of anticoagulants may be decreased; monitoring of blood clotting time may be necessary during and after carbamazepine treatment
- Cimetidine (e.g., Tagamet)—Blood levels of carbamazepine may be increased, leading to an increase in serious side effects
- Diltiazem (e.g., Cardizem) or
- Erythromycin (e.g., E-Mycin, Erythrocin, Ilosone) or
- Propoxyphene (e.g., Darvon) or
- Verapamil (e.g., Calan)—Blood levels of carbamazepine may be increased; these medicines should not be used with carbamazepine
- Estrogens (female hormones) or
- Quinidine or
- Oral contraceptives (birth control pills), containing estrogen—The effects of these medicines may be decreased; use of a nonhormonal method of birth control or an oral contraceptive containing only a progestin may be necessary
- Isoniazid (e.g., INH)—The risk of serious side effects may be increased

- Monoamine oxidase (MAO) inhibitors (furazolidone [e.g., Furoxone], isocarboxazid [e.g., Marplan], phenelzine [e.g., Nardil], procarbazine [e.g., Matulane], tranylcypromine [e.g., Parnate])—Taking carbamazepine while you are taking or within 2 weeks of taking monoamine oxidase (MAO) inhibitors may cause sudden high body temperature, extremely high blood pressure, and severe convulsions; at least 14 days should be allowed between stopping treatment with one medicine and starting treatment with the other
- Other anticonvulsants (seizure medicine)—The effects of these medicines may be decreased; in addition, if these medicines and carbamazepine are used together during pregnancy, the risk of birth defects may be increased
- Tricyclic antidepressants (amitriptyline [e.g., Elavil], amoxapine [e.g., Asendin], clomipramine [e.g., Anafranil], desipramine [e.g., Pertofrane], doxepin [e.g., Sinequan], imipramine [e.g., Tofranil], nortriptyline [e.g., Aventyl], protriptyline [e.g., Vivactil], trimipramine [e.g., Surmontil])—Central nervous system depressant effects of carbamazepine may be increased while the anticonvulsant effects of carbamazepine may be decreased; seizures may occur more frequently

Other medical problems—The presence of other medical problems may affect the use of carbamazepine. Make sure you tell your doctor if you have any other medical problems, especially:

- Alcohol abuse (or history of) or
- Anemia or other blood problems or
- Behavioral problems or
- Diabetes mellitus (sugar diabetes) or
- Glaucoma or
- Heart or blood vessel disease or
- Problems with urination—Carbamazepine may make the condition worse
- Kidney disease or
- Liver disease—Higher blood levels of carbamazepine may result, increasing the chance of side effects

Before you begin using any new medicine (prescription or nonprescription) or if you develop any new medical problem while you are using this medicine, check with your doctor, nurse, or pharmacist.

Proper Use of This Medicine

Carbamazepine should be taken with meals to lessen the chance of stomach upset (nausea and vomiting).

It is very important that you take this medicine exactly as directed by your doctor to obtain the best results and lessen the chance of serious side effects. Do not take more of it, do not take it more often, and do not take it for a longer time than your doctor ordered.

If you are taking this medicine for pain relief:

- Carbamazepine is *not* an ordinary pain reliever. It should be used only when a doctor prescribes it for certain kinds of pain. *Do not take carbamazepine for any other aches or pains.*

If you are taking this medicine for epilepsy:

- *Do not suddenly stop taking this medicine without first checking with your doctor.* To keep your seizures under control, it is usually best to gradually reduce the amount of carbamazepine you are taking before stopping completely.

Missed dose—If you miss a dose of this medicine, take it as soon as possible. However, if it is almost time for your next dose, skip the missed dose and go back to your regular dosing schedule. Do not double doses. However, if you miss more than one dose a day, check with your doctor.

Storage—To store this medicine:

- Keep out of the reach of children.
- Store away from heat and direct light.
- *Do not store the tablet forms of carbamazepine in the bathroom, near the kitchen sink, or in other damp places. Heat or moisture may cause the medicine to break down and become less effective.*
- Keep the liquid form of this medicine from freezing.
- Do not keep outdated medicine or medicine no longer needed. Be sure that any discarded medicine is out of the reach of children.

Precautions While Using This Medicine

It is very important that your doctor check your progress at regular visits. Your doctor may want to have certain tests done to see if you are receiving the right amount of medicine or if certain side effects may be occurring without your knowing it. Also, the amount of medicine you are taking may have to be changed often.

This medicine will add to the effects of alcohol and other CNS depressants (medicines that slow down the nervous system, possibly causing drowsiness). Some examples of CNS depressants are antihistamines or medicine for hay fever, other allergies, or colds; sedatives, tranquilizers, or sleeping medicine; prescription pain medicine or narcotics; barbiturates; medicine for seizures; muscle relaxants; or anesthetics, including some dental anesthetics. *Check with your doctor before taking any of the above while you are using this medicine.*

This medicine may cause some people to become drowsy, dizzy, lightheaded, or less alert than they are normally, especially when they are starting treatment or increasing the dose. It may also cause blurred or double vision, weakness, or loss of muscle control in some people. *Make sure you know how you react to this medicine before you drive, use machines, or do anything else that could be dangerous if you are not alert and well-coordinated or able to see well.*

Some people who take carbamazepine may become more sensitive to sunlight than they are normally. Exposure to sunlight, even for brief periods of time, may cause a skin rash, itching, redness or other discoloration of the skin, or a severe sunburn. When you begin taking this medicine:

- Stay out of direct sunlight, especially between the hours of 10:00 a.m. and 3:00 p.m., if possible.
- Wear protective clothing, including a hat. Also, wear sunglasses.
- Apply a sun block product that has a skin protection factor (SPF) of at least 15. Some patients may require a product with a higher SPF number, especially if they

have a fair complexion. If you have any questions about this, check with your doctor or pharmacist.

- Apply a sun block lipstick that has an SPF of at least 15 to protect your lips.
- Do not use a sunlamp or tanning bed or booth.

If you have a severe reaction from the sun, check with your doctor.

For diabetic patients:

- Carbamazepine may affect urine sugar levels. While you are using this medicine, be especially careful when testing for sugar in your urine. If you notice a change in the results of your urine sugar tests or have any questions about this, check with your doctor.

Before having any medical tests, tell the medical doctor in charge that you are taking this medicine. The results of some pregnancy tests and the metyrapone test may be affected by this medicine.

Before having any kind of surgery, dental treatment, or emergency treatment, tell the medical doctor or dentist in charge that you are taking this medicine.

Your doctor may want you to carry a medical identification card or bracelet stating that you are taking this medicine.

Side Effects of This Medicine

Along with its needed effects, a medicine may cause some unwanted effects. Although not all of these side effects may occur, if they do occur they may need medical attention.

Check with your doctor immediately if any of the following side effects occur:

Rare

Black, tarry stools; blood in urine or stools; bone or joint pain; cough or hoarseness; darkening of urine; lower back or side pain; nosebleeds or other unusual bleeding or bruising; painful or difficult urination; pain, tenderness, swelling, or bluish color in leg or foot; pale stools; pinpoint red spots on skin; shortness of breath or cough; sores, ulcers, or white spots on lips or in the mouth; sore throat, chills, and fever; swollen or painful glands; unusual tiredness or weakness; wheezing, tightness in chest, or troubled breathing; yellow eyes or skin

Symptoms of overdose

Body spasm in which head and heels are bent backward and body is bowed forward; clumsiness or unsteadiness; convulsions (seizures)—especially in small children; dizziness (severe) or fainting; drowsiness (severe); fast or irregular heartbeat; high or low blood pressure (hypertension or hypotension); irregular, slow, or shallow breathing; large pupils; nausea or vomiting (severe); overactive reflexes followed by underactive reflexes; poor control in body movements (for example, when reaching or stepping); sudden decrease in amount of urine; trembling, twitching, or abnormal body movements

In addition, check with your doctor as soon as possible if any of the following side effects occur:

More common

Blurred vision or double vision; continuous back-and-forth eye movements

Less common

Behavioral changes (especially in children); confusion, agitation, or hostility (especially in the elderly); diarrhea (severe); headache (continuing); increase in seizures; nausea and vomiting (severe); skin rash, hives, or itching; unusual drowsiness

Rare

Chest pain; difficulty in speaking or slurred speech; fainting; frequent urination; irregular, pounding, or unusually slow heartbeat; mental depression with restlessness and nervousness or other mood or mental changes; numbness, tingling, pain, or weakness in hands and feet; rapid weight gain; rigidity; ringing, buzzing, or other unexplained sounds in the ears; sudden decrease in amount of urine; swelling of face, hands, feet, or lower legs; trembling; uncontrolled body movements; visual hallucinations (seeing things that are not there)

Other side effects may occur that usually do not need medical attention. These side effects may go away during treat-

ment as your body adjusts to the medicine. However, check with your doctor if any of the following side effects continue or are bothersome:

More common

Clumsiness or unsteadiness; dizziness (mild); drowsiness (mild); lightheadedness; nausea or vomiting (mild)

Less common or rare

Aching joints or muscles; constipation; diarrhea; dryness of mouth; headache; increased sensitivity of skin to sunlight (skin rash, itching, redness or other discoloration of skin, or severe sunburn); increased sweating; irritation or soreness of tongue or mouth; loss of appetite; loss of hair; muscle or abdominal cramps; sexual problems in males; stomach pain or discomfort

Other side effects not listed above may also occur in some patients. If you notice any other effects, check with your doctor.

Additional Information

Once a medicine has been approved for marketing for a certain use, experience may show that it is also useful for other medical problems. Although these uses are not included in product labeling, carbamazepine is used in certain patients with the following medical conditions:

- Neurogenic pain (a type of continuing pain)
- Bipolar disorder (manic-depressive illness)
- Central partial diabetes insipidus (water diabetes)
- Alcohol withdrawal
- Psychotic disorders (severe mental illness)

Other than the above information, there is no additional information relating to proper use, precautions, or side effects for these uses.

CEPHALOSPORINS   Systemic

This information applies to the following medicines:

Cefaclor (SEF-a-klor)
Cefadroxil (sef-a-DROX-ill)
Cefamandole (sef-a-MAN-dole)
Cefazolin (sef-A-zoe-lin)
Cefixime (sef-IX-eem)
Cefmetazole (sef-MET-a-zole)
Cefonicid (se-FON-i-sid)
Cefoperazone (sef-oh-PER-a-zone)
Ceforanide (se-FOR-a-nide)
Cefotaxime (sef-oh-TAKS-eem)
Cefotetan (sef-oh-TEE-tan)
Cefoxitin (se-FOX-i-tin)
Cefprozil (sef-PROE-zil)
Ceftazidime (sef-TAY-zi-deem)
Ceftizoxime (sef-ti-ZOX-eem)
Ceftriaxone (sef-try-AX-one)
Cefuroxime (se-fyoor-OX-eem)
Cephalexin (sef-a-LEX-in)
Cephalothin (sef-A-loe-thin)
Cephapirin (sef-a-PYE-rin)
Cephradine (SEF-ra-deen)
Moxalactam (MOX-a-lak-tam)

Some commonly used brand names are:

For Cefaclor
In the U.S.
Ceclor

In Canada
Ceclor

For Cefadroxil
In the U.S.
Duricef   Ultracef

Generic name product may also be available.

In Canada
Duricef

For Cefamandole
In the U.S.
Mandol

In Canada
Mandol

For Cefazolin
In the U.S.
 Ancef   Zolicef
 Kefzol

 Generic name product may also be available.

In Canada
 Ancef   Kefzol

For Cefixime
In the U.S.
 Suprax
In Canada
 Suprax

For Cefmetazole†
In the U.S.
 Zefazone

For Cefonicid
In the U.S.
 Monocid
In Canada
 Monocid

For Cefoperazone
In the U.S.
 Cefobid
In Canada
 Cefobid

For Ceforanide†
In the U.S.
 Precef

For Cefotaxime
In the U.S.
 Claforan
In Canada
 Claforan

For Cefotetan
In the U.S.
 Cefotan
In Canada
 Cefotan

For Cefoxitin
In the U.S.
 Mefoxin
In Canada
 Mefoxin

For Cefprozil†
  In the U.S.
    Cefzil

For Ceftazidime
  In the U.S.
    Ceptaz   Tazicef
    Fortaz   Tazidime
  In Canada
    Ceptaz   Fortaz

For Ceftizoxime
  In the U.S.
    Cefizox
  In Canada
    Cefizox

For Ceftriaxone
  In the U.S.
    Rocephin
  In Canada
    Rocephin

For Cefuroxime
  In the U.S.
    Ceftin   Zinacef
    Kefurox
  In Canada
    Zinacef

For Cephalexin
  In the U.S.
    Cefanex   Keflex
    C-Lexin   Keftab
    Keflet
    Generic name product may also be available.
  In Canada
    Apo-Cephalex   Novolexin
    Ceporex   Nu-Cephalex
    Keflex

For Cephalothin
  In the U.S.
    Keflin
    Generic name product may also be available
  In Canada
    Ceporacin   Keflin

For Cephapirin
  In the U.S.
    Cefadyl
    Generic name product may also be available.

In Canada
Cefadyl

For Cephradine
In the U.S.
Anspor   Velosef
Generic name product may also be available.
In Canada
Velosef

For Moxalactam†
In the U.S.
Moxam

---

†Not commercially available in Canada.

Description

Cephalosporins (sef-a-loe-SPOR-ins) are used in the treatment of infections caused by bacteria. They work by killing bacteria or preventing their growth.

Cephalosporins are used to treat infections in many different parts of the body. They are sometimes given with other antibiotics. Some cephalosporins are also given by injection to prevent infections before, during, and after surgery. However, cephalosporins will not work for colds, flu, or other virus infections.

Cephalosporins are available only with your doctor's prescription, in the following dosage forms:

Oral
Cefaclor
• Capsules (U.S. and Canada)
• Oral suspension (U.S. and Canada)
Cefadroxil
• Capsules (U.S. and Canada)
• Oral suspension (U.S. and Canada)
• Tablets (U.S.)
Cefixime
• Oral suspension (U.S. and Canada)
• Tablets (U.S. and Canada)
Cefprozil
• Oral suspension (U.S.)
• Tablets (U.S.)

Cefuroxime
- Tablets (U.S.)

Cephalexin
- Capsules (U.S. and Canada)
- Oral suspension (U.S. and Canada)
- Tablets (U.S. and Canada)

Cephradine
- Capsules (U.S. and Canada)
- Oral suspension (U.S.)

Parenteral

Cefamandole
- Injection (U.S. and Canada)

Cefazolin
- Injection (U.S. and Canada)

Cefmetazole
- Injection (U.S.)

Cefonicid
- Injection (U.S. and Canada)

Cefoperazone
- Injection (U.S. and Canada)

Ceforanide
- Injection (U.S.)

Cefotaxime
- Injection (U.S. and Canada)

Cefotetan
- Injection (U.S. and Canada)

Cefoxitin
- Injection (U.S. and Canada)

Ceftazidime
- Injection (U.S. and Canada)

Ceftizoxime
- Injection (U.S. and Canada)

Ceftriaxone
- Injection (U.S. and Canada)

Cefuroxime
- Injection (U.S. and Canada)

Cephalothin
- Injection (U.S. and Canada)

Cephapirin
- Injection (U.S. and Canada)

Cephradine
- Injection (U.S.)

Moxalactam
- Injection (U.S.)

It is very important that you read and understand the following information. If any of it causes you special concern, check with your doctor. Also, *if you have any questions* or if you want more information about this medicine or your medical problem, *ask your doctor, nurse, or pharmacist.*

Before Using This Medicine

In deciding to use a medicine, the risks of taking the medicine must be weighed against the good it will do. This is a decision you and your doctor will make. For the cephalosporins, the following should be considered:

Allergies—Tell your doctor if you have ever had any unusual or allergic reaction to any of the cephalosporins, penicillins, penicillin-like medicines, or penicillamine. Also tell your doctor and pharmacist if you are allergic to any other substances, such as foods, preservatives, or dyes.

Pregnancy—Studies have not been done in humans. However, most cephalosporins have not been reported to cause birth defects or other problems in animal studies. Studies in rabbits have shown that cefoxitin may increase the risk of miscarriages and cause other problems. Studies in rats and mice have shown that moxalactam causes a decrease in the animal's ability to live after birth. Moxalactam has not been shown to cause birth defects or other problems in rats and mice given up to 20 times the usual human dose.

Breast-feeding—Most cephalosporins pass into human breast milk, usually in small amounts. However, cephalosporins have not been reported to cause problems in nursing babies.

Children—Many cephalosporins have been tested in children and, in effective doses, have not been shown to cause different side effects or problems than they do in adults. However, there are some cephalosporins that have not been tested in children up to 1 year of age.

Older adults—Cephalosporins have been used in the elderly, and they are not expected to cause different side effects or problems in older people than they do in younger adults.

Other medicines—Although certain medicines should not be used together at all, in other cases 2 different medicines may be used together even if an interaction might occur. In these cases, your doctor may want to change the dose, or other precautions may be necessary. When you are taking a cephalosporin, it is especially important that your doctor and pharmacist know if you are taking any of the following:

- Alcohol and alcohol-containing medicine (cefamandole, cefmetazole, cefoperazone, cefotetan, and moxalactam only)—Using alcohol and these cephalosporins together may cause abdominal or stomach cramps, nausea, vomiting, headache, dizziness or lightheadedness, shortness of breath, sweating, or facial flushing; this reaction usually begins within 15 to 30 minutes after alcohol is consumed and usually goes away over several hours
- Anticoagulants (blood thinners) or
- Carbenicillin by injection (e.g., Geopen) or
- Dipyridamole (e.g., Persantine) or
- Divalproex (e.g., Depakote) or
- Heparin (e.g., Panheprin) or
- Pentoxifylline (e.g., Trental) or
- Plicamycin (e.g., Mithracin) or
- Sulfinpyrazone (e.g., Anturane) or
- Ticarcillin (e.g., Ticar) or
- Thrombolytic agents or
- Valproic acid (e.g., Depakene)—Any of these medicines may increase the chance of bleeding, especially when used with cefamandole, cefmetazole, cefoperazone, cefotetan, or moxalactam
- Probenecid (e.g., Benemid) (except cefoperazone, ceforanide, ceftazidime, ceftriaxone, moxalactam)—Probenecid increases the blood level of many cephalosporins. Although probenecid may be given with a cephalosporin by your doctor to purposely increase the blood level to treat some infections, in other cases, this effect may be unwanted and may increase the chance of side effects

Other medical problems—The presence of other medical problems may affect the use of cephalosporins. Make sure you tell your doctor if you have any other medical problems, especially:

- Bleeding problems, history of (cefamandole, cefmetazole, cefoperazone, cefotetan, and moxalactam only)—These medicines may increase the chance of bleeding

- Kidney disease—Some cephalosporins need to be given at a lower dose to people with kidney disease. Also, cephalothin, especially, may increase the chance of kidney damage
- Liver disease (cefoperazone only)—Cefoperazone needs to be given at a lower dose to people with liver and kidney disease
- Phenylketonuria—Cefprozil oral suspension contains phenylalanine
- Stomach or intestinal disease, history of (especially colitis, including colitis caused by antibiotics, or enteritis)—Cephalosporins may cause colitis in some patients

Proper Use of This Medicine

Cephalosporins may be taken on a full or empty stomach. If this medicine upsets your stomach, it may help to take it with food. Cefuroxime axetil tablets should be taken with food to increase absorption of the medicine.

For patients taking the *oral liquid* form of this medicine:

- This medicine is to be taken by mouth even if it comes in a dropper bottle. If this medicine does not come in a dropper bottle, use a specially marked measuring spoon or other device to measure each dose accurately. The average household teaspoon may not hold the right amount of liquid.
- Do not use after the expiration date on the label since the medicine may not work properly after that date. Check with your pharmacist if you have any questions about this.

For patients unable to swallow *cefuroxime axetil tablets* whole:

- Cefuroxime axetil tablets may be crushed and mixed with food (e.g., applesauce, ice cream) or drinks (apple, orange, or grape juice, or chocolate milk) to cover up the strong, lasting, bitter taste.

To help clear up your infection completely, *keep taking this medicine for the full time of treatment,* even if you begin to feel better after a few days. *If you have a "strep" infection, you should keep taking this medicine for at least 10 days. This is especially important in "strep" infections since serious heart or kidney problems could develop later* if your infection is not cleared up completely. Also, if you stop taking this medicine too soon, your symptoms may return.

This medicine works best when there is a constant amount in the blood or urine. *To help keep the amount constant, do not miss any doses. Also, it is best to take the doses at evenly spaced times, day and night.* For example, if you are to take 4 doses a day, the doses should be spaced about 6 hours apart. If this interferes with your sleep or other daily activities, or if you need help in planning the best times to take your medicine, check with your doctor, nurse, or pharmacist.

Missed dose—If you do miss a dose of this medicine, take it as soon as possible. This will help to keep a constant amount of medicine in the blood or urine. However, if it is almost time for your next dose, skip the missed dose and go back to your regular dosing schedule. Do not double doses.

Storage—To store this medicine:
- Keep out of the reach of children.
- Store away from heat and direct light.
- Do not store the capsule or tablet form of this medicine in the bathroom, near the kitchen sink, or in other damp places. Heat or moisture may cause the medicine to break down.
- Store the oral liquid form of most cephalosporins in the refrigerator because heat will cause this medicine to break down. However, keep the medicine from freezing. Follow the directions on the label. Cefixime oral suspension and Ceporex oral suspension do not need to be refrigerated.
- Do not keep outdated medicine or medicine no longer needed. Be sure that any discarded medicine is out of the reach of children.

Precautions While Using This Medicine

If your symptoms do not improve within a few days, or if they become worse, check with your doctor.

For diabetic patients:
- *This medicine may cause false test results with some urine sugar tests.* Check with your doctor before changing your diet or the dosage of your diabetes medicine.

For patients with phenylketonuria (PKU):
- Cefprozil oral suspension contains phenylalanine. Check with your doctor before taking this medicine.

In some patients, cephalosporins may cause diarrhea:
- Severe diarrhea may be a sign of a serious side effect. *Do not take any diarrhea medicine without first checking with your doctor.* Diarrhea medicines may make your diarrhea worse or make it last longer.
- For mild diarrhea, diarrhea medicine containing kaolin or attapulgite (e.g., Kaopectate tablets, Diasorb) may be taken. However, other kinds of diarrhea medicine should not be taken. They may make your diarrhea worse or make it last longer.
- If you have any questions about this or if mild diarrhea continues or gets worse, check with your doctor or pharmacist.

For patients receiving *cefamandole, cefmetazole, cefoperazone, cefotetan, or moxalactam by injection:*
- Drinking alcoholic beverages or taking other alcohol-containing preparations (for example, elixirs, cough syrups, tonics, or injections of alcohol) while receiving these medicines may cause problems. The problems may occur if you consume alcohol even several days after you stop taking the cephalosporin. Drinking alcoholic beverages may result in increased side effects such as abdominal or stomach cramps, nausea, vomiting, headache, fainting, fast or irregular heartbeat, difficult breathing, sweating, or redness of the face or skin. These effects usually start within 15 to 30 minutes after you drink alcohol and may not go away for up to several hours. Therefore, *you should not drink alcoholic beverages or take other alcohol-containing preparations while you are receiving these medicines and for several days after stopping them.*

Side Effects of This Medicine

Along with its needed effects, a medicine may cause some
unwanted effects. Although not all of these side effects may
occur, if they do occur they may need medical attention.

Check with your doctor immediately if any of the following
side effects occur:

> *Less common or rare*
>> Abdominal or stomach cramps and pain (severe); watery and
>> severe diarrhea, which may also be bloody; fever (these
>> side effects may also occur up to several weeks after you
>> stop taking this medicine); unusual bleeding or bruising
>> (more common for cefamandole, cefmetazole, cefopera-
>> zone, cefotetan, and moxalactam)
>
> *Rare*
>> Blistering, peeling, or loosening of skin; convulsions (sei-
>> zures); decrease in urine output; dizziness or lighthead-
>> edness; fever; joint pain; loss of appetite; pain, redness,
>> and swelling at place of injection; skin rash, itching, red-
>> ness, or swelling; trouble in breathing

Other side effects may occur that usually do not need medical attention. These side effects may go away during treatment as your body adjusts to the medicine. However, check
with your doctor if any of the following side effects continue
or are bothersome:

> *More common (less common with some cephalosporins)*
>> Diarrhea (mild); nausea and vomiting; sore mouth or tongue;
>> stomach cramps (mild)
>
> *Less common or rare*
>> Vaginal itching or discharge

Other side effects not listed above may also occur in some
patients. If you notice any other effects, check with your
doctor.

CHENODIOL   Systemic†

A commonly used brand name in the U.S. is Chenix.
Another commonly used name is chenodeoxycholic acid.

†Not commercially available in Canada.

Description

Chenodiol (kee-noe-DYE-ole) is used in the treatment of gallstone disease. It is taken by mouth to dissolve the gallstones.

Chenodiol is used in patients who do not need to have their gallbladder removed or in those in whom surgery is best avoided because of other medical problems. However, chenodiol works only in those patients who have a working gallbladder and whose gallstones are made of cholesterol. Chenodiol works best when these stones are small and of the "floating" type.

Chenodiol is available only with your doctor's prescription, in the following dosage form:

Oral
- Tablets (U.S.)

It is very important that you read and understand the following information. If any of it causes you special concern, check with your doctor. Also, *if you have any questions* or if you want more information about this medicine or your medical problem, *ask your doctor, nurse, or pharmacist.*

Before Using This Medicine

In deciding to use a medicine, the risks of taking the medicine must be weighed against the good it will do. This is a decision you and your doctor will make. For chenodiol, the following should be considered:

Allergies—Tell your doctor if you have ever had any unusual or allergic reaction to chenodiol or to other bile acid products.

Diet—If you have gallstones, your doctor may prescribe chenodiol and a personal high-fiber diet for you. Some foods that are high in fiber are whole grain breads and cereals, bran, fruit, and green, leafy vegetables. It has been found that such a diet may help dissolve the stones faster and may keep new stones from forming.

It may also be important for you to go on a reducing diet. However, check with your doctor before going on any diet.

Pregnancy—Chenodiol is not recommended for use during pregnancy. It has been shown to cause liver and kidney problems in animals when given in doses many times the human dose. Be sure you have discussed this with your doctor.

Breast-feeding—It is not known whether chenodiol passes into the breast milk. However, this medicine has not been reported to cause problems in nursing babies.

Children—Studies on this medicine have been done only in adult patients, and there is no specific information comparing use of chenodiol in children with use in other age groups.

Older adults—Many medicines have not been studied specifically in older people. Therefore, it may not be known whether they work exactly the same way they do in younger adults. Although there is no specific information comparing use of chenodiol in the elderly with use in other age groups, this medicine is not expected to cause different side effects or problems in older people than it does in younger adults.

Other medicines—Although certain medicines should not be used together at all, in other cases two different medicines may be used together even if an interaction might occur. In these cases, your doctor may want to change the dose, or other precautions may be necessary. Tell your doctor and pharmacist if you are taking any other prescription or nonprescription (over-the-counter [OTC]) medicine.

Other medical problems—The presence of other medical problems may affect the use of chenodiol. Make sure you tell your doctor if you have any other medical problems, especially:
- Biliary tract problems or
- Blood vessel disease or
- Pancreatitis (inflammation of pancreas)—These conditions may make it necessary to have surgery since treatment with chenodiol would take too long
- Liver disease—Liver disease may become worse with use of chenodiol

Before you begin using any new medicine (prescription or nonprescription) or if you develop any new medical problem while you are using this medicine, check with your doctor, nurse, or pharmacist.

Proper Use of This Medicine

Take chenodiol with food or milk for best results, unless otherwise directed by your doctor.

Take chenodiol for the full time of treatment, even if you begin to feel better. If you stop taking this medicine too soon, the gallstones may not dissolve as fast or may not dissolve at all.

Missed dose—If you miss a dose of this medicine, take it as soon as possible. However, if it is almost time for your next dose, skip the missed dose and go back to your regular dosing schedule. Do not double doses.

Storage—To store this medicine:
- Keep out of the reach of children.
- Store away from heat and direct light.
- Do not store in the bathroom, near the kitchen sink, or in other damp places. Heat or moisture may cause the medicine to break down.
- Do not keep outdated medicine or medicine no longer needed. Be sure that any discarded medicine is out of the reach of children.

Precautions While Using This Medicine

Do not take aluminum-containing antacids (e.g., ALternaGel, Maalox) while taking chenodiol. To do so may keep the chenodiol from working properly.

It is important that your doctor check your progress at regular visits. Laboratory tests will have to be done every few months while you are taking this medicine to make sure that the gallstones are dissolving and your liver is working properly.

Check with your doctor immediately if severe abdominal or stomach pain, especially toward the upper right side, and severe nausea and vomiting occur. These symptoms may mean that you have other medical problems or that your gallstone condition needs your doctor's attention.

Side Effects of This Medicine

Along with its needed effects, a medicine may cause some unwanted effects. Although not all of these side effects may occur, if they do occur they may need medical attention.

Check with your doctor as soon as possible if the following side effect occurs:

Less common or rare
Diarrhea (severe)

Other side effects may occur that usually do not need medical attention. These side effects may go away during treatment as your body adjusts to the medicine. However, check with your doctor if any of the following side effects continue or are bothersome:

More common
Diarrhea (mild)

Less common or rare
Constipation; frequent urge for bowel movement; gas or indigestion (usually disappears within 2 to 4 weeks after the beginning of treatment); loss of appetite; nausea or vomiting; stomach cramps or pain

Other side effects not listed above may also occur in some patients. If you notice any other effects, check with your doctor.

CHOLESTYRAMINE   Oral

Some commonly used brand names are:
In the U.S.
Cholybar   Questran Light
Questran

In Canada
Questran   Questran Light

Description

Cholestyramine (koe-less-TEAR-a-meen) is used to remove substances called bile acids from your body. With some liver problems, there is too much bile acid in your body and this can cause severe itching. Cholestyramine is also used to lower high cholesterol levels in the blood. This may help prevent medical problems caused by cholesterol clogging the blood vessels.

Cholestyramine works by attaching to certain substances in the intestine. Since cholestyramine is not absorbed into the body, these substances also pass out of the body without being absorbed.

Cholestyramine may also be used for other conditions as determined by your doctor.

Cholestyramine is available only with your doctor's prescription, in the following dosage forms:

Oral
- Chewable bar (U.S.)
- Powder (U.S. and Canada)

It is very important that you read and understand the following information. If any of it causes you special concern, check with your doctor. Also, *if you have any questions* or if you want more information about this medicine or your medical problem, *ask your doctor, nurse, or pharmacist.*

Before Using This Medicine

In deciding to use a medicine, the risks of taking the medicine must be weighed against the good it will do. This is a decision you and your doctor will make. For cholestyramine, the following should be considered:

Allergies—Tell your doctor if you have ever had any unusual or allergic reaction to cholestyramine. Also tell your doctor and pharmacist if you are allergic to any other substances, such as foods, preservatives, or dyes.

Pregnancy—Cholestyramine is not absorbed into the body and is not likely to cause problems. However, it may reduce absorption of vitamins into the body. Ask your doctor whether you need to take extra vitamins.

Breast-feeding—Cholestyramine is not absorbed into the body and is not likely to cause problems. However, the reduced absorption of vitamins by the mother may affect the nursing infant.

Children—There is no specific information comparing use of cholestyramine in children with use in other age groups. However, use is not recommended in children under 2 years of age since cholesterol is needed for normal development.

Older adults—Side effects may be more likely to occur in patients over 60 years of age, who are usually more sensitive to the effects of cholestyramine.

Other medicines—Although certain medicines should not be used together at all, in other cases two different medicines may be used together even if an interaction might occur. In these cases, your doctor may want to change the dose, or other precautions may be necessary. When you are taking cholestyramine it is especially important that your doctor and pharmacist know if you are taking any of the following:

- Anticoagulants (blood thinners)—The effects of the anticoagulant may be altered
- Digitalis glycosides (heart medicine) or
- Diuretics (water pills) or
- Penicillin G, taken by mouth or
- Phenylbutazone or
- Propranolol (e.g., Inderal) or
- Tetracyclines, taken by mouth (medicine for infection) or
- Thyroid hormones or
- Vancomycin, taken by mouth—Cholestyramine may prevent these medicines from working properly

Other medical problems—The presence of other medical problems may affect the use of cholestyramine. Make sure you tell your doctor if you have any other medical problems, especially:

- Bleeding problems or
- Constipation or
- Gallstones or
- Heart or blood vessel disease or

- Hemorrhoids or
- Stomach ulcer or other stomach problems or
- Underactive thyroid—Cholestyramine may make these conditions worse
- Kidney disease—There is an increased risk of the developing electrolyte problems
- Phenylketonuria—The sugar-free brand of cholestyramine powder contains aspartame, which can cause problems in people with this condition. It is best if you avoid using this product. Phenylalanine in aspartame is included in sugar-free preparations and should be avoided

Before you begin using any new medicine (prescription or nonprescription) or if you develop any new medical problem while you are using this medicine, check with your doctor, nurse, or pharmacist.

Proper Use of This Medicine

Take this medicine exactly as directed by your doctor. Try not to miss any doses and do not take more medicine than your doctor ordered.

For patients taking *the powder form* of this medicine:

- *This medicine should never be taken in its dry form, since it could cause you to choke.* Instead, always mix as follows:

    —Place the medicine in 2 ounces of any beverage and mix thoroughly. Then add an additional 2 to 4 ounces of beverage and again mix thoroughly (it will not dissolve) before drinking. After drinking all the liquid containing the medicine, rinse the glass with a little more liquid and drink that also, to make sure you get all the medicine.

    —You may also mix this medicine with milk in hot or regular breakfast cereals, or in thin soups such as tomato or chicken noodle soup. Or you may add it to some pulpy fruits such as crushed pineapple, pears, peaches, or fruit cocktail.

For patients taking *the chewable bar form* of this medicine:
- Chew each bite well before swallowing.

For patients taking this medicine *for high cholesterol*:
- Importance of diet—Before prescribing medicine for your condition, your doctor will probably try to control your condition by prescribing a personal diet for you. Such a diet may be low in fats, sugars, and/or cholesterol. Many people are able to control their condition by carefully following their doctor's orders for proper diet and exercise. Medicine is prescribed only when additional help is needed. *Follow carefully the special diet your doctor gave you,* since the medicine is effective only when a schedule of diet and exercise is properly followed.
- Also, this medicine is less effective if you are greatly overweight. It may be very important for you to go on a reducing diet. However, check with your doctor before going on any diet.
- Remember that this medicine will not cure your cholesterol problem but it will help control it. Therefore, you must continue to take it as directed if you expect to lower your cholesterol level.

Missed dose—If you miss a dose of this medicine, take it as soon as possible. Then go back to your regular dosing schedule. However, if it is almost time for your next dose, skip the missed dose and go back to your regular dosing schedule. Do not double doses.

Storage—To store this medicine:
- Keep out of the reach of children.
- Store away from heat and direct light.
- Do not store in the bathroom, near the kitchen sink, or in other damp places. Heat or moisture may cause the medicine to break down.
- Do not keep outdated medicine or medicine no longer needed. Be sure that any discarded medicine is out of the reach of children.

Precautions While Using This Medicine

It is very important that your doctor check your progress at regular visits. This will allow your doctor to see if the medicine is working properly and to decide if you should continue to take it.

Do not take any other medicine unless prescribed by your doctor since cholestyramine may change the effect of other medicines.

Do not stop taking this medicine without first checking with your doctor. When you stop taking this medicine, your blood cholesterol levels may increase again. Your doctor may want you to follow a special diet to help prevent this from happening.

Side Effects of This Medicine

In some animal studies, cholestyramine was found to cause tumors. It is not known whether cholestyramine causes tumors in humans.

Along with its needed effects, a medicine may cause some unwanted effects. Although not all of these side effects may occur, if they do occur they may need medical attention.

Check with your doctor immediately if either of the following side effects occurs:

Rare

   Black, tarry stools; stomach pain (severe) with nausea and
      vomiting

Check with your doctor as soon as possible if either of the following side effects occurs:

More common
   Constipation
Rare
   Loss of weight (sudden)

Other side effects may occur that usually do not need medical attention. These side effects may go away during treat-

ment as your body adjusts to the medicine. However, check with your doctor if any of the following side effects continue or are bothersome:

More common
 Heartburn or indigestion; nausea or vomiting; stomach pain
Less common
 Belching; bloating; diarrhea; dizziness; headache

Other side effects not listed above may also occur in some patients. If you notice any other effects, check with your doctor.

Additional Information

Once a medicine has been approved for marketing for a certain use, experience may show that it is also useful for other medical problems. Although these uses are not included in product labeling, cholestyramine is used in certain patients with the following medical conditions:

- Digitalis glycoside overdose
- Excess oxalate in the urine

Other than the above information, there is no additional information relating to proper use, precautions, or side effects for these uses.

CIPROFLOXACIN   Systemic

Some commonly used brand names are:
In the U.S.
 Cipro   Cipro IV
In Canada
 Cipro

Description

Ciprofloxacin (sip-roe-FLOX-a-sin) is used to treat bacterial infections in many different parts of the body. It works by killing bacteria or preventing their growth. However, this medicine will not work for colds, flu, or other virus infections.

Ciprofloxacin may be used for other problems as determined by your doctor.

Ciprofloxacin is available only with your doctor's prescription, in the following dosage form:
Oral
 • Tablets (U.S. and Canada)
Parenteral
 • Injection (U.S.)

It is very important that you read and understand the following information. If any of it causes you special concern, check with your doctor. Also, *if you have any questions* or if you want more information about this medicine or your medical problem, *ask your doctor, nurse, or pharmacist.*

Before Using This Medicine
In deciding to use a medicine, the risks of taking the medicine must be weighed against the good it will do. This is a decision you and your doctor will make. For ciprofloxacin, the following should be considered:

Allergies—Tell your doctor if you have ever had any unusual or allergic reaction to ciprofloxacin or to any related medicines such as cinoxacin (e.g., Cinobac), nalidixic acid (e.g., NegGram), norfloxacin (e.g., Noroxin), or ofloxacin (e.g., Floxin). Also tell your doctor and pharmacist if you are allergic to any other substances, such as foods, preservatives, or dyes.

Pregnancy—Studies have not been done in humans. However, use is not recommended during pregnancy since ciprofloxacin has been reported to cause bone development problems in young animals.

Breast-feeding—Ciprofloxacin does pass into human breast milk. Since ciprofloxacin has been reported to cause bone development problems in young animals, breast-feeding is not recommended during treatment with this medicine.

Children—Use is not recommended for infants, children, or adolescents since ciprofloxacin has been shown to cause bone development problems in young animals.

Older adults—This medicine has been tested and has not been shown to cause different side effects or problems in older people than it does in younger adults.

Other medicines—Although certain medicines should not be used together at all, in other cases two different medicines may be used together even if an interaction might occur. In these cases, your doctor may want to change the dose, or other precautions may be necessary. Tell your doctor and pharmacist if you are taking any of the following:

- Antacids, aluminum- or magnesium-containing or
- Iron supplements or
- Sucralfate—Antacids, iron, or sucralfate may keep ciprofloxacin from working properly
- Theophylline (e.g., Somophyllin-T, Theodur, Elixophyllin)— Ciprofloxacin may increase the chance of side effects of theophylline
- Warfarin (e.g., Coumadin)—Ciprofloxacin may increase the effect of warfarin, increasing the chance of bleeding

Other medical problems—The presence of other medical problems may affect the use of ciprofloxacin. Make sure you tell your doctor if you have any other medical problems, especially:

- Brain or spinal cord disease, including hardening of the arteries in the brain or epilepsy or other seizures—Ciprofloxacin may cause nervous system side effects
- Kidney disease or
- Kidney disease and liver disease—Patients with kidney disease (alone) or kidney disease and liver disease (together) may have an increased chance of side effects

Before you begin using any new medicine (prescription or nonprescription) or if you develop any new medical problem while you are using this medicine, check with your doctor, nurse, or pharmacist.

Proper Use of This Medicine

Do not give ciprofloxacin to infants, children, adolescents, or pregnant women unless otherwise directed by your doctor. This medicine has been shown to cause bone development problems in young animals.

Ciprofloxacin is best taken with a full glass (8 ounces) of water. Several additional glasses of water should be taken every day, unless you are otherwise directed by your doctor. Drinking extra water will help to prevent some unwanted effects of ciprofloxacin.

Ciprofloxacin may be taken with meals or on an empty stomach.

To help clear up your infection completely, *keep taking ciprofloxacin for the full time of treatment,* even if you begin to feel better after a few days. If you stop taking this medicine too soon, your symptoms may return.

This medicine works best when there is a constant amount in the blood or urine. *To help keep the amount constant, do not miss any doses. Also, it is best to take the doses at evenly spaced times, day and night.* For example, if you are to take 2 doses a day, the doses should be spaced about 12 hours apart. If this interferes with your sleep or other daily activities, or if you need help in planning the best times to take your medicine, check with your doctor, nurse, or pharmacist.

Missed dose—If you do miss a dose of this medicine, take it as soon as possible. This will help to keep a constant amount of medicine in the blood or urine. However, if it is almost time for your next dose, skip the missed dose and go back to your regular dosing schedule. Do not double doses.

Storage—To store this medicine:
- Keep out of the reach of children.
- Store away from heat and direct light.
- Do not store in the bathroom, near the kitchen sink, or in other damp places. Heat or moisture may cause the medicine to break down.
- Do not keep outdated medicine or medicine no longer needed. Be sure that any discarded medicine is out of the reach of children.

Precautions While Using This Medicine

If your symptoms do not improve within a few days, or if they become worse, check with your doctor.

If you are taking aluminum- or magnesium-containing antacids, or sucralfate do not take them at the same time that you take ciprofloxacin. It is best to take these medicines at least 4 hours before or 2 hours after taking ciprofloxacin. These medicines may keep ciprofloxacin from working properly.

Some people who take ciprofloxacin may become more sensitive to sunlight than they are normally. Exposure to sunlight, even for brief periods of time, may cause severe sunburn; skin rash, redness, itching, or discoloration; or vision changes. When you begin taking this medicine:

- Stay out of direct sunlight, especially between the hours of 10:00 a.m. and 3:00 p.m., if possible.
- Wear protective clothing, including a hat and sunglasses.
- Apply a sun block product that has a skin protection factor (SPF) of at least 15. Some patients may require a product with a higher SPF number, especially if they have a fair complexion. If you have any questions about this, check with your doctor or pharmacist.
- Do not use a sunlamp or tanning bed or booth.

If you have a severe reaction from the sun, check with your doctor.

Ciprofloxacin may also cause some people to become dizzy, lightheaded, drowsy, or less alert than they are normally. *Make sure you know how you react to this medicine before you drive, use machines, or do anything else that could be dangerous if you are dizzy or are not alert.* If these reactions are especially bothersome, check with your doctor.

Side Effects of This Medicine

Along with its needed effects, a medicine may cause some unwanted effects. Although not all of these side effects may occur, if they do occur they may need medical attention.

Check with your doctor immediately if any of the following side effects occur:

Rare

Agitation; confusion; fever; hallucinations (seeing, hearing, or feeling things that are not there); pain at site of injection; shakiness or tremors; skin rash, itching, or redness; swelling of face or neck

In addition to the side effects listed above, check with your doctor as soon as possible if the following side effect occurs:

Rare

Increased sensitivity of skin to sunlight

Other side effects may occur that usually do not need medical attention. These side effects may go away during treatment as your body adjusts to the medicine. However, check with your doctor if any of the following side effects continue or are bothersome:

More common

Abdominal or stomach pain or discomfort; diarrhea; dizziness; drowsiness; headache; lightheadedness; nausea or vomiting; nervousness; trouble in sleeping

Other side effects not listed above may also occur in some patients. If you notice any other effects, check with your doctor.

CLARITHROMYCIN   Systemic†

A commonly used brand name in the U.S. is Biaxin.

†Not commercially available in Canada.

Description

Clarithromycin (kla-RITH-roe-mye-sin) is used to treat bacterial infections in many different parts of the body. It works by killing bacteria or preventing their growth. However, this medicine will not work for colds, flu, or other virus infections. Clarithromycin may be used for other problems as determined by your doctor.

Clarithromycin is available only with your doctor's prescription, in the following dosage form:

Oral
- Tablets (U.S.)

It is very important that you read and understand the following information. If any of it causes you special concern, check with your doctor. Also, *if you have any questions* or if you want more information about this medicine or your medical problem, *ask your doctor, nurse, or pharmacist.*

Before Using This Medicine

In deciding to use a medicine, the risks of taking the medicine must be weighed against the good it will do. This is a decision you and your doctor will make. For clarithromycin, the following should be considered:

Allergies—Tell your doctor if you have ever had any unusual or allergic reaction to clarithromycin or to any related medicines such as erythromycin. Also tell your doctor and pharmacist if you are allergic to any other substances, such as foods, preservatives, or dyes.

Pregnancy—Clarithromycin has not been studied in pregnant women. However, studies in animals have shown that clarithromycin causes birth defects and other problems. Before taking this medicine, make sure your doctor knows if you are pregnant or if you may become pregnant.

Breast-feeding—Clarithromycin passes into breast milk.

Children—Studies on this medicine have not been done in children up to 12 years of age. In effective doses, the medicine has not been shown to cause different side effects or problems in children over the age of 12 than it does in adults.

Older adults—This medicine has been tested in a limited number of elderly patients and has not been shown to cause different side effects or problems in older people than it does in younger adults.

Other medicines—Although certain medicines should not be used together at all, in other cases two different medicines may be used together even if an interaction might occur. In these cases, your doctor may want to change the dose, or

other precautions may be necessary. When you are taking clarithromycin, it is especially important that your doctor and pharmacist know if you are taking any of the following:

- Theophylline (e.g., Theodur, Slo-Bid)—Clarithromycin may increase the chance of side effects of theophylline
- Zidovudine (e.g., Retrovir)—Clarithromycin may decrease the amount of zidovudine in the blood

Other medical problems—The presence of other medical problems may affect the use of clarithromycin. Make sure you tell your doctor if you have any other medical problems, especially:

- Kidney disease—Patients with severe kidney disease may have an increased chance of side effects

Before you begin using any new medicine (prescription or nonprescription) or if you develop any new medical problem while you are using this medicine, check with your doctor, nurse, or pharmacist.

Proper Use of This Medicine

Clarithromycin may be taken with meals or on an empty stomach.

To help clear up your infection completely, *keep taking clarithromycin for the full time of treatment,* even if you begin to feel better after a few days. If you stop taking this medicine too soon, your symptoms may return.

Dosing—The dose of clarithromycin will be different for different patients. *Follow your doctor's orders or the directions on the label.* The following information includes only the average doses of clarithromycin. Your dose may be different if you have kidney disease. *If your dose is different, do not change it* unless your doctor tells you to do so:

- Adults and children 12 years of age and older: 250 mg to 500 mg every twelve hours.
- Children up to 12 years of age: To be determined by doctor.

Missed dose—If you miss a dose of this medicine, take it as soon as possible. However, if it is almost time for your

next dose, skip the missed dose and go back to your regular
dosing schedule. Do not double doses.

Storage—To store this medicine:

- Keep out of the reach of children.
- Store away from heat and direct light.
- Do not store in the bathroom, near the kitchen sink, or
  in other damp places. Heat or moisture may cause the
  medicine to break down.
- Do not keep outdated medicine or medicine no longer
  needed. Be sure that any discarded medicine is out of
  the reach of children.

Precautions While Using This Medicine

If your symptoms do not improve within a few days, or if
they become worse, check with your doctor.

Side Effects of This Medicine

Side effects may occur that usually do not need medical
attention. These side effects may go away during treatment
as your body adjusts to the medicine. However, check with
your doctor if any of the following side effects continue or
are bothersome:

Less common

Abnormal taste; diarrhea; headache; nausea; stomach pain
or discomfort

Other side effects not listed above may also occur in some
patients. If you notice any other effects, check with your
doctor.

Additional Information

Once a medicine has been approved for marketing for a
certain use, experience may show that it is also useful for
other medical problems. Although these uses are not specifically included in product labeling, clarithromycin is used
in certain patients with the following medical conditions:

- Legionnaires' disease
- *Mycobacterium avium* complex (MAC)

Other than the above information, there is no additional
information relating to proper use, precautions, or side effects for these uses.

CLINDAMYCIN   Systemic

Some commonly used brand names are:
> *In the U.S.*
>> Cleocin
>> Cleocin Pediatric
>
> Generic name product may also be available.
>
> *In Canada*
>> Dalacin C   Dalacin C Phosphate
>> Dalacin C Palmitate

Description

Clindamycin is used to treat bacterial infections. It will not work for colds, flu, or other virus infections.

Clindamycin is available only with your doctor's prescription, in the following dosage forms:
> *Oral*
> - Capsules (U.S. and Canada)
> - Oral solution (U.S. and Canada)
>
> *Parenteral*
> - Injection (U.S. and Canada)

It is very important that you read and understand the following information. If any of it causes you special concern, check with your doctor. Also, *if you have any questions* or if you want more information about this medicine or your medical problem, *ask your doctor, nurse, or pharmacist.*

Before Using This Medicine

In deciding to use a medicine, the risks of taking the medicine must be weighed against the good it will do. This is a decision you and your doctor will make. For clindamycin, the following should be considered:

Allergies—Tell your doctor if you have ever had any unusual or allergic reaction to clindamycin, lincomycin, or doxorubicin. Also tell your doctor and pharmacist if you are allergic to any other substances, such as foods, preservatives, or dyes.

Pregnancy—Clindamycin has not been reported to cause birth defects or other problems in humans.

Breast-feeding—Clindamycin passes into the breast milk. However, clindamycin has not been reported to cause problems in nursing babies.

Children—This medicine has been tested in children and, in effective doses, has not been reported to cause different side effects or problems than it does in adults.

Older adults—Many medicines have not been studied specifically in older people. Therefore, it may not be known whether they work exactly the same way they do in younger adults or if they cause different side effects or problems in older people. There is no specific information comparing use of clindamycin in the elderly with use in other age groups.

Other medicines—Although certain medicines should not be used together at all, in other cases two different medicines may be used together even if an interaction might occur. In these cases, your doctor may want to change the dose, or other precautions may be necessary. When you are taking clindamycin, it is especially important that your doctor and pharmacist know if you are taking any of the following:

- Chloramphenicol (e.g., Chloromycetin) or
- Diarrhea medicine containing kaolin or attapulgite or
- Erythromycins (medicine for infection)—Taking these medicines along with clindamycin may decrease the effects of clindamycin

Other medical problems—The presence of other medical problems may affect the use of clindamycin. Make sure you tell your doctor if you have any other medical problems, especially:

- Kidney disease (severe) or
- Liver disease (severe)—Severe kidney or liver disease may increase blood levels of this medicine, increasing the chance of side effects
- Stomach or intestinal disease, history of (especially colitis, including colitis caused by antibiotics, or enteritis)—Patients with a history of stomach or intestinal disease may have an increased chance of side effects

Before you begin using any new medicine (prescription or nonprescription) or if you develop any new medical problem while you are using this medicine, check with your doctor, nurse, or pharmacist.

Proper Use of This Medicine

For patients taking the *capsule form* of clindamycin:

- *The capsule form of clindamycin should be taken with a full glass (8 ounces) of water or with meals* to prevent irritation of the esophagus (tube between the throat and stomach).

For patients taking the *oral liquid form* of clindamycin:

- Use a specially marked measuring spoon or other device to measure each dose accurately. The average household teaspoon may not hold the right amount of liquid.
- Do not use after the expiration date on the label. The medicine may not work properly after this date. Check with your pharmacist if you have any questions about this.

To help clear up your infection completely, *keep taking this medicine for the full time of treatment,* even if you begin to feel better after a few days. *If you have a "strep" infection, you should keep taking this medicine for at least 10 days. This is especially important in "strep" infections. Serious heart problems could develop later* if your infection is not cleared up completely. Also, if you stop taking this medicine too soon, your symptoms may return.

This medicine works best when there is a constant amount in the blood. *To help keep the amount constant, do not miss any doses. Also, it is best to take each dose at evenly spaced times day and night.* For example, if you are to take 4 doses a day, doses should be spaced about 6 hours apart. If this interferes with your sleep or other daily activities, or if you need help in planning the best times to take your medicine, check with your doctor, nurse, or pharmacist.

Missed dose—If you do miss a dose of this medicine, take it as soon as possible. This will help to keep a constant amount of medicine in the blood. However, if it is almost time for your next dose, skip the missed dose and go back to your regular dosing schedule. Do not double doses.

Storage—To store this medicine:
- Keep out of the reach of children.
- Store away from heat and direct light.
- Do not store the capsule form of this medicine in the bathroom, near the kitchen sink, or in other damp places. Heat or moisture may cause the medicine to break down.
- Do not refrigerate the oral liquid form of clindamycin. If chilled, the liquid may thicken and be difficult to pour. Follow the directions on the label.
- Do not keep outdated medicine or medicine no longer needed. Be sure that any discarded medicine is out of the reach of children.

Precautions While Using This Medicine

It is important that your doctor check your progress at regular visits.

If your symptoms do not improve within a few days, or if they become worse, check with your doctor.

In some patients, clindamycin may cause diarrhea.
- Severe diarrhea may be a sign of a serious side effect. *Do not take any diarrhea medicine without first checking with your doctor.* Diarrhea medicines, such as loperamide (Imodium A-D) or diphenoxylate and atropine (Lomotil), may make your diarrhea worse or make it last longer.
- For mild diarrhea, diarrhea medicine containing attapulgite (e.g., Kaopectate tablets, Diasorb) may be taken. However, attapulgite may keep clindamycin from being absorbed into the body. Therefore, these diarrhea medicines should be taken at least 2 hours before or 3 to 4 hours after you take clindamycin by mouth. Other kinds of diarrhea medicine should not be taken. They may make your diarrhea worse or make it last longer.

- If you have any questions about this or if mild diarrhea continues or gets worse, check with your doctor or pharmacist.

Before having surgery (including dental surgery) with a general anesthetic, tell the medical doctor or dentist in charge that you are taking clindamycin.

Side Effects of This Medicine

Along with its needed effects, a medicine may cause some unwanted effects. Although not all of these side effects may occur, if they do occur they may need medical attention.

Check with your doctor immediately if any of the following side effects occur:

More common

Abdominal or stomach cramps and pain (severe); abdominal tenderness; diarrhea (watery and severe), which may also be bloody; fever
(the above side effects may also occur up to several weeks after you stop taking this medicine)

Less common

Sore throat and fever; skin rash, redness, and itching; unusual bleeding or bruising

Other side effects may occur that usually do not need medical attention. These side effects may go away during treatment as your body adjusts to the medicine. However, check with your doctor if any of the following side effects continue or are bothersome:

More common

Diarrhea (mild); nausea and vomiting; stomach pain

Less common

Itching of rectal, or genital (sex organ) areas

Other side effects not listed above may also occur in some patients. If you notice any other effects, check with your doctor.

CLOFIBRATE   Systemic

Some commonly used brand names are:
In the U.S.
    Abitrate
    Atromid-S
    Generic name product may also be available.

In Canada
    Atromid-S
    Claripex
    Novofibrate

Description

Clofibrate (kloe-FYE-brate) is used to lower cholesterol and triglyceride (fat-like substances) levels in the blood. This may help prevent medical problems caused by such substances clogging the blood vessels.

Clofibrate may also be used for other conditions as determined by your doctor.

Clofibrate is available only with your doctor's prescription, in the following dosage form:
    Oral
    • Capsules (U.S. and Canada)

It is very important that you read and understand the following information. If any of it causes you special concern, check with your doctor. Also, *if you have any questions* or if you want more information about this medicine or your medical problem, *ask your doctor, nurse, or pharmacist.*

Before Using This Medicine

In addition to its helpful effects in treating your medical problem, this medicine may have some harmful effects.

You may have read or heard about a study called the World Health Organization (WHO) Study. This study compared the effects in patients who used clofibrate with effects in those who used a placebo (sugar pill). The results of this study suggested that clofibrate might increase the patient's risk of cancer, liver disease, and pancreatitis (inflammation of the pancreas), although it might also decrease the risk of heart attack. It may also increase the risk of gallstones and problems from gallbladder surgery. Other studies have not found all of these effects. Be sure you have discussed this with your doctor before taking this medicine.

In deciding to use a medicine, the risks of taking the medicine must be weighed against the good it will do. This is a decision you and your doctor will make. For clofibrate, the following should be considered:

Allergies—Tell your doctor if you have ever had any unusual or allergic reaction to clofibrate. Also tell your doctor and pharmacist if you are allergic to any other substances, such as foods, preservatives, or dyes.

Diet—Before prescribing medicine for your condition, your doctor will probably try to control your condition by prescribing a personal diet for you. Such a diet may be low in fats, sugars, and/or cholesterol. Many people are able to control their condition by carefully following their doctors' orders for proper diet and exercise. *Medicine is prescribed only when additional help is needed* and is effective only when a schedule of diet and exercise is properly followed.

Also, this medicine is less effective if you are greatly overweight. It may be very important for you to go on a reducing diet. However, check with your doctor before going on any diet.

Make certain your doctor and pharmacist know if you are on a low-sodium, low-sugar, or any other special diet. Most medicines contain more than their active ingredient.

Pregnancy—Use of clofibrate is not recommended during pregnancy. Although studies have not been done in pregnant women, studies in rabbits have shown that the fetus may not be able to break down and get rid of this medicine as well as the mother. Because of this, it is possible that clofibrate may be harmful to the fetus if you take it while you are pregnant or for up to several months before you become pregnant. Be sure that you have discussed this with your doctor before taking this medicine, especially if you plan to become pregnant in the near future.

Breast-feeding—Clofibrate passes into breast milk. This medicine is not recommended during breast-feeding because it may cause unwanted effects in nursing babies.

Children—There is no specific information comparing the use of clofibrate in children with use in other age groups. However, use is not recommended in children under 2 years of age since cholesterol is needed for normal development.

Older adults—Many medicines have not been studied specifically in older people. Therefore, it may not be known whether they work exactly the same way they do in younger adults. Although there is no specific information comparing use of clofibrate in the elderly with use in other age groups, this medicine is not expected to cause different side effects or problems in older people than it does in younger adults.

Other medicines—Although certain medicines should not be used together at all, in other cases two different medicines may be used together even if an interaction might occur. In these cases, your doctor may want to change the dose, or other precautions may be necessary. When you are taking clofibrate, it is especially important that your doctor and pharmacist know if you are taking the following:

- Anticoagulants (blood thinners)—Use with clofibrate may increase the effects of the anticoagulant

Other medical problems—The presence of other medical problems may affect the use of clofibrate. Make sure you tell your doctor if you have any other medical problems, especially:

- Gallstones or
- Stomach or intestinal ulcer—May make these conditions worse
- Heart disease or
- Kidney disease or
- Liver disease—Higher blood levels may result and increase the risk of side effects
- Underactive thyroid—Clofibrate may cause or worsen muscle disease

Before you begin using any new medicine (prescription or nonprescription) or if you develop any new medical problem while you are using this medicine, check with your doctor, nurse, or pharmacist.

Proper Use of This Medicine

Use this medicine only as directed by your doctor. Do not use more or less of it, and do not use it more often or for a longer time than your doctor ordered.

Follow carefully the special diet your doctor gave you. This is the most important part of controlling your condition and is necessary if the medicine is to work properly.

Stomach upset may occur but usually lessens after a few doses. Take this medicine with food or immediately after meals to lessen possible stomach upset.

Missed dose—If you miss a dose of this medicine, take it as soon as possible. However, if it is almost time for your next dose, skip the missed dose and go back to your regular dosing schedule. Do not double doses.

Storage—To store this medicine:
- Keep out of the reach of children.
- Store away from heat and direct light.
- Do not store in the bathroom, near the kitchen sink, or in other damp places. Heat or moisture may cause the medicine to break down.
- Do not keep outdated medicine or medicine no longer needed. Be sure that any discarded medicine is out of the reach of children.

Precautions While Using This Medicine

It is very important that your doctor check your progress at regular visits. This will allow your doctor to see if the medicine is working properly to lower your cholesterol and triglyceride levels and to decide if you should continue to take it.

Do not stop taking this medicine without first checking with your doctor. When you stop taking this medicine, your blood fat levels may increase again. Your doctor may want you to follow a special diet to help prevent that.

Side Effects of This Medicine

Along with its needed effects, a medicine may cause some unwanted effects. Although not all of these side effects may occur, if they do occur they may need medical attention.

Check with your doctor immediately if you think you have taken an overdose or if any of the following side effects occur:

Rare

Chest pain; irregular heartbeat; shortness of breath; stomach pain (severe) with nausea and vomiting

Check with your doctor as soon as possible if any of the following side effects occur:

Rare

Blood in urine; cough or hoarseness; decrease in urination; fever or chills; lower back or side pain; painful or difficult urination; swelling of feet or lower legs

Other side effects may occur that usually do not need medical attention. These side effects may go away during treatment as your body adjusts to the medicine. However, check with your doctor if any of the following side effects continue or are bothersome:

More common

Diarrhea; nausea

Less common or rare

Decreased sexual ability; headache; increased appetite or weight gain (slight); muscle aches or cramps; sores in mouth and on lips; stomach pain, gas, or heartburn; unusual tiredness or weakness; vomiting

Other side effects not listed above may also occur in some patients. If you notice any other effects, check with your doctor.

Additional Information

Once a medicine has been approved for marketing for a certain use, experience may show that it is also useful for other medical problems. Although this use is not included in product labeling, clofibrate is used in certain patients with the following medical condition:

• Certain types of diabetes insipidus (water diabetes)

Other than the above information, there is no additional information relating to proper use, precautions, or side effects for this use.

CLONIDINE   Systemic

Some commonly used brand names are:
> *In the U.S.*
> > Catapres
> > Catapres-TTS
> > Generic name product may also be available.

> *In Canada*
> > Catapres
> > Dixarit

Description

Clonidine (KLOE-ni-deen) belongs to the general class of medicines called antihypertensives. It is used to treat high blood pressure (hypertension).

High blood pressure adds to the workload of the heart and arteries. If it continues for a long time, the heart and arteries may not function properly. This can damage the blood vessels of the brain, heart, and kidneys, resulting in a stroke, heart failure, or kidney failure. Hypertension may also increase the risk of heart attacks. These problems may be less likely to occur if blood pressure is controlled.

Clonidine works by controlling nerve impulses along certain nerve pathways. As a result, it relaxes blood vessels so that blood passes through them more easily. This helps to lower blood pressure.

Clonidine may also be used for other conditions as determined by your doctor.

Clonidine is available only with your doctor's prescription, in the following dosage forms:

Oral
- Tablets (U.S. and Canada)

Transdermal
- Skin patch (U.S.)

It is very important that you read and understand the following information. If any of it causes you special concern, check with your doctor. Also, *if you have any questions* or if you want more information about this medicine or your medical problem, *ask your doctor, nurse, or pharmacist.*

Before Using This Medicine

In deciding to use a medicine, the risks of taking the medicine must be weighed against the good it will do. This is a decision you and your doctor will make. For clonidine, the following should be considered:

Allergies—Tell your doctor if you have ever had any unusual or allergic reaction to clonidine. Also tell your doctor and pharmacist if you are allergic to any other substance, such as foods, preservatives, or dyes.

Pregnancy—Studies have not been done in humans. Although clonidine has not been shown to cause birth defects in animals, it has been shown to cause toxic or harmful effects in the animal fetus, even at doses of only one-third the maximum human dose. Be sure you have discussed this with your doctor before taking this medicine.

Breast-feeding—Although clonidine passes into breast milk, it has not been reported to cause problems in nursing babies.

Children—There is no specific information about the use of clonidine in children.

Older adults—Dizziness or faintness may be more likely to occur in the elderly, who are more sensitive to the effects of clonidine.

Other medicines—Although certain medicines should not be used together at all, in other cases two different medicines may be used together even if an interaction might occur. In these cases, your doctor may want to change the dose, or other precautions may be necessary. When you are taking clonidine, it is especially important that your doctor and pharmacist know if you are taking any of the following:

- Beta-blockers (acebutolol [e.g., Sectral], atenolol [e.g., Tenormin], betaxolol [e.g., Kerlone], carteolol [e.g., Cartrol], labetalol [e.g., Normodyne], metoprolol [e.g., Lopressor], nadolol [e.g., Corgard], oxprenolol [e.g., Trasicor], penbutolol [e.g., Levatol], pindolol [e.g., Visken], propranolol [e.g., Inderal], sotalol [e.g., Sotacor], timolol [e.g., Blocadren])— May increase the risk of harmful effects when clonidine treatment is stopped suddenly
- Tricyclic antidepressants (amitriptyline [e.g., Elavil], amoxapine [e.g., Asendin], clomipramine [e.g., Anafranil], desipramine [e.g., Pertofrane], doxepin [e.g., Sinequan], imipramine [e.g., Tofranil], nortriptyline [e.g., Aventyl], protriptyline [e.g., Vivactil], trimipramine [e.g., Surmontil])—May decrease the effects of clonidine on blood pressure

Other medical problems—The presence of other medical problems may affect the use of clonidine. Make sure you tell your doctor if you have any other medical problems, especially:

- Heart or blood vessel disease
- Irritated or scraped skin (with transdermal system [skin patch] only)—Effects of clonidine may be increased because more is absorbed into the body
- Kidney disease—Effects may be increased because of slower removal of clonidine from the body
- Mental depression (history of)
- Raynaud's syndrome
- Systemic lupus erythematosus (SLE)—with transdermal system (skin patch) only—Effects of clonidine may be decreased because absorption of this medicine into the body is blocked

Before you begin using any new medicine (prescription or nonprescription) or if you develop any new medical problem while you are using this medicine, check with your doctor, nurse, or pharmacist.

Proper Use of This Medicine

For patients taking this medicine *for high blood pressure*:

- Importance of diet—When prescribing medicine for your condition, your doctor may also prescribe a personal diet for you. Such a diet may be low in sodium (salt). Most people eat much more sodium than they need and too much sodium in the diet may increase blood pressure. Some foods that contain large amounts of sodium are canned soup, pickles, ketchup, green and ripe olives, relish, frankfurters, soy sauce, and carbonated beverages. Your doctor may want you to limit the amounts of these and other high-sodium foods in your diet. High blood pressure medicine is usually more effective when such a diet is properly followed.

  Also, it may be very important for you to go on a reducing diet. However, check with your doctor before changing your diet.

- Many patients who have high blood pressure will not notice any signs of the problem. In fact, many may feel normal. It is very important that you *take your medicine exactly as directed* and that you keep your appointments with your doctor even if you feel well.

- Remember that this medicine will not cure your high blood pressure but it does help control it. Therefore, you must continue to use it as directed if you expect to lower your blood pressure and keep it down. *You may have to take high blood pressure medicine for the rest of your life.* If high blood pressure is not treated, it can cause serious problems such as heart failure, blood vessel disease, stroke, or kidney disease.

For patients using the *transdermal system (skin patch)*:

- *Use this medicine exactly as directed by your doctor.* It will work only if applied correctly. *This medicine usually comes with patient instructions. Read them carefully before using.*

- Do not try to trim or cut the adhesive patch to adjust the dosage. Check with your doctor if you think the medicine is not working as it should.

- Apply the patch to a clean, dry area of skin on your upper arm or chest. Choose an area with little or no hair and free of scars, cuts, or irritation.
- The system should stay in place even during showering, bathing, or swimming. If the patch becomes loose, cover it with the extra adhesive overlay provided. Apply a new patch if the first one becomes too loose or falls off.
- Each dose is best applied to a different area of skin to prevent skin problems or other irritation.
- After removing a used patch, fold the patch in half with the sticky sides together. Make sure to dispose of it out of the reach of children.

To help you remember to use your medicine, try to get into the habit of using it at regular times. If you are taking the tablets, take them at the same time each day. If you are using the transdermal system (skin patch), try to change it at the same time and day of the week.

Missed dose—If you miss a dose of this medicine, take it or use it as soon as possible. Then go back to your regular dosing schedule. *If you miss two or more doses of the tablets in a row or if you miss changing the transdermal patch for three or more days, check with your doctor right away.* If your body goes without this medicine for too long, your blood pressure may go up to a dangerously high level and some unpleasant effects may occur.

Storage—To store this medicine:

- Keep out of the reach of children.
- Store away from heat and direct light.
- Do not store in the bathroom, near the kitchen sink, or in other damp places. Heat or moisture may cause the medicine to break down.
- Do not keep outdated medicine or medicine no longer needed. Be sure that any discarded medicine is out of the reach of children.

Precautions While Using This Medicine

It is important that your doctor check your progress at regular visits to make sure that this medicine is working properly.

Check with your doctor before you stop using this medicine. Your doctor may want you to reduce gradually the amount you are using before stopping completely.

Make sure that you have enough clonidine on hand to last through weekends, holidays, or vacations. You should not miss any doses. You may want to ask your doctor for another written prescription for clonidine to carry in your wallet or purse. You can then have it filled if you run out of medicine when you are away from home.

For patients taking this medicine *for high blood pressure*:
* *Do not take other medicines unless they have been discussed with your doctor.* This especially includes over-the-counter (nonprescription) medicines for appetite control, asthma, colds, cough, hay fever, or sinus problems, since they may tend to increase your blood pressure.

Clonidine will add to the effects of alcohol and other CNS depressants (medicines that slow down the nervous system, possibly causing drowsiness). Some examples of CNS depressants are antihistamines or medicine for hay fever, other allergies, or colds; sedatives, tranquilizers, or sleeping medicine; prescription pain medicine or narcotics; barbiturates; medicine for seizures; muscle relaxants; or anesthetics, including some dental anesthetics. *Check with your doctor before taking any of the above while you are using this medicine.*

Clonidine may cause some people to become drowsy or less alert than they are normally. This is more likely to happen when you begin to take it or when you increase the amount of medicine you are taking. *Make sure you know how you react to this medicine before you drive, use machines, or do anything else that could be dangerous if you are not alert.*

Before having any kind of surgery (including dental surgery) or emergency treatment, *tell the medical doctor or dentist in charge that you are using this medicine.*

Dizziness, lightheadedness, or fainting may occur, especially when you get up from a lying or sitting position. Getting up slowly may help but if the problem continues or gets worse, check with your doctor.

The dizziness, lightheadedness, or fainting is also more likely to occur if you drink alcohol, stand for long periods of time, exercise, or if the weather is hot. While you are taking clonidine, be careful in the amount of alcohol you drink. Also, use extra care during exercise or hot weather or if you must stand for long periods of time.

Clonidine may cause dryness of the mouth. For temporary relief, use sugarless candy or gum, melt bits of ice in your mouth, or use a saliva substitute. However, if dry mouth continues for more than 2 weeks, check with your medical doctor or dentist. Continuing dryness of the mouth may increase the chance of dental disease, including tooth decay, gum disease, and fungus infections.

Side Effects of This Medicine

Along with its needed effects, a medicine may cause some unwanted effects. Although not all of these side effects may occur, if they do occur they may need medical attention.

Check with your doctor immediately if any of the following side effects occur:

> *Signs and symptoms of overdose*
>> Difficulty in breathing; dizziness (extreme) or faintness; pinpoint pupils of eyes; slow heartbeat; unusual tiredness or weakness (extreme)

Check with your doctor as soon as possible if any of the following side effects occur:

> *More common—with transdermal system (skin patch) only*
>> Itching or redness of skin
>
> *Less common*
>> Mental depression; swelling of feet and lower legs

Rare
> Paleness or cold feeling in fingertips and toes; vivid dreams or nightmares

Other side effects may occur that usually do not need medical attention. These side effects may go away during treatment as your body adjusts to the medicine. However, check with your doctor if any of the following side effects continue or are bothersome:

More common
> Constipation; dizziness; drowsiness; dry mouth; unusual tiredness or weakness

Less common
> Darkening of skin—with transdermal system (skin patch) only; decreased sexual ability; dizziness, lightheadedness, or fainting, especially when getting up from a lying or sitting position; dry, itching, or burning eyes; loss of appetite; nausea or vomiting; nervousness

After you have been using this medicine for a while, it may cause unpleasant or even harmful effects if you stop taking it too suddenly. After you stop taking this medicine, *check with your doctor immediately* if any of the following occur:

> Anxiety or tenseness; chest pain; fast or irregular heartbeat; headache; increased salivation; nausea; nervousness; restlessness; shaking or trembling of hands and fingers; stomach cramps; sweating; trouble in sleeping; vomiting

Other side effects not listed above may also occur in some patients. If you notice any other effects, check with your doctor.

CLOZAPINE   Systemic

Some commonly used brand names are:

In the U.S. and Canada
> Clozaril

Other
> Leponex

Description

Clozapine (KLOE-za-peen) is used to treat schizophrenia in patients who have not been helped by or are unable to take other medicines.

Clozapine is only available from pharmacies that agree to participate with your doctor in a plan to monitor your blood tests. You will need to have blood tests done every week, and you will receive a 7-day supply of clozapine only if the results of your blood tests show that it is safe for you to take this medicine.

Clozapine is available in the following dosage form:
Oral
- Tablets (U.S. and Canada)

It is very important that you read and understand the following information. If any of it causes you special concern, check with your doctor. Also, *if you have any questions* or if you want more information about this medicine or your medical problem, *ask your doctor, nurse, or pharmacist.*

Before Using This Medicine

In deciding to use a medicine, the risks of taking the medicine must be weighed against the good it will do. This is a decision you and your doctor will make. For clozapine, the following should be considered:

Allergies—Tell your doctor if you have ever had any unusual or allergic reaction to clozapine. Also tell your doctor and pharmacist if you are allergic to any other substance, such as foods, preservatives, or dyes.

Pregnancy—Clozapine has not been studied in pregnant women. However, clozapine has not been shown to cause birth defects or other problems in animal studies.

Breast-feeding—Clozapine may pass into breast milk and cause sedation, decreased suckling, restlessness or irritability, seizures, or heart or blood vessel problems in nursing babies.

Children—Studies on this medicine have been done only in adult patients, and there is no specific information comparing use of clozapine in children with use in other age groups.

Older adults—Many medicines have not been tested in older people. Therefore, it may not be known whether they work exactly the same way they do in younger adults. Clozapine may be more likely to cause side effects in the elderly, including dizziness and fainting, low blood pressure, and confusion or excitement.

Other medicines—Although certain medicines should not be used together at all, in other cases 2 different medicines may be used together even if an interaction might occur. In these cases, your doctor may want to change the dose, or other precautions may be necessary. When you are taking clozapine, it is especially important that your doctor and pharmacist know if you are taking any of the following:

- Alcohol or
- Central nervous system (CNS) depressants (medicines that cause drowsiness) or
- Tricyclic antidepressants (medicine for depression)—Clozapine may cause an increase in sedation or effects on the heart, or increase the risk of seizures
- Amphotericin B by injection (e.g., Fungizone) or
- Antineoplastics (cancer medicine) or
- Antithyroid agents (medicine for overactive thyroid) or
- Azathioprine (e.g., Imuran) or
- Chlorambucil (e.g., Leukeran) or
- Chloramphenicol (e.g., Chloromycetin) or
- Colchicine or
- Cyclophosphamide (e.g., Cytoxan) or
- Flucytosine (e.g., Ancobon) or
- Interferon (e.g., Intron A, Roferon-A) or
- Mercaptopurine (e.g., Purinethol) or
- Methotrexate (e.g., Mexate) or
- Plicamycin (e.g., Mithracin) or
- Zidovudine (e.g., Retrovir)—Taking clozapine with any of these medicines may cause increased blood problems
- Lithium—Using clozapine with lithium may increase the risk of seizures, or cause confusion or body movement disorders

Other medical problems—The presence of other medical problems may affect the use of clozapine. Make sure you

tell your doctor if you have any other medical problems, especially:

- Blood diseases or
- Enlarged prostate or difficult urination or
- Gastrointestinal problems or
- Heart or blood vessel problems—Clozapine may make the condition worse
- Epilepsy or other seizure disorder—Clozapine may increase the risk of seizures
- Kidney or liver disease—Higher blood levels of clozapine may occur, increasing the chance of side effects

Before you begin using any new medicine (prescription or nonprescription) or if you develop any new medical problem while you are using this medicine, check with your doctor, nurse, or pharmacist.

Proper Use of This Medicine

Take this medicine exactly as directed. Do not take more of this medicine and do not take it more often than your doctor ordered. Do not miss any doses.

This medicine has been prescribed for your current medical problem only. It must not be given to other people or used for other problems unless you are directed to do so by your doctor.

Missed dose—If you miss a dose of this medicine, take it as soon as possible. However, if it is almost time for your next dose, skip the missed dose and go back to your regular dosing schedule. Do not double doses.

Storage—To store this medicine:

- Keep out of the reach of children.
- Store away from heat and direct light.
- Do not store in the bathroom, near the kitchen sink, or in other damp places. Heat or moisture may cause the medicine to break down.
- Do not keep outdated medicine or medicine no longer needed. Be sure that any discarded medicine is out of the reach of children.

Precautions While Using This Medicine

It is important that you have your blood tests done weekly and that your doctor check your progress at regular visits. This will allow your doctor to make sure the medicine is working properly and to change the dosage if needed.

If you have been using this medicine regularly, do not stop taking it without first checking with your doctor. Your doctor may want you to reduce gradually the amount you are taking before stopping completely.

This medicine will add to the effects of alcohol and other CNS depressants (medicines that slow down the nervous system, possibly causing drowsiness). Some examples of CNS depressants are antihistamines or medicine for hay fever, other allergies, or colds; sedatives, tranquilizers, or sleeping medicine; prescription pain medicine or narcotics; barbiturates; medicine for seizures; muscle relaxants; or anesthetics, including some dental anesthetics. *Check with your doctor before taking any of the above while you are using this medicine.*

Clozapine may cause drowsiness, blurred vision or convulsions (seizures). *Do not drive, climb, swim, operate machines or do anything else that could be dangerous* while you are taking this medicine.

Dizziness, lightheadedness, or fainting may occur, especially when you get up from a lying or sitting position. Getting up slowly may help. If this problem continues or gets worse, check with your doctor.

In some patients, clozapine may cause increased watering of the mouth. Other patients, however, may get dryness of the mouth. For temporary relief of mouth dryness, use sugarless gum or candy, melt bits of ice in your mouth, or use a saliva substitute. However, if your mouth continues to feel dry for more than 2 weeks, check with your medical doctor or dentist. Continuing dryness of the mouth may increase the chance of dental disease, including tooth decay, gum disease, and fungus infections.

Side Effects of This Medicine

Along with its needed effects, a medicine may cause some unwanted effects. Although not all of these side effects may occur, if they do occur they may need medical attention.

Check with your doctor immediately if any of the following side effects occur:

More common

Fast or irregular heartbeat; fever; low blood pressure

Less common

High blood pressure

Rare

Chills; convulsions (seizures); difficult or fast breathing; increased sweating; loss of bladder control; muscle stiffness (severe); sore throat; sores, ulcers, or white spots on lips or in mouth; unusual bleeding or bruising; unusual tiredness or weakness; unusually pale skin

Check with your doctor as soon as possible if any of the following side effects occur:

More common

Dizziness or fainting

Less common

Blurred vision; confusion; restlessness or need to keep moving; trembling; unusual anxiety, nervousness, or irritability

Rare

Absence of or decrease in movement; decreased sexual ability; difficulty in sleeping; difficulty in urinating; headache (severe or continuing); lip smacking or puckering; mental depression; puffing of cheeks; rapid or worm-like movements of tongue; uncontrolled chewing movements; uncontrolled movements of arms and legs

Symptoms of overdose

Dizziness or fainting; drowsiness (severe); fast, slow, or irregular heartbeat; hallucinations (seeing, hearing, or feeling things that are not there); increased watering of mouth (severe); slow, irregular, or troubled breathing; unusual excitement, nervousness, or restlessness

Other side effects may occur that usually do not need medical attention. These side effects may go away during treatment as your body adjusts to the medicine. However, check with your doctor if any of the following side effects continue or are bothersome:

More common
Constipation; dizziness or lightheadedness (mild); drowsiness; headache (mild); increased watering of mouth; nausea or vomiting; unusual weight gain

Less common
Abdominal discomfort or heartburn; dryness of mouth

Other side effects not listed above may also occur in some patients. If you notice any other effects, check with your doctor.

COLESTIPOL   Oral

A commonly used brand name is:
In the U.S.
Colestid
In Canada
Colestid

Description

Colestipol (koe-LES-ti-pole) is used to lower high cholesterol levels in the blood. This may help prevent medical problems caused by cholesterol clogging the blood vessels.

Colestipol works by attaching to certain substances in the intestine. Since colestipol is not absorbed into the body, these substances also pass out of the body without being absorbed.

Colestipol may also be used for other conditions as determined by your doctor.

Colestipol is available only with your doctor's prescription, in the following dosage form:

Oral
- Powder (U.S. and Canada)

It is very important that you read and understand the following information. If any of it causes you special concern, check with your doctor. Also, *if you have any questions* or if you want more information about this medicine or your medical problem, *ask your doctor, nurse, or pharmacist.*

Before Using This Medicine

In deciding to use a medicine, the risks of taking the medicine must be weighed against the good it will do. This is a decision you and your doctor will make. For colestipol, the following should be considered:

Allergies—Tell your doctor if you have ever had any unusual or allergic reaction to colestipol. Also tell your doctor and pharmacist if you are allergic to any substances, such as foods, preservatives, or dyes.

Diet—Before prescribing medicine for your condition, your doctor will probably try to control your condition by prescribing a personal diet for you. Such a diet may be low in fats, sugars, and/or cholesterol. Many people are able to control their condition by carefully following their doctor's orders for proper diet and exercise. Medicine is prescribed only when additional help is needed and is effective only when a schedule of diet and exercise is properly followed.

Also, this medicine is less effective if you are greatly overweight. It may be very important for you to go on a reducing diet. However, check with your doctor before going on any diet.

Make certain your doctor and pharmacist know if you are on a low-sodium, low-sugar, or any other special diet.

Pregnancy—Colestipol is not absorbed into the body and is not likely to cause problems. However, it may reduce absorption of vitamins into the body. Ask your doctor whether you need to take extra vitamins.

Breast-feeding—Colestipol is not absorbed into the body and is not likely to cause problems.

Children—There is no specific information comparing use of colestipol in children with use in other age groups. However, use is not recommended in children under 2 years of age since cholesterol is needed for normal development.

Older adults—Side effects may be more likely to occur in patients over 60 years of age, who are usually more sensitive to the effects of colestipol.

Other medicines—Although certain medicines should not be used together at all, in other cases two different medicines may be used together even if an interaction might occur. In these cases, your doctor may want to change the dose, or other precautions may be necessary. When taking colestipol it is especially important that your doctor and pharmacist know if you are taking any of the following:
- Anticoagulants (blood thinners)—The effects of the anticoagulant may be altered
- Digitalis glycosides (heart medicine) or
- Diuretics (water pills) or
- Penicillin G, taken by mouth, or
- Propranolol, taken by mouth, or
- Tetracyclines (medicine for infection), taken by mouth, or
- Thyroid hormone or
- Vancomycin, taken by mouth—Colestipol may cause these medicines to be less effective

Other medical problems—The presence of other medical problems may affect the use of colestipol. Make sure you tell your doctor if you have any other medical problems, especially:
- Bleeding problems or
- Constipation or
- Gallstones or
- Heart or blood vessel disease or
- Hemorrhoids or
- Stomach ulcer or other stomach problems or
- Underactive thyroid—Colestipol may make these conditions worse
- Kidney disease—There is an increased risk of developing electrolyte problems
- Liver disease—Cholesterol levels may be raised

Before you begin using any new medicine (prescription or nonprescription) or if you develop any new medical problem while you are using this medicine, check with your doctor, nurse, or pharmacist.

Proper Use of This Medicine

Take this medicine exactly as directed by your doctor. Try not to miss any doses and do not take more medicine than your doctor ordered.

Follow carefully the special diet your doctor gave you. This is the most important part of controlling your condition and is necessary if the medicine is to work properly.

This medicine should never be taken in its dry form, since it could cause you to choke. Instead, always mix as follows:

- Add this medicine to 3 ounces or more of water, milk, flavored drink, or your favorite juice or carbonated drink. If you use a carbonated drink, slowly mix in the powder in a large glass to prevent too much foaming. Stir until it is completely mixed (it will *not* dissolve) before drinking. After drinking all the liquid containing the medicine, rinse the glass with a little more liquid and drink that also, to make sure you get all the medicine.
- You may also mix this medicine with milk in hot or regular breakfast cereals, or in thin soups such as tomato or chicken noodle soup. Or you may add it to some pulpy fruits such as crushed pineapple, pears, peaches, or fruit cocktail.

Missed dose—If you miss a dose of this medicine, take it as soon as possible. Then go back to your regular dosing schedule. However, if it is almost time for your next dose, skip the missed dose and go back to your regular dosing schedule. Do not double doses.

Storage—To store this medicine:

- Keep out of the reach of children.
- Store away from heat and direct light.

- Do not store in the bathroom, near the kitchen sink or in other damp places. Heat or moisture may cause the medicine to break down.
- Do not keep outdated medicine or medicine no longer needed. Be sure that any discarded medicine is out of the reach of children.

Precautions While Using This Medicine

It is very important that your doctor check your progress at regular visits. This will allow your doctor to see if the medicine is working properly to lower your cholesterol levels and to decide if you should continue to take it.

Do not stop taking this medicine without first checking with your doctor. When you stop taking this medicine, your blood cholesterol levels may increase again. Your doctor may want you to follow a special diet to help prevent this from happening.

Do not take any other medicine unless prescribed by your doctor since colestipol may interfere with other medicines.

Side Effects of This Medicine

Along with its needed effects, a medicine may cause some unwanted effects. Although not all of these side effects may occur, if they do occur they may need medical attention.

Check with your doctor immediately if either of the following side effects occurs:

> *Rare*
>> Black, tarry stools; stomach pain (severe) with nausea and vomiting

Check with your doctor as soon as possible if either of the following side effects occurs:

> *More common*
>> Constipation
>
> *Rare*
>> Loss of weight (sudden)

Other side effects may occur that usually do not need medical attention. These side effects may go away during treat-

ment as your body adjusts to the medicine. However, check with your doctor if any of the following side effects continue or are bothersome:

Less common

Belching; bloating; diarrhea; dizziness; headache; nausea or vomiting; stomach pain

Other side effects not listed above may also occur in some patients. If you notice any other effects, check with your doctor.

Additional Information

Once a medicine has been approved for marketing for a certain use, experience may show that it is also useful for other medical problems. Although these uses are not included in product labeling, colestipol is used in certain patients with the following medical conditions:

- Diarrhea caused by bile acids
- Digitalis glycoside overdose
- Excess oxalate in the urine
- Itching (pruritus) associated with partial biliary obstruction

Other than the above information, there is no additional information relating to proper use, precautions, or side effects for these uses.

CORTICOSTEROIDS   Inhalation

This information applies to the following medicines:

Beclomethasone (be-kloe-METH-a-sone)
Dexamethasone (dex-a-METH-a-sone)
Flunisolide (floo-NISS-oh-lide)
Triamcinolone (trye-am-SIN-oh-lone)

Some commonly used brand names are:

For Beclomethasone

In the U.S.
Beclovent   Vanceril

In Canada
Beclovent   Vanceril
Beclovent Rotacaps

Another commonly used name is beclometasone.

For Dexamethasone†
> *In the U.S.*
>> Decadron Respihaler

For Flunisolide
> *In the U.S.*
>> AeroBid
>
> *In Canada*
>> Bronalide

For Triamcinolone
> *In the U.S.*
>> Azmacort
>
> *In Canada*
>> Azmacort

---

†Not commercially available in Canada.

Description

Inhalation adrenocorticoids (a-dree-noe-KOR-ti-koids) are used to help prevent asthma attacks. However, they will not relieve an asthma attack that has already started. They are cortisone-like medicines. Adrenocorticoids also belong to the general family of medicines called steroids.

Inhalation adrenocorticoids are available only with your doctor's prescription, in the following dosage forms:

> *Oral Inhalation*
>> Beclomethasone
>> - Aerosol (U.S. and Canada)
>> - Capsules (Canada)
>> Dexamethasone
>> - Aerosol (U.S.)
>> Flunisolide
>> - Aerosol (U.S. and Canada)
>> Triamcinolone
>> - Aerosol (U.S. and Canada)

It is very important that you read and understand the following information. If any of it causes you special concern, check with your doctor. Also, *if you have any questions* or if you want more information about this medicine or your medical problem, *ask your doctor, nurse, or pharmacist.*

Before Using This Medicine

In deciding to use a medicine, the risks of taking the medicine must be weighed against the good it will do. This is a decision you and your doctor will make. For adrenocorticoids, the following should be considered:

Allergies—Tell your doctor if you have ever had any unusual or allergic reaction to adrenocorticoids. Also tell your doctor and pharmacist if you are allergic to any other substances, such as foods, preservatives, or dyes.

Pregnancy—In one human study, use of beclomethasone inhalation did not cause birth defects or other problems. Studies on birth defects with dexamethasone, flunisolide, or triamcinolone inhalations have not been done in humans.

In animal studies, adrenocorticoids taken by mouth or injection during pregnancy were shown to cause birth defects. Also, too much use of adrenocorticoids during pregnancy may cause other unwanted effects in the infant, such as slower growth and reduced adrenal gland function.

If adrenocorticoids are medically necessary during pregnancy to control asthma, inhaled adrenocorticoids are generally considered safer than adrenocorticoids taken by mouth or injection. Also, use of inhaled adrenocorticoids may allow some patients to stop using or decrease the amount of adrenocorticoids taken by mouth or injection.

Breast-feeding—Dexamethasone passes into the breast milk and may cause problems in nursing babies. It may be necessary to take another medicine or to stop breast-feeding during treatment.

It is not known whether beclomethasone, flunisolide, or triamcinolone passes into the breast milk. However, these medicines have not been shown to cause problems in nursing babies.

Children—Adrenocorticoids taken by mouth or injection have been shown to slow or stop growth in children and cause reduced adrenal gland function. If adrenocorticoids are medically necessary to control asthma in a child, inhaled adre-

nocorticoids are generally considered to be safer than adrenocorticoids taken by mouth or injection. Most inhaled
adrenocorticoids have not been shown to affect growth. Also,
use of most inhaled adrenocorticoids may allow some children to stop using or decrease the amount of adrenocorticoids
taken by mouth or injection.

Before this medicine is given to a child, you and your child's
doctor should talk about the good this medicine will do as
well as the risks of using it. Follow the doctor's directions
very carefully to lessen the chance that these unwanted effects will occur.

Older adults—Although there is no specific information about
the use of adrenocorticoids in the elderly, they are not expected to cause different side effects or problems in older
people than they do in younger adults.

Other medicines—Although certain medicines should not be
used together at all, in other cases two different medicines
may be used together even if an interaction might occur. In
these cases, your doctor may want to change the dose, or
other precautions may be necessary. When you are using
adrenocorticoids, it is especially important that your doctor
and pharmacist know if you are taking any of the following:

- Antidiabetics, oral (diabetes medicine taken by mouth) or
- Insulin—Long-term use of dexamethasone or triamcinolone
  may interfere with the effects of oral antidiabetic medicines
  or insulin by increasing blood glucose (sugar) levels, leading
  to a loss of control of diabetes mellitus (sugar diabetes)

Other medical problems—The presence of other medical
problems may affect the use of adrenocorticoids. Make sure
you tell your doctor if you have any other medical problems,
especially:

For all adrenocorticoid aerosols

- Certain types of lung disease
- Infection of the mouth, throat, or lungs—Signs of an infection
  may be covered up by the use of adrenocorticoids, or healing
  of the infection may be delayed

For long-term use of dexamethasone or triamcinolone aerosols

- Bone disease or
- Colitis or
- Diabetes mellitus (sugar diabetes) or
- Diverticulitis or
- Fungus or other infection or
- Glaucoma or
- Heart disease or
- High blood pressure or
- High cholesterol levels or
- Kidney disease or kidney stones or
- Stomach ulcer or other stomach problems—These conditions may be worsened by certain side effects of dexamethasone and triamcinolone
- Heart attack (recent)—Very rarely, a serious heart condition has been reported with the use of dexamethasone or triamcinolone shortly after a heart attack
- Herpes simplex virus infection of the eye—Use of dexamethasone or triamcinolone while the eye is infected may cause a hole to form in the cornea
- Liver disease
- Myasthenia gravis—Dexamethasone or triamcinolone may cause problems in breathing
- Tuberculosis (history of)—Use of dexamethasone may cause a new tuberculosis infection
- Underactive thyroid—This condition may cause an increased effect from the dexamethasone or triamcinolone, possibly leading to toxic effects

Before you begin using any new medicine (prescription or nonprescription) or if you develop any new medical problem while you are using this medicine, check with your doctor, nurse, or pharmacist.

Proper Use of This Medicine

Inhalation adrenocorticoids are used with a special inhaler and usually come with patient directions. *Read the directions carefully before using.* If you do not understand the directions, or if you are not sure how to use the inhaler, check with your doctor, nurse, or pharmacist.

Do not use more of this medicine, and do not use it more often, than your doctor ordered. To do so may increase the chance of absorption into the body and the chance of unwanted effects.

In order for this medicine to help prevent asthma attacks, it must be taken every day in regularly spaced doses as ordered by your doctor. Up to four weeks may pass before you feel its full effects. However, this may take less time if you have been taking certain other medicines for your asthma.

Do not use this medicine to treat an asthma attack that has already started, because it will not work. However, continue to take this medicine at the usual time, even if you use another medicine to relieve the asthma attack.

The inhaler should be cleaned every day as directed. If you do not receive instructions with the inhaler, or if you are not certain how to clean it, check with your pharmacist.

Gargling and rinsing your mouth with water after each dose may help prevent hoarseness, throat irritation, and infection in the mouth. However, do not swallow the water after you rinse. Your doctor may also want you to use a spacer to decrease these problems. A spacer is a tube that fits on the mouthpiece of the inhaler. It makes the inhaler easier to use and allows more of the medicine to reach your lungs, rather than staying in the mouth and throat.

Missed dose—If you miss a dose of this medicine, use it as soon as possible. However, if it is almost time for your next dose, skip the missed dose and go back to your regular dosing schedule. Do not double doses.

Check with your pharmacist to see if you should save the inhaler piece that comes with this medicine. Refill units may be available at lower cost. However, remember that the inhaler is meant to be used only for the medicine that comes with it. Do not use the inhaler for any other inhalation aerosol medicine, even if the cartridge fits.

Storage—To store this medicine:
   • Keep out of the reach of children.
   • Store away from heat and direct light.

- Keep the medicine from getting too cold or freezing. This medicine may be less effective if the container is cold when you use it.
- Do not puncture, break, or burn the aerosol container, even after it is empty.
- Do not keep outdated medicine or medicine no longer needed. Be sure that any discarded medicine is out of the reach of children.

Precautions While Using This Medicine

Check with your doctor:
- *if you go through a period of unusual stress.*
- *if you have an asthma attack* that does not improve after you take a bronchodilator medicine.
- *if signs of mouth, throat, or lung infection occur.*
- *if your symptoms do not improve.*
- *if your condition gets worse.*

Also, *check with your doctor immediately if any of the following side effects occur* while you are using this medicine:

Abdominal or back pain
Dizziness or fainting
Fever
Muscle or joint pain
Nausea or vomiting
Prolonged loss of appetite
Shortness of breath
Unusual tiredness or weakness
Unusual weight loss

Your doctor may want you to carry a medical identification card stating that you are using this medicine and may need additional medicine during times of emergency, a severe asthma attack or other illness, or unusual stress.

Before you have any kind of surgery (including dental surgery) or emergency treatment, tell the medical doctor or dentist in charge that you are using this medicine.

For patients who are also using a bronchodilator inhalation aerosol:

- Unless otherwise directed by your doctor, use the bronchodilator aerosol first, then wait about 5 minutes before using this medicine. This allows the adrenocorticoid aerosol to better reach the passages of the lungs (bronchioles) because the bronchodilator opens up the bronchioles.

For patients who are also regularly taking an adrenocorticoid in tablet or liquid form:

- *Do not stop taking the other adrenocorticoid without your doctor's advice, even if your asthma seems better.* Your doctor may want you to reduce gradually the amount you are taking before stopping completely to lessen the chance of unwanted effects.
- When your doctor tells you to reduce the dose, or to stop taking the other adrenocorticoid, follow the directions carefully. Your body may need time to adjust to the change. The length of time this takes may depend on the amount of medicine you were taking and how long you took it. *It is especially important that your doctor check your progress at regular visits during this time.* Also, ask your doctor if there are special directions you should follow if you have a severe asthma attack, if you need any other medical or surgical treatment, or if certain side effects occur. Be certain that you understand these directions, and follow them carefully.

Side Effects of This Medicine

Along with its needed effects, a medicine may cause some unwanted effects. Although not all of these side effects may occur, if they do occur they may need medical attention.

Check with your doctor immediately if any of the following side effects occur just after you use this medicine:

Rare

Shortness of breath, troubled breathing, tightness in chest, or wheezing

Also, check with your doctor as soon as possible if any of the following side effects occur:

More common

Any sign of possible infection, such as chest pain, chills, fever, cough, congestion, ear pain, eye pain, red or teary eyes, runny nose, sneezing, or sore throat; creamy white, curd-like patches inside the mouth; fast or pounding heartbeat; increased susceptibility to infection; nausea or vomiting; skin rash or itching

Less common or rare

Decreased or blurred vision; difficulty in swallowing; hives; increased blood pressure; increased thirst; mental depression or other mood or mental changes; swelling of face; swelling of feet or lower legs; unusual weight gain

Additional side effects may occur after you have been using this medicine for a long time. Check with your doctor as soon as possible if any of the following side effects occur:

Acne or other skin problems; back or rib pain; bloody or black, tarry stools; fullness or rounding out of the face (moon face); frequent urination; increased thirst; irregular heartbeat; menstrual problems; muscle weakness, cramps, or pains; stomach pain or burning (severe and continuing); unusual tiredness or weakness; wounds that will not heal

Other side effects may occur that usually do not need medical attention. These side effects may go away during treatment as your body adjusts to the medicine. However, check with your doctor if any of the following side effects continue or are bothersome:

More common

Abdominal or stomach pain (mild); bloated feeling or gas; constipation; cough without other signs of infection; diarrhea; dizziness or lightheadedness; headache; heartburn or indigestion; hoarseness or other voice changes without other signs of infection; loss of appetite; loss of smell or taste sense; nervousness or restlessness; unpleasant taste

Less common or rare
> Dry or irritated nose, mouth, tongue, or throat; false sense of well-being; general feeling of discomfort, illness, shakiness, or faintness; increase in appetite; increased sweating; trouble in sleeping; unexplained nosebleeds

Some of the above side effects have been reported for dexamethasone or flunisolide, but not for beclomethasone or triamcinolone. All of the inhalation adrenocorticoids are similar, so any of the above side effects may occur with beclomethasone or triamcinolone also, especially if large amounts are used for a long time.

Other side effects not listed above may also occur in some patients. If you notice any other effects, check with your doctor.

CORTICOSTEROIDS   Nasal

This information applies to the following medicines:
  Beclomethasone (be-kloe-METH-a-sone)
  Dexamethasone (dex-a-METH-a-sone)†
  Flunisolide (floo-NISS-oh-lide)
Some commonly used brand names are:
For Beclomethasone
  In the U.S.

Beconase	Vancenase
Beconase AQ	Vancenase AQ

  In Canada

Beconase	Vancenase
Beconase AQ	

  Another commonly used name is beclometasone.

For Dexamethasone†
  In the U.S.
    Decadron Turbinaire

For Flunisolide
  In the U.S.
    Nasalide
  In Canada
    Rhinalar

†Not commercially available in Canada.

Description

Nasal adrenocorticoids (a-dree-noe-KOR-ti-koids) are cortisone-like medicines. They belong to the family of medicines called steroids. These medicines are sprayed into the nose to help relieve the stuffy nose, irritation, and discomfort of hay fever, other allergies, and other nasal problems. These medicines are also used to prevent nasal polyps from growing back after they have been removed by surgery.

These medicines are available only with your doctor's prescription, in the following dosage forms:

Nasal

Beclomethasone
- Aerosol (U.S. and Canada)
- Spray (U.S. and Canada)

Dexamethasone
- Aerosol (U.S.)

Flunisolide
- Solution (U.S. and Canada)

It is very important that you read and understand the following information. If any of it causes you special concern, check with your doctor. Also, *if you have any questions* or if you want more information about this medicine or your medical problem, *ask your doctor, nurse, or pharmacist.*

Before Using This Medicine

In deciding to use a medicine, the risks of taking the medicine must be weighed against the good it will do. This is a decision you and your doctor will make. For adrenocorticoids, the following should be considered:

Allergies—Tell your doctor if you have ever had any unusual or allergic reaction to adrenocorticoids. Also tell your doctor and pharmacist if you are allergic to any other substances, such as foods, preservatives, or dyes.

Pregnancy—In one human study, use of beclomethasone oral inhalation by pregnant women did not cause birth defects or other problems. Studies on birth defects with dexamethasone or flunisolide have not been done in humans.

In animal studies, adrenocorticoids taken by mouth or injection during pregnancy were shown to cause birth defects. Also, too much use of adrenocorticoids during pregnancy may cause other unwanted effects in the infant, such as slower growth and reduced adrenal gland function.

If adrenocorticoids are medically necessary during pregnancy to control nasal problems, nasal adrenocorticoids are generally considered safer than adrenocorticoids taken by mouth or injection. Also, use of nasal adrenocorticoids may allow some patients to stop using or decrease the amount of adrenocorticoids taken by mouth or injection.

Breast-feeding—Use of dexamethasone is not recommended in nursing mothers since dexamethasone passes into the breast milk and may affect the infant's growth.

It is not known whether beclomethasone or flunisolide passes into the breast milk. However, these medicines have not been reported to cause problems in nursing babies.

Children—Adrenocorticoids taken by mouth or injection have been shown to slow or stop growth in children and cause reduced adrenal gland function. If adrenocorticoids are medically necessary to control nasal problem in a child, nasal adrenocorticoids are generally considered to be safer than adrenocorticoids taken by mouth or injection. Most nasal adrenocorticoids have not been shown to affect growth. Also, use of most nasal adrenocorticoids may allow some children to stop using or decrease the amount of adrenocorticoids taken by mouth or injection.

Before this medicine is given to a child, you and your child's doctor should talk about the good this medicine will do as well as the risks of using it. Follow the doctor's directions very carefully to lessen the chance that these unwanted effects will occur.

Older adults—Although there is no specific information about the use of nasal adrenocorticoids in the elderly, they are not expected to cause different side effects or problems in older people than they do in younger adults.

Other medicines—Although certain medicines should not be used together at all, in other cases two different medicines

may be used together even if an interaction might occur. In these cases, your doctor may want to change the dose, or other precautions may be necessary. When you are using nasal adrenocorticoids, it is especially important that your doctor and pharmacist know if you are taking any prescription or nonprescription (over-the-counter [OTC]) medicines.

Other medical problems—The presence of other medical problems may affect the use of adrenocorticoids. Make sure you tell your doctor if you have any other medical problems, especially:

- Glaucoma—Long-term use of nasal adrenocorticoids may worsen glaucoma by increasing the pressure within the eye
- Herpes simplex (virus) infection of the eye
- Infections
- Injury to the nose (recent) or
- Nose surgery (recent) or
- Sores in the nose—Nasal adrenocorticoids may prevent proper healing of these conditions
- Liver disease
- Tuberculosis (active or history of)
- Underactive thyroid

Before you begin using any new medicine (prescription or nonprescription) or if you develop any new medical problem while you are using this medicine, check with your doctor, nurse, or pharmacist.

Proper Use of This Medicine

This medicine usually comes with patient directions. *Read them carefully before using the medicine.* Beclomethasone and dexamethasone are used with a special inhaler. If you do not understand the directions, or if you are not sure how to use the inhaler, check with your doctor, nurse, or pharmacist.

In order for this medicine to help you, it must be used regularly as ordered by your doctor. This medicine usually begins to work in about 1 week, but up to 3 weeks may pass before you feel its full effects.

Use this medicine only as directed. Do not use more of it and do not use it more often than your doctor ordered. To do so may increase the chance of absorption through the lining of the nose and the chance of unwanted effects.

Check with your doctor before using this medicine for nasal problems other than the one for which it was prescribed, since it should not be used on many bacterial, virus, or fungus nasal infections.

Save the inhaler that comes with beclomethasone or dexamethasone, since refill units may be available at lower cost.

Missed dose—If you miss a dose of this medicine and remember within an hour or so, use it right away. However, if you do not remember until later, skip the missed dose and go back to your regular dosing schedule. Do not double doses.

Storage—To store this medicine:
  • Keep out of the reach of children.
  • Store away from heat and direct light.
  • Keep the medicine from getting too cold or freezing. This medicine may be less effective if it is too cold when you use it.
  • Do not puncture, break, or burn the beclomethasone or dexamethasone aerosol container, even after it is empty.
  • Do not keep outdated medicine or medicine no longer needed. Also, discard any unused flunisolide or beclomethasone solution 3 months after you open the package. Be sure that any discarded medicine is out of the reach of children.

Precautions While Using This Medicine

If you will be using this medicine for more than a few weeks, your doctor should check your progress at regular visits.

Check with your doctor:
  • *if signs of a nose, sinus, or throat infection occur.*
  • *if your symptoms do not improve within 7 days (for dexamethasone) or within 3 weeks (for beclomethasone or flunisolide).*
  • *if your condition gets worse.*

Side Effects of This Medicine

Along with its needed effects, a medicine may cause some unwanted effects. Although not all of these side effects may occur, if they do occur they may need medical attention.

Check with your doctor as soon as possible if any of the following side effects occur:

Less common or rare

Bloody mucus or unexplained nosebleeds; crusting, white patches, or sores inside the nose; eye pain; gradual loss of vision; headache; hives; lightheadedness or dizziness; loss of sense of taste or smell; nausea or vomiting; shortness of breath, troubled breathing, tightness in chest, or wheezing; skin rash; sore throat, cough, or hoarseness; stomach pains; stuffy nose or watery eyes (continuing); swellings on face; unusual tiredness or weakness; white patches in throat

Symptoms of overdose

Acne; fullness or rounding of the face; menstrual changes

Other side effects may occur that usually do not need medical attention. These side effects may go away during treatment as your body adjusts to the medicine. However, check with your doctor if any of the following side effects continue or are bothersome:

More common

Burning, dryness, or other irritation inside the nose (mild, lasting only a short time); increase in sneezing; irritation of throat

Not all of the side effects listed above have been reported for each of these medicines, but they have been reported for at least one of them. All of the nasal adrenocorticoids are very similar, so any of the above side effects may occur with any of these medicines.

Other side effects not listed above may also occur in some patients. If you notice any other effects, check with your doctor.

CORTICOSTEROIDS/CORTICOTROPIN—
Glucocorticoid Effects   Systemic

This information applies to the following medicines:

Betamethasone (bay-ta-METH-a-sone)
Corticotropin (kor-ti-koe-TROE-pin)
Cortisone (KOR-ti-sone)
Dexamethasone (dex-a-METH-a-sone)
Hydrocortisone (hye-droe-KOR-ti-sone)
Methylprednisolone (meth-ill-pred-NISS-oh-lone)
Paramethasone (par-a-METH-a-sone)
Prednisolone (pred-NISS-oh-lone)
Prednisone (PRED-ni-sone)
Triamcinolone (trye-am-SIN-oh-lone)

The following information does *not* apply to desoxycorticosterone or flu-
drocortisone.

Some commonly used brand names are:

For Betamethasone
In the U.S.
    Celestone   Celestone Soluspan
    Celestone Phosphate   Selestoject
    Generic name product may also be available.

In Canada
    Betnelan   Celestone
    Betnesol   Celestone Soluspan

For Corticotropin
In the U.S.
    Acthar   H.P. Acthar Gel
    Cortrophin-Zinc
    Generic name product may also be available.

In Canada
    Acthar   Acthar Gel (H.P.)

Another commonly used name is ACTH.

For Cortisone
In the U.S.
    Cortone Acetate
    Generic name product may also be available.

In Canada
    Cortone
    Generic name product may also be available.

For Dexamethasone

In the U.S.

AK-Dex	Dexasone
Dalalone	Dexasone-LA
Dalalone D.P.	Dexone
Dalalone L.A.	Dexone 0.5
Decadrol	Dexone 0.75
Decadron	Dexone 1.5
Decadron-LA	Dexone 4
Decadron Phosphate	Dexone LA
Decaject	Hexadrol
Decaject-L.A.	Hexadrol Phosphate
Deronil	Mymethasone
Dexacen-4	Solurex
Dexacen LA-8	Solurex-LA
Dexamethasone Intensol	

Generic name product may also be available.

In Canada

Decadron	Dexasone
Decadron Phosphate	Hexadrol
Deronil	Oradexon

Generic name product may also be available.

For Hydrocortisone

In the U.S.

A-hydroCort	Hydrocortone
Cortef	Hydrocortone Acetate
Cortenema	Hydrocortone Phosphate
Cortifoam	Solu-Cortef

In Canada

Cortef	Cortifoam
Cortenema	Solu-Cortef

Another commonly used name is cortisol.

For Methylprednisolone

In the U.S.

A-methaPred	Duralone-40
depMedalone 40	Duralone-80
depMedalone 80	Medralone-40
Depoject-40	Medralone-80
Depoject-80	Medrol
Depo-Medrol	Medrol Enpak
Depopred-40	Meprolone
Depopred-80	Rep-Pred 40
Depo-Predate 40	Rep-Pred 80
Depo-Predate 80	Solu-Medrol

Generic name product may also be available.

In Canada

Depo-Medrol	Solu-Medrol
Medrol	

For Paramethasone
In the U.S.
    Haldrone

For Prednisolone
In the U.S.

Articulose-50	Predalone T.B.A.
Delta-Cortef	Predate 50
Hydeltrasol	Predate S
Hydeltra-T.B.A.	Predate TBA
Key-Pred 25	Predcor-25
Key-Pred 50	Predcor-50
Key-Pred SP	Predcor-TBA
Nor-Pred T.B.A.	Predicort-50
Pediapred	Predicort-RP
Predaject-50	Prelone
Predalone 50	

Generic name product may also be available.

For Prednisone
In the U.S.

Deltasone	Orasone 20
Liquid Pred	Orasone 50
Meticorten	Prednicen-M
Orasone 1	Prednisone Intensol
Orasone 5	Sterapred
Orasone 10	Sterapred DS

Generic name product may also be available.

In Canada

Apo-Prednisone	Winpred
Deltasone	

Generic name product may also be available.

For Triamcinolone
In the U.S.

Amcort	Kenaject-40
Aristocort	Kenalog-10
Aristocort Forte	Kenalog-40
Artistocort Intralesional	Tac-3
Artistospan Intra-articular	Triam-A
Aristospan Intralesional	Triam-Forte
Articulose-L.A.	Triamolone 40
Cenocort A-40	Triamonide 40
Cenocort Forte	Tri-Kort
Cinalone 40	Trilog
Cinonide 40	Trilone
Kenacort	Tristoject
Kenacort Diacetate	

Generic name product may also be available.

In Canada
Aristocort	Kenacort
Artistocort Forte	Kenalog-10
Aristocort Intralesional	Kenalog-40
Aristospan Intra-articular	

Generic name product may also be available.

Description

Adrenocorticoids (a-dree-noe-KOR-ti-koids) (cortisone-like medicines) are used to provide relief for inflamed areas of the body. They lessen swelling, redness, itching, and allergic reactions. They are often used as part of the treatment for a number of different diseases, such as severe allergies or skin problems, asthma, or arthritis. Adrenocorticoids may also be used for other conditions as determined by your doctor.

Your body naturally produces certain cortisone-like hormones that are necessary to maintain good health. If your body does not produce enough, your doctor may have prescribed this medicine to help make up the difference.

Corticotropin is not an adrenocorticoid. It is a hormone that occurs naturally in the body. Corticotropin is known as an adrenocorticotropic hormone, which means it causes the adrenal glands to produce cortisone-like hormones. Corticotropin is used as a test to determine whether your adrenal glands are producing enough hormones. Also, it is sometimes used instead of adrenocorticoids to treat many of the same medical problems.

Adrenocorticoids and corticotropin are very strong medicines. In addition to their helpful effects in treating your medical problem, they have side effects that can be very serious. If your adrenal glands are not producing enough cortisone-like hormones, taking this medicine is not likely to cause problems unless you take too much of it. If you are taking this medicine to treat another medical problem, be sure that you discuss the risks and benefits of this medicine with your doctor.

These medicines are available only with your doctor's prescription, in the following dosage forms:

Oral

Betamethasone
- Syrup (U.S.)
- Tablets (U.S. and Canada)
- Effervescent tablets (Canada)
- Extended-release tablets (Canada)

Cortisone
- Tablets (U.S. and Canada)

Dexamethasone
- Elixir (U.S.)
- Oral solution (U.S.)
- Tablets (U.S. and Canada)

Hydrocortisone
- Oral suspension (U.S.)
- Tablets (U.S. and Canada)

Methylprednisolone
- Tablets (U.S. and Canada)

Paramethasone
- Tablets (U.S.)

Prednisolone
- Oral solution (U.S.)
- Syrup (U.S.)
- Tablets (U.S.)

Prednisone
- Oral solution (U.S.)
- Syrup (U.S.)
- Tablets (U.S. and Canada)

Triamcinolone
- Syrup (U.S. and Canada)
- Tablets (U.S. and Canada)

Parenteral

Betamethasone
- Injection (U.S. and Canada)

Corticotropin
- Injection (U.S. and Canada)

Cortisone
- Injection (U.S. and Canada)

Dexamethasone
- Injection (U.S. and Canada)

Hydrocortisone
- Injection (U.S. and Canada)

Methylprednisolone
- Injection (U.S. and Canada)

Prednisolone
* Injection (U.S.)
Triamcinolone
* Injection (U.S. and Canada)

Rectal

Betamethasone
* Enema (Canada)
Hydrocortisone
* Aerosol foam (U.S. and Canada)
* Enema (U.S. and Canada)
Methylprednisolone
* Enema (U.S.)

It is very important that you read and understand the following information. If any of it causes you special concern, check with your doctor. Also, *if you have any questions* or if you want more information about this medicine or your medical problem, *ask your doctor, nurse, or pharmacist.*

Before Using This Medicine

In deciding to use a medicine, the risks of taking the medicine must be weighed against the good it will do. This is a decision you and your doctor will make. For adrenocorticoids and corticotropin, the following should be considered:

Allergies—Tell your doctor if you have ever had any unusual or allergic reaction to adrenocorticoids or corticotropin. Also tell your doctor and pharmacist if you are allergic to any other substances, such as foods, preservatives, or dyes.

Diet—If you will be using this medicine for a long time, your doctor may want you to:

* Follow a low-salt diet and/or a potassium-rich diet.

* Watch your calories to prevent weight gain.

* Add extra protein to your diet. Make certain your doctor and pharmacist know if you are already on any special diet, such as a low-sodium or low-sugar diet.

Pregnancy—Studies on birth defects with adrenocorticoids or with corticotropin have not been done in humans. However, too much use of adrenocorticoids during pregnancy may cause the baby to have problems after birth, such as slower growth. Also, studies in animals have shown that adrenocorticoids cause birth defects and that corticotropin may cause other unwanted effects in the fetus.

Breast-feeding—Adrenocorticoids pass into breast milk and may cause problems with growth or other unwanted effects in nursing babies. Depending on the amount of medicine you are taking every day, it may be necessary for you to take another medicine or to stop breast-feeding during treatment. Corticotropin has not been shown to cause problems in nursing babies.

Children—Adrenocorticoids or corticotropin may slow or stop growth in children and in growing teenagers, especially when they are used for a long time. Before this medicine is given to children or teenagers, you should discuss its use with your child's doctor and then carefully follow the doctor's instructions.

Older adults—Older patients may be more likely to develop high blood pressure or bone disease from adrenocorticoids. Women are especially at risk of developing bone disease.

Athletes—The U.S. Olympic Committee (USOC) has restrictions on the use of adrenocorticoids and corticotropin. Certain ways of taking these medicines are banned. Other ways (such as injection into a joint or other tissues) are accepted as long as your doctor notifies the USOC, International Olympic Committee, or National Governing Body in writing. The National Collegiate Athletic Association (NCAA) allows the use of adrenocorticoids or corticotropin but requires that your doctor notify them. The NCAA doctor must then approve of their use.

Other medicines—Although certain medicines should not be used together at all, in other cases two different medicines may be used together even if an interaction might occur. In these cases, your doctor may want to change the dose, or other precautions may be necessary. When you are taking adrenocorticoids or corticotropin, it is especially important that your doctor and pharmacist know if you are taking any of the following:

- Aminoglutethimide or
- Antacids (in large amounts) or

- Barbiturates, except butalbital, or
- Carbamazepine (e.g., Tegretol) or
- Griseofulvin (e.g., Fulvicin) or
- Mitotane (e.g., Lysodren) or
- Phenylbutazone (e.g., Butazolidin) or
- Phenytoin (e.g., Dilantin) or
- Primidone (e.g., Mysoline) or
- Rifampin (e.g., Rifadin)—Use of these medicines may make corticotropin or certain adrenocorticoids less effective
- Amphotericin B by injection (e.g., Fungizone)—Adrenocorticoids and this medicine decrease the amount of potassium in the blood. Serious side effects could occur if the level of potassium gets too low
- Antidiabetics, oral (diabetes medicine taken by mouth) or
- Insulin—Adrenocorticoids may increase blood glucose (sugar) levels
- Digitalis glycosides (heart medicine)—Adrenocorticoids decrease the amount of potassium in the blood. Digitalis can cause an irregular heartbeat or other problems more commonly if the blood potassium gets too low
- Diuretics (water pills) or
- Medicine containing potassium—Using adrenocorticoids with diuretics may cause the diuretic to be less effective. Also, adrenocorticoids may increase the risk of low blood potassium, which is also a problem with certain diuretics. Potassium supplements or a different type of diuretic is used in treating high blood pressure in those people who have problems keeping their blood potassium at a normal level. Adrenocorticoids may make these medicines less able to do this
- Immunizations (vaccinations)—While you are being treated with this medicine, and even after you stop taking it, do not have any immunizations without your doctor's approval. Also, other people living in your home should not receive oral polio vaccine, since there is a chance they could pass the polio virus on to you. In addition, you should avoid close contact with other people at school or work who have recently taken oral polio vaccine
- Skin test injections—Adrenocorticoids may cause false results in skin tests
- Sodium-containing medicine—Adrenocorticoids and corticotropin cause the body to retain (keep) more salt and water. Too much sodium may cause high blood sodium, high blood pressure, and excess body water

Other medical problems—The presence of other medical problems may affect the use of adrenocorticoids and corticotropin. Make sure you tell your doctor if you have any other medical problems, especially:

- Bone disease—These medicines may worsen bone disease because they cause the body to lose more calcium

- Colitis or
- Diverticulitis or
- Stomach ulcer or other stomach or intestine problems—These medicines may cover up symptoms of a worsening stomach or intestinal condition. A patient would not know if his/her condition was getting worse and would not get medical help when needed

- Diabetes mellitus (sugar diabetes)—Adrenocorticoids may cause a loss of control of diabetes by increasing blood glucose (sugar)

- Fungus infection or any other infection or
- Herpes simplex infection of the eye or
- Infection at the place of treatment or
- Recent surgery or serious injury or
- Tuberculosis (active TB, nonactive TB, or past history of)—These medicines can cause slower healing, worsen existing infections, or cause new infections

- Glaucoma—Adrenocorticoids may cause the pressure within the eye to increase

- Heart disease or
- High blood pressure or
- Kidney disease (especially if you are receiving dialysis) or
- Kidney stones—These medicines cause the body to retain (keep) more salt and water. These conditions may be made worse by this extra body water

- High cholesterol levels—Adrenocorticoids may increase blood cholesterol levels

- Liver disease or
- Overactive thyroid or
- Underactive thyroid—With these conditions, the body may not eliminate the adrenocorticoid at the usual rate, which may change the medicine's effect

- Myasthenia gravis—When these medicines are first started, muscle weakness may occur. Your doctor may want to take special precautions because this could cause problems with breathing

- Systemic lupus erythematosus (SLE)—This condition may cause certain side effects of adrenocorticoids to occur more easily

Before you begin using any new medicine (prescription or nonprescription) or if you develop any new medical problem while you are using this medicine, check with your doctor, nurse, or pharmacist.

Proper Use of This Medicine

For patients taking this medicine by mouth:

- *Take this medicine with food* to help prevent stomach upset. If stomach upset, burning, or pain continues, check with your doctor.
- Stomach problems may be more likely to occur if you drink alcoholic beverages while being treated with this medicine. You should not drink alcoholic beverages while taking this medicine, unless you have first checked with your doctor.

For patients using this medicine rectally:

- This medicine usually comes with patient directions. Read them carefully before using this medicine.
- For patients using hydrocortisone enema:

—Each bottle contains a single dose. Use it all, unless otherwise directed by your doctor.

—For best results, use this medicine right after a bowel movement. Lie down on your left side when giving the enema.

—Insert the rectal tip of the enema applicator gently to prevent damage to the rectal wall.

—Stay on your left side for at least 30 minutes after the enema is given so the medicine can work. If you can, keep the medicine inside the rectum all night.

- For patients using hydrocortisone acetate rectal aerosol foam:

—This medicine is used with a special applicator. Do not insert any part of the aerosol container into the rectum.

- For patients using methylprednisolone acetate for enema:

    —Each bottle contains a single dose. Use it all, unless otherwise directed by your doctor.

    —Insert the rectal tip of the enema applicator gently to prevent damage to the rectal wall.

    —If you have been directed to use this enema slowly (not all at once), shake the bottle once in a while while you are giving the enema.

    —Save your applicator. Refill units of this medicine may be available at a lower cost.

Use this medicine only as directed by your doctor. Do not use more or less of it, do not use it more often, and do not use it for a longer time than your doctor ordered. To do so may increase the chance of side effects.

Missed dose—If you miss a dose of this medicine and your dosing schedule is:

- One dose every other day—Take the missed dose as soon as possible if you remember it the same morning, then go back to your regular dosing schedule. If you do not remember the missed dose until later, wait and take it the following morning. Then skip a day and start your regular dosing schedule again.

- One dose a day—Take the missed dose as soon as possible, then go back to your regular dosing schedule. If you do not remember until the next day, skip the missed dose and do not double the next one.

- Several doses a day—Take the missed dose as soon as possible, then go back to your regular dosing schedule. If you do not remember until your next dose is due, double the next dose.

If you have any questions about this, check with your doctor, nurse, or pharmacist.

Storage—To store this medicine:

- Keep out of the reach of children.
- Store away from heat and direct light.

- Do not store tablets in the bathroom, near the kitchen sink, or in other damp places. Heat or moisture may cause the medicine to break down.
- Keep the liquid dosage forms of this medicine, including enemas, and hydrocortisone rectal aerosol foam from freezing.
- Do not puncture, break, or burn the hydrocortisone rectal aerosol foam container, even when it is empty.
- Do not keep outdated medicine or medicine no longer needed. Be sure that any discarded medicine is out of the reach of children.

Precautions While Using This Medicine

Your doctor should check your progress at regular visits. Also, your progress may have to be checked after you have stopped using this medicine, since some of the effects may continue.

Do not stop using this medicine without first checking with your doctor. Your doctor may want you to reduce gradually the amount you are using before stopping completely.

Check with your doctor if your condition reappears or worsens after the dose has been reduced or treatment with this medicine is stopped.

If you will be using adrenocorticoids or corticotropin for a long time:

- *Your doctor may want you to follow a low-salt diet and/or a potassium-rich diet.*
- Your doctor may want you to watch your calories to prevent weight gain.
- Your doctor may want you to add extra protein to your diet.
- Your doctor may want you to have your eyes examined by an ophthalmologist (eye doctor) before and also sometime later during treatment.
- Your doctor may want you to carry a medical identification card stating that you are using this medicine.

Tell the doctor in charge that you are using this medicine:

- *Before having skin tests.*
- *Before having any kind of surgery (including dental surgery) or emergency treatment.*
- *If you get a serious infection or injury.*

While you are being treated with this medicine, and after you stop taking it, *do not have any immunizations without your doctor's approval.* Also, other people living in your home should not receive oral polio vaccine, since there is a chance they could pass the polio virus on to you. In addition, you should avoid close contact with other people at school or work who have recently taken oral polio vaccine.

For diabetic patients:

- This medicine may affect blood sugar levels. If you notice a change in the results of your blood or urine sugar tests or if you have any questions, check with your doctor.

For patients having this medicine injected into their joints:

- If this medicine is injected into one of your joints, you should be careful not to put too much stress or strain on that joint for a while, even if it begins to feel better. Make sure your doctor has told you how much you are allowed to move this joint while it is healing.
- If redness or swelling occurs at the place of injection, and continues or gets worse, check with your doctor.

For patients using this medicine rectally:

- Check with your doctor if you notice rectal bleeding, pain, burning, itching, blistering, or any other sign of irritation not present before you started using this medicine, or if signs of infection occur.

Side Effects of This Medicine

Adrenocorticoids or corticotropin may lower your resistance to infections. Also, any infection you get may be harder to treat. Always check with your doctor as soon as possible if you notice any signs of a possible infection, such as sore throat, fever, sneezing, or coughing.

Along with its needed effects, a medicine may cause some
unwanted effects. Although not all of these side effects may
occur, if they do occur they may need medical attention.
When this medicine is used for short periods of time, side
effects usually are rare. However, check with your doctor
as soon as possible if any of the following side effects occur:

> *Less common*
>
>> Decreased or blurred vision; frequent urination; increased
>> thirst; rectal bleeding, blistering, burning, itching, or pain
>> not present before use of this medicine (when used rec-
>> tally)
>
> *Rare*
>
>> Blindness (sudden, when injected in the head or neck area);
>> confusion; excitement; false sense of well-being; halluci-
>> nations (seeing, hearing, or feeling things that are not
>> there); mental depression; mood swings (sudden and wide);
>> mistaken feelings of self-importance or being mistreated;
>> redness, swelling, pain, or other sign of allergy or infection
>> at place of injection; restlessness

Additional side effects may occur if you take this medicine
for a long time. Check with your doctor if any of the following side effects occur:

> Abdominal or stomach pain or burning (continuing); acne or
> other skin problems; bloody or black, tarry stools; filling or
> rounding out of the face; irregular heartbeat; menstrual prob-
> lems; muscle cramps or pain; muscle weakness; nausea; pain
> in back, hips, ribs, arms, shoulders, or legs; pitting, scarring,
> or depression of skin at place of injection; reddish purple
> lines on arms, face, legs, trunk, or groin; swelling of feet or
> lower legs; thin, shiny skin; unusual bruising; unusual tired-
> ness or weakness; vomiting; weight gain (rapid); wounds that
> will not heal

Other side effects may occur that usually do not need medical attention. These side effects may go away during treatment as your body adjusts to the medicine. However, check

with your doctor if any of the following side effects continue or are bothersome:

More common

Increased appetite; indigestion; loss of appetite (for triamcinolone only); nervousness or restlessness; trouble in sleeping

Less common or rare

Darkening or lightening of skin color; dizziness; flushing of face or cheeks (after injection into the nose); headache; increased joint pain (after injection into a joint); increased sweating; lightheadedness; nosebleeds (after injection into the nose); unusual increase in hair growth on body or face

After you stop using this medicine, your body may need time to adjust. The length of time this takes depends on the amount of medicine you were using and how long you used it. If you have taken large doses of this medicine for a long time, your body may need one year to adjust. During this time, *check with your doctor immediately if any of the following side effects occur:*

Abdominal, stomach, or back pain; dizziness; fainting; fever; loss of appetite (continuing); muscle or joint pain; nausea; reappearance of disease symptoms; shortness of breath; unexplained headaches (frequent or continuing); unusual tiredness or weakness; vomiting; weight loss (rapid)

Other side effects not listed above may also occur in some patients. If you notice any other effects, check with your doctor.

COUGH/COLD COMBINATIONS Systemic

Some commonly used brand names are:

In the U.S.—

Actagen-C Cough[41]
Actifed with Codeine Cough[41]
Adatuss D.C. Expectorant[97]
Alamine-C Liquid[28]
Alamine Expectorant[113]
Allerfrin with Codeine[41]
Ambay Cough[1]
Ambenyl Cough[1]
Ambenyl-D Decongestant
    Cough Formula[114]
Ambophen Expectorant[9]
Ami-Tex LA[121]
Anamine HD[23]
Anatuss[74]
Anatuss with Codeine[75]
Anti-Tuss DM Expectorant[94]
Banex[120]
Banex-LA[121]
Banex Liquid[120]
Bayaminic Expectorant[121]
Bayaminicol[27]
Baycodan[89]
Baycomine[103]
Baycomine Pediatric[103]
BayCotussend Liquid[106]
Baydec DM Drops[20]
Bayhistine DH[28]
Bayhistine Expectorant[113]
Baytussin AC[91]
Baytussin DM[94]
Benylin Expectorant
    Cough Formula[94]
Biphetane DC Cough[19]
Brexin[81]
Bromanate DC Cough[19]
Bromfed-AT[19b]
Bromfed-DM[19b]
Bromphen DC with Codeine
    Cough[19]
Broncholate[118]
Bronkotuss Expectorant[82]
Brotane DX Cough[19b]
Calcidrine[90]
Carbinoxamine Compound[20]
Carbodec DM Drops[20]
Cerose-DM[22]
Cheracol[91]

Cheracol D Cough[94]
Cheracol Plus[27]
Children's NyQuil Nighttime
    Cold Medicine[29]
Chlorgest-HD[23]
Citra Forte[15 44]
Co-Apap[50]
Codamine[103]
Codamine Pediatric[103]
Codan[89]
Codegest Expectorant[111]
Codehist DH[28]
Codiclear DH[97]
Codimal DH[40]
Codimal DM[39]
Codimal Expectorant[121]
Codimal PH[38]
Codistan No. 1[94]
Comtrex Multi-Symptom
    Cold Reliever[48]
Comtrex Daytime Caplets[108]
Comtrex Multi-Symptom
    Non-Drowsy Caplets[108]
Comtrex Nighttime[50]
Conar[100]
Conar-A[116]
Conar Expectorant[109]
Concentrin[114]
Conex[121]
Conex with Codeine
    Liquid[111]
Congess JR[122]
Congess SR[122]
Contac Jr. Children's Cold
    Medicine[107]
Contac Severe Cold
    Formula[50]
Contac Severe Cold Formula
    Night Strength[51]
Cophene-S[26]
Cophene-X[64]
Cophene-XP[64]
Coricidin Cough[112]
CoTylenol Cold Medication[50]
C-Tussin Expectorant[113]
DayCare[117]

Deproist Expectorant with Codeine[113]
De-Tuss[106]
Detussin Expectorant[115]
Detussin Liquid[106]
Dihistine DH[28]
Dilaudid Cough[99]
Dimacol[114]
Dimetane-DC Cough[19]
Dimetane-DX Cough[19b]
Dimetapp DM Cold and Cough[19a]
Donatussin[62]
Donatussin DC[110]
Donatussin Drops[83]
Dondril[22]
Dorcol Children's Cough[114]
Dura-Vent[121]
Efficol Cough Whip (Cough Suppressant/Decongestant)[102]
Efficol Cough Whip (Cough Suppressant/Decongestant/Antihistamine)[27]
Efficol Cough Whip (Cough Suppressant/Expectorant)[94]
Efricon Expectorant Liquid[60]
Endal-HD[23]
Entex[120]
Entex LA[121]
Entex Liquid[120]
Entex PSE[122]
Entuss-D[106 115]
Entuss Expectorant[97 98]
Entuss Pediatric Expectorant[115]
Extra Action Cough[94]
Father John's Medicine Plus[63]
Fedahist Expectorant[122]
Fedahist Expectorant Pediatric Drops[122]
Fendol[123]
2/G-DM Cough[94]
Gentab-LA[121]
Glycotuss-dM[94]
Glydeine Cough[91]
Guaifed[122]

Guaifed-PD[122]
Guaipax[121]
Guaitab[122]
Guiamid D.M. Liquid[94]
Guiatuss A.C.[91]
Guiatuss-DM[94]
Guiatussin with Codeine Liquid[91]
Halotussin-DM Expectorant[94]
Histafed C[41]
Histalet X[122]
Histatuss Pediatric[21]
Hold (Children's Formula)[102]
Hycodan[89]
Hycomine[103]
Hycomine Compound[47]
Hycomine Pediatric[103]
Hycotuss Expectorant[97]
Hydromine[103]
Hydromine Pediatric[103]
Hydropane[89]
Hydrophen[103]
Improved Sino-Tuss[46]
Iophen-C Liquid[92]
Iotuss[92]
Iotuss-DM[95]
Ipsatol Cough Formula for Children[112]
Isoclor Expectorant[113]
Kiddy Koff[112]
KIE[119]
Kolephrin/DM[49]
Kolephrin GG/DM[94]
Kolephrin NN Liquid[54]
Kophane[65]
Kophane Cough and Cold Formula[27]
Kwelcof Liquid[97]
Lanatuss Expectorant[85]
Mallergan-VC with Codeine[37]
Meda Syrup Forte[62]
Medatussin[94a]
Medatussin Plus[67a]
Medi-Flu[50]
Medi-Flu Caplets[50]
Mediquell Decongestant Formula[105]

Midahist DH[28]
Mycotussin[106]
Myhistine DH[28]
Myhistine Expectorant[113]
Myhydromine[103]
Myhydromine Pediatric[103]
Myphetane DC Cough[19]
Mytussin AC[91]
Mytussin DAC[113]
Mytussin DM[94]
Naldecon-CX Adult
  Liquid[111]
Naldecon-DX Adult
  Liquid[112]
Naldecon-DX
  Children's Syrup[112]
Naldecon-DX Pediatric
  Drops[112]
Naldecon-EX[121]
Naldecon Senior DX[94]
Nolex LA[121]
Noratuss II Liquid[114]
Normatane DC[19]
Nortussin with Codeine[91]
Novahistine DH Liquid[28]
Novahistine DMX Liquid[114]
Novahistine Expectorant[113]
Nucochem[104]
Nucochem Expectorant[113]
Nucochem Pediatric
  Expectorant[113]
Nucofed[104]
Nucofed Expectorant[113]
Nucofed Pediatric
  Expectorant[113]
NyQuil Liquicaps[50a]
NyQuil Nighttime Colds
  Medicine[51]
Nytime Cold Medicine
  Liquid[51]
Omnicol[43]
Orthoxicol Cough[27]
Par Glycerol C[92]
Par Glycerol DM[95]
PediaCare Children's Cold
  Relief Night Rest Cough-
  Cold Formula[29]

PediaCare Children's Cough-
  Cold Formula[29]
Pediacof Cough[61]
Pertussin AM[114]
Pertussin CS[94]
Pertussin PM[51]
Phanadex[72a]
Phanatuss[94a]
Phenameth VC with
  Codeine[37]
Phenergan with Codeine[5]
Phenergan with
  Dextromethorphan[6]
Phenergan VC with
  Codeine[37]
Phenhist Expectorant[113]
Phenylfenesin L.A.[121]
Pherazine VC with Codeine[37]
Polaramine Expectorant[87]
Poly-Histine-CS[19]
Poly-Histine-DM[19a]
Prometh VC with Codeine[37]
Prominic Expectorant[121]
Prominicol Cough[69]
Promist HD Liquid[30]
Pseudo-Car DM[20]
Pseudodine C Cough[41]
P-V-Tussin[13 58]
Quelidrine Cough[57]
Queltuss[94]
Remcol-C[8]
Rentamine
  Pediatric[21]
Rescaps-D S.R.[101]
Respaire-60 SR[122]
Respaire-120 SR[122]
Respinol-G[120]
Rhinosyn-DM[29]
Rhinosyn-DMX
  Expectorant[94]
Rhinosyn-X[114]
Robitussin A-C[91]
Robitussin-CF[112]
Robitussin-DAC[113]
Robitussin-DM[94]
Robitussin Night Relief[53]
Robitussin Night Relief
  Colds Formula Liquid[53]

Robitussin-PE[122]
Rondec-DM[20]
Rondec-DM Drops[20]
Ru-Tuss DE[122]
Ru-Tuss Expectorant[114]
Ru-Tuss with Hydrocodone Liquid[34]
Rymed[120]
Rymed Liquid[120]
Rymed-TR[122]
Ryna-C Liquid[28]
Ryna-CX Liquid[113]
Rynatuss[21]
Rynatuss Pediatric[21]
Saleto-CF[107]
Silexin Cough[94]
Sinufed Timecelles[122]
Snaplets-DM[102]
Snaplets-EX[121]
Snaplets-Multi[27]
SRC Expectorant[115]
Sudafed Cough[114]
Sudafed Severe Cold Formula Caplets[108]
Syracol Liquid[102]
TheraFlu/Flu, Cold and Cough Medicine[50]
T-Koff[24]
Tolu-Sed Cough[91]
Tolu-Sed DM Cough[94]
Triacin C Cough[41]
Triaminic-DM Cough Formula[102]
Triaminic Expectorant[121]
Triaminic Expectorant with Codeine[111]
Triaminic Nite Light[29]
Triaminicol Multi-Symptom Relief[27]
Tricodene Forte[27]
Tricodene NN[27]
Tricodene Pediatric[102]
Trifed-C Cough[41]
Trimedine Liquid[22]
Trind DM Liquid[27]

Trinex[86]
Triphenyl Expectorant[121]
Tusquelin[25]
Tuss-Ade[101]
Tussafed[20]
Tuss Allergine Modified T.D.[101]
Tussanil DH[23 76]
Tussar-2[10]
Tussar DM[29]
Tussar SF[10]
Tuss-DM[94]
Tussigon[89]
Tussionex[3a 4]
Tussi-Organidin DM Liquid[95]
Tussi-Organidin Liquid[92]
Tussirex with Codeine Liquid[78]
Tuss-LA[122]
Tusso-DM[95]
Tussogest[101]
Tuss-Ornade Liquid[101]
Tuss-Ornade Spansules[101]
Ty-Cold Cold Formula[50]
Tylenol Cold and Flu[50]
Tylenol Cold Medication[50]
Tylenol Cold Medication, Non-Drowsy[108]
Tylenol Cold Night Time[50a]
Tylenol Cough[108]
Unproco[94]
Utex-S.R.[121]
Vanex Expectorant[115]
Vanex-HD[23]
Vicks Children's Cough[94]
Vicks Formula 44 Cough Mixture[3]
Vicks Formula 44D Decongestant Cough Mixture[114]
Vicks Formula 44M Multi-symptom Cough Mixture[117]
Viro-Med[77]
Zephrex[122]
Zephrex-LA[122]

In Canada—

Actifed DM[42]
Benylin with Codeine[11]
Benylin-DM[12]
Caldomine-DH Forte[36]
Caldomine-DH Pediatric[36]
Calmylin with Codeine[11]
CoActifed[41]
CoActifed Expectorant[73]
Coricidin with Codeine[7]
Coristex-DH[33]
Coristine-DH[33]
Dimetane Expectorant[80]
Dimetane Expectorant-C[55]
Dimetane Expectorant-DC[56]
Dimetapp with Codeine[17]
Dimetapp-DM[18]
Dorcol DM[112]
Entex LA[121]
Hycomine[72]
Hycomine-S Pediatric[72]
Novahistex C[31]
Novahistex DH[33]
Novahistex DH
  Expectorant[68]
Novahistex DM[32]

Novahistine DH[33]
Novahistine DH
  Expectorant[68]
Omni-Tuss[67]
Ornade-DM 10[27]
Ornade-DM 15[27]
Ornade-DM 30[27]
Ornade Expectorant[84]
Robitussin A-C[14]
Robitussin with Codeine[14]
Sudafed DM[105]
Sudafed Expectorant[122]
Triaminic-DM Expectorant[70]
Triaminic Expectorant[88]
Triaminic Expectorant DH[71]
Triaminicin with Codeine[52]
Triaminicol DM[35]
Tylenol Cold Medication[50]
Tylenol Cold Medication,
  Non-Drowsy[108]
Tussaminic C Forte[34a]
Tussaminic C Pediatric[34a]
Tussaminic DH Forte[36]
Tussaminic DH Pediatric[36]
Tussionex[4]
Tuss-Ornade Spansules[26a]

Note: For quick reference the following cough/cold combinations are numbered to match the preceding corresponding brand names.

Antihistamine and antitussive combinations—

1. Bromodiphenhydramine (broe-moe-dye-fen-HYE-dra-meen) and Codeine (KOE-deen)
2. No product available
3. Chlorpheniramine (klor-fen-EER-a-meen) and Dextromethorphan (dex-troe-meth-OR-fan)
3a. Chlorpheniramine and Hydrocodone (hye-droe-KOE-done)
4. Phenyltoloxamine (fen-ill-tole-OX-a-meen) and Hydrocodone
5. Promethazine (proe-METH-a-zeen) and Codeine†
6. Promethazine and Dextromethorphan

Antihistamine, antitussive, and analgesic combinations—

7. Chlorpheniramine (klor-fen-EER-a-meen), Codeine (KOE-deen), Aspirin, and Caffeine (kaf-EEN)
8. Chlorpheniramine, Dextromethorphan (dex-troe-meth-OR-fan), and Acetaminophen (a-seat-a-MIN-oh-fen)

Antihistamine, antitussive, and expectorant combinations—

9. Bromodiphenhydramine (broe-moe-dye-fen-HYE-dra-meen), Diphenhydramine (dye-fen-HYE-dra-meen), Codeine (KOE-deen), Ammonium Chloride (a-MOE-nee-um KLOR-ide), and Potassium Guaiacolsulfonate (poe-TAS-ee-um gwye-a-kol-SUL-fon-ate)

10. Chlorpheniramine (klor-fen-EER-a-meen), Codeine, and Guaifenesin (gwye-FEN-e-sin)
11. Diphenhydramine, Codeine, and Ammonium Chloride
12. Diphenhydramine, Dextromethorphan (dex-troe-meth-OR-fan), and Ammonium Chloride
13. Phenindamine (fen-IN-da-meen), Hydrocodone (hye-droe-KOE-done), and Guaifenesin
14. Pheniramine (fen-EER-a-meen), Codeine, and Guaifenesin
15. Pheniramine, Pyrilamine (peer-ILL-a-meen), Hydrocodone, and Potassium Citrate (poe-TAS-ee-um SI-trate)
16. No product available.

Antihistamine, decongestant, and antitussive combinations—

17. Brompheniramine (brome-fen-EER-a-meen), Phenylephrine (fen-ill-EF-rin), Phenylpropanolamine (fen-ill-proe-pa-NOLE-a-meen), and Codeine (KOE-deen)
18. Brompheniramine, Phenylephrine, Phenylpropanolamine, and Dextromethorphan (dex-troe-meth-OR-fan)
19. Brompheniramine, Phenylpropanolamine, and Codeine
19a. Brompheniramine, Phenylpropanolamine, and Dextromethorphan
19b. Brompheniramine, Pseudoephedrine (soo-doe-e-FED-rin), and Dextromethorphan
20. Carbinoxamine (kar-bi-NOX-a-meen), Pseudoephedrine, and Dextromethorphan
21. Chlorpheniramine (klor-fen-EER-a-meen), Ephedrine (e-FED-rin), Phenylephrine, and Carbetapentane (kar-bay-ta-PEN-tane)
22. Chlorpheniramine, Phenylephrine, and Dextromethorphan
23. Chlorpheniramine, Phenylephrine, and Hydrocodone (hye-droe-KOE-done)
24. Chlorpheniramine, Phenylephrine, Phenylpropanolamine, and Codeine
25. Chlorpheniramine, Phenylephrine, Phenylpropanolamine, and Dextromethorphan
26. Chlorpheniramine, Phenylephrine, Phenylpropanolamine, and Dihydrocodeine (dye-hye-droe-KOE-deen)
26a. Chlorpheniramine, Phenylpropanolamine, and Caramiphen (kar-AM-i-fen)
27. Chlorpheniramine, Phenylpropanolamine, and Dextromethorphan
28. Chlorpheniramine, Pseudoephedrine, and Codeine
29. Chlorpheniramine, Pseudoephedrine, and Dextromethorphan
30. Chlorpheniramine, Pseudoephedrine, and Hydrocodone
31. Diphenylpyraline (dye-fen-il-PEER-a-leen), Phenylephrine, and Codeine
32. Diphenylpyraline, Phenylephrine, and Dextromethorphan
33. Diphenylpyraline, Phenylephrine, and Hydrocodone
34. Pheniramine (fen-EER-a-meen), Pyrilamine (peer-ILL-a-meen), Phenylephrine, Phenylpropanolamine, and Hydrocodone
34a. Pheniramine, Pyrilamine, Phenylpropanolamine, and Codeine
35. Pheniramine, Pyrilamine, Phenylpropanolamine, and Dextromethorphan
36. Pheniramine, Pyrilamine, Phenylpropanolamine, and Hydrocodone

37. Promethazine (proe-METH-a-zeen), Phenylephrine, and Codeine
38. Pyrilamine, Phenylephrine, and Codeine
39. Pyrilamine, Phenylephrine, and Dextromethorphan
40. Pyrilamine, Phenylephrine, and Hydrocodone
41. Triprolidine (trye-PROE-li-deen), Pseudoephedrine, and Codeine
42. Triprolidine, Pseudoephedrine, and Dextromethorphan

Antihistamine, decongestant, antitussive, and analgesic combinations—

43. Chlorpheniramine (klor-fen-EER-a-meen), Phenindamine (fen-IN-da-meen), Phenylephrine (fen-ill-EF-rin), Dextromethorphan (dex-troe-meth-OR-fan), Acetaminophen (a-seat-a-MIN-oh-fen), Salicylamide (sal-i-SILL-a-mide), Caffeine (kaf-EEN), and Ascorbic (a-SKOR-bik) Acid
44. Chlorpheniramine, Pheniramine (fen-EER-a-meen), Pyrilamine (peer-ILL-a-meen), Phenylephrine, Hydrocodone (hye-droe-KOE-done), Salicylamide, Caffeine, and Ascorbic Acid
45. No product available
46. Chlorpheniramine, Phenylephrine, Dextromethorphan, Acetaminophen, and Salicylamide
47. Chlorpheniramine, Phenylephrine, Hydrocodone (hye-droe-KOE-done), Acetaminophen, and Caffeine
48. Chlorpheniramine, Phenylpropanolamine (fen-ill-proe-pa-NOLE-a-meen), Dextromethorphan, and Acetaminophen
49. Chlorpheniramine, Phenylpropanolamine, Dextromethorphan, Acetaminophen, and Caffeine
50. Chlorpheniramine, Pseudoephedrine (soo-doe-e-FED-rin), Dextromethorphan, and Acetaminophen
50a. Diphenhydramine (dye-fen-HYE-dra-meen), Pseudoephedrine, Dextromethorphan, and Acetaminophen
51. Doxylamine (dox-ILL-a-meen), Pseudoephedrine, Dextromethorphan, and Acetaminophen
52. Pheniramine, Pyrilamine, Phenylpropanolamine, Codeine, Acetaminophen, and Caffeine
53. Pyrilamine, Phenylephrine, Dextromethorphan, and Acetaminophen
54. Pyrilamine, Phenylpropanolamine, Dextromethorphan, and Sodium Salicylate (sa-LI-si-late)

Antihistamine, decongestant, antitussive, and expectorant combinations—

55. Brompheniramine (brome-fen-EER-a-meen), Phenylephrine (fen-ill-EF-rin), Phenylpropanolamine (fen-ill-proe-pa-NOLE-a-meen), Codeine (KOE-deen), and Guaifenesin (gwye-FEN-e-sin)
56. Brompheniramine, Phenylephrine, Phenylpropanolamine, Hydrocodone (hye-droe-KOE-done), and Guaifenesin
57. Chlorpheniramine, Ephedrine, Phenylephrine, Dextromethorphan (dex-troe-meth-OR-fan), Ammonium Chloride, and Ipecac (IP-e-kak)
58. Chlorpheniramine, Phenindamine (fen-IN-da-meen), Pyrilamine (peer-ILL-a-meen), Phenylephrine, Hydrocodone, and Ammonium Chloride
59. No product available

60. Chlorpheniramine, Phenylephrine, Codeine, Ammonium Chloride, Potassium Guaiacolsulfonate (poe-TAS-ee-um gwye-a-kol-SUL-fon-ate), and Sodium Citrate (SOE-dee-um SI-trate)

61. Chlorpheniramine, Phenylephrine, Codeine, and Potassium Iodide (EYE-oh-dyed)

62. Chlorpheniramine, Phenylephrine, Dextromethorphan, and Guaifenesin

63. Chlorpheniramine, Phenylephrine, Dextromethorphan, Guaifenesin, and Ammonium Chloride

64. Chlorpheniramine, Phenylephrine, Phenylpropanolamine, Carbetapentane (kar-bay-ta-PEN-tane), and Potassium Guaiacolsulfonate

65. Chlorpheniramine, Phenylpropanolamine, Dextromethorphan, and Ammonium Chloride

66. No product available

67. Chlorpheniramine, Phenyltoloxamine (fen-ill-tole-OX-a-meen), Ephedrine, Codeine, and Guaiacol Carbonate (GYWE-a-kole KAR-bone-ate)

67a. Chlorpheniramine, Phenyltoloxamine, Phenylpropanolamine, Dextromethorphan, and Guaifenesin

68. Diphenylpyraline (dye-fen-il-PEER-a-leen), Phenylephrine, Hydrocodone, and Guaifenesin

69. Pheniramine (fen-EER-a-meen), Pyrilamine, Phenylpropanolamine, Dextromethorphan, and Ammonium Chloride

70. Pheniramine, Pyrilamine, Phenylpropanolamine, Dextromethorphan, and Guaifenesin

71. Pheniramine, Pyrilamine, Phenylpropanolamine, Hydrocodone, and Guaifenesin

72. Pyrilamine, Phenylephrine, Hydrocodone, and Ammonium Chloride

72a. Pyrilamine, Phenylpropanolamine, Dextromethorphan, Guaifenesin, Potassium Citrate, and Citric Acid

73. Triprolidine (trye-PROE-li-deen), Pseudoephedrine (soo-doe-e-FED-rin), Codeine, and Guaifenesin

Antihistamine, decongestant, antitussive, expectorant, and analgesic combinations—

74. Chlorpheniramine (klor-fen-EER-a-meen), Phenylephrine (fen-ill-EF-rin), Phenylpropanolamine (fen-ill-proe-pa-NOLE-a-meen), Dextromethorphan (dex-troe-meth-OR-fan), Guaifenesin (gwye-FEN-e-sin), and Acetaminophen (a-seat-a-MIN-oh-fen)

75. Chlorpheniramine, Phenylpropanolamine, Codeine (KOE-deen), Guaifenesin, and Acetaminophen

76. Chlorpheniramine, Phenylpropanolamine, Hydrocodone (hye-droe-KOE-done), Guaifenesin, and Salicylamide (sal-i-SILL-a-mide)

77. Chlorpheniramine, Pseudoephedrine (soo-doe-e-FED-rin), Dextromethorphan, Guaifenesin, and Aspirin

78. Pheniramine (fen-EER-a-meen), Phenylephrine, Codeine, Sodium Citrate (SOE-dee-um SI-trate), Sodium Salicylate (sa-LI-sill-ate), and Caffeine (kaf-EEN)

79. No product available

Antihistamine, decongestant, and expectorant combinations—

80. Brompheniramine (brome-fen-EER-a-meen), Phenylephrine (fen-ill-EF-rin), Phenylpropanolamine (fen-ill-proe-pa-NOLE-a-meen), and Guaifenesin (gwye-FEN-e-sin)
81. Carbinoxamine (kar-bi-NOX-a-meen), Pseudoephedrine (soo-doe-e-FED-rin), and Guaifenesin
82. Chlorpheniramine (klor-fen-EER-a-meen), Ephedrine (e-FED-rin), and Guaifenesin
83. Chlorpheniramine, Phenylephrine, and Guaifenesin
84. Chlorpheniramine, Phenylpropanolamine, and Guaifenesin
85. Chlorpheniramine, Phenylpropanolamine, Guaifenesin, Sodium Citrate (SOE-dee-um SI-trate), and Citric (SI-trik) Acid
86. Chlorpheniramine, Pseudoephedrine, and Guaifenesin
87. Dexchlorpheniramine (dex-klor-fen-EER-a-meen), Pseudoephedrine, and Guaifenesin
88. Pheniramine (fen-EER-a-meen), Pyrilamine (peer-ILL-a-meen), Phenylpropanolamine, and Guaifenesin

Antitussive and anticholinergic combination—

89. Hydrocodone (hye-droe-KOE-done) and Homatropine (hoe-MA-troe-peen)†

Antitussive and expectorant combinations—

90. Codeine (KOE-deen) and Calcium Iodide (KAL-see-um EYE-oh-dyed)
91. Codeine and Guaifenesin (gwye-FEN-e-sin)
92. Codeine and Iodinated Glycerol (EYE-oh-di-nay-ted GLI-ser-ole)
93. No product available.
94. Dextromethorphan and Guaifenesin
94a. Dextromethorphan, Guaifenesin, Potassium Citrate, and Citric Acid
95. Dextromethorphan and Iodinated Glycerol
96. No product available.
97. Hydrocodone (hye-droe-KOE-done) and Guaifenesin
98. Hydrocodone and Potassium Guaiacolsulfonate
99. Hydromorphone (hye-droe-MOR-fone) and Guaifenesin

Decongestant and antitussive combinations—

100. Phenylephrine (fen-ill-EF-rin) and Dextromethorphan (dex-troe-meth-OR-fan)
101. Phenylpropanolamine (fen-ill-proe-pa-NOLE-a-meen) and Caramiphen (kar-AM-i-fen)
102. Phenylpropanolamine and Dextromethorphan
103. Phenylpropanolamine and Hydrocodone (hye-droe-KOE-done)
104. Pseudoephedrine (soo-doe-e-FED-rin) and Codeine (KOE-deen)
105. Pseudoephedrine and Dextromethorphan
106. Pseudoephedrine and Hydrocodone

Decongestant, antitussive, and analgesic combinations—

107. Phenylpropanolamine (fen-ill-proe-pa-NOLE-a-meen), Dextromethorphan (dex-troe-meth-OR-fan), and Acetaminophen (a-seat-a-MIN-oh-fen)
108. Pseudoephedrine (soo-doe-e-FED-rin), Dextromethorphan, and Acetaminophen

Decongestant, antitussive, and expectorant combinations—
109. Phenylephrine (fen-ill-EF-rin), Dextromethorphan (dex-troe-meth-OR-fan), and Guaifenesin (gwye-FEN-e-sin)
110. Phenylephrine, Hydrocodone (hye-droe-KOE-done), and Guaifenesin
111. Phenylpropanolamine (fen-ill-proe-pa-NOLE-a-meen), Codeine (KOE-deen), and Guaifenesin
112. Phenylpropanolamine, Dextromethorphan, and Guaifenesin
113. Pseudoephedrine (soo-doe-e-FED-rin), Codeine, and Guaifenesin
114. Pseudoephedrine, Dextromethorphan, and Guaifenesin
115. Pseudoephedrine, Hydrocodone, and Guaifenesin

Decongestant, antitussive, expectorant, and analgesic combinations—
116. Phenylephrine (fen-ill-EF-rin), Dextromethorphan (dex-troe-meth-OR-fan), Guaifenesin (gwye-FEN-e-sin), and Acetaminophen (a-seat-a-MIN-oh-fen)
117. Pseudoephedrine (soo-doe-e-FED-rin), Dextromethorphan, Guaifenesin, and Acetaminophen

Decongestant and expectorant combinations—
118. Ephedrine (e-FED-rin) and Guaifenesin (gwye-FEN-e-sin)
119. Ephedrine and Potassium Iodide (poe-TAS-ee-um EYE-oh-dyed)
120. Phenylephrine (fen-ill-EF-rin), Phenylpropanolamine (fen-ill-proe-pa-NOLE-a-meen), and Guaifenesin
121. Phenylpropanolamine and Guaifenesin
122. Pseudoephedrine (soo-doe-e-FED-rin) and Guaifenesin

Decongestant, expectorant, and analgesic combination—
123. Phenylephrine (fen-ill-EF-rin), Guaifenesin (gwye-FEN-e-sin), Acetaminophen (a-seat-a-MIN-oh-fen), Salicylamide and Caffeine

---

†Generic name product available in the U.S.

Description

Cough/cold combinations are used mainly to relieve the cough due to colds, influenza, or hay fever. They are not to be used for the chronic cough that occurs with smoking, asthma, or emphysema or when there is an unusually large amount of mucus or phlegm (pronounced flem) with the cough.

Cough/cold combination products contain more than one ingredient. For example, some products may contain an antihistamine, a decongestant, and an analgesic, in addition to a medicine for coughing. If you are treating yourself, it is important to select a product that is best for your symptoms. Also, in general, it is best to buy a product that includes only those medicines you really need. If you have questions about which product to buy, check with your pharmacist.

Since different products contain ingredients that will have different precautions and side effects, it is important that you know the ingredients of the medicine you are taking. The different kinds of ingredients that may be found in cough/cold combinations include:

Antihistamines—Antihistamines are used to relieve or prevent the symptoms of hay fever and other types of allergy. They also help relieve some symptoms of the common cold, such as sneezing and runny nose. They work by preventing the effects of a substance called histamine, which is produced by the body. Some examples of antihistamines contained in these combinations are: chlorpheniramine, diphenhydramine, pheniramine, promethazine, and triprolidine.

Decongestants—Decongestants, such as ephedrine, phenylephrine, phenylpropanolamine (also known as PPA), and pseudoephedrine, produce a narrowing of blood vessels. This leads to clearing of nasal congestion. However, this effect may also increase blood pressure in patients who have high blood pressure.

Antitussives—To help relieve coughing these combinations contain either a narcotic (codeine, dihydrocodeine, hydrocodone or hydromorphone) or a non-narcotic (carbetapentane, dextromethorphan, or noscapine) antitussive. These antitussives act directly on the cough center in the brain. Narcotics may become habit-forming, causing mental or physical dependence, if used for a long time. Physical dependence may lead to withdrawal side effects when you stop taking the medicine.

Expectorants—Guaifenesin works by loosening the mucus or phlegm in the lungs. Other ingredients added as expectorants (for example, ammonium chloride, calcium iodide, iodinated glycerol, ipecac, potassium guaiacolsulfonate, potassium iodide, and sodium citrate) have not been proven to be effective. In general, the best thing you can do to loosen mucus or phlegm is to drink plenty of water.

Analgesics—Analgesics, such as acetaminophen, aspirin, and other salicylates (such as salicylamide and sodium salicylate), are used in these combination medicines to help relieve the aches and pain that may occur with the common cold.

The use of too much acetaminophen and salicylates at the same time may cause kidney damage or cancer of the kidney or urinary bladder. This may occur if large amounts of both medicines are taken together for a long time. However, taking the recommended amounts of combination medicines that contain both acetaminophen and a salicylate for short periods of time has not been shown to cause these unwanted effects.

Anticholinergics—Anticholinergics such as homatropine may help produce a drying effect in the nose and chest.

Some of these combinations are available only with your doctor's prescription. Others are available without a prescription; however, your doctor or pharmacist may have special instructions on the proper dose of the medicine for your medical condition.

Cough/cold combinations are available in the following dosage forms:

Antihistamine and antitussive combinations—
Oral
  Bromodiphenhydramine and Codeine
  • Syrup (U.S.)
  Chlorpheniramine and Dextromethorphan
  • Oral solution (U.S.)
  Chlorpheniramine and Hydrocodone
  • Oral suspension (U.S.)
  Phenyltoloxamine and Hydrocodone
  • Capsules (Canada)
  • Oral suspension (U.S. and Canada)
  Promethazine and Codeine
  • Syrup (U.S.)
  Promethazine and Dextromethorphan
  • Syrup (U.S.)

Antihistamine, antitussive, and analgesic combinations—
Oral

Chlorpheniramine, Codeine, Aspirin, and Caffeine
  • Tablets (Canada)
Chlorpheniramine, Dextromethorphan, and Acetaminophen
  • Capsules (U.S.)

Antihistamine, antitussive, and expectorant combinations—
Oral

Bromodiphenhydramine, Diphenhydramine, Codeine, Ammonium Chloride, and Potassium Guaiacolsulfonate
  • Oral solution (U.S.)
Chlorpheniramine, Codeine, and Guaifenesin
  • Syrup (U.S.)
Diphenhydramine, Codeine, and Ammonium Chloride
  • Syrup (Canada)
Diphenhydramine, Dextromethorphan, and Ammonium Chloride
  • Syrup (Canada)
Phenindamine, Hydrocodone, and Guaifenesin
  • Tablets (U.S.)
Pheniramine, Codeine, and Guaifenesin
  • Syrup (Canada)
Pheniramine, Pyrilamine, Hydrocodone, and Potassium Citrate
  • Syrup (U.S.)

Antihistamine, decongestant, and antitussive combinations—
Oral

Brompheniramine, Phenylephrine, Phenylpropanolamine, and Codeine
  • Tablets (Canada)
Brompheniramine, Phenylephrine, Phenylpropanolamine, and Dextromethorphan
  • Elixir (Canada)
  • Tablets (Canada)
Brompheniramine, Phenylpropanolamine, and Codeine
  • Syrup (U.S.)
Brompheniramine, Phenylpropanolamine, and Dextromethorphan
  • Syrup (U.S.)
Brompheniramine, Pseudoephedrine, and Dextromethorphan
  • Syrup (U.S.)

Carbinoxamine, Pseudoephedrine, and Dextromethorphan
- Oral solution (U.S.)
- Syrup (U.S.)

Chlorpheniramine, Ephedrine, Phenylephrine, and Carbetapentane
- Oral suspension (U.S.)
- Tablets (U.S.)

Chlorpheniramine, Phenylephrine, and Dextromethorphan
- Oral solution (U.S.)
- Tablets (U.S.)

Chlorpheniramine, Phenylephrine, and Hydrocodone
- Syrup (U.S.)

Chlorpheniramine, Phenylephrine, Phenylpropanolamine, and Codeine
- Syrup (U.S.)

Chlorpheniramine, Phenylephrine, Phenylpropanolamine, and Dextromethorphan
- Syrup (U.S.)

Chlorpheniramine, Phenylephrine, Phenylpropanolamine, and Dihydrocodeine
- Syrup (U.S.)

Chlorpheniramine, Phenylpropanolamine, and Caramiphen
- Extended-release capsules (Canada)

Chlorpheniramine, Phenylpropanolamine, and Dextromethorphan
- Granules (U.S.)
- Oral gel (U.S.)
- Oral solution (U.S. and Canada)
- Syrup (U.S.)
- Tablets (U.S.)

Chlorpheniramine, Pseudoephedrine, and Codeine
- Elixir (U.S.)
- Oral solution (U.S.)
- Syrup (U.S.)

Chlorpheniramine, Pseudoephedrine, and Dextromethorphan
- Oral solution (U.S.)
- Syrup (U.S.)

Chlorpheniramine, Pseudoephedrine, and Hydrocodone
- Oral solution (U.S.)

Diphenylpyraline, Phenylephrine, and Codeine
- Oral solution (Canada)

Diphenylpyraline, Phenylephrine, and Dextromethorphan
- Syrup (Canada)

Diphenylpyraline, Phenylephrine, and Hydrocodone
- Oral solution (Canada)
- Syrup (Canada)

Pheniramine, Pyrilamine, Phenylephrine, Phenylpropanolamine, and Hydrocodone
- Oral solution (U.S.)

Pheniramine, Pyrilamine, Phenylpropanolamine, and Codeine
- Syrup (Canada)

Pheniramine, Pyrilamine, Phenylpropanolamine, and Dextromethorphan
- Syrup (Canada)

Pheniramine, Pyrilamine, Phenylpropanolamine, and Hydrocodone
- Oral solution (Canada)

Promethazine, Phenylephrine, and Codeine
- Syrup (U.S.)

Pyrilamine, Phenylephrine, and Codeine
- Syrup (U.S.)

Pyrilamine, Phenylephrine, and Dextromethorphan
- Oral solution (U.S.)

Pyrilamine, Phenylephrine, and Hydrocodone
- Syrup (U.S.)

Triprolidine, Pseudoephedrine, and Codeine
- Syrup (U.S. and Canada)
- Tablets (Canada)

Triprolidine, Pseudoephedrine, and Dextromethorphan
- Oral solution (Canada)

Antihistamine, decongestant, antitussive, and analgesic combinations—
Oral

Chlorpheniramine, Phenindamine, Phenylephrine, Dextromethorphan, Acetaminophen, Salicylamide, Caffeine, and Ascorbic Acid
- Tablets (U.S.)

Chlorpheniramine, Pheniramine, Pyrilamine, Phenylephrine, Hydrocodone, Salicylamide, Caffeine, and Ascorbic Acid
- Capsules (U.S.)

Chlorpheniramine, Phenylephrine, Dextromethorphan, Acetaminophen, and Salicylamide
- Tablets (U.S.)

Chlorpheniramine, Phenylephrine, Hydrocodone, Acetaminophen, and Caffeine
- Tablets (U.S.)

Chlorpheniramine, Phenylpropanolamine, Dextromethorphan, and Acetaminophen
  • Capsules (U.S.)
  • Oral solution (U.S.)
  • Tablets (U.S.)
Chlorpheniramine, Phenylpropanolamine, Dextromethorphan, Acetaminophen, and Caffeine
  • Capsules (U.S.)
Chlorpheniramine, Pseudoephedrine, Dextromethorphan, and Acetaminophen
  • Capsules (U.S.)
  • Oral solution (U.S.)
  • Tablets (U.S./Canada)
Diphenhydramine, Pseudoephedrine, Dextromethorphan, and Acetaminophen
  • Capsules (U.S.)
  • Oral solution (U.S.)
Doxylamine, Pseudoephedrine, Dextromethorphan, and Acetaminophen
  • Oral solution (U.S.)
Pheniramine, Pyrilamine, Phenylpropanolamine, Codeine, Acetaminophen, and Caffeine
  • Tablets (Canada)
Pyrilamine, Phenylephrine, Dextromethorphan, and Acetaminophen
  • Oral solution (U.S.)
Pyrilamine, Phenylpropanolamine, Dextromethorphan, and Sodium Salicylate
  • Oral solution (U.S.)

Antihistamine, decongestant, antitussive, and expectorant combinations—
Oral

Brompheniramine, Phenylephrine, Phenylpropanolamine, Codeine, and Guaifenesin
  • Syrup (Canada)
Brompheniramine, Phenylephrine, Phenylpropanolamine, Hydrocodone, and Guaifenesin
  • Oral solution (Canada)
Chlorpheniramine, Ephedrine, Phenylephrine, Dextromethorphan, Ammonium Chloride, and Ipecac
  • Syrup (U.S.)
Chlorpheniramine, Phenindamine, Pyrilamine, Phenylephrine, Hydrocodone, and Ammonium Chloride
  • Syrup (U.S.)

Chlorpheniramine, Phenylephrine, Codeine, Ammonium Chloride, Potassium Guaiacolsulfonate, and Sodium Citrate
- Oral solution (U.S.)

Chlorpheniramine, Phenylephrine, Codeine, and Potassium Iodide
- Syrup (U.S.)

Chlorpheniramine, Phenylephrine, Dextromethorphan, and Guaifenesin
- Syrup (U.S.)

Chlorpheniramine, Phenylephrine, Dextromethorphan, Guaifenesin, and Ammonium Chloride
- Oral solution (U.S.)

Chlorpheniramine, Phenylephrine, Phenylpropanolamine, Carbetapentane, and Potassium Guaiacolsulfonate
- Capsules (U.S.)
- Syrup (U.S.)

Chlorpheniramine, Phenylpropanolamine, Dextromethorphan, and Ammonium Chloride
- Syrup (U.S.)

Chlorpheniramine, Phenyltoloxamine, Ephedrine, Codeine, and Guaiacol Carbonate
- Oral suspension (Canada)

Chlorpheniramine, Phenyltoloxamine, Phenylpropanolamine, Dextromethorphan, and Guaifenesin
- Syrup (U.S.)

Diphenylpyraline, Phenylephrine, Hydrocodone, and Guaifenesin
- Oral solution (Canada)

Pheniramine, Pyrilamine, Phenylpropanolamine, Dextromethorphan, and Ammonium Chloride
- Syrup (U.S.)

Pheniramine, Pyrilamine, Phenylpropanolamine, Dextromethorphan, and Guaifenesin
- Oral solution (Canada)

Pheniramine, Pyrilamine, Phenylpropanolamine, Hydrocodone, and Guaifenesin
- Oral solution (U.S.)

Pyrilamine, Phenylephrine, Hydrocodone, and Ammonium Chloride
- Syrup (Canada)

Pyrilamine, Phenylpropanolamine, Dextromethorphan, Guaifenesin, Potassium Citrate, and Citric Acid
- Syrup (U.S.)

Triprolidine, Pseudoephedrine, Codeine, and Guaifenesin
- Oral solution (Canada)

Antihistamine, decongestant, antitussive, expectorant, and analgesic combinations—
Oral

Chlorpheniramine, Phenylephrine, Phenylpropanolamine, Dextromethorphan, Guaifenesin, and Acetaminophen
- Syrup (U.S.)
- Tablets (U.S.)

Chlorpheniramine, Phenylpropanolamine, Codeine, Guaifenesin, and Acetaminophen
- Syrup (U.S.)
- Tablets (U.S.)

Chlorpheniramine, Phenylpropanolamine, Hydrocodone, Guaifenesin, and Salicylamide
- Tablets (U.S.)

Chlorpheniramine, Pseudoephedrine, Dextromethorphan, Guaifenesin, and Aspirin
- Tablets (U.S.)

Pheniramine, Phenylephrine, Codeine, Sodium Citrate, Sodium Salicylate, and Caffeine
- Syrup (U.S.)

Antihistamine, decongestant, and expectorant combinations—
Oral

Brompheniramine, Phenylephrine, Phenylpropanolamine, and Guaifenesin
- Syrup (Canada)

Carbinoxamine, Pseudoephedrine, and Guaifenesin
- Capsules (U.S.)
- Oral solution (U.S.)

Chlorpheniramine, Ephedrine, and Guaifenesin
- Oral solution (U.S.)

Chlorpheniramine, Phenylephrine, and Guaifenesin
- Oral solution (U.S.)

Chlorpheniramine, Phenylpropanolamine, and Guaifenesin
- Oral solution (Canada)

Chlorpheniramine, Phenylpropanolamine, Guaifenesin, Sodium Citrate, and Citric Acid
- Oral solution (U.S.)

Chlorpheniramine, Pseudoephedrine, and Guaifenesin
- Extended-release tablets (U.S.)

Dexchlorpheniramine, Pseudoephedrine, and Guaifenesin
- Oral solution (U.S.)

Pheniramine, Pyrilamine, Phenylpropanolamine, and Guaifenesin
- Oral solution (Canada)

Antitussive and anticholinergic combination—
Oral

Hydrocodone and Homatropine
- Syrup (U.S.)
- Tablets (U.S.)

Antitussive and expectorant combinations—
Oral

Codeine and Calcium Iodide
- Syrup (U.S.)

Codeine and Guaifenesin
- Oral solution (U.S.)
- Syrup (U.S.)

Codeine and Iodinated Glycerol
- Oral solution (U.S.)

Dextromethorphan and Guaifenesin
- Capsules (U.S.)
- Oral gel (U.S.)
- Lozenges (U.S.)
- Oral solution (U.S.)
- Syrup (U.S.)
- Tablets (U.S.)

Dextromethorphan, Guaifenesin, Potassium Citrate, and Citric Acid
- Syrup (U.S.)

Dextromethorphan and Iodinated Glycerol
- Oral solution (U.S.)

Hydrocodone and Guaifenesin
- Oral solution (U.S.)
- Syrup (U.S.)
- Tablets (U.S.)

Hydrocodone and Potassium Guaiacolsulfonate
- Syrup (U.S.)

Hydromorphone and Guaifenesin
- Syrup (U.S.)

Decongestant and antitussive combinations—
Oral

Phenylephrine and Dextromethorphan
- Oral suspension (U.S.)

Phenylpropanolamine and Caramiphen
- Extended-release capsules (U.S.)
- Oral solution (U.S.)

Phenylpropanolamine and Dextromethorphan
- Oral gel (U.S.)
- Granules (U.S.)
- Lozenges (U.S.)
- Oral solution (U.S.)
- Syrup (U.S.)

Phenylpropanolamine and Hydrocodone
- Oral solution (U.S.)
- Syrup (U.S.)

Pseudoephedrine and Codeine
- Capsules (U.S.)
- Syrup (U.S.)

Pseudoephedrine and Dextromethorphan
- Oral solution (Canada)
- Chewable tablets (U.S.)

Pseudoephedrine and Hydrocodone
- Oral solution (U.S.)
- Syrup (U.S.)

Decongestant, antitussive, and analgesic combinations—
Oral

Phenylpropanolamine, Dextromethorphan, and Acetaminophen
- Oral solution (U.S.)
- Tablets (U.S.)

Pseudoephedrine, Dextromethorphan, and Acetaminophen
- Oral solution (U.S.)
- Tablets (U.S./Canada)

Decongestant, antitussive, and expectorant combinations—
Oral

Phenylephrine, Dextromethorphan, and Guaifenesin
- Syrup (U.S.)

Phenylephrine, Hydrocodone, and Guaifenesin
- Syrup (U.S.)

Phenylpropanolamine, Codeine, and Guaifenesin
- Oral solution (U.S.)
- Oral suspension (U.S.)
- Syrup (U.S.)

Phenylpropanolamine, Dextromethorphan, and Guaifenesin
- Oral solution (U.S.)
- Syrup (U.S.)

Pseudoephedrine, Codeine, and Guaifenesin
- Oral solution (U.S.)
- Syrup (U.S.)

Pseudoephedrine, Dextromethorphan, and Guaifenesin
- Capsules (U.S.)
- Oral solution (U.S.)
- Syrup (U.S.)

Pseudoephedrine, Hydrocodone, and Guaifenesin
- Oral solution (U.S.)
- Tablets (U.S.)

Decongestant, antitussive, expectorant, and analgesic combinations—
Oral

Phenylephrine, Dextromethorphan, Guaifenesin, and Acetaminophen
- Tablets (U.S.)

Pseudoephedrine, Dextromethorphan, Guaifenesin, and Acetaminophen
- Oral solution (U.S.)
- Tablets (U.S.)

Decongestant and expectorant combinations—
Oral

Ephedrine and Guaifenesin
- Capsules (U.S.)
- Syrup (U.S.)

Ephedrine and Potassium Iodide
- Syrup (U.S.)

Phenylephrine, Phenylpropanolamine, and Guaifenesin
- Capsules (U.S.)
- Oral solution (U.S.)
- Tablets (U.S.)

Phenylpropanolamine and Guaifenesin
- Oral solution (U.S.)
- Syrup (U.S.)
- Extended-release tablets (U.S. and Canada)

Pseudoephedrine and Guaifenesin
- Extended-release capsules (U.S.)
- Oral solution (U.S.)
- Syrup (U.S.)
- Tablets (U.S.)
- Extended-release tablets (U.S.)

Decongestant, expectorant, and analgesic combination—
Oral

Phenylephrine, Guaifenesin, Acetaminophen, Salicylamide and Caffeine
- Tablets (U.S.)

It is very important that you read and understand the following information. If any of it causes you special concern, check with your doctor or pharmacist. Also, *if you have any questions* or if you want more information about this medicine or your medical problem, *ask your doctor, nurse, or pharmacist.*

Before Using This Medicine

If you are taking this medicine without a prescription, carefully read and follow any precautions on the label. For cough/cold combinations, the following should be considered:

Allergies—Tell your doctor if you have ever had any unusual or allergic reaction to any of the ingredients contained in this medicine. Also tell your doctor and pharmacist if you are allergic to any other substances, such as foods, preservatives, or dyes. In addition, if this medicine contains *aspirin or other salicylates*, before taking it, check with your doctor if you have ever had any unusual or allergic reaction to any of the following medicines:

    Aspirin or other salicylates
    Diclofenac (e.g., Voltaren)
    Diflunisal (e.g., Dolobid)
    Fenoprofen (e.g., Nalfon)
    Floctafenine
    Flurbiprofen, by mouth (e.g., Ansaid)
    Ibuprofen (e.g., Motrin)
    Indomethacin (e.g., Indocin)
    Ketoprofen (e.g., Orudis)
    Ketorolac (e.g., Toradol)
    Meclofenamate (e.g., Meclomen)
    Mefenamic acid (e.g., Ponstel)
    Methyl salicylate (oil of wintergreen)
    Naproxen (e.g., Naprosyn)
    Oxyphenbutazone (e.g., Tandearil)
    Phenylbutazone (e.g., Butazolidin)
    Piroxicam (e.g., Feldene)
    Sulindac (e.g., Clinoril)
    Suprofen (e.g., Suprol)
    Tiaprofenic acid (e.g., Surgam)
    Tolmetin (e.g., Tolectin)
    Zomepirac (e.g., Zomax)

Diet—Make certain your doctor and pharmacist know if you are on any special diet, such as a low-sodium or low-sugar diet.

Pregnancy—The occasional use of a cough/cold combination is not likely to cause problems in the fetus or in the newborn baby. However, when these medicines are used at higher doses and/or for a long time, the chance that problems might occur may increase. For the individual ingredients of these combinations, the following information should be considered before you decide to use a particular cough/cold combination:

- *Acetaminophen*—Studies on birth defects have not been done in humans. However, acetaminophen has not been shown to cause birth defects or other problems in humans.

- *Alcohol*—Some of these combination medicines contain a large amount of alcohol. Too much use of alcohol during pregnancy may cause birth defects.

- *Antihistamines*—Antihistamines have not been shown to cause problems in humans.

- *Caffeine*—Studies in humans have not shown that caffeine causes birth defects. However, studies in animals have shown that caffeine causes birth defects when given in very large doses (amounts equal to the amount of caffeine contained in 12 to 24 cups of coffee a day).

- *Codeine*—Although studies on birth defects with codeine have not been done in humans, it has not been reported to cause birth defects in humans. Codeine has not been shown to cause birth defects in animal studies, but it caused other unwanted effects. Also, regular use of narcotics during pregnancy may cause the baby to become dependent on the medicine. This may lead to withdrawal side effects after birth. In addition, narcotics may cause breathing problems in the newborn baby if taken by the mother just before delivery.

- *Hydrocodone*—Although studies on birth defects with hydrocodone have not been done in humans, it has not been reported to cause birth defects in humans. However, hydrocodone has been shown to cause birth defects in animals when given in very large doses. Also, regular use of narcotics during pregnancy may cause the baby to become dependent on the medicine. This may lead to withdrawal side effects after birth. In addition, narcotics may cause breathing problems in the newborn baby if taken by the mother just before delivery.

• *Iodides (e.g., calcium iodide and iodinated glycerol)*—Not recommended during pregnancy. Iodides have caused enlargement of the thyroid gland in the fetus and resulted in breathing problems in newborn babies whose mothers took iodides in large doses for a long period of time.

• *Phenylephrine*—Studies on birth defects with phenylephrine have not been done in either humans or animals.

• *Phenylpropanolamine*—Studies on birth defects with phenylpropanolamine have not been done in either humans or animals. However, it seems that women who take phenylpropanolamine in the weeks following delivery are more likely to suffer mental or mood changes.

• *Pseudoephedrine*—Studies on birth defects with pseudoephedrine have not been done in humans. In animal studies pseudoephedrine did not cause birth defects but did cause a decrease in average weight, length, and rate of bone formation in the animal fetus when given in high doses.

• *Salicylates (e.g., aspirin)*—Studies on birth defects in humans have been done with aspirin, but not with salicylamide or sodium salicylate. Salicylates have not been shown to cause birth defects in humans. However, salicylates have been shown to cause birth defects in animals.

Some reports have suggested that too much use of aspirin late in pregnancy may cause a decrease in the newborn's weight and possible death of the fetus or newborn infant. However, the mothers in these reports had been taking much larger amounts of aspirin than are usually recommended. Studies of mothers taking aspirin in the doses that are usually recommended did not show these unwanted effects. However, there is a chance that regular use of salicylates late in pregnancy may cause unwanted effects on the heart or blood flow in the fetus or newborn baby.

Use of salicylates, especially aspirin, during the last 2 weeks of pregnancy may cause bleeding problems in the fetus before or during delivery, or in the newborn baby. Also, too much use of salicylates during the last 3 months of pregnancy may increase the length of pregnancy, prolong labor, cause other problems during delivery, or cause severe bleeding in the mother before, during, or after delivery. *Do not take aspirin during the last 3 months of pregnancy unless it has been ordered by your doctor.*

Breast-feeding—If you are breast-feeding, the chance that problems might occur depends on the ingredients of the combination. For the individual ingredients of these combinations, the following apply:

- *Acetaminophen*—Acetaminophen passes into the breast milk. However, it has not been reported to cause problems in nursing babies.

- *Alcohol*—Alcohol passes into the breast milk. However, the amount of alcohol in recommended doses of this medicine does not usually cause problems in nursing babies.

- *Antihistamines*—Small amounts of antihistamines pass into the breast milk. Antihistamine-containing medicine is not recommended for use while breast-feeding since most antihistamines are especially likely to cause side effects, such as unusual excitement or irritability, in the baby. Also, since antihistamines tend to decrease the secretions of the body, the flow of breast milk may be reduced in some patients.

- *Caffeine*—Small amounts of caffeine pass into the breast milk and may build up in the nursing baby. However, the amount of caffeine in recommended doses of this medicine does not usually cause problems in nursing babies.

- *Decongestants (e.g., ephedrine, phenylephrine, phenylpropanolamine, pseudoephedrine)*—Phenylephrine and phenylpropanolamine have not been reported to cause problems in nursing babies. Ephedrine and pseudo-ephedrine pass into the breast milk and may cause unwanted effects in nursing babies (especially newborn and premature babies).

- *Iodides (e.g., calcium iodide and iodinated glycerol)*—These medicines pass into the breast milk and may cause unwanted effects, such as underactive thyroid, in the baby.

- *Narcotic antitussives (e.g., codeine, dihydrocodeine, hydrocodone, and hydromorphone)*—Small amounts of codeine have been shown to pass into the breast milk. However, the amount of codeine or other narcotic antitussives in recommended doses of this medicine has not been reported to cause problems in nursing babies.

- *Salicylates (e.g., aspirin)*—Salicylates pass into the breast milk. Although salicylates have not been reported to cause problems in nursing babies, it is possible that problems may occur if large amounts are taken regularly.

Children—Very young children are usually more sensitive to the effects of this medicine. *Before giving any of these combination medicines to a child, check the package label very carefully. Some of these medicines are too strong for use in children.* If you are not certain whether a specific product can be given to a child, or if you have any questions about the amount to give, check with your doctor or pharmacist, especially if it contains:

- *Antihistamines*—Nightmares, unusual excitement, nervousness, restlessness, or irritability may be more likely to occur in children taking antihistamines.

- *Decongestants (e.g., ephedrine, phenylephrine, phenylpropanolamine, pseudoephedrine)*—Increases in blood pressure may be more likely to occur in children taking decongestants. Also, mental changes may be more likely to occur in young children taking phenylpropanolamine-containing combinations.

- *Narcotic antitussives (e.g., codeine, hydrocodeine, hydrocodone, and hydromorphone)*—Breathing problems may be especially likely to occur in children younger than 2 years of age taking narcotic antitussives. Also, unusual excitement or restlessness may be more likely to occur in children receiving these medicines.

- *Salicylates (e.g., aspirin)—Do not give medicines containing aspirin or other salicylates to a child with a fever or other symptoms of a virus infection, especially flu or chickenpox, without first discussing its use with your child's doctor.* This is very important because salicylates may cause a serious illness called Reye's syndrome in children with fever caused by a virus infection, especially flu or chickenpox. Also, children may be more sensitive to the aspirin or other salicylates contained in some of these medicines, especially if they have a fever or have lost large amounts of body fluid because of vomiting, diarrhea, or sweating.

Teenagers—*Do not give medicines containing aspirin or other salicylates to a teenager with a fever or other symptoms of a virus infection, especially flu or chickenpox, without first discussing its use with your child's doctor.* This is very important because salicylates may cause a serious illness called Reye's syndrome in teenagers with fever caused by a virus infection, especially flu or chickenpox.

Older adults—The elderly are usually more sensitive to the effects of this medicine, especially if it contains:

- *Antihistamines*—Confusion, difficult or painful urination, dizziness, drowsiness, feeling faint, or dryness of mouth, nose, or throat may be more likely to occur in elderly patients. Also, nightmares or unusual excitement, nervousness, restlessness, or irritability may be more likely to occur in the elderly taking antihistamines.

- *Decongestants (e.g., ephedrine, phenylephrine, phenylpropanolamine, pseudoephedrine)*—Confusion, hallucinations, drowsiness, or convulsions (seizures) may be more likely to occur in the elderly, who are usually more sensitive to the effects of this medicine. Also, increases in blood pressure may be more likely to occur in elderly persons taking decongestants.

Athletes—Caffeine is tested for by the U.S. Olympic Committee (USOC) and the National Collegiate Athletic Association (NCAA). In addition, the USOC tests for narcotic antitussives (e.g., codeine, dihydrocodeine, hydrocodone, and hydromorphone) and sympathomimetic stimulants (e.g., ephedrine, phenylephrine, phenylpropanolamine, pseudo-ephedrine). The USOC and the NCAA have set limits on the amount of caffeine, and the USOC on the amount of narcotic antitussives and sympathomimetics, they consider to be acceptable in the urine. An athlete will be disqualified for competition if the amount of these substances in the urine is above those limits.

Other medicines—Although certain medicines should not be used together at all, in other cases two different medicines may be used together even if an interaction might occur. In these cases, your doctor may want to change the dose, or other precautions may be necessary. Tell your doctor and pharmacist if you are taking *any* other prescription or non-prescription (over-the-counter [OTC]) medicine, for example, aspirin or other medicine for allergies. Some medicines may change the way this medicine affects your body. Also, the effect of other medicines may be increased or reduced by some of the ingredients in this medicine. Check with your doctor or pharmacist about which medicines you should not take with this medicine.

Other medical problems—The presence of other medical problems may affect the use of the cough/cold combination medicine. Make sure you tell your doctor if you have any other medical problems, especially:

- Alcohol abuse (or history of)—Acetaminophen-containing medicines increase the chance of liver damage; also, some of the liquid medicines contain a large amount of alcohol
- Anemia or
- Gout or
- Hemophilia or other bleeding problems or
- Stomach ulcer or other stomach problems—These conditions may become worse if you are taking a combination medicine containing aspirin or another salicylate
- Brain disease or injury or
- Colitis or

- Convulsions (seizures) (history of) or
- Diarrhea or
- Gallbladder disease or gallstones—These conditions may become worse if you are taking a combination medicine containing codeine, dihydrocodeine, hydrocodone, or hydromorphone
- Cystic fibrosis (in children)—Side effects of iodinated glycerol may be more likely in children with cystic fibrosis
- Diabetes mellitus (sugar diabetes)—Decongestants may put diabetic patients at greater risk of having heart or blood vessel disease
- Emphysema, asthma, or chronic lung disease (especially in children)—Salicylate-containing medicine may cause an allergic reaction in which breathing becomes difficult
- Enlarged prostate or
- Urinary tract blockage or difficult urination—Some of the effects of anticholinergics (e.g., homatropine) or antihistamines may make urinary problems worse
- Glaucoma—A slight increase in inner eye pressure may occur with the use of anticholinergics (e.g., homatropine) or antihistamines, which may make the condition worse
- Heart or blood vessel disease or
- High blood pressure—Decongestant-containing medicine may increase the blood pressure and speed up the heart rate; also, caffeine-containing medicine, if taken in large amounts, may speed up the heart rate
- Kidney disease—This condition may increase the chance of side effects of this medicine because the medicine may build up in the body
- Liver disease—Liver disease increases the chance of side effects because the medicine may build up in the body; also, if liver disease is severe, there is a greater chance that aspirin-containing medicine may cause bleeding
- Thyroid disease—If an overactive thyroid has caused a fast heart rate, the decongestant in this medicine may cause the heart rate to speed up further; also, if the medicine contains narcotic antitussives (e.g., codeine), iodides (e.g., iodinated glycerol), or salicylates, the thyroid problem may become worse

Proper Use of This Medicine

To help loosen mucus or phlegm in the lungs, *drink a glass of water after each dose of this medicine*, unless otherwise directed by your doctor.

Take this medicine only as directed. Do not take more of it and do not take it more often than recommended on the label, unless otherwise directed by your doctor. To do so may increase the chance of side effects.

For patients *taking the extended-release capsule or tablet form of this medicine:*
- Swallow the capsule or tablet whole.
- Do not crush, break, or chew before swallowing.
- If the capsule is too large to swallow, you may mix the contents of the capsule with applesauce, jelly, honey, or syrup and swallow without chewing.

For patients *taking a combination medicine containing an antihistamine and/or aspirin or other salicylate:*
- Take with food or a glass of water or milk to lessen stomach irritation, if necessary.

If a combination medicine containing aspirin has a strong vinegar-like odor, do not use it. This odor means the medicine is breaking down. If you have any questions about this, check with your pharmacist.

Missed dose—If you must take this medicine regularly and you miss a dose, take it as soon as possible. However, if it is almost time for your next dose, skip the missed dose and go back to your regular dosing schedule. Do not double doses.

Storage—To store this medicine:
- Keep this medicine out of the reach of children. Overdose is very dangerous in young children.
- Store away from heat and direct light.
- Do not store the capsule or tablet form of this medicine in the bathroom, near the kitchen sink, or in other damp places. Heat or moisture may cause the medicine to break down.

- Keep the liquid form of this medicine from freezing. Do not refrigerate the syrup.
- Do not keep outdated medicine or medicine no longer needed. Be sure that any discarded medicine is out of the reach of children.

Precautions While Using This Medicine

If your cough has not improved after 7 days or if you have a high fever, skin rash, continuing headache, or sore throat with the cough, check with your doctor. These signs may mean that you have other medical problems.

For patients *taking antihistamine-containing medicine:*

- Before you have any skin tests for allergies, tell the doctor in charge that you are taking this medicine. The results of the test may be affected by the antihistamine in this medicine.
- This medicine will add to the effects of alcohol and other CNS depressants (medicines that slow down the nervous system, possibly causing drowsiness). Some examples of CNS depressants are antihistamines or medicine for hay fever, other allergies, or colds; sedatives, tranquilizers, or sleeping medicine; prescription pain medicine or narcotics; barbiturates; medicine for seizures; muscle relaxants; or anesthetics, including some dental anesthetics. *Check with your doctor before taking any of the above while you are taking this medicine.*
- This medicine may cause some people to become drowsy, dizzy, or less alert than they are normally. *Make sure you know how you react to this medicine before you drive, use machines, or do anything else that could be dangerous if you are dizzy or are not alert.*
- When taking antihistamines on a regular basis, make sure your doctor knows if you are taking large amounts of aspirin at the same time (as in arthritis or rheumatism). Effects of too much aspirin, such as ringing in the ears, may be covered up by the antihistamine.
- Antihistamines may cause dryness of the mouth. For temporary relief, use sugarless candy or gum, melt bits of ice in your mouth, or use a saliva substitute. How-

ever, if your mouth continues to feel dry for more than 2 weeks, check with your medical doctor or dentist. Continuing dryness of the mouth may increase the chance of dental disease, including tooth decay, gum disease, and fungus infections.

For patients *taking decongestant-containing medicine:*

- This medicine may add to the central nervous system (CNS) stimulant and other effects of phenylpropanolamine (PPA)-containing diet aids. *Do not use medicines for diet or appetite control while taking this medicine unless you have checked with your doctor.*

- This medicine may cause some people to be nervous or restless or to have trouble in sleeping. If you have trouble in sleeping, *take the last dose of this medicine for each day a few hours before bedtime.* If you have any questions about this, check with your doctor.

- Before having any kind of surgery (including dental surgery) or emergency treatment, tell the medical doctor or dentist in charge that you are taking this medicine.

For patients *taking narcotic antitussive (codeine, dihydrocodeine, hydrocodone, or hydromorphone)-containing medicine:*

- This medicine will add to the effects of alcohol and other CNS depressants (medicines that slow down the nervous system, possibly causing drowsiness). Some examples of CNS depressants are antihistamines or medicine for hay fever, other allergies, or colds; sedatives, tranquilizers, or sleeping medicine; prescription pain medicine or narcotics; barbiturates; medicine for seizures; muscle relaxants; or anesthetics, including some dental anesthetics. *Check with your doctor before taking any of the above while you are taking this medicine.*

- This medicine may cause some people to become drowsy, dizzy, less alert than they are normally, or to feel a false sense of well-being. *Make sure you know how you react to this medicine before you drive, use machines, or do anything else that could be dangerous if you are dizzy or are not alert and clearheaded.*

- Nausea or vomiting may occur after taking a narcotic antitussive. This effect may go away if you lie down for a while. However, if nausea or vomiting continues, check with your doctor.
- Dizziness, lightheadedness, or fainting may be especially likely to occur when you get up suddenly from a lying or sitting position. Getting up slowly may help lessen this problem.
- Before having any kind of surgery (including dental surgery) or emergency treatment, tell the medical doctor or dentist in charge that you are taking this medicine.

For patients *taking iodide (calcium iodide, iodinated glycerol, or potassium iodide)-containing medicine:*

- Make sure your doctor knows if you are planning to have any future thyroid tests. The results of the thyroid test may be affected by the iodine in this medicine.

For patients *taking analgesic-containing medicine:*

- *Check the label of all nonprescription (over-the-counter [OTC]), and prescription medicines you now take.* If any contain acetaminophen or aspirin or other salicylates, including diflunisal or bismuth subsalicylate, be especially careful. Taking them while taking a cough/cold combination medicine that already contains them may lead to overdose. If you have any questions about this, check with your doctor or pharmacist.
- Do not take aspirin-containing medicine for 5 days before any surgery, including dental surgery, unless otherwise directed by your medical doctor or dentist. Taking aspirin during this time may cause bleeding problems.

For *diabetic patients taking aspirin- or sodium salicylate–containing medicine:*

- False urine sugar test results may occur:

—If you take 8 or more 325-mg (5-grain) doses of aspirin every day for several days in a row.

—If you take 8 or more 325-mg (5-grain), or 4 or more 500-mg (10-grain) doses of sodium salicylate.

- Smaller doses or occasional use of aspirin or sodium salicylate usually will not affect urine sugar tests. If you have any questions about this, check with your doctor, nurse, or pharmacist, especially if your diabetes is not well controlled.

For patients *taking homatropine-containing medicine:*

- This medicine may make you sweat less, causing your body temperature to increase. *Use extra care not to become overheated during exercise or hot weather while you are taking this medicine,* since overheating may result in heat stroke. Also, hot baths or saunas may make you feel dizzy or faint while you are taking this medicine.

Side Effects of This Medicine

Along with its needed effects, a medicine may cause some unwanted effects. Although serious side effects occur rarely when this medicine is taken as recommended, they may be more likely to occur if:

- too much medicine is taken.
- it is taken in large doses.
- it is taken for a long period of time.

Get emergency help immediately if any of the following symptoms of overdose occur:

For narcotic antitussive (codeine, dihydrocodeine, hydrocodone, or hydromorphone)–containing

Cold, clammy skin; confusion (severe); convulsions (seizures); drowsiness or dizziness (severe); nervousness or restlessness (severe); pinpoint pupils of eyes; slow heartbeat; slow or troubled breathing; weakness (severe)

For acetaminophen-containing

Diarrhea; increased sweating; loss of appetite; nausea or vomiting; stomach cramps or pain; swelling or tenderness in the upper abdomen or stomach area

For salicylate-containing

Any loss of hearing; bloody urine; confusion; convulsions (seizures); diarrhea (severe or continuing); dizziness or lightheadedness; drowsiness (severe); excitement or nervousness (severe); fast or deep breathing; fever; hallucinations (seeing, hearing, or feeling things that are not there); increased sweating; nausea or vomiting (severe or continuing); shortness of breath or troubled breathing (for salicylamide only); stomach pain (severe or continuing); uncontrollable flapping movements of the hands, especially in elderly patients; unusual thirst; vision problems

For decongestant-containing

Fast, pounding, or irregular heartbeat; headache (continuing and severe); nausea or vomiting (severe); nervousness or restlessness (severe); shortness of breath or troubled breathing (severe or continuing)

Also, check with your doctor as soon as possible if any of the following side effects occur:

For all combinations

Skin rash, hives, and/or itching

For antihistamine- or anticholinergic-containing

Clumsiness or unsteadiness; convulsions (seizures); drowsiness (severe); dryness of mouth, nose, or throat (severe); flushing or redness of face; hallucinations (seeing, hearing, or feeling things that are not there); restlessness (severe); shortness of breath or troubled breathing; slow or fast heartbeat

For iodine-containing

Headache (continuing); increased watering of mouth; loss of appetite; metallic taste; skin rash, hives, or redness; sore throat; swelling of face, lips, or eyelids

For acetaminophen-containing

Unexplained sore throat and fever; unusual tiredness or weakness; yellow eyes or skin

Other side effects may occur that usually do not need medical attention. These side effects may go away during treatment as your body adjusts to the medicine. However, check with your doctor if any of the following side effects continue or are bothersome:

Constipation; decreased sweating; difficult or painful urination; dizziness or lightheadedness; drowsiness; dryness of mouth, nose, or throat; false sense of well-being; increased sensitivity of skin to sun; nausea or vomiting; nightmares; stomach pain; thickening of mucus; trouble in sleeping; unusual excitement,

nervousness, restlessness, or irritability; unusual tiredness or
weakness

Not all of the side effects listed above have been reported
for each of these medicines, but they have been reported for
at least one of them. There are some similarities among these
combination medicines, so many of the above side effects
may occur with any of these medicines.

Other side effects not listed above may also occur in some
patients. If you notice any other effects, check with your
doctor.

CROMOLYN   Inhalation

Some commonly used brand names are:
In the U.S.
Intal
In Canada
Fivent
Intal
Another commonly used name is sodium cromoglycate.

Description

Cromolyn (KROE-moe-lin) is used to prevent asthma attacks. It is also used before and during exposure to substances that cause reactions, to prevent bronchospasm
(wheezing or difficulty in breathing). In addition, this medicine is used to prevent bronchospasm caused by exercise.

Cromolyn inhalation works by acting on certain cells in the
body, called mast cells, to prevent them from releasing substances that cause the asthma or bronchospasm attack.

Cromolyn will not help an asthma attack that has already
started. If this medicine is used during a severe attack, it
may cause irritation and make the attack worse.

This medicine is available only with your doctor's prescription, in the following dosage forms:

Inhalation
- Capsules for inhalation (U.S. and Canada)
- Inhalation aerosol (U.S. and Canada)
- Inhalation solution (U.S. and Canada)

It is very important that you read and understand the following information. If any of it causes you special concern, check with your doctor. Also, *if you have any questions* or if you want more information about this medicine or your medical problem, *ask your doctor, nurse, or pharmacist.*

Before Using This Medicine

In deciding to use a medicine, the risks of taking the medicine must be weighed against the good it will do. This is a decision you and your doctor will make. For cromolyn inhalation, the following should be considered:

Allergies—Tell your doctor if you have ever had any unusual or allergic reaction to cromolyn or to inhalation aerosols. Also tell your doctor and pharmacist if you are allergic to any other substances, such as foods, preservatives, or dyes.

Diet—Make certain your doctor and pharmacist know if you are on any special diet, such as a low-sodium or low-sugar diet.

Pregnancy—Cromolyn has not been studied in pregnant women. However, studies in animals have shown that cromolyn causes a decrease in successful pregnancies and a decrease in the weight of the animal fetus when given by injection in very large amounts.

Breast-feeding—It is not known whether cromolyn passes into the breast milk. However, this medicine has not been reported to cause problems in nursing babies.

Children—Although there is no specific information about the use of cromolyn inhalation in children, it is not expected to cause different side effects or problems in children than it does in adults.

Older adults—Many medicines have not been tested in older people. Therefore, it may not be known whether they work exactly the same way they do in younger adults. Although there is no specific information about the use of cromolyn inhalation in the elderly, it is not expected to cause different side effects or problems in older people than it does in younger adults.

Other medical problems—The presence of other medical problems may affect the use of cromolyn. Make sure you tell your doctor if you have any other medical problems, especially:

- Heart disease (or history of)—The inhalation aerosol form of cromolyn may make the condition worse
- Kidney disease or
- Liver disease—The effects of cromolyn may be increased, which may increase the chance of side effects

Before you begin using any new medicine (prescription or nonprescription) or if you develop any new medical problem while you are using this medicine, check with your doctor, nurse, or pharmacist.

Proper Use of This Medicine

Cromolyn oral inhalation is used to prevent asthma or bronchospasm (wheezing or difficulty in breathing) attacks. It will not relieve an attack that has already started. If this medicine is used during a severe attack, it may cause irritation and make the attack worse.

For patients using *cromolyn aerosol:*

- This medicine usually comes with patient directions. Read them carefully before using this medicine.
- Keep the spray away from the eyes because it may cause irritation.

For patients using *cromolyn capsules for inhalation:*

- This medicine is used with a special inhaler and usually comes with patient directions. Read the directions carefully before using.
- *Do not swallow the capsules because the medicine will not work if you swallow it.*

For patients using *cromolyn solution for inhalation:*
- Use this medicine only in a power-operated nebulizer with an adequate flow rate and equipped with a face mask or mouthpiece. Make sure you understand exactly how to use it. Hand-operated nebulizers are not suitable for use with this medicine. If you have any questions about this, check with your doctor.

Use cromolyn oral inhalation only as directed. Do not use more of it and do not use it more often than your doctor ordered. To do so may increase the chance of side effects.

For patients using *cromolyn oral inhalation* regularly (for example, every day):
- *In order for cromolyn to work properly, it must be inhaled every day in regularly spaced doses as ordered by your doctor.* Up to 4 weeks may pass before you feel the full effects of the medicine.
- **Missed dose**—If you miss a dose of this medicine, take it as soon as possible. Then take any remaining doses for that day at regularly spaced intervals. Do not double doses.

Storage—To store this medicine:
- Keep out of the reach of children.
- Store away from heat.
- Store the capsule or solution form of this medicine away from direct light. Store the aerosol form of this medicine away from direct sunlight.
- Do not store the capsule form of this medicine in the bathroom, near the kitchen sink, or in other damp places. Heat or moisture may cause the medicine to break down.
- Keep the aerosol or solution form of this medicine from freezing.
- Do not puncture, break, or burn the aerosol container, even if it is empty.
- Do not keep outdated medicine or medicine no longer needed. Be sure that any discarded medicine is out of the reach of children.

Precautions While Using This Medicine

If your symptoms do not improve or if your condition becomes worse, check with your doctor.

If you are also taking an adrenocorticoid (cortisone-like medicine, such as cortisone or prednisone) for your asthma along with this medicine, do not stop taking the adrenocorticoid even if your asthma seems better, unless you are told to do so by your doctor.

Dryness of the mouth or throat, throat irritation, and hoarseness may occur after using this medicine. Gargling and rinsing the mouth after each dose may help prevent these effects.

Side Effects of This Medicine

Along with its needed effects, a medicine may cause some unwanted effects. Although not all of these side effects may occur, if they do occur they may need medical attention.

Check with your doctor as soon as possible if any of the following side effects occur:

Less common

Difficult or painful urination; dizziness; frequent urge to urinate; headache (severe or continuing); increased wheezing, tightness in chest, or difficulty in breathing; joint pain or swelling; muscle pain or weakness; nausea or vomiting; skin rash, hives, or itching; swelling of the face, lips, eyelids, hands, feet, or inside of mouth

Rare

Chest pain; chills; difficulty in swallowing; sweating; wheezing or difficulty in breathing (severe)

Other side effects may occur that usually do not need medical attention. These side effects may go away during treatment as your body adjusts to the medicine. However, check with your doctor if any of the following side effects continue or are bothersome:

More common

Cough; hoarseness

Less common
> Dryness of the mouth or throat; sneezing; stuffy nose; throat irritation; watering of the eyes

If you are using cromolyn aerosol, you may notice an unpleasant taste. This may be expected and will go away when you stop using the medicine.

Other side effects not listed above may also occur in some patients. If you notice any other effects, check with your doctor.

CYCLOBENZAPRINE   Systemic

Some commonly used brand names are:
In the U.S.
> Cycoflex
> Flexeril
> Generic name product may also be available.

In Canada
> Flexeril

Description

Cyclobenzaprine (sye-kloe-BEN-za-preen) is used to help relax certain muscles in your body. It helps relieve the pain, stiffness, and discomfort caused by strains, sprains, or injuries to your muscles. However, this medicine does not take the place of rest, exercise or physical therapy, or other treatment that your doctor may recommend for your medical problem. Cyclobenzaprine acts on the central nervous system (CNS) to produce its muscle relaxant effects. Its actions on the CNS may also cause some of this medicine's side effects.

Cyclobenzaprine may also be used for other conditions as determined by your doctor.

Cyclobenzaprine is available only with your doctor's prescription, in the following dosage form:

Oral
- Tablets (U.S. and Canada)

It is very important that you read and understand the following information. If any of it causes you special concern, check with your doctor or pharmacist. Also, *if you have any questions* or if you want more information about this medicine or your medical problem, *ask your doctor, nurse, or pharmacist.*

Before Using This Medicine

In deciding to use a medicine, the risks of taking the medicine must be weighed against the good it will do. This is a decision you and your doctor will make. For cyclobenzaprine, the following should be considered:

Allergies—Tell your doctor if you have ever had any unusual or allergic reaction to cyclobenzaprine. Also tell your doctor and pharmacist if you are allergic to any other substances, such as foods, preservatives, or dyes.

Pregnancy—Studies on birth defects with cyclobenzaprine have not been done in humans. However, cyclobenzaprine has not been shown to cause birth defects or other problems in animal studies.

Breast-feeding—Although it is not known whether cyclobenzaprine passes into the breast milk, cyclobenzaprine has not been reported to cause problems in nursing babies.

Children—Studies on this medicine have been done only in adult patients, and there is no specific information comparing use of cyclobenzaprine in children with use in other age groups.

Teenagers—Studies on this medicine have been done only in adult patients, and there is no specific information comparing use of cyclobenzaprine in teenagers up to 15 years of age with use in other age groups.

Older adults—Many medicines have not been studied specifically in older people. Therefore, it may not be known whether they work exactly the same way they do in younger adults or if they cause different side effects or problems in older people. There is no specific information comparing use of cyclobenzaprine in the elderly with use in other age groups.

Athletes—Cyclobenzaprine is banned in competitors in biathlon and modern pentathlon by the U.S. Olympic Committee (USOC). Cyclobenzaprine use can lead to disqualification in these events.

Other medicines—Although certain medicines should not be used together at all, in other cases two different medicines may be used together even if an interaction might occur. In these cases, your doctor may want to change the dose, or other precautions may be necessary. When you are taking cyclobenzaprine, it is especially important that your doctor and pharmacist know if you are taking any of the following:

- Central nervous system (CNS) depressants or
- Tricyclic antidepressants (amitriptyline [e.g., Elavil], amoxapine [e.g., Asendin], clomipramine [e.g., Anafranil], desipramine [e.g., Pertofrane], doxepin [e.g., Sinequan], imipramine [e.g., Tofranil], nortriptyline [e.g., Aventyl], protriptyline [e.g., Vivactil], trimipramine [e.g., Surmontil])—The chance of side effects may be increased
- Monoamine oxidase (MAO) inhibitors (furazolidone [e.g., Furoxone], isocarboxazid [e.g., Marplan], phenelzine [e.g., Nardil], procarbazine [e.g., Matulane], tranylcypromine [e.g., Parnate])—Taking cyclobenzaprine while you are taking or within 2 weeks of taking monoamine oxidase (MAO) inhibitors may increase the chance of side effects

Other medical problems—The presence of other medical problems may affect the use of cyclobenzaprine. Make sure you tell your doctor if you have any other medical problems, especially:

- Glaucoma or
- Problems with urination—Cyclobenzaprine can make your condition worse
- Heart or blood vessel disease or
- Overactive thyroid—The chance of side effects may be increased

Before you begin using any new medicine (prescription or nonprescription) or if you develop any new medical problem while you are using this medicine, check with your doctor, nurse, or pharmacist.

Proper Use of This Medicine

Take this medicine only as directed by your doctor. Do not take more of it and do not take it more often than your doctor ordered. To do so may increase the chance of serious side effects.

Missed dose—If you miss a dose of this medicine and remember within an hour or so of the missed dose, take it right away. Then go back to your regular dosing schedule. But if you do not remember until later, skip the missed dose and go back to your regular dosing schedule. Do not double doses.

Storage—To store this medicine:
- Keep out of the reach of children.
- Store away from heat and direct light.
- Do not store this medicine in the bathroom, near the kitchen sink, or in other damp places. Heat or moisture may cause the medicine to break down.
- Do not keep outdated medicine or medicine no longer needed. Be sure that any discarded medicine is out of the reach of children.

Precautions While Using This Medicine

This medicine will add to the effects of alcohol and other CNS depressants (medicines that slow down the nervous system, possibly causing drowsiness). Some examples of CNS depressants are antihistamines or medicine for hay fever, other allergies, or colds; sedatives, tranquilizers, or sleeping medicine; prescription pain medicine or narcotics; barbiturates; medicine for seizures; other muscle relaxants; or anesthetics, including some dental anesthetics. *Check with your doctor before taking any of the above while you are using this medicine.*

This medicine may cause some people to have blurred vision or to become drowsy, dizzy, or less alert than they are normally. *Make sure you know how you react to this medicine before you drive, use machines, or do anything else that could be dangerous if you are dizzy or are not alert and able to see well.*

Cyclobenzaprine may cause dryness of the mouth. For temporary relief, use sugarless candy or gum, melt bits of ice in your mouth, or use a saliva substitute. However, if your mouth continues to feel dry for more than 2 weeks, check with your medical doctor or dentist. Continuing dryness of the mouth may increase the chance of dental disease, including tooth decay, gum disease, and fungus infections.

Side Effects of This Medicine

Along with its needed effects, a medicine may cause some unwanted effects. Although not all of these side effects may occur, if they do occur they may need medical attention.

Check with your doctor immediately if any of the following side effects occur:

Rare

Fainting; swelling of face, lips, or tongue

Symptoms of overdose

Convulsions (seizures); drowsiness (severe); dry, hot, flushed skin; fast or irregular heartbeat; hallucinations (seeing, hearing, or feeling things that are not there); increase or decrease in body temperature; troubled breathing; unexplained muscle stiffness; unusual nervousness or restlessness (severe); vomiting

Also, check with your doctor as soon as possible if any of the following side effects occur:

Rare

Clumsiness or unsteadiness; confusion; mental depression or other mood or mental changes; problems in urinating; ringing or buzzing in the ears; skin rash, hives, or itching; unusual thoughts or dreams; yellow eyes or skin

Other side effects may occur that usually do not need medical attention. These side effects may go away during treat-

ment as your body adjusts to the medicine. However, check with your doctor if any of the following side effects continue or are bothersome:

More common

Dizziness or lightheadedness; drowsiness; dryness of mouth

Less common or rare

Bloated feeling or gas, indigestion, nausea or vomiting, or stomach cramps or pain; blurred vision; constipation; decrease in blood pressure; diarrhea; excitement or nervousness; frequent urination; general feeling of discomfort or illness; headache; muscle twitching; numbness, tingling, pain, or weakness in hands or feet; pounding heartbeat; problems in speaking; trembling; trouble in sleeping; unpleasant taste or other taste changes; unusual muscle weakness; unusual tiredness

Other side effects not listed above may also occur in some patients. If you notice any other effects, check with your doctor.

Additional Information

Once a medicine has been approved for marketing for a certain use, experience may show that it is also useful for other medical problems. Although this use is not included in product labeling, cyclobenzaprine is used in certain patients with fibromyalgia syndrome (also called fibrositis or fibrositis syndrome).

There is no additional information relating to proper use, precautions, or side effects for this use of cyclobenzaprine.

DIDANOSINE   Systemic

A commonly used brand name in the U.S. and Canada is Videx.
Another commonly used name is ddI.

Description

Didanosine (di-DAN-oe-seen) (also known as ddI) is used in the treatment of the infection caused by the human immunodeficiency virus (HIV). HIV is the virus responsible for acquired immune deficiency syndrome (AIDS).

Didanosine (ddI) will not cure or prevent HIV infection or AIDS. It appears to slow down the destruction of the immune system caused by HIV. This may help delay the development of symptoms related to advanced HIV disease. However, it will not keep you from spreading the virus to other people. People who receive this medicine may continue to have the problems usually related to AIDS or HIV disease.

HIV infection can result in a very serious, usually fatal, disease. An estimated 1 to 1.5 million persons in the United States are currently infected with HIV. It has become one of the leading causes of death in men and women under the age of 45 and in children between 1 and 5 years of age.

HIV primarily attacks certain white blood cells and slowly, over several years, breaks down the body's immune system. When this happens, the person may develop other serious infections as well. These include fungus infections, *Pneumocystis* (noo-moe-SISS-tis) *carinii* pneumonia (PCP), and cytomegalovirus (CMV) infections, which can affect the retina of the eyes, the lungs, and the stomach and intestines. The person may also develop certain kinds of cancer, such as non-Hodgkin's lymphoma and Kaposi's sarcoma, a form of cancer usually causing purplish tumors of the skin or mouth. Didanosine may be given with other medicines to treat these problems.

Although most cases of HIV infection in the U.S. have occurred in homosexual and bisexual men, HIV infection has increased most rapidly in people exposed to the virus through heterosexual contact. Other people at risk of contracting HIV are intravenous drug users and their sexual partners, and people who received transfusions with blood or blood products contaminated with the AIDS virus and their sexual partners. Children born to mothers infected with HIV are also at risk of getting the virus.

This virus is spread from person to person by infected body fluids, such as blood, semen, vaginal fluids (including menstrual blood), and breast milk. HIV is almost always spread by the intimate exchange of these fluids that occurs during unprotected sex (vaginal, anal, and possibly oral) with someone who is infected with the virus and/or by sharing contaminated needles and syringes when injecting drugs. HIV is also spread from an infected mother to her fetus during pregnancy or childbirth, and, rarely, through breast-feeding. It is not spread by casual contact, such as touching, shaking hands, coughing, sneezing, or by routine everyday contact, such as working in the same office, going to the same school, or eating in the same restaurant.

HIV can infect people of any age, sex, race, or sexual orientation. Because symptoms may take months, or more often years, to appear, an infected person may look and feel fine. During this time a person may spread the infection to others without knowing it.

The early symptoms of HIV infection may include fever; night sweats; swollen glands in the neck, armpit, and/or groin; unexplained weight loss; profound tiredness; yeast infections in the mouth; diarrhea; continuing cough; weakness; loss of appetite; or, in women, vaginal yeast infections.

Didanosine may cause some serious side effects, including pancreatitis (inflammation of the pancreas). Symptoms of pancreatitis include stomach pain, and nausea and vomiting. Didanosine may also cause peripheral neuropathy. Symptoms of peripheral neuropathy include tingling, burning, numbness, and pain in the hands or feet. *Check with your doctor if any new health problems or symptoms occur while you are taking didanosine.*

Didanosine is available only with your doctor's prescription, in the following dosage forms:

Oral

- Oral solution (U.S.)
- Oral suspension (U.S. and Canada)
- Tablets (U.S. and Canada)

It is very important that you read and understand the following information. If any of it causes you special concern, check with your doctor. Also, *if you have any questions* or if you want more information about this medicine or your medical problem, *ask your doctor, nurse, or pharmacist.*

Before Using This Medicine

In deciding to use a medicine, the risks of taking the medicine must be weighed against the good it will do. This is a decision you and your doctor will make. For didanosine, the following should be considered:

Allergies—Tell your doctor if you have ever had any unusual or allergic reaction to didanosine. Also tell your doctor and pharmacist if you are allergic to any other substances, such as foods, preservatives, or dyes.

Diet—Make certain your doctor and pharmacist know if you are on any special diet, such as a low-sodium or low-phenylalanine diet. Didanosine chewable tablets and the oral solution packets contain a large amount of sodium.

Pregnancy—Didanosine crosses the placenta. Studies in pregnant women have not been done. However, didanosine has not been shown to cause birth defects or other problems in animal studies.

Breast-feeding—It is not known whether didanosine passes into the breast milk. However, if your baby does not already have the AIDS virus, there is a chance that you could pass it to your baby by breast-feeding. Talk to your doctor first if you are thinking about breast-feeding your baby.

Children—Didanosine can cause serious side effects in any patient. Therefore, it is especially important that you discuss with your child's doctor the good that this medicine may do as well as the risks of using it. Your child must be carefully followed, and frequently seen, by the doctor while taking didanosine.

Older adults—Didanosine has not been studied specifically in older people. Therefore, it is not known whether it causes different side effects or problems in the elderly than it does in younger adults.

Other medicines—Although certain medicines should not be used together at all, in other cases 2 different medicines may be used together even if an interaction might occur. In these cases, your doctor may want to change the dose, or other

precautions may be necessary. When you are taking didanosine, it is especially important that your doctor and pharmacist know if you are taking any of the following:

- Alcohol or
- Asparaginase (e.g., Elspar) or
- Azathioprine (e.g., Imuran) or
- Estrogens (female hormones) or
- Furosemide (e.g., Lasix) or
- Methyldopa (e.g., Aldomet) or
- Pentamidine (e.g., Pentam, Pentacarinat) or
- Sulfonamides (e.g., Bactrim, Septra) or
- Sulindac (e.g., Clinoril) or
- Thiazide diuretics (e.g., Diuril, Hydrodiuril) or
- Valproic acid (e.g., Depakote)—Use of these medicines with didanosine may increase the chance of pancreatitis (inflammation of the pancreas)
- Chloramphenicol (e.g., Chloromycetin) or
- Cisplatin (e.g., Platinol) or
- Ethambutol (e.g., Myambutol) or
- Ethionamide (e.g., Trecator-SC) or
- Hydralazine (e.g., Apresoline) or
- Isoniazid (e.g., Nydrazid) or
- Lithium (e.g., Eskalith, Lithobid) or
- Metronidazole (e.g., Flagyl) or
- Nitrous oxide or
- Phenytoin (e.g., Dilantin) or
- Vincristine (e.g., Oncovin)—Use of these medicines with didanosine may increase the chance of peripheral neuropathy (tingling, burning, numbness, or pain in your hands or feet)
- Ciprofloxacin (e.g., Cipro) or
- Ketoconazole (e.g., Nizoral) or
- Norfloxacin (e.g., Noroxin) or
- Ofloxacin (e.g., Floxin) or
- Trimethoprim (e.g., Proloprim, Trimpex)—Use of these medicines with didanosine may keep these medicines from working properly; these medicines should be taken at least 2 hours before or 2 hours after taking didanosine
- Dapsone (e.g., Avlosulfon)—Use of dapsone with didanosine may increase the chance of peripheral neuropathy (tingling, burning, numbness, or pain in your hands or feet); it may also keep dapsone from working properly; dapsone should be taken at least 2 hours before or 2 hours after taking didanosine

- Nitrofurantoin (e.g., Macrodantin)—Use of nitrofurantoin with didanosine may increase the chance of pancreatitis (inflammation of the pancreas) and peripheral neuropathy (tingling, burning, numbness, or pain in your hands or feet)
- Tetracyclines (e.g., Achromycin, Minocin)—Use of tetracyclines with didanosine may increase the chance of pancreatitis (inflammation of the pancreas); it may also keep the tetracycline from working properly; tetracyclines should be taken at least 2 hours before or 2 hours after taking didanosine

Other medical problems—The presence of other medical problems may affect the use of didanosine. Make sure you tell your doctor if you have any other medical problems, especially:

- Alcoholism, active, or
- Increased blood triglycerides or
- Pancreatitis (or a history of)—Patients with these medical problems may be at increased risk of pancreatitis (inflammation of the pancreas)
- Edema or
- Heart disease or
- High blood pressure or
- Kidney disease or
- Liver disease or
- Toxemia of pregnancy—The salt contained in the didanosine tablets and the oral solution packets may make these conditions worse
- Gout—Didanosine may cause an attack or worsen gout
- Peripheral neuropathy—Didanosine may make this condition worse
- Phenyketonuria (PKU)—Didanosine tablets contain phenylalanine, which must be restricted in patients with PKU

Before you begin using any new medicine (prescription or nonprescription) or if you develop any new medical problem while you are using this medicine, check with your doctor, nurse, or pharmacist.

Proper Use of This Medicine

Take this medicine exactly as directed by your doctor. Do not take more of it, do not take it more often, and do not take it for a longer time than your doctor ordered. Also, do not stop taking this medicine without checking with your doctor first.

Keep taking didanosine for the full time of treatment, even if you begin to feel better.

For patients taking *didanosine pediatric oral suspension:*
- Use a specially marked measuring spoon or other device to measure each dose accurately. The average household teaspoon may not hold the right amount of liquid.

For patients taking *didanosine oral solution:*
- Open the foil packet and pour its contents into approximately 1/2 glass (4 ounces) of water. Do not mix with fruit juice or other acid-containing drinks.
- Stir for approximately 2 to 3 minutes until the powder is dissolved.
- Drink at once.

For patients taking *didanosine tablets:*
- Tablets should be thoroughly chewed or crushed or mixed in 1 ounce of water before swallowing. The tablets are hard and some people may find them difficult to chew. If the tablets are mixed in water, stir well until a uniform suspension is formed and taken at once.
- Two tablets must be taken together by patients over 1 year of age. These tablets contain a special buffer to keep didanosine from being destroyed in the stomach. In order to get the correct amount of buffer, 2 tablets always need to be taken together. Infants from 6 to 12 months of age will get enough buffer from just 1 tablet.

Didanosine should be taken on an empty stomach since food may decrease the absorption in the stomach and keep it from working properly. Didanosine should be taken at least 2 hours before or 2 hours after you eat.

This medicine works best when there is a constant amount in the blood. *To help keep the amount constant, do not miss any doses.* If you need help in planning the best times to take your medicine, check with your doctor, nurse, or pharmacist.

Missed dose—If you do miss a dose of this medicine, take it as soon as possible. However, if it is almost time for your next dose, skip the missed dose and go back to your regular dosing schedule. Do not double doses.

Only take medicine that your doctor has prescribed specifically for you. Do not share your medicine with others.

Storage—To store this medicine:
- Keep out of the reach of children.
- Store away from heat and direct light.
- Do not store in the bathroom, near the kitchen sink, or in other damp places. Heat or moisture may cause the medicine to break down.
- Do not keep outdated medicine or medicine no longer needed. Be sure that any discarded medicine is out of the reach of children.

Precautions While Using This Medicine

It is very important that your doctor check your progress at regular visits.

Do not take any other medicines without checking with your doctor first. To do so may increase the chance of side effects from didanosine.

HIV may be acquired from or spread to other people through infected body fluids, including blood, vaginal fluid, or semen. *If you are infected, it is best to avoid any sexual activity involving an exchange of body fluids with other people. If you do have sex, always wear (or have your partner wear) a condom ("rubber").* Only use condoms made of latex, and *use them every time you have vaginal, anal, or oral sex.* The use of a spermicide (such as nonoxynol-9) may also help prevent transmission of HIV if it is not irritating to the vagina, rectum, or mouth. Spermicides have been shown to kill HIV in lab tests. Do not use oil-based Jelly, cold cream, baby oil, or shortening as a lubricant—these products can cause the rubber to break. Lubricants without oil, such as *K-Y jelly* or *CondomMate*, are recommended. Women may wish to carry their own condoms. Birth control pills and diaphragms will help protect against pregnancy, but they will not prevent someone from giving or getting the AIDS virus. *If you inject drugs*, get help to stop. *Do not share needles or equipment with anyone.* In some cities, more than half of the drug users are infected and sharing even 1 needle or syringe can spread the virus. If you have any questions about this, check with your doctor, nurse, or pharmacist.

Side Effects of This Medicine

Along with its needed effects, a medicine may cause some unwanted effects. Although not all of these side effects may occur, if they do occur they may need medical attention.

Check with your doctor immediately if any of the following side effects occur:

> *Less common*
>> Nausea and vomiting; stomach pain; tingling, burning, numbness, and pain in the hands or feet
>
> *Rare*
>> Convulsions (seizures); fever and chills; sore throat; skin rash and itching; unusual bleeding and bruising; unusual tiredness and weakness

Other side effects may occur that usually do not need medical attention. These side effects may go away during treatment as your body adjusts to the medicine. However, check with your doctor if any of the following side effects continue or are bothersome:

> *More common*
>> Anxiety; diarrhea; difficulty in sleeping; headache; irritability; restlessness

Other side effects not listed above may also occur in some patients. If you notice any other effects, check with your doctor.

DIGITALIS MEDICINES   Systemic

This information applies to the following medicines:

Deslanoside (des-LAN-oh-side)
Digitoxin (di-ji-TOX-in)
Digoxin (di-JOX-in)

Some commonly used brand names are:

For Deslanoside
In the U.S.
Cedilanid-D

In Canada
Cedilanid

For Digitoxin†
In the U.S.
Crystodigin
Generic name product may also be available.

For Digoxin
In the U.S.
Lanoxicaps
Lanoxin
Generic name product may also be available.

In Canada
Lanoxin
Novodigoxin
Generic name product may also be available.

†Not commercially available in Canada.

Description

Digitalis medicines are used to improve the strength and efficiency of the heart, or to control the rate and rhythm of the heartbeat. This leads to better blood circulation and reduced swelling of hands and ankles in patients with heart problems.

Although digitalis has been prescribed to help some patients lose weight, it should *never* be used in this way. When used improperly, digitalis can cause serious problems.

Digitalis medicines are available only with your doctor's prescription, in the following dosage forms:

Oral
> Digitoxin
> > • Tablets (U.S.)
> Digoxin
> > • Capsules (U.S.)
> > • Elixir (U.S. and Canada)
> > • Tablets (U.S. and Canada)

Parenteral
> Deslanoside
> > • Injection (U.S. and Canada)
> Digoxin
> > • Injection (U.S. and Canada)

It is very important that you read and understand the following information. If any of it causes you special concern, check with your doctor. Also, *if you have any questions* or if you want more information about this medicine or your medical problem, *ask your doctor, nurse, or pharmacist.*

Before Using This Medicine

In deciding to use a medicine, the risks of taking the medicine must be weighed against the good it will do. This is a decision you and your doctor will make. For digitalis medicines, the following should be considered:

Allergies—Tell your doctor if you have ever had any unusual or allergic reaction to digitalis medicines. Also tell your doctor and pharmacist if you are allergic to any other substances, such as foods, preservatives, or dyes.

Diet—Make certain your doctor and pharmacist know if you are on a low-sodium, low-sugar, or any other special diet. Most medicines contain more than their active ingredient, and many liquid medicines contain alcohol.

Pregnancy—Digitalis medicines have not been studied in pregnant women or animals. However, these medicines pass from the mother to the fetus. Make sure your doctor knows if you are pregnant or if you may become pregnant before taking digitalis medicines.

Breast-feeding—Although small amounts of digitalis medicines pass into the breast milk, they have not been reported to cause problems in nursing babies.

Children—This medicine has been tested in children and, in effective doses, has not been shown to cause different side effects or problems than it does in adults. However, the dose is very different for babies and children, and it is important to follow your doctor's instructions exactly.

Older adults—Signs and symptoms of overdose may be especially likely to occur in elderly patients, who are usually more sensitive than younger adults to the effects of digitalis medicines.

Other medicines—Although certain medicines should not be used together at all, in other cases 2 different medicines may be used together even if an interaction might occur. In these cases, your doctor may want to change the dose, or other precautions may be necessary. When taking or receiving digitalis medicines it is especially important that your doctor and pharmacist know if you are taking any of the following:

- Adrenocorticoids (cortisone-like medicine) or
- Amphotericin B by injection (e.g., Fungizone) or
- Diuretics (water pills)—These medicines can cause hypokalemia (low levels of potassium in the body), which can increase the unwanted effects of digitalis medicines
- Amiodarone (e.g., Cordarone)—May cause levels of digitalis medicines in the body to be higher than usual, which could lead to signs or symptoms of overdose
- Amphetamines or
- Appetite suppressants (diet pills) or
- Digitalis medicines (other) or other heart medicine or
- Medicine for asthma or other breathing problems or
- Medicine for colds, sinus problems, or hay fever or other allergies (including nose drops or sprays)—May increase the risk of heart rhythm problems
- Cholestyramine (e.g., Questran) or
- Colestipol (e.g., Colestid) or
- Diarrhea medicine or
- If your diet contains large amounts of fiber, such as bran— May decrease effects of digitalis medicines by blocking them from being absorbed into the body
- Diltiazem (e.g., Cardizem) or
- Verapamil (e.g., Calan)—May cause levels of digitalis medicines in the body to be higher than usual, which could lead to signs or symptoms of overdose

- Potassium-containing medicines or supplements—If levels of potassium in the body become too high, there is a serious risk of heart rhythm problems being caused by digitalis medicines
- Quinidine (e.g., Quinidex)—May cause levels of digitalis medicines in the body to be higher than usual, which could lead to signs or symptoms of overdose

Other medical problems—The presence of other medical problems may affect the use of digitalis medicines. Make sure you tell your doctor if you have any other medical problems, especially:

- Kidney disease or
- Liver disease—Effects may be increased because of slower removal of digitalis medicines from the body
- Lung disease (severe) or
- Rheumatic fever (history of)—The heart may be more sensitive to the effects of digitalis medicines

Before you begin using any new medicine (prescription or nonprescription) or if you develop any new medical problem while you are using this medicine, check with your doctor, nurse, or pharmacist.

Proper Use of This Medicine

To keep your heart working properly, *take this medicine exactly as directed even though you may feel well.* Do not take more of it than your doctor ordered and do not miss any doses.

For patients taking the *liquid form of digoxin:*

- This medicine is to be taken by mouth even if it comes in a dropper bottle. The amount you should take is to be measured only with the specially marked dropper.

To help you remember to take your dose of medicine, try to take it at the same time every day.

Ask your doctor about checking your pulse rate. Then, while you are taking this medicine, check your pulse regularly. If it is much slower, or faster, than your usual rate (or less than 60 beats per minute), or if it changes in rhythm or force, check with your doctor. Such changes may mean that side effects are developing.

Missed dose—If you do miss a dose of this medicine, and you remember it within 12 hours, take it as soon as you remember. However, if you do not remember until later, do not take the missed dose at all and do not double the next one. Instead, go back to your regular dosing schedule. If you have any questions about this or if you miss doses for 2 or more days in a row, check with your doctor.

Storage—To store this medicine:
- Keep out of the reach of children.
- Store away from heat and direct light.
- Do not store in the bathroom, near the kitchen sink, or in other damp places. Heat or moisture may cause the medicine to break down.
- Keep the oral liquid form of this medicine from freezing.
- Do not keep outdated medicine or medicine no longer needed. Be sure that any discarded medicine is out of the reach of children.

Precautions While Using This Medicine

It is important that your doctor check your progress at regular visits to make sure the medicine is working properly. This will allow your doctor to make any changes in directions for taking it, if necessary.

Do not stop taking this medicine without first checking with your doctor. Stopping suddenly may cause a serious change in heart function.

Keep this medicine out of the reach of children. Digitalis medicines are a major cause of accidental poisoning in children.

Watch for signs and symptoms of overdose while you are taking digitalis medicine. Follow your doctor's directions carefully. The amount of this medicine needed to help most people is very close to the amount that could cause serious problems from overdose. Some early warning signs of overdose are loss of appetite, nausea, vomiting, diarrhea, or extremely slow heartbeat. In infants and small children, the earliest signs of overdose are changes in the rate and rhythm of the heartbeat. Children may not show the other symptoms as soon as adults.

Before having any kind of surgery (including dental surgery) or emergency treatment, tell the medical doctor or dentist in charge that you are using this medicine.

Your doctor may want you to carry a medical identification card or bracelet stating that you are taking this medicine.

Do not take any other medicine unless ordered by your doctor. Many over-the-counter (OTC) or nonprescription medicines contain ingredients that interfere with digitalis medicines or that may make your condition worse. These medicines include antacids; laxatives; asthma remedies; cold, cough, or sinus preparations; medicine for diarrhea; and reducing or diet medicines.

For patients taking the *tablet or capsule* form of this medicine:

- This medicine may look like other tablets or capsules you now take. It is very important that you do not get the medicines mixed up since this may have serious results. Ask your pharmacist for ways to avoid mix-ups with medicines that look alike.

Side Effects of This Medicine

Along with its needed effects, a medicine may cause some unwanted effects. Although not all of these side effects may occur, if they do occur they may need medical attention.

Check with your doctor as soon as possible if any of the following side effects or symptoms of overdose occur:

Rare
    Skin rash or hives

Signs and symptoms of overdose (in the order in which they may occur)

> Loss of appetite; nausea or vomiting; lower stomach pain; diarrhea;. unusual tiredness or weakness (extreme); slow or irregular heartbeat (may be fast heartbeat in children); blurred vision or "yellow, green, or white vision" (yellow, green, or white halo seen around objects); drowsiness; confusion or mental depression; headache; fainting

Note: Overdose symptoms in infants and small children may occur at first only as changes in the heartbeat rate or rhythm, while in adults and older children the first symptoms may be mostly stomach upset, stomach pain, loss of appetite, or unusually slow heartbeat.

Other side effects not listed above may also occur in some patients. If you notice any other effects, check with your doctor.

DISOPYRAMIDE   Systemic

Some commonly used brand names are:
> *In the U.S.*
>> Norpace
>> Norpace CR
>> Generic name product may also be available.
>
> *In Canada*
>> Norpace   Rythmodan
>> Norpace CR   Rythmodan-LA

Description

Disopyramide (dye-soe-PEER-a-mide) is used to correct irregular heartbeats to a normal rhythm and to slow an overactive heart. This allows the heart to work more efficiently.

Disopyramide is available only with your doctor's prescription, in the following dosage forms:
> *Oral*
> - Capsules (U.S. and Canada)
> - Extended-release capsules (U.S.)
> - Extended-release tablets (Canada)

It is very important that you read and understand the following information. If any of it causes you special concern, check with your doctor. Also, *if you have any questions* or if you want more information about this medicine or your medical problem, *ask your doctor, nurse, or pharmacist.*

Before Using This Medicine

In deciding to use a medicine, the risks of taking the medicine must be weighed against the good it will do. This is a decision you and your doctor will make. For disopyramide, the following should be considered:

Allergies—Tell your doctor if you have ever had any unusual or allergic reaction to disopyramide. Also tell your doctor and pharmacist if you are allergic to any other substance, such as foods, sulfites or other preservatives, or dyes.

Pregnancy—Studies have not been done in humans. Although use in pregnant patients is limited, there are some reports that disopyramide when taken during pregnancy caused contractions of the uterus.

Breast-feeding—Although disopyramide passes into breast milk, this medicine has not been reported to cause problems in nursing babies.

Children—This medicine has been tested in children and has not been shown to cause different side effects or problems than it does in adults.

Older adults—Some side effects, such as difficult urination and dry mouth, may be especially likely to occur in elderly patients, who are usually more sensitive than younger adults to the effects of disopyramide.

Other medicines—Although certain medicines should not be used together at all, in other cases two different medicines may be used together even if an interaction might occur. In these cases, your doctor may want to change the dose, or other precautions may be necessary. When you are taking disopyramide, it is especially important that your doctor and pharmacist know if you are taking any of the following:

- Other heart medicine—Effects on the heart may be increased
- Pimozide (e.g., Orap)—Risk of heart rhythm problems may be increased

Other medical problems—The presence of other medical problems may affect the use of disopyramide. Make sure you tell your doctor if you have any other medical problems, especially:

- Diabetes mellitus (sugar diabetes)—Disopyramide may cause low blood sugar
- Difficult urination or
- Enlarged prostate—Disopyramide may cause difficult urination
- Glaucoma (history of)—May be worsened by disopyramide
- Kidney disease or
- Liver disease—Effects may be increased because of slower removal from the body
- Myasthenia gravis—May be worsened by disopyramide

Before you begin using any new medicine (prescription or nonprescription) or if you develop any new medical problem while you are using this medicine, check with your doctor, nurse, or pharmacist.

Proper Use of This Medicine

Take disopyramide exactly as directed by your doctor even though you may feel well. Do not take more medicine than ordered.

For patients taking the *extended-release capsules:*

- Swallow the capsule whole without breaking, crushing, or chewing.

For patients taking the *extended-release tablets:*

- Do not crush or chew the tablet.

This medicine works best when there is a constant amount in the blood. *To help keep the amount constant, do not miss any doses. Also, it is best to take the doses at evenly spaced times day and night.* For example, if you are to take 4 doses a day, the doses should be spaced about 6 hours apart. If this interferes with your sleep or other daily activities, or if you need help in planning the best times to take your medicine, check with your doctor, nurse, or pharmacist.

Missed dose—*If you do miss a dose of this medicine, take it as soon as possible unless the next scheduled dose is in less than 4 hours.* If you do not remember until later, skip the missed dose and go back to your regular dosing schedule. Do not double doses.

Storage—To store this medicine:
- Keep out of the reach of children.
- Store away from heat and direct light.
- Do not store in the bathroom, near the kitchen sink, or in other damp places. Heat or moisture may cause the medicine to break down.
- Do not keep outdated medicine or medicine no longer needed. Be sure that any discarded medicine is out of the reach of children.

Precautions While Using This Medicine

Your doctor should check your progress at regular visits to make sure the medicine is working properly.

Do not stop taking this medicine without first checking with your doctor. Stopping suddenly may cause a serious change in heart function.

Dizziness, lightheadedness, or fainting may occur, especially when you get up from a lying or sitting position. This is due to lowered blood pressure. Getting up slowly may help. This effect does not occur often at doses of disopyramide usually used; however, *make sure you know how you react to this medicine before you drive, use machines, or do anything else that could be dangerous if you are not alert.* If the problem continues or gets worse, check with your doctor.

Avoid alcoholic beverages until you have discussed their use with your doctor. Alcohol may make the low blood sugar effect worse and/or increase the possibility of dizziness or fainting.

Disopyramide may cause hypoglycemia (low blood sugar) in some people. Patients with congestive heart disease or diabetes especially should be aware of the signs of hypoglycemia. (See Side Effects of This Medicine.) If these signs appear, eat or drink a food containing sugar and call your doctor right away.

This medicine may cause blurred vision or other vision problems. If any of these occur, *do not drive, use machines, or do anything else that could be dangerous if you are not able to see well.*

Disopyramide may cause dryness of the mouth, nose, and throat. For temporary relief of mouth dryness, use sugarless candy or gum, melt bits of ice in your mouth, or use a saliva substitute. However, if dry mouth continues for more than 2 weeks, check with your medical doctor or dentist. Continuing dryness of the mouth may increase the chance of dental disease, including tooth decay, gum disease, and fungus infections.

This medicine will often make you sweat less, allowing your body temperature to increase. *Use extra care not to become overheated during exercise or hot weather while you are taking this medicine*, since overheating could possibly result in heat stroke.

Side Effects of This Medicine

Along with its needed effects, a medicine may cause some unwanted effects. Although not all of these side effects may occur, if they do occur they may need medical attention.

Check with your doctor as soon as possible if any of the following side effects occur:

More common
    Difficult urination

Less common

Chest pains; dizziness, lightheadedness, or fainting; fast or slow heartbeat; muscle weakness; shortness of breath (unexplained); swelling of feet or lower legs; weight gain (rapid)

Rare

Eye pain; mental depression; sore throat and fever; yellow eyes or skin

Signs and symptoms of hypoglycemia (low blood sugar)

Anxious feeling; chills; cold sweats; confusion; cool, pale skin; drowsiness; fast heartbeat; headache; hunger (excessive); nausea; nervousness; shakiness; unsteady walk; unusual tiredness or weakness

Other side effects may occur that usually do not need medical attention. These side effects may go away during treatment as your body adjusts to the medicine. However, check with your doctor or nurse if any of the following side effects continue or are bothersome:

More common

Dry mouth and throat

Less common

Bloating or stomach pain; blurred vision; constipation; decreased sexual ability; dry eyes and nose; frequent urge to urinate; loss of appetite

Other side effects not listed above may also occur in some patients. If you notice any other effects, check with your doctor.

DIURETICS, LOOP   Systemic

This information applies to the following medicines:

Bumetanide (byoo-MET-a-nide)
Ethacrynic Acid (eth-a-KRIN-ik AS-id)
Furosemide (fur-OH-se-mide)

Some commonly used brand names are:

For Bumetanide†
In the U.S.
Bumex

For Ethacrynic Acid
> *In the U.S.*
> > Edecrin
> *In Canada*
> > Edecrin

For Furosemide
> *In the U.S.*
> > Lasix
> > Myrosemide
>
> > Generic name product may also be available.
>
> *In Canada*
> > Apo-Furosemide   Lasix Special
> > Furoside   Novosemide
> > Lasix   Uritol
>
> > Generic name product may also be available.

---

†Not commercially available in Canada.

Description

Loop diuretics are given to help reduce the amount of water in the body. They work by acting on the kidneys to increase the flow of urine.

Furosemide is also used to treat high blood pressure (hypertension) in those patients who are not helped by other medicines or in those patients who have kidney problems.

High blood pressure adds to the workload of the heart and arteries. If it continues for a long time, the heart and arteries may not function properly. This can damage the blood vessels of the brain, heart, and kidneys, resulting in a stroke, heart failure, or kidney failure. High blood pressure may also increase the risk of heart attacks. These problems may be less likely to occur if blood pressure is controlled.

Loop diuretics may also be used for other conditions as determined by your doctor.

This medicine is available only with your doctor's prescription, in the following dosage forms:
> *Oral*
> > Bumetanide
> > > • Tablets (U.S.)

Ethacrynic Acid
- Oral solution (U.S. and Canada)
- Tablets (U.S. and Canada)

Furosemide
- Oral solution (U.S. and Canada)
- Tablets (U.S. and Canada)

Parenteral

Bumetanide
- Injection (U.S.)

Ethacrynic Acid
- Injection (U.S. and Canada)

Furosemide
- Injection (U.S. and Canada)

It is very important that you read and understand the following information. If any of it causes you special concern, check with your doctor. Also, *if you have any questions* or if you want more information about this medicine or your medical problem, *ask your doctor, nurse, or pharmacist.*

Before Using This Medicine

In deciding to use a medicine, the risks of taking the medicine must be weighed against the good it will do. This is a decision you and your doctor will make. For loop diuretics, the following should be considered:

Allergies—Tell your doctor if you have ever had any unusual or allergic reaction to bumetanide, ethacrynic acid, furosemide, sulfonamides (sulfa drugs), or thiazide diuretics (water pills). Also tell your doctor and pharmacist if you are allergic to any other substances, such as foods, preservatives, or dyes.

Pregnancy—Studies have not been done in pregnant women. However, studies in animals have shown this medicine to cause harmful effects.

In general, diuretics are not useful for normal swelling of feet and hands that occurs during pregnancy. Diuretics should not be taken during pregnancy unless recommended by your doctor.

Breast-feeding—This medicine has not been reported to cause problems in nursing babies. Furosemide passes into breast milk; it is not known whether bumetanide or ethacrynic acid passes into breast milk.

Children—Although there is no specific information comparing the use of loop diuretics in children with use in any other age group, they are not expected to cause different side effects in children than they do in adults.

Older adults—Dizziness, lightheadedness, or signs of too much potassium loss may be more likely to occur in the elderly, who are more sensitive to the effects of this medicine. Elderly patients may also be more likely to develop blood clots.

Athletes—Diuretics are banned and tested for by the U.S. Olympic Committee (USOC) and the National Collegiate Athletic Association (NCAA). Diuretic use can lead to disqualification in all athletic events.

Other medicines—Although certain medicines should not be used together at all, in other cases two different medicines may be used together even if an interaction might occur. In these cases, your doctor may want to change the dose, or other precautions may be necessary. When you are taking loop diuretics, it is especially important that your doctor and pharmacist know if you are taking *any* other medicines.

Other medical problems—The presence of other medical problems may affect the use of loop diuretics. Make sure you tell your doctor if you have any other medical problems, especially:

- Diabetes mellitus (sugar diabetes)—Loop diuretics may increase the amount of sugar in the blood
- Diarrhea or
- Gout or
- Hearing problems or
- Pancreatitis (inflammation of the pancreas)—Loop diuretics may make these conditions worse
- Heart attack, recent—Use of loop diuretics after a recent heart attack may increase the chance of side effects

- Kidney disease (severe) or
- Liver disease—Higher blood levels of the loop diuretic may occur, which may increase the chance of side effects
- Lupus erythematosus (history of)—Ethacrynic acid and furosemide may make this condition worse

Before you begin using any new medicine (prescription or nonprescription) or if you develop any new medical problem while you are using this medicine, check with your doctor, nurse, or pharmacist.

Proper Use of This Medicine

This medicine may cause you to have an unusual feeling of tiredness when you begin to take it. You may also notice an increase in the amount of urine or in your frequency of urination. After you have taken the medicine for a while, these effects should lessen. In general, to keep the increase in urine from affecting your sleep:

- If you are to take a single dose a day, take it in the morning after breakfast.
- If you are to take more than one dose a day, take the last dose no later than 6 p.m., unless otherwise directed by your doctor.

However, it is best to plan your dose or doses according to a schedule that will least affect your personal activities and sleep. Ask your doctor, nurse, or pharmacist to help you plan the best time to take this medicine.

To help you remember to take your medicine, try to get into the habit of taking it at the same time each day.

For patients taking the *oral liquid form* of furosemide:

- This medicine is to be taken by mouth even if it comes in a dropper bottle. If this medicine does not come in a dropper bottle, use a specially marked measuring spoon or other device to measure each dose accurately, since the average household teaspoon may not hold the right amount of liquid.

For patients taking this medicine for *high blood pressure:*

- Importance of diet—When prescribing medicine for your condition, your doctor may prescribe a personal

diet for you. Such a diet may be low in sodium (salt).
Most people eat much more sodium than they need and
too much sodium in the diet may increase blood pressure. Some foods that contain large amounts of sodium
are canned soup, pickles, ketchup, green and ripe olives,
relish, frankfurters, soy sauce, and carbonated beverages. Your doctor may want you to limit the amounts
of these and other high-sodium foods in your diet. High
blood pressure medicine is usually more effective when
such a diet is properly followed.

Also, it may be very important for you to go on a reducing diet. However, check with your doctor before
changing your diet.

- Many patients who have high blood pressure will not
notice any signs of the problem. In fact, many may feel
normal. It is very important that you *take your medicine exactly as directed* and that you keep your appointments with your doctor even if you feel well.

- Remember that this medicine will not cure your high
blood pressure but it does help control it. Therefore,
you must continue to take it as directed if you expect
to lower your blood pressure and keep it down. *You
may have to take high blood pressure medicine for the
rest of your life.* If high blood pressure is not treated,
it can cause serious problems such as heart failure,
blood vessel disease, stroke, or kidney disease.

If this medicine upsets your stomach, it may be taken with
meals or milk. If stomach upset (nausea, vomiting, or stomach pain) continues or gets worse, or if you suddenly get
severe diarrhea, check with your doctor.

Missed dose—If you miss a dose of this medicine, take it
as soon as possible. However, if it is almost time for your
next dose, skip the missed dose and go back to your regular
dosing schedule. Do not double doses.

Storage—To store this medicine:

- Keep out of the reach of children.
- Store away from heat and direct light.

- Do not store in the bathroom, near the kitchen sink, or in other damp places. Heat or moisture may cause the medicine to break down.
- Keep the oral liquid form of this medicine from freezing.
- Do not keep outdated medicine or medicine no longer needed. Be sure that any discarded medicine is out of the reach of children.

Precautions While Using This Medicine

It is important that your doctor check your progress at regular visits to make sure that this medicine is working properly.

This medicine may cause a loss of potassium from your body:

- To help prevent this, your doctor may want you to:
  —eat or drink foods that have a high potassium content (for example, orange or other citrus fruit juices), or
  —take a potassium supplement, or
  —take another medicine to help prevent the loss of the potassium in the first place.
- It is very important to follow these directions. Also, it is important not to change your diet on your own. This is more important if you are already on a special diet (as for diabetes), or if you are taking a potassium supplement or a medicine to reduce potassium loss. Extra potassium may not be necessary and, in some cases, too much potassium could be harmful.

To prevent the loss of too much water and potassium, tell your doctor if you become sick, especially with severe or continuing nausea and vomiting or diarrhea.

Before having any kind of surgery (including dental surgery) or emergency treatment, make sure the medical doctor or dentist in charge knows that you are taking this medicine.

Dizziness, lightheadedness, or fainting may occur, especially when you get up from a lying or sitting position. This is more likely to occur in the morning. *Getting up slowly may help.* When you get up from lying down, sit on the edge of the bed with your feet dangling for 1 or 2 minutes. Then stand up slowly. If the problem continues or gets worse, check with your doctor.

The dizziness, lightheadedness, or fainting is also more likely to occur if you drink alcohol, stand for long periods of time, exercise, or if the weather is hot. *While you are taking this medicine, be careful to limit the amount of alcohol you drink. Also, use extra care during exercise or hot weather or if you must stand for long periods of time.*

For *diabetic patients:*

• This medicine may affect blood sugar levels. While you are using this medicine, be especially careful in testing for sugar in your blood or urine.

For patients taking this medicine for *high blood pressure:*

• *Do not take other medicines unless they have been discussed with your doctor.* This especially includes over-the-counter (nonprescription) medicines for appetite control, asthma, colds, cough, hay fever, or sinus problems, since they may tend to increase your blood pressure.

For patients taking *furosemide:*

• Furosemide may cause your skin to be more sensitive to sunlight than it is normally. Exposure to sunlight, even for brief periods of time, may cause a skin rash, itching, redness or other discoloration of the skin, or a severe sunburn. When you begin taking this medicine:

—Stay out of direct sunlight, especially between the hours of 10:00 a.m. and 3:00 p.m., if possible.

—Wear protective clothing, including a hat. Also, wear sunglasses.

—Apply a sun block product that has a skin protection factor (SPF) of at least 15. Some patients may require a product with a higher SPF number, especially if they have a fair complexion. If you have any questions about this, check with your doctor or pharmacist.

—Apply a sun block lipstick that has an SPF of at least 15 to protect your lips.

—Do not use a sunlamp or tanning bed or booth.

If you have a severe reaction from the sun, check with your doctor.

Side Effects of This Medicine

Along with its needed effects, a medicine may cause some unwanted effects. Although not all of these side effects may occur, if they do occur they may need medical attention.

Check with your doctor as soon as possible if any of the following side effects occur:

Rare

Black, tarry stools; blood in urine or stools; cough or hoarseness; fever or chills; joint pain; lower back or side pain; painful or difficult urination; pinpoint red spots on skin; ringing or buzzing in ears or any loss of hearing—more common with ethacrynic acid; skin rash or hives; stomach pain (severe) with nausea and vomiting; unusual bleeding or bruising; yellow eyes or skin; yellow vision—for furosemide only

Signs and symptoms of too much potassium loss

Dryness of mouth; increased thirst; irregular heartbeat; mood or mental changes; muscle cramps or pain; nausea or vomiting; unusual tiredness or weakness; weak pulse

Other side effects may occur that usually do not need medical attention. These side effects may go away during treatment as your body adjusts to the medicine. However, check with your doctor if any of the following side effects continue or are bothersome:

More common

Dizziness or lightheadedness when getting up from a lying or sitting position

Less common or rare

Blurred vision; chest pain—with bumetanide only; confusion—with ethacrynic acid only; diarrhea—more common with ethacrynic acid; headache; increased sensitivity of skin to sunlight—with furosemide only; loss of appetite—more common with ethacrynic acid; nervousness—

with ethacrynic acid only; premature ejaculation or difficulty in keeping an erection—with bumetanide only; redness or pain at place of injection; stomach cramps or pain

Other side effects not listed above may also occur in some patients. If you notice any other effects, check with your doctor.

Additional Information

Once a medicine has been approved for marketing for a certain use, experience may show that it is also useful for other medical problems. Although these uses are not included in product labeling, loop diuretics are used in certain patients with the following medical conditions:

- Hypercalcemia (too much calcium in the blood)
- Diagnostic aid for kidney disease

Other than the above information, there is no additional information relating to proper use, precautions, or side effects for these uses.

DIURETICS, POTASSIUM-SPARING Systemic

This information applies to the following medicines:

Amiloride (a-MILL-oh-ride)
Spironolactone (speer-on-oh-LAK-tone)
Triamterene (trye-AM-ter-een)

Some commonly used brand names are:

For Amiloride
In the U.S.
Midamor
Generic name product may also be available.

In Canada
Midamor

For Spironolactone
In the U.S.
Aldactone
Generic name product may also be available.

In Canada
  Aldactone
  Novospiroton

For Triamterene
  In the U.S.
    Dyrenium
  In Canada
    Dyrenium

Description

Potassium-sparing diuretics are commonly used to help reduce the amount of water in the body. Unlike some other diuretics, these medicines do not cause your body to lose potassium.

Amiloride and spironolactone are also used to treat high blood pressure (hypertension). High blood pressure adds to the workload of the heart and arteries. If the condition continues for a long time, the heart and arteries may not function properly. This can damage the blood vessels of the brain, heart, and kidneys, resulting in a stroke, heart failure, or kidney failure. High blood pressure may also increase the risk of heart attacks. These problems may be less likely to occur if blood pressure is controlled.

Spironolactone is also used to help increase the amount of potassium in the body when it is getting too low.

Potassium-sparing diuretics help to reduce the amount of water in the body by acting on the kidneys to increase the flow of urine. This also helps to lower blood pressure.

These medicines can also be used for other conditions as determined by your doctor.

Potassium-sparing diuretics are available only with your doctor's prescription, in the following dosage forms:

Oral
  Amiloride
    • Tablets (U.S. and Canada)
  Spironolactone
    • Tablets (U.S. and Canada)

Triamterene
- Capsules (U.S.)
- Tablets (Canada)

It is very important that you read and understand the following information. If any of it causes you special concern, check with your doctor. Also, *if you have any questions* or if you want more information about this medicine or your medical problem, *ask your doctor, nurse, or pharmacist.*

Before Using This Medicine

In deciding to use a medicine, the risks of taking the medicine must be weighed against the good it will do. This is a decision you and your doctor will make. For potassium-sparing diuretics, the following should be considered:

Allergies—Tell your doctor if you have ever had any unusual or allergic reaction to amiloride, spironolactone, or triamterene. Also tell your doctor and pharmacist if you are allergic to any other substances, such as foods, preservatives, or dyes.

Pregnancy—Studies have not been done in pregnant women. However, this medicine has not been shown to cause birth defects or other problems in animals.

In general, diuretics are not useful for normal swelling of feet and hands that occurs during pregnancy. Diuretics should not be taken during pregnancy unless recommended by your doctor.

Breast-feeding—Although amiloride, spironolactone, and triamterene may pass into breast milk, these medicines have not been reported to cause problems in nursing babies.

Children—This medicine has been tested in children and, in effective doses, has not been shown to cause different side effects or problems in children than it does in adults.

Older adults—Signs and symptoms of too much potassium are more likely to occur in the elderly, who are more sensitive than younger adults to the effects of this medicine.

Athletes—Diuretics are banned and tested for by the U.S. Olympic Committee (USOC) and the National Collegiate Athletic Association (NCAA). Diuretic use can lead to disqualification in all athletic events.

Other medicines—Although certain medicines should not be used together at all, in other cases two different medicines may be used together even if an interaction might occur. In these cases, your doctor may want to change the dose, or other precautions may be necessary. When you are taking potassium-sparing diuretics, it is especially important that your doctor and pharmacist know if you are taking any of the following:

- Captopril (e.g., Capoten) or
- Cyclosporine (e.g., Sandimmune) or
- Enalapril (e.g., Vasotec) or
- Lisinopril (e.g., Prinivil, Zestril) or
- Potassium-containing medicines or supplements—Use with potassium-sparing diuretics may cause high blood levels of potassium, which may increase the chance of side effects
- Digoxin—Use with spironolactone may cause high blood levels of digoxin, which may increase the chance of side effects
- Lithium (e.g., Lithane)—Use with potassium-sparing diuretics may cause high blood levels of lithium, which may increase the chance of side effects

Other medical problems—The presence of other medical problems may affect the use of potassium-sparing diuretics. Make sure you tell your doctor if you have any other medical problems, especially:

- Diabetes mellitus (sugar diabetes) or
- Kidney disease or
- Liver disease—Higher blood levels of potassium may occur, which may increase the chance of side effects
- Gout or
- Kidney stones (history of)—Triamterene may make these conditions worse
- Menstrual problems or breast enlargement—Spironolactone may make these conditions worse

Before you begin using any new medicine (prescription or nonprescription) or if you develop any new medical problem while you are using this medicine, check with your doctor, nurse, or pharmacist.

Proper Use of This Medicine

This medicine may cause you to have an unusual feeling of tiredness when you begin to take it. You may also notice an increase in the amount of urine or in your frequency of urination. After you have taken the medicine for a while, these effects should lessen. In general, to keep the increase in urine from affecting your sleep:

- If you are to take a single dose a day, take it in the morning after breakfast.
- If you are to take more than one dose a day, take the last dose no later than 6 p.m., unless otherwise directed by your doctor.

However, it is best to plan your dose or doses according to a schedule that will least affect your personal activities and sleep. Ask your doctor, nurse, or pharmacist to help you plan the best time to take this medicine.

To help you remember to take your medicine, try to get into the habit of taking it at the same time each day.

If this medicine upsets your stomach, it may be taken with meals or milk. If stomach upset (nausea, vomiting, stomach pain or cramps) continues, check with your doctor.

For patients taking this medicine for *high blood pressure:*

- Importance of diet—When prescribing medicine for your condition, your doctor may also prescribe a personal diet for you. Such a diet may be low in sodium (salt). Most people eat much more sodium than they need and too much sodium in the diet may increase blood pressure. Some foods that contain large amounts of sodium are canned soup, pickles, ketchup, green and ripe olives, relish, frankfurters, soy sauce, and carbonated beverages. Your doctor may want you to limit the amounts of these and other high-sodium foods in your diet. High blood pressure medicine is usually more effective when such a diet is properly followed.

  Also, it may be very important for you to go on a reducing diet. However, check with your doctor before changing your diet.

- Many patients who have high blood pressure will not notice any signs of the problem. In fact, many may feel normal. It is very important that you *take your medicine exactly as directed* and that you keep your appointments with your doctor even if you feel well.
- Remember that this medicine will not cure your high blood pressure but it does help control it. Therefore, you must continue to take it as directed if you expect to lower your blood pressure and keep it down. *You may have to take high blood pressure medicine for the rest of your life.* If high blood pressure is not treated, it can cause serious problems such as heart failure, blood vessel disease, stroke, or kidney disease.

Missed dose—If you miss a dose of this medicine, take it as soon as possible. However, if it is almost time for your next dose, skip the missed dose and go back to your regular dosing schedule. Do not double doses.

Storage—To store this medicine:

- Keep out of the reach of children.
- Store away from heat and direct light.
- Do not store in the bathroom, near the kitchen sink, or in other damp places. Heat or moisture may cause the medicine to break down.
- Do not keep outdated medicine or medicine no longer needed. Be sure that any discarded medicine is out of the reach of children.

Precautions While Using This Medicine

It is important that your doctor check your progress at regular visits to make sure that this medicine is working properly.

This medicine does not cause a loss of potassium from your body as some other diuretics (water pills) do. Therefore, it is not necessary for you to get extra potassium in your diet, and too much potassium could even be harmful. Since salt substitutes and low-sodium milk may contain potassium, do not use them unless told to do so by your doctor.

Check with your doctor if you become sick and have severe or continuing nausea, vomiting, or diarrhea. These problems may cause you to lose additional water, which could be harmful, or to lose potassium, which could lessen the medicine's helpful effects.

Before having any kind of surgery (including dental surgery) or emergency treatment, tell the medical doctor or dentist in charge that you are taking this medicine.

For patients taking this medicine for *high blood pressure:*
- *Do not take other medicines unless they have been discussed with your doctor.* This especially includes over-the-counter (nonprescription) medicines for appetite control, asthma, colds, cough, hay fever, or sinus problems, since these medicines may tend to increase your blood pressure.

For patients taking *triamterene:*
- For *diabetic patients*—This medicine may raise blood sugar levels. While you are using triamterene, be especially careful in testing for sugar in your urine. If you have any questions about this, check with your doctor.

Potassium-sparing diuretics may cause your skin to be more sensitive to sunlight than it is normally. Exposure to sunlight, even for brief periods of time, may cause a skin rash, itching, redness or other discoloration of the skin, or a severe sunburn. When you begin taking this medicine:
- Stay out of direct sunlight, especially between the hours of 10:00 a.m. and 3:00 p.m., if possible.
- Wear protective clothing, including a hat. Also, wear sunglasses.
- Apply a sun block product that has a skin protection factor (SPF) of at least 15. Some patients may require a product with a higher SPF number, especially if they have a fair complexion. If you have any questions about this, check with your doctor or pharmacist.

- Apply a sun block lipstick that has an SPF of at least 15 to protect your lips.
- Do not use a sunlamp or tanning bed or booth.

If you have a severe reaction from the sun, check with your doctor.

Before you have any medical tests, tell the doctor in charge that you are taking this medicine. The results of some tests may be affected by this medicine.

Side Effects of This Medicine

In rats, spironolactone has been found to increase the risk of tumors. It is not known if spironolactone increases the chance of tumors in humans.

Along with its needed effects, a medicine may cause some unwanted effects. Although not all of these side effects may occur, if they do occur they may need medical attention.

Check with your doctor as soon as possible if any of the following side effects occur:

Rare

For amiloride, spironolactone, and triamterene

Skin rash or itching

For spironolactone and triamterene only (in addition to effects listed above)

Cough or hoarseness; fever or chills; lower back or side pain; painful or difficult urination

For triamterene only (in addition to effects listed above)

Black, tarry stools; blood in urine or stools; bright red tongue; burning, inflamed feeling in tongue; cracked corners of mouth; pinpoint red spots on skin; unusual bleeding or bruising; weakness

Signs and symptoms of too much potassium

Confusion; irregular heartbeat; nervousness; numbness or tingling in hands, feet, or lips; shortness of breath or difficult breathing; unusual tiredness or weakness; weakness or heaviness of legs

Other side effects may occur that usually do not need medical attention. These side effects may go away during treat-

ment as your body adjusts to the medicine. However, check with your doctor if any of the following side effects continue or are bothersome:

More common (less common with amiloride and triamterene)
> Nausea and vomiting; stomach cramps and diarrhea

Less common
> *For amiloride, spironolactone, and triamterene*
>> Dizziness; headache

> *For amiloride and spironolactone only (in addition to effects listed above)*
>> Decreased sexual ability

> *For amiloride only (in addition to effects listed above)*
>> Constipation; muscle cramps

> *For spironolactone only (in addition to effects listed above for spironolactone)*
>> Breast tenderness in females; clumsiness; deepening of voice in females; enlargement of breasts in males; inability to have or keep an erection; increased hair growth in females; irregular menstrual periods; sweating

> *For triamterene only (in addition to effects listed above for triamterene)*
>> Increased sensitivity of skin to sunlight

Signs and symptoms of too little sodium
> Drowsiness; dryness of mouth; increased thirst; lack of energy

For *male patients:*
- Spironolactone sometimes causes enlarged breasts in males, especially when they take large doses of it for a long time. Breasts usually decrease in size gradually over several months after this medicine is stopped. If you have any questions about this, check with your doctor.

Other side effects not listed above may also occur in some patients. If you notice any other effects, check with your doctor.

Additional Information

Once a medicine has been approved for marketing for a certain use, experience may show that it is also useful for other medical problems. Although these uses are not specifically included in product labeling, spironolactone is used in certain patients with the following medical conditions:

- Polycystic ovary syndrome
- Hirsutism, female (increased hair growth)

Other than the above information, there is no additional information relating to proper use, precautions, or side effects for this use.

DIURETICS, THIAZIDE   Systemic

This information applies to the following medicines:

    Bendroflumethiazide (ben-droe-floo-meth-EYE-a-zide)
    Benzthiazide (benz-THYE-a-zide)
    Chlorothiazide (klor-oh-THYE-a-zide)
    Chlorthalidone (klor-THAL-i-doan)
    Cyclothiazide (sye-kloe-THYE-a-zide)
    Hydrochlorothiazide (hye-droe-klor-oh-THYE-a-zide)
    Hydroflumethiazide (hye-droe-floo-meth-EYE-a-zide)
    Methyclothiazide (meth-ee-kloe-THYE-a-zide)
    Metolazone (me-TOLE-a-zone)
    Polythiazide (pol-i-THYE-a-zide)
    Quinethazone (kwin-ETH-a-zone)
    Trichlormethiazide (trye-klor-meth-EYE-a-zide)

Some commonly used brand names are:

For Bendroflumethiazide
    In the U.S.
        Naturetin
    In Canada
        Naturetin

For Benzthiazide†
    In the U.S.
        Exna
        Hydrex
        Generic name product may also be available.

For Chlorothiazide†
    In the U.S.
        Diuril
        Generic name product may also be available.

For Chlorthalidone
In the U.S.
    Hygroton
    Thalitone
    Generic name product may also be available.
In Canada
    Apo-Chlorthalidone   Novo-Thalidone
    Hygroton   Uridon
    Generic name product may also be available.
Another commonly used name is chlortalidone.

For Cyclothiazide†
In the U.S.
    Anhydron

For Hydrochlorothiazide
In the U.S.
    Esidrix   HydroDIURIL
    Hydro-chlor   Oretic
    Hydro-D
    Generic name product may also be available.
In Canada
    Apo-Hydro   Neo-Codema
    Diuchlor H   Novo-Hydrazide
    HydroDIURIL   Urozide
    Generic name product may also be available.

For Hydroflumethiazide†
In the U.S.
    Diucardin
    Saluron
    Generic name product may also be available.

For Methyclothiazide
In the U.S.
    Aquatensen
    Enduron
    Generic name product may also be available.
In Canada
    Duretic

For Metolazone
In the U.S.
    Diulo   Zaroxolyn
    Mykrox
In Canada
    Zaroxolyn

For Polythiazide†
  In the U.S.
    Renese

For Quinethazone†
  In the U.S.
    Hydromox

For Trichlormethiazide†
  In the U.S.
    Metahydrin   Trichlorex
    Naqua
    Generic name product may also be available.

---

†Not commercially available in Canada.

Description

Thiazide or thiazide-like diuretics are commonly used to treat high blood pressure (hypertension). High blood pressure adds to the workload of the heart and arteries. If it continues for a long time, the heart and arteries may not function properly. This can damage the blood vessels of the brain, heart, and kidneys, resulting in a stroke, heart failure, or kidney failure. High blood pressure may also increase the risk of heart attacks. These problems may be less likely to occur if blood pressure is controlled.

Thiazide diuretics are also used to help reduce the amount of water in the body by increasing the flow of urine. They may also be used for other conditions as determined by your doctor.

Thiazide diuretics are available only with your doctor's prescription, in the following dosage forms:
  Oral
    Bendroflumethiazide
      • Tablets (U.S. and Canada)
    Benzthiazide
      • Tablets (U.S.)
    Chlorothiazide
      • Oral suspension (U.S.)
      • Tablets (U.S.)
    Chlorthalidone
      • Tablets (U.S. and Canada)

Cyclothiazide
- Tablets (U.S.)

Hydrochlorothiazide
- Oral solution (U.S.)
- Tablets (U.S. and Canada)

Hydroflumethiazide
- Tablets (U.S.)

Methyclothiazide
- Tablets (U.S. and Canada)

Metolazone
- Tablets (U.S. and Canada)

Polythiazide
- Tablets (U.S.)

Quinethazone
- Tablets (U.S.)

Trichlormethiazide
- Tablets (U.S.)

Parenteral

Chlorothiazide
- Injection (U.S.)

It is very important that you read and understand the following information. If any of it causes you special concern, check with your doctor. Also, *if you have any questions* or if you want more information about this medicine or your medical problem, *ask your doctor, nurse, or pharmacist.*

Before Using This Medicine

In deciding to use a medicine, the risks of taking the medicine must be weighed against the good it will do. This is a decision you and your doctor will make. For thiazide diuretics, the following should be considered:

Allergies—Tell your doctor if you have ever had any unusual or allergic reaction to sulfonamides (sulfa drugs), bumetanide, furosemide, acetazolamide, dichlorphenamide, methazolamide, or to any of the thiazide diuretics. Also tell your doctor and pharmacist if you are allergic to any other substances, such as foods, preservatives, or dyes.

Pregnancy—When this medicine is used during pregnancy, it may cause side effects including jaundice, blood problems, and low potassium in the newborn infant. In addition, although this medicine has not been shown to cause birth defects or other problems in animals, studies have not been done in humans.

In general, diuretics are not useful for normal swelling of feet and hands that occurs during pregnancy. They should not be taken during pregnancy unless recommended by your doctor.

Breast-feeding—Thiazide diuretics pass into breast milk. These medicines also may decrease the flow of breast milk. Therefore, you should avoid use of thiazide diuretics during the first month of breast-feeding.

Children—Although there is no specific information comparing the use of thiazide diuretics in children with use in other age groups, these medicines are not expected to cause different side effects or problems in children than they do in adults. However, extra caution may be necessary in infants with jaundice, because these medicines can make the condition worse.

Older adults—Dizziness or lightheadedness and signs of too much potassium loss may be more likely to occur in the elderly, who are more sensitive than younger adults to the effects of thiazide diuretics.

Athletes—Diuretics are banned and tested for by the U.S. Olympic Committee (USOC), the International Olympic Committee (IOC), and the National Collegiate Athletic Association (NCAA). Diuretic use can lead to disqualification in all athletic events.

Other medicines—Although certain medicines should not be used together at all, in other cases two different medicines may be used together even if an interaction might occur. In these cases, your doctor may want to change the dose, or other precautions may be necessary. When you are taking thiazide diuretics, it is especially important that your doctor and pharmacist know if you are taking any of the following:

- Cholestyramine or
- Colestipol—Use with thiazide diuretics may prevent the diuretic from working properly; take the diuretic at least 1 hour before or 4 hours after cholestyramine or colestipol

- Digitalis glycosides (heart medicine)—Use with thiazide diuretics may cause high blood levels of digoxin, which may increase the chance of side effects
- Lithium (e.g., Lithane)—Use with thiazide diuretics may cause high blood levels of lithium, which may increase the chance of side effects

Other medical problems—The presence of other medical problems may affect the use of thiazide diuretics. Make sure you tell your doctor if you have any other medical problems, especially:

- Diabetes mellitus (sugar diabetes)—Thiazide diuretics may increase the amount of sugar in the blood
- Gout (history of) or
- Lupus erythematosus (history of) or
- Pancreatitis (inflammation of the pancreas)—Thiazide diuretics may make these conditions worse
- Heart or blood vessel disease—Thiazide diuretics may cause high cholesterol levels or high triglyceride levels
- Liver disease or
- Kidney disease (severe)—Higher blood levels of the thiazide diuretic may occur, which may prevent the thiazide diuretic from working properly

Before you begin using any new medicine (prescription or nonprescription) or if you develop any new medical problem while you are using this medicine, check with your doctor, nurse, or pharmacist.

Proper Use of This Medicine

This medicine may cause you to have an unusual feeling of tiredness when you begin to take it. You may also notice an increase in the amount of urine or in your frequency of urination. After you have taken the medicine for a while, these effects should lessen. In general, to keep the increase in urine from affecting your sleep:

- If you are to take a single dose a day, take it in the morning after breakfast.
- If you are to take more than one dose a day, take the last dose no later than 6 p.m., unless otherwise directed by your doctor.

However, it is best to plan your dose or doses according to a schedule that will least affect your personal activities and sleep. Ask your doctor, nurse, or pharmacist to help you plan the best time to take this medicine.

To help you remember to take your medicine, try to get into the habit of taking it at the same time each day.

For patients taking this medicine for *high blood pressure:*
- In addition to the use of the medicine your doctor has prescribed, appropriate treatment for your high blood pressure may include weight control and care in the types of foods you eat, especially foods high in sodium. Your doctor will tell you which factors are most important for you. You should check with your doctor before changing your diet.
- Many patients who have high blood pressure will not notice any signs of the problem. In fact, many may feel normal. It is very important that you *take your medicine exactly as directed* and that you keep your appointments with your doctor even if you feel well.
- Remember that this medicine will not cure your high blood pressure but it does help control it. Therefore, you must continue to take it as directed if you expect to lower your blood pressure and keep it down. *You may have to take high blood pressure medicine for the rest of your life.* If high blood pressure is not treated, it can cause serious problems such as heart failure, blood vessel disease, stroke, or kidney disease.

For patients taking the *oral liquid form of hydrochlorothiazide,* which comes in a dropper bottle:
- This medicine is to be taken by mouth. The amount you should take is to be measured only with the specially marked dropper.

Missed dose—If you miss a dose of this medicine, take it as soon as possible. However, if it is almost time for your next dose, skip the missed dose and go back to your regular dosing schedule. Do not double doses.

Storage—To store this medicine:
- Keep out of the reach of children.
- Store away from heat and direct light.
- Do not store in the bathroom, near the kitchen sink, or in other damp places. Heat or moisture may cause the medicine to break down.
- Keep the oral liquid form of this medicine from freezing.
- Do not keep outdated medicine or medicine no longer needed. Be sure that any discarded medicine is out of the reach of children.

Precautions While Using This Medicine

It is important that your doctor check your progress at regular visits to make sure that this medicine is working properly.

This medicine may cause a loss of potassium from your body:
- To help prevent this, your doctor may want you to:
   —eat or drink foods that have a high potassium content (for example, orange or other citrus fruit juices), or
   —take a potassium supplement, or
   —take another medicine to help prevent the loss of the potassium in the first place.
- It is very important to follow these directions. Also, it is important not to change your diet on your own. This is more important if you are already on a special diet (as for diabetes), or if you are taking a potassium supplement or a medicine to reduce potassium loss. Extra potassium may not be necessary and, in some cases, too much potassium could be harmful.

Check with your doctor if you become sick and have severe or continuing vomiting or diarrhea. These problems may cause you to lose additional water and potassium.

For *diabetic patients:*
- Thiazide diuretics may raise blood sugar levels. While you are using this medicine, be especially careful in testing for sugar in your blood or urine.

Thiazide diuretics may cause your skin to be more sensitive to sunlight than it is normally. Exposure to sunlight, even for brief periods of time, may cause a skin rash, itching, redness or other discoloration of the skin, or a severe sunburn. When you begin taking this medicine:
- Stay out of direct sunlight, especially between the hours of 10:00 a.m. and 3:00 p.m., if possible.
- Wear protective clothing, including a hat. Also, wear sunglasses.
- Apply a sun block product that has a skin protection factor (SPF) of at least 15. Some patients may require a product with a higher SPF number, especially if they have a fair complexion. If you have any questions about this, check with your doctor or pharmacist.
- Apply a sun block lipstick that has an SPF of at least 15 to protect your lips.
- Do not use a sunlamp or tanning bed or booth.

If you have a severe reaction from the sun, check with your doctor.

For patients taking this medicine for *high blood pressure:*
- *Do not take other medicines unless they have been discussed with your doctor.* This especially includes over-the-counter (nonprescription) medicines for appetite control, asthma, colds, cough, hay fever, or sinus problems, since they may tend to increase your blood pressure.

Side Effects of This Medicine

Along with its needed effects, a medicine may cause some unwanted effects. Although not all of these side effects may occur, if they do occur they may need medical attention.

Check with your doctor as soon as possible if any of the following side effects occur:

Rare

Black, tarry stools; blood in urine or stools; cough or hoarseness; fever or chills; joint pain; lower back or side pain; painful or difficult urination; pinpoint red spots on skin; skin rash or hives; stomach pain (severe) with nausea and vomiting; unusual bleeding or bruising; yellow eyes or skin

Signs and symptoms of too much potassium loss

Dryness of mouth; increased thirst; irregular heartbeat; mood or mental changes; muscle cramps or pain; nausea or vomiting; unusual tiredness or weakness; weak pulse

Signs and symptoms of too much sodium loss

Confusion; convulsions; decreased mental activity; irritability; muscle cramps; unusual tiredness or weakness

Other side effects may occur that usually do not need medical attention. These side effects may go away during treatment as your body adjusts to the medicine. However, check with your doctor if any of the following side effects continue or are bothersome:

Less common

Decreased sexual ability; diarrhea; dizziness or lightheadedness when getting up from a lying or sitting position; increased sensitivity of skin to sunlight; loss of appetite; upset stomach

Other side effects not listed above may also occur in some patients. If you notice any other effects, check with your doctor.

Additional Information

Once a medicine has been approved for marketing for a certain use, experience may show that it is also useful for other medical problems. Although these uses are not specifically included in product labeling, thiazide diuretics are used in certain patients with the following medical conditions:

- Diabetes insipidus (water diabetes)
- Kidney stones (calcium-containing)

For patients taking this medicine for *diabetes insipidus (water diabetes):*

- Some thiazide diuretics are used in the treatment of diabetes insipidus (water diabetes). In patients with water diabetes, this medicine causes a decrease in the flow of urine and helps the body hold water. Thus, the information given above about increased urine flow will not apply to you.

Other than the above information, there is no additional information relating to proper use, precautions, or side effects for these uses.

DOXAZOSIN   Systemic

A commonly used brand name in the U.S. and Canada is Cardura.

Description

Doxazosin (dox-AY-zoe-sin) belongs to the general class of medicines called antihypertensives. It is used to treat high blood pressure (hypertension).

High blood pressure adds to the workload of the heart and arteries. If it continues for a long time, the heart and arteries may not function properly. This can damage the blood vessels of the brain, heart, and kidneys, resulting in a stroke, heart failure, or kidney failure. High blood pressure may also increase the risk of heart attacks. These problems may be less likely to occur if blood pressure is controlled.

Doxazosin works by relaxing blood vessels so that blood passes through them more easily. This helps to lower blood pressure.

Doxazosin is available only with your doctor's prescription, in the following dosage form:

   Oral
- Tablets (U.S. and Canada)

It is very important that you read and understand the following information. If any of it causes you special concern,

check with your doctor. Also, *if you have any questions* or if you want more information about this medicine or your medical problem, *ask your doctor, nurse, or pharmacist.*

Before Using This Medicine

In deciding to use a medicine, the risks of taking the medicine must be weighed against the good it will do. This is a decision you and your doctor will make. For doxazosin, the following should be considered:

Allergies—Tell your doctor if you have ever had any unusual or allergic reaction to doxazosin, prazosin, or terazosin. Also tell your doctor and pharmacist if you are allergic to any other substances, such as foods, preservatives, or dyes.

Pregnancy—Doxazosin has not been studied in pregnant women. However, studies in rats receiving oral doses of 75 times the highest recommended human dose have not shown that doxazosin causes harm to the fetus.

Breast-feeding—It is not known whether doxazosin passes into breast milk. However, this medicine has not been reported to cause problems in nursing babies.

Children—Studies on this medicine have been done only in adult patients, and there is no specific information comparing use of doxazosin in children with use in other age groups.

Older adults—Dizziness, lightheadedness, or fainting may be especially likely to occur in elderly patients, who are usually more sensitive than younger adults to the effects of doxazosin.

Other medicines—Although certain medicines should not be used together at all, in other cases two different medicines may be used together even if an interaction might occur. In these cases, your doctor may want to change the dose, or other precautions may be necessary. Tell your doctor and pharmacist if you are using any other prescription or non-prescription (over-the-counter [OTC]) medicine.

Other medical problems—The presence of other medical problems may affect the use of doxazosin. Make sure you

tell your doctor if you have any other medical problems, especially:

- Liver disease—The effects of doxazosin may be increased, which may increase the chance of side effects
- Kidney disease—Possible increased sensitivity to the effects of doxazosin

Before you begin using any new medicine (prescription or nonprescription) or if you develop any new medical problem while you are using this medicine, check with your doctor, nurse, or pharmacist.

Proper Use of This Medicine

For patients *taking this medicine for high blood pressure:*

- In addition to the use of the medicine your doctor has prescribed, treatment for your high blood pressure may include weight control and care in the types of foods you eat, especially foods high in sodium. Your doctor will tell you which of these are most important for you. You should check with your doctor before changing your diet.
- Many patients who have high blood pressure will not notice any signs of the problem. In fact, many may feel normal. It is very important that you *take your medicine exactly as directed* and that you keep your appointments with your doctor even if you feel well.
- Remember that doxazosin will not cure your high blood pressure but it does help control it. Therefore, you must continue to take it as directed if you expect to lower your blood pressure and keep it down. *You may have to take high blood pressure medicine for the rest of your life.* If high blood pressure is not treated, it can cause serious problems such as heart failure, blood vessel disease, stroke, or kidney disease.

To help you remember to take your medicine, try to get into the habit of taking it at the same time each day.

Missed dose—If you miss a dose of this medicine, take it as soon as possible. However, if it is almost time for your next dose, skip the missed dose and go back to your regular dosing schedule. Do not double doses.

Storage—To store this medicine:
- Keep out of the reach of children.
- Store away from heat and direct light.
- Do not store in the bathroom, near the kitchen sink, or in other damp places. Heat or moisture may cause the medicine to break down.
- Do not keep outdated medicine or medicine no longer needed. Be sure that any discarded medicine is out of the reach of children.

Precautions While Using This Medicine

It is important that your doctor check your progress at regular visits to make sure that this medicine is working properly. This is especially important for elderly patients, who may be more sensitive to the effects of this medicine.

Do not take other medicines unless they have been discussed with your doctor. This especially includes over-the-counter (nonprescription) medicines for appetite control, asthma, colds, cough, hay fever, or sinus problems, since they may tend to increase your blood pressure.

Dizziness, lightheadedness, or sudden fainting may occur after you take this medicine, especially when you get up from a lying or sitting position. These effects are more likely to occur when you take the first dose of this medicine. Taking the first dose at bedtime may prevent problems. However, *be especially careful if you need to get up during the night*. These effects may also occur with any doses you take after the first dose. Getting up slowly may help lessen this problem. *If you feel dizzy, lie down so that you do not faint*. Then sit for a few moments before standing to prevent the dizziness from returning.

The dizziness, lightheadedness, or sudden fainting is more likely to occur if you drink alcohol, stand for a long time, exercise, or if the weather is hot. *While you are taking this medicine, be careful to limit the amount of alcohol you drink. Also, use extra care during exercise or hot weather or if you must stand for a long time.*

Doxazosin may cause some people to become drowsy or less alert than they are normally. *Make sure you know how you react to this medicine before you drive, use machines, or do anything else that could be dangerous if you are dizzy, drowsy, or are not alert.* After you have taken several doses of this medicine, these effects should lessen.

Side Effects of This Medicine

Along with its needed effects, a medicine may cause some unwanted effects. Although not all of these side effects may occur, if they do occur they may need medical attention.

Check with your doctor as soon as possible if any of the following side effects occur:

More common

Dizziness or lightheadedness

Less common

Dizziness or lightheadedness when getting up from a lying or sitting position; fainting (sudden); fast and pounding heartbeat; irregular heartbeat; shortness of breath; swelling of feet or lower legs

Other side effects may occur that usually do not need medical attention. These side effects may go away during treatment as your body adjusts to the medicine. However, check with your doctor if any of the following side effects continue or are bothersome:

More common

Headache; unusual tiredness

Less common

Nausea; nervousness, restlessness, unusual irritability; runny nose; sleepiness or drowsiness

Other side effects not listed above may also occur in some patients. If you notice any other effects, check with your doctor.

Additional Information

Once a medicine has been approved for marketing for a certain use, experience may show that it is also useful for other medical problems. Although this use is not included in product labeling, doxazosin is used in certain patients with the following medical condition:

- Benign enlargement of the prostate

Other than the above information, there is no additional information relating to proper use, precautions, or side effects for this use.

ERYTHROMYCINS Systemic

This information applies to the following medicines:

    Erythromycin Base
    Erythromycin Estolate
    Erythromycin Ethylsuccinate
    Erythromycin Gluceptate
    Erythromycin Lactobionate
    Erythromycin Stearate

Some commonly used brand names are:

For Erythromycin Base
  In the U.S.

E-Mycin	PCE Dispertab
ERYC	Robimycin
Ery-Tab	

    Generic name product may also be available.

  In Canada

Apo-Erythro	ERYC-250
Apo-Erythro-EC	Erythromid
E-Mycin	Novorythro
Erybid	PCE Dispertab
ERYC-125	

    Generic name product may also be available.

For Erythromycin Estolate
  In the U.S.

Erythrozone	Ilosone

    Generic name product may also be available.

  In Canada

Ilosone	Novorythro

For Erythromycin Ethylsuccinate
In the U.S.
  E.E.S.   Erythro
  EryPed

  Generic name product may also be available.

In Canada
  Apo-Erythro-ES   E.E.S.

For Erythromycin Gluceptate
In the U.S.
  Ilotycin
In Canada
  Ilotycin

For Erythromycin Lactobionate
In the U.S.
  Erythrocin

  Generic name product may also be available.

In Canada
  Erythrocin

For Erythromycin Stearate
In the U.S.
  Erythrocin   Wintrocin
  Erythrocot   Wyamycin-S
  My-E

  Generic name product may also be available.

In Canada
  Apo-Erythro-S   Novorythro
  Erythrocin

Description

Erythromycins (eh-rith-roe-MYE-sins) are used to treat infections. Erythromycins are also used to prevent "strep" infections in patients with a history of rheumatic heart disease who may be allergic to penicillin.

These medicines may also be used to treat Legionnaires' disease and for other problems as determined by your doctor. They will not work for colds, flu, or other virus infections.

Erythromycins are available only with your doctor's prescription, in the following dosage forms:
Oral
  Erythromycin Base
  • Delayed-release capsules (U.S. and Canada)
  • Delayed-release tablets (U.S. and Canada)
  • Tablets (U.S. and Canada)

Erythromycin Estolate
- Capsules (U.S. and Canada)
- Chewable tablets (U.S.)
- Oral suspension (U.S. and Canada)
- Tablets (U.S. and Canada)

Erythromycin Ethylsuccinate
- Chewable tablets (U.S. and Canada)
- Oral suspension (U.S. and Canada)
- Tablets (U.S. and Canada)

Erythromycin Stearate
- Oral suspension (Canada)
- Tablets (U.S. and Canada)

Parenteral

Erythromycin Gluceptate
- Injection (U.S. and Canada)

Erythromycin Lactobionate
- Injection (U.S. and Canada)

It is very important that you read and understand the following information. If any of it causes you special concern, check with your doctor. Also, *if you have any questions* or if you want more information about this medicine or your medical problem, *ask your doctor, nurse, or pharmacist.*

Before Using This Medicine

In deciding to use a medicine, the risks of taking the medicine must be weighed against the good it will do. This is a decision you and your doctor will make. For erythromycins, the following should be considered:

Allergies—Tell your doctor if you have ever had any unusual or allergic reaction to erythromycins. Also tell your doctor and pharmacist if you are allergic to any other substances, such as foods, preservatives, or dyes.

Pregnancy—Erythromycin estolate has caused side effects involving the liver in some pregnant women. However, none of the erythromycins has been shown to cause birth defects or other problems in humans.

Breast-feeding—Erythromycins pass into the breast milk. However, erythromycins have not been shown to cause problems in nursing babies.

Children—This medicine has been tested in children and has not been shown to cause different side effects or problems in children than it does in adults.

Older adults—This medicine has been tested and has not been shown to cause different side effects or problems in older people than it does in younger adults.

Other medicines—Although certain medicines should not be used together at all, in other cases two different medicines may be used together even if an interaction might occur. In these cases, your doctor may want to change the dose, or other precautions may be necessary. When you are taking or receiving erythromycins, it is especially important that your doctor and pharmacist know if you are taking any of the following:

- Acetaminophen (e.g., Tylenol) (with long-term, high-dose use) or
- Amiodarone (e.g., Cordarone) or
- Anabolic steroids (nandrolone [e.g., Anabolin], oxandrolone [e.g., Anavar], oxymetholone [e.g., Anadrol], stanozolol [e.g., Winstrol]) or
- Androgens (male hormones) or
- Antithyroid agents (medicine for overactive thyroid) or
- Carmustine (e.g., BiCNU) or
- Chloroquine (e.g., Aralen) or
- Dantrolene (e.g., Dantrium) or
- Daunorubicin (e.g., Cerubidine) or
- Disulfiram (e.g., Antabuse) or
- Divalproex (e.g., Depakote) or
- Estrogens (female hormones) or
- Etretinate (e.g., Tegison) or
- Gold salts (medicine for arthritis) or
- Hydroxychloroquine (e.g., Plaquenil) or
- Mercaptopurine (e.g., Purinethol) or
- Methotrexate (e.g., Mexate) or
- Methyldopa (e.g., Aldomet) or
- Naltrexone (e.g., Trexan) (with long-term, high-dose use) or
- Oral contraceptives (birth control pills) containing estrogen or
- Other anti-infectives by mouth or by injection (medicine for infection) or
- Phenothiazines (acetophenazine [e.g., Tindal], chlorpromazine [e.g., Thorazine], fluphenazine [e.g., Prolixin], mesoridazine [e.g., Serentil], perphenazine [e.g., Trilafon], pro-

chlorperazine [e.g., Compazine], promazine [e.g., Sparine], promethazine [e.g., Phenergan], thioridazine [e.g., Mellaril], trifluoperazine [e.g., Stelazine], triflupromazine [e.g., Vesprin], trimeprazine [e.g., Temaril]) or

- Phenytoin (e.g., Dilantin) or
- Plicamycin (e.g., Mithracin) or
- Valproic acid (e.g., Depakene)—Use of these medicines with erythromycins, especially erythromycin estolate, may increase the chance of liver problems
- Aminophylline (e.g., Somophyllin) or
- Caffeine (e.g., NoDoz) or
- Oxtriphylline (e.g., Choledyl) or
- Theophylline (e.g., Somophyllin-T, Theo-Dur)—Use of these medicines with erythromycins may increase the chance of side effects from aminophylline, caffeine, oxtriphylline, or theophylline
- Carbamazepine (e.g., Tegretol)—Use of carbamazepine with erythromycin may increase the side effects of carbamazepine or increase the chance of liver problems
- Chloramphenicol (e.g., Chloromycetin) or
- Clindamycin (e.g., Cleocin) or
- Lincomycin (e.g., Lincocin)—Use of these medicines with erythromycins may decrease their effectiveness
- Cyclosporine (e.g., Sandimmune) or
- Warfarin (e.g., Coumadin)—Use of any of these medicines with erythromycins may increase the side effects of these medicines
- Terfenadine (e.g., Seldane)—Use of terfenadine with erythromycins may cause heart problems, such as an irregular heartbeat; these medicines should not be used together

Other medical problems—The presence of other medical problems may affect the use of erythromycins. Make sure you tell your doctor if you have any other medical problems, especially:

- Heart disease—High doses of erythromycin may increase the chance of side effects in patients with a history of an irregular heartbeat
- Liver disease—Erythromycins, especially erythromycin estolate, may increase the chance of side effects involving the liver
- Loss of hearing—High doses of erythromycins may, on rare occasion, cause hearing loss

Before you begin using any new medicine (prescription or nonprescription) or if you develop any new medical problem while you are using this medicine, check with your doctor, nurse, or pharmacist.

Proper Use of This Medicine

Erythromycins may be taken with food if they upset your stomach.

For patients taking the *oral liquid form* of this medicine:

- This medicine is to be taken by mouth even if it comes in a dropper bottle. If this medicine does not come in a dropper bottle, use a specially marked measuring spoon or other device to measure each dose accurately. The average household teaspoon may not hold the right amount of liquid.

- Do not use after the expiration date on the label. The medicine may not work properly after that date. Check with your pharmacist if you have any questions about this.

For patients taking the *chewable tablet form* of this medicine:

- Tablets must be chewed or crushed before they are swallowed.

For patients taking the *delayed-release capsule form (with enteric-coated pellets) or the delayed-release tablet form* of this medicine:

- Swallow capsules or tablets whole. Do not break or crush. If you are not sure about which type of capsule or tablet you are taking, check with your pharmacist.

To help clear up your infection completely, *keep taking this medicine for the full time of treatment,* even if you begin to feel better after a few days. *If you have a "strep" infection, you should keep taking this medicine for at least 10 days. This is especially important in "strep" infections. Serious heart problems could develop later* if your infection is not cleared up completely. Also, if you stop taking this medicine too soon, your symptoms may return.

This medicine works best when there is a constant amount in the blood. *To help keep the amount constant, do not miss any doses. Also, it is best to take the doses at evenly spaced times day and night.* For example, if you are to take 4 doses a day, the doses should be spaced about 6 hours apart. If this interferes with your sleep or other daily activities, or if you need help in planning the best times to take your medicine, check with your doctor, nurse, or pharmacist.

Missed dose—If you do miss a dose of this medicine, take it as soon as possible. This will help to keep a constant amount of medicine in the blood. However, if it is almost time for your next dose, skip the missed dose and go back to your regular dosing schedule. Do not double doses.

Storage—To store this medicine:
- Keep out of the reach of children.
- Store away from heat and direct light.
- Do not store the capsule or tablet form of erythromycins in the bathroom, near the kitchen sink, or in other damp places. Heat or moisture may cause the medicine to break down.
- Store the oral liquid form of some erythromycins in the refrigerator because heat will cause this medicine to break down. However, keep the medicine from freezing. Follow the directions on the label.
- Do not keep outdated medicine or medicine no longer needed. Be sure that any discarded medicine is out of the reach of children.

Precautions While Using This Medicine

If your symptoms do not improve within a few days, or if they become worse, check with your doctor.

Side Effects of This Medicine

Along with its needed effects, a medicine may cause some unwanted effects. Although not all of these side effects may occur, if they do occur they may need medical attention.

Check with your doctor immediately if any of the following side effects occur:

Less common–with all erythromycins
Skin rash, hives, itching

Less common–with erythromycin injection
Pain, swelling, or redness at place of injection

Less common–with erythromycin estolate (rare with other erythromycins)
Dark or amber urine; pale stools; stomach pain (severe); unusual tiredness or weakness; yellow eyes or skin

Rare (with liver or kidney disease and high doses)
Fainting (recurrent); loss of hearing (temporary)

Other side effects may occur that usually do not need medical attention. These side effects may go away during treatment as your body adjusts to the medicine. However, check with your doctor if any of the following side effects continue or are bothersome:

More common
Abdominal or stomach cramping and discomfort; diarrhea; nausea or vomiting

Less common
Sore mouth or tongue

Other side effects not listed above may also occur in some patients. If you notice any other effects, check with your doctor.

ESTROGENS Systemic

This information applies to the following medicines:
Chlorotrianisene (klor-oh-trye-AN-i-seen)
Diethylstilbestrol (dye-eth-il-stil-BESS-trole)

Estradiol (ess-tra-DYE-ole)
Estrogens, Conjugated (ESS-troe-jenz, CON-ju-gate-ed)
Estrogens, Esterified (ess-TAIR-i-fyed)
Estrone (ESS-trone)
Estropipate (ess-troe-PI-pate)
Ethinyl Estradiol (ETH-in-il ess-tra-DYE-ole)
Quinestrol (quin-ESS-trole)

Some commonly used brand names are:

For Chlorotrianisene
In the U.S. and Canada
TACE

For Diethylstilbestrol
In the U.S.
Stilphostrol

Generic name product may also be available.

In Canada
Honvol

Another commonly used name is DES.

For Estradiol
In the U.S.

Deladiol-40	Estradiol L.A. 20
Delestrogen	Estradiol L.A. 40
depGynogen	Estra-L 20
Depo-Estradiol	Estra-L 40
Depogen	Estraval
Dioval	Estro-Cyp
Dioval 40	Estrofem
Dioval XX	Estroject-LA
Dura-Estrin	Estronol-LA
Duragen-10	Gynogen L.A. 10
Duragen-20	Gynogen L.A. 20
Duragen-40	Gynogen L.A. 40
E-Cypionate	Hormogen Depot
Estrace	L.A.E. 20
Estra-D	Valergen-10
Estraderm	Valergen-20
Estradiol L.A.	

Generic name product may also be available.

In Canada

Delestrogen	Estrace
Estraderm	Femogex

For Estrogens, Conjugated
In the U.S.
Premarin
Premarin Intravenous

In Canada
C.E.S.   Premarin
Conjugated Estrogens C.S.D.   Premarin Intravenous

For Estrogens, Esterified
In the U.S.
Estratab   Menest
In Canada
Neo-Estrone

For Estrone
In the U.S.
Estroject-2   Kestrin Aqueous
Estrone '5'   Kestrone-5
Estrone-A   Theelin Aqueous
Estronol   Unigen
Foygen Aqueous   Wehgen
Gynogen

Generic name product may also be available.

In Canada
Femogen Forte

For Estropipate
In the U.S.
Ogen .625   Ogen 2.5
Ogen 1.25   Ogen 5
In Canada
Ogen

Another commonly used name is piperazine estrone sulfate.

For Ethinyl Estradiol
In the U.S.
Estinyl   Feminone
In Canada
Estinyl

For Quinestrol
In the U.S.
Estrovis

Description

Estrogens (ESS-troe-jenz) are female hormones. They are produced by the body and are necessary for the normal sexual development of the female and for the regulation of the menstrual cycle during the childbearing years.

The ovaries begin to produce less estrogen after menopause (the change of life). This medicine is prescribed to make up for the lower amount of estrogen. This should relieve signs of menopause, such as hot flashes and unusual sweating, chills, faintness, or dizziness.

Estrogens are prescribed for several reasons:
- to provide additional hormone when the body does not produce enough of its own, as during the menopause or following certain kinds of surgery.
- in the treatment of selected cases of breast cancer in men and women.
- in the treatment of men with certain kinds of cancer of the prostate.
- to help prevent weakening of bones (osteoporosis) in women past menopause.

Estrogens may also be used for other conditions as determined by your doctor.

There is *no* medical evidence to support the belief that the use of estrogens will keep the patient feeling young, keep the skin soft, or delay the appearance of wrinkles. Nor has it been proven that the use of estrogens during the menopause will relieve emotional and nervous symptoms, unless these symptoms are caused by other menopausal symptoms, such as hot flashes or hot flushes.

Estrogens are very useful medicines. However, in addition to their helpful effects in treating your medical problem, they sometimes have side effects that could be very serious. *A paper called "Information for the Patient" should be given to you with your prescription. Read this carefully.* Also, before you use an estrogen, you and your doctor should discuss the good that it will do as well as the risks of using it.

Estrogens are available only with your doctor's prescription, in the following dosage forms:

Oral

Chlorotrianisene
- Capsules (U.S. and Canada)

Diethylstilbestrol
- Tablets (U.S. and Canada)

Estradiol
  • Tablets (U.S. and Canada)
Estrogens, Conjugated
  • Tablets (U.S. and Canada)
Estrogens, Esterified
  • Tablets (U.S. and Canada)
Estropipate
  • Tablets (U.S. and Canada)
Ethinyl Estradiol
  • Tablets (U.S. and Canada)
Quinestrol
  • Tablets (U.S.)

Parenteral

Diethylstilbestrol
  • Injection (U.S. and Canada)
Estradiol
  • Injection (U.S. and Canada)
Estrogens, Conjugated
  • Injection (U.S. and Canada)
Estrone
  • Injection (U.S. and Canada)

Topical

Estradiol
  • Transdermal system (stick-on patch) (U.S. and Canada)

It is very important that you read and understand the following information. If any of it causes you special concern, check with your doctor. Also, *if you have any questions* or if you want more information about this medicine or your medical problem, *ask your doctor, nurse, or pharmacist.*

Before Using This Medicine

In deciding to use a medicine, the risks of taking the medicine must be weighed against the good it will do. This is a decision you and your doctor will make. For estrogens, the following should be considered:

Allergies—Tell your doctor if you have ever had any unusual or allergic reaction to estrogens. Also tell your doctor and pharmacist if you are allergic to any other substances, such as foods, preservatives, or dyes.

Pregnancy—Estrogens are not recommended for use during pregnancy, since some have been shown to cause serious birth defects in humans and animals. Some daughters of women who took diethylstilbestrol (DES) during pregnancy have developed reproductive (genital) tract problems and, rarely, cancer of the vagina or cervix (opening to the uterus) when they reached childbearing age. Some sons of women who took DES during pregnancy have developed urinary-genital tract problems.

Breast-feeding—Use of this medicine is not recommended in nursing mothers. Estrogens pass into the breast milk and their possible effect on the baby is not known.

Older adults—This medicine has been tested and has not been shown to cause different side effects or problems in older women than it does in younger women.

Other medicines—Although certain medicines should not be used together at all, in other cases two different medicines may be used together even if an interaction might occur. In these cases, your doctor may want to change the dose, or other precautions may be necessary. When you are taking estrogens, it is especially important that your doctor and pharmacist know if you are taking any of the following:

- Acetaminophen (e.g., Tylenol) (with long-term, high-dose use) or
- Amiodarone (e.g., Cordarone) or
- Anabolic steroids (nandrolone [e.g., Anabolin], oxandrolone [e.g., Anavar], oxymetholone [e.g., Anadrol], stanozolol [e.g., Winstrol]) or
- Androgens (male hormones) or
- Anti-infectives by mouth or by injection (medicine for infection) or
- Antithyroid agents (medicine for overactive thyroid) or
- Carbamazepine (e.g., Tegretol) or
- Carmustine (e.g., BiCNU) or
- Chloroquine (e.g., Aralen) or
- Dantrolene (e.g., Dantrium) or
- Daunorubicin (e.g., Cerubidine) or
- Disulfiram (e.g., Antabuse) or
- Divalproex (e.g., Depakote) or
- Etretinate (e.g., Tegison) or
- Gold salts or

- Hydroxychloroquine (e.g., Plaquenil) or
- Mercaptopurine (e.g., Purinethol) or
- Methotrexate (e.g., Mexate) or
- Methyldopa (e.g., Aldomet) or
- Naltrexone (e.g., Trexan) (with long-term, high-dose use) or
- Oral contraceptives (birth control pills) containing estrogen or
- Phenothiazines (acetophenazine [e.g., Tindal], chlorproma-
  zine [e.g., Thorazine], fluphenazine [e.g., Prolixin], meso-
  ridazine [e.g., Serentil], perphenazine [e.g., Trilafon], prochlorperazine [e.g., Compazine], promazine [e.g., Sparine],
  promethazine [e.g., Phenergan], thioridazine [e.g., Mellaril],
  trifluoperazine [e.g., Stelazine], triflupromazine [e.g., Ves-
  prin], trimeprazine [e.g., Temaril]) or
- Phenytoin (e.g., Dilantin) or
- Plicamycin (e.g., Mithracin) or
- Valproic acid (e.g., Depakene)—Estrogens and all of these
  medicines can cause liver damage. Your doctor may want
  you to have extra blood tests that tell about your liver, if
  you must take any of these medicines with estrogens
- Bromocriptine (e.g., Parlodel)—Estrogens may interfere with
  the effects of bromocriptine
- Cyclosporine (e.g., Sandimmune)—Estrogens can increase the
  chance of toxic effects to the kidney or liver from cyclosporine because estrogens can interfere with the body's ability to get the cyclosporine out of the bloodstream as it normally would

Other medical problems—The presence of other medical
problems may affect the use of estrogens. Make sure you
tell your doctor if you have any other medical problems,
especially:

For all patients

- Blood clots (or history of during previous estrogen therapy)—
  Estrogens may worsen blood clots or cause new clots to form
- Breast cancer (active or suspected)—Estrogens may cause
  growth of the tumor in some cases
- Changes in vaginal bleeding of unknown causes—Some irregular vaginal bleeding is a sign that the lining of the uterus
  is growing too much or is a sign of cancer of the uterus
  lining; estrogens may make these conditions worse
- Endometriosis—Estrogens may worsen endometriosis by causing growth of endometriosis implants
- Fibroid tumors of the uterus—Estrogens may cause fibroid
  tumors to increase in size

- Gallbladder disease or gallstones (or history of)—Estrogens may possibly increase the risk of gallbladder disease or gallstones
- Jaundice (or history of during pregnancy)—Estrogens may worsen or cause jaundice in these patients
- Liver disease—Toxic drug effects may occur in patients with liver disease because the body is not able to get this medicine out of the bloodstream as it normally would
- Porphyria—Estrogens can worsen porphyria

For males treated for breast or prostate cancer

- Blood clots or
- Heart or circulation disease or
- Stroke—Males with these medical problems may be more likely to have clotting problems while taking estrogens; the doses of estrogens used to treat male breast or prostate cancer have been shown to increase the chances of heart attack, phlebitis (inflamed veins) caused by a blood clot, or blood clots in the lungs

Before you begin using any new medicine (prescription or nonprescription) or if you develop any new medical problem while you are using this medicine, check with your doctor, nurse, or pharmacist.

Proper Use of This Medicine

For patients taking any of the estrogens by mouth:

- *Take this medicine only as directed by your doctor. Do not take more of it and do not take it for a longer time than your doctor ordered.* Try to take the medicine at the same time each day to reduce the possibility of side effects and to allow it to work better.
- Nausea may occur during the first few weeks after you start taking estrogens. This effect usually disappears with continued use. If the nausea is bothersome, it can usually be prevented or reduced by taking each dose with food or immediately after food.

For patients using the transdermal (stick-on patch) form of estradiol:

- This medicine comes with patient directions. Read them carefully before using this medicine.

- Wash and dry your hands thoroughly before and after handling.
- Apply the patch to a clean, dry, non-oily skin area of your abdomen (stomach) or buttocks that has little or no hair and is free of cuts or irritation.
- *Do not apply to the breasts.* Also, do not apply to the waistline or anywhere else where tight clothes may rub the patch loose.
- Press the patch firmly in place with the palm of your hand for about 10 seconds. Make sure there is good contact, especially around the edges.
- If a patch becomes loose or falls off, you may reapply it or discard it and apply a new patch.
- Each dose is best applied to a different area of skin on your abdomen so that at least 1 week goes by before the same area is used again. This will help prevent skin irritation.

Missed dose—

- For patients taking any of the estrogens by mouth: If you miss a dose of this medicine, take it as soon as possible. However, if it is almost time for your next dose, skip the missed dose and go back to your regular dosing schedule. Do not double doses.
- For patients using the transdermal (stick-on patch) form of estradiol: If you forget to apply a new patch when you are supposed to, apply it as soon as possible. However, if it is almost time for the next patch, skip the missed one and go back to your regular schedule. Do not apply more than one patch at a time.

Storage—To store this medicine:

- Keep out of the reach of children.
- Store away from heat and direct light.
- Do not store in the bathroom medicine cabinet because the heat or moisture may cause the medicine to break down.
- Keep the injectable form of this medicine from freezing.

- Do not keep outdated medicine or medicine no longer needed. Be sure that any discarded medicine is out of the reach of children.

Precautions While Using This Medicine

It is very important that your doctor check your progress at regular visits to make sure this medicine does not cause unwanted effects. These visits will usually be every year, but some doctors require them more often.

It is not yet known whether the use of estrogens increases the risk of breast cancer in women. Therefore, it is very important that you regularly check your breasts for any unusual lumps or discharge. You should also have a mammogram (x-ray pictures of the breasts) done if your doctor recommends it. Because breast cancer has occurred in men taking estrogens, regular self-breast exams and exams by your doctor for any unusual lumps or discharge should be done.

In some patients using estrogens, tenderness, swelling, or bleeding of the gums may occur. Brushing and flossing your teeth carefully and regularly and massaging your gums may help prevent this. See your dentist regularly to have your teeth cleaned. Check with your medical doctor or dentist if you have any questions about how to take care of your teeth and gums, or if you notice any tenderness, swelling, or bleeding of your gums.

If you think that you may be pregnant, stop using the medicine immediately and check with your doctor. Continued use of some estrogens during pregnancy may cause birth defects in the child. DES may also increase the risk of vaginal cancer developing in daughters when they reach child-bearing age.

Do not give this medicine to anyone else. Your doctor has prescribed it only for you after studying your health record and the results of your physical examination. Estrogens may be dangerous for other people because of differences in their health and body make-up.

Side Effects of This Medicine

Discuss these possible effects with your doctor:

- The prolonged use of estrogens has been reported to increase the risk of endometrial cancer (cancer of the lining of the uterus) in women after the menopause. This risk seems to increase as the dose and the length of use increase. When estrogens are used in low doses for less than 1 year, there is less risk. The risk is also reduced if a progestin (another female hormone) is added to, or replaces part of, your estrogen dose. If the uterus has been removed by surgery (total hysterectomy), there is no risk of endometrial cancer.

- It is not yet known whether the use of estrogens increases the risk of breast cancer in women. Although some large studies show an increased risk, most studies and information gathered to date do not support this idea. Breast cancer has been reported in men taking estrogens.

- In studies with oral contraceptives (birth control pills) containing estrogens, cigarette smoking was shown to cause an increased risk of serious side effects affecting the heart or blood circulation, such as dangerous blood clots, heart attack, or stroke. The risk increased as the amount of smoking and the age of the smoker increased. Women aged 35 and over were at greatest risk when they smoked while using oral contraceptives containing estrogens. It is not known if this risk exists with the use of estrogens for symptoms of menopause. However, smoking may make estrogens less effective.

The following side effects may be caused by blood clots, which could lead to stroke, heart attack, or death. These side effects rarely occur, and, when they do occur, they occur in men treated for cancer using high doses of estrogens. *Get emergency help immediately* if any of the following side effects occur:

Rare—For males being treated for breast or prostate cancer only

Headache (sudden or severe); loss of coordination (sudden); loss of vision or change of vision (sudden); pains in chest, groin, or leg, especially in calf of leg; shortness of breath (sudden and unexplained); slurring of speech (sudden); weakness or numbness in arm or leg

Also, check with your doctor as soon as possible if any of the following side effects occur:

More common

Breast pain (in females and males); increased breast size (in females and males); swelling of feet and lower legs; weight gain (rapid)

Less common or rare

Changes in vaginal bleeding (spotting, breakthrough bleeding, prolonged or heavier bleeding, or complete stoppage of bleeding); lumps in, or discharge from, breast (in females and males); pains in stomach, side, or abdomen; uncontrolled jerky muscle movements; yellow eyes or skin

Other side effects may occur that usually do not need medical attention. These side effects may go away during treatment as your body adjusts to the medicine. However, check with your doctor if any of the following side effects continue or are bothersome:

More common

Bloating of stomach; cramps of lower stomach; loss of appetite; nausea; skin irritation or redness where skin patch was worn

Less common

Diarrhea (mild); dizziness (mild); headaches (mild); migraine headaches; problems in wearing contact lenses; unusual decrease in sexual desire (in males); unusual increase in sexual desire (in females); vomiting (usually with high doses)

Also, many women who are taking estrogens with a progestin (another female hormone) will start having monthly vaginal bleeding, similar to menstrual periods again. This effect will continue for as long as the medicine is taken. However, monthly bleeding will not occur in women who have had the uterus removed by surgery (total hysterectomy).

Other side effects not listed above may also occur in some patients. If you notice any other effects, check with your doctor.

ESTROGENS AND PROGESTINS   Oral Contraceptives   Systemic

This information applies to the following medicines:

Ethynodiol (e-thye-noe-DYE-ole) Diacetate and Ethinyl Estradiol (ETH-in-il ess-tra-DYE-ole)

Ethynodiol Diacetate and Mestranol* (MES-tra-nole)

Levonorgestrel (LEE-voe-nor-jess-trel) and Ethinyl Estradiol

Norethindrone (nor-eth-IN-drone) Acetate and Ethinyl Estradiol

Norethindrone and Ethinyl Estradiol

Norethindrone and Mestranol

Norethynodrel (nor-e-THYE-noe-drel) and Mestranol

Norgestrel (nor-JESS-trel) and Ethinyl Estradiol

For information about Norethindrone (e.g., Micronor) or Norgestrel (e.g., Ovrette) when used as single-ingredient oral contraceptives, see *Progestins (Systemic)*.

Some commonly used brand names are:

For Ethynodiol Diacetate and Ethinyl Estradiol
Demulen

For Ethynodiol Diacetate and Mestranol*
Ovulen*

For Levonorgestrel and Ethinyl Estradiol

Levlen	Tri-Levlen
Nordette	Triphasil

For Norethindrone Acetate and Ethinyl Estradiol

Loestrin	Norlestrin
Minestrin*	

For Norethindrone and Ethinyl Estradiol

Brevicon	Norinyl 1+35
Genora 1/35	Norquest
ModiCon	Ortho*
N.E.E. 1/35	Ortho-Novum 1/35
Nelova 0.5/35E	Ortho-Novum 7/7/7
Nelova 1/35E	Ortho-Novum 10/11
Nelova 10/11	Ovcon
Norcept-E 1/35	Synphasic*
Norethin 1/35E	Tri-Norinyl

For Norethindrone and Mestranol

Genora 1/50	Ortho-Novum 0.5*
Nelova 1/50M	Ortho-Novum 1/50
Norethin 1/50M	Ortho-Novum 1/80*
Norinyl 1+50	Ortho-Novum 2*
Norinyl 1+80*	Program*
Norinyl 2*	

For Norethynodrel and Mestranol
    Enovid

For Norgestrel and Ethinyl Estradiol
    Lo/Ovral   Ovral
    Min-Ovral*

---

*Not commercially available in the U.S.

Description

Oral contraceptives are known also as the Pill, OC's, BC's, BC tablets, or birth control pills. They usually contain two types of female hormones, estrogens (ESS-troe-jenz) and progestins (proe-JESS-tins). When taken by mouth on a regular schedule, they change the hormone balance of the body, which prevents pregnancy.

Sometimes these preparations can be used in the treatment of conditions that are helped by added hormones. Oral contraceptives do not prevent or cure venereal diseases (VD), however.

Before you take an oral contraceptive, you and your doctor should discuss the benefits and risks of using these medicines. Besides surgery or not having intercourse, these medicines are the most effective method of preventing pregnancy. However, oral contraceptives sometimes have side effects that could be very serious.

To make the use of oral contraceptives as safe and reliable as possible, you should understand how and when to take them and what effects may be expected. *A paper with information for the patient will be given to you with your filled prescription, and will provide many details concerning the use of oral contraceptives. Read this paper carefully* and ask your doctor, nurse, or pharmacist if you need additional information or explanation.

Oral contraceptives are available only with your doctor's prescription, in the following dosage forms:
    Oral
        Ethynodiol Diacetate and Ethinyl Estradiol
            • Tablets

Ethynodiol Diacetate and Mestranol
  • Tablets
Levonorgestrel and Ethinyl Estradiol
  • Tablets
Norethindrone Acetate and Ethinyl Estradiol
  • Tablets
Norethindrone and Ethinyl Estradiol
  • Tablets
Norethindrone and Mestranol
  • Tablets
Norethynodrel and Mestranol
  • Tablets
Norgestrel and Ethinyl Estradiol
  • Tablets

It is very important that you read and understand the following information. If any of it causes you special concern, check with your doctor. Also, *if you have any questions* or if you want more information about this medicine or your medical problem, *ask your doctor, nurse, or pharmacist.*

Before Using This Medicine

In deciding to use a medicine, the risks of taking the medicine must be weighed against the good it will do. This is a decision you and your doctor will make. For estrogen and progestin birth control pills, the following should be considered:

Allergies—Tell your doctor if you have ever had any unusual or allergic reaction to estrogens or progestins. Also tell your doctor and pharmacist if you are allergic to any other substances, such as foods, preservatives, or dyes.

Pregnancy—Oral contraceptives are not recommended for use during pregnancy.

Breast-feeding—The estrogens in oral contraceptives pass into the breast milk. It is not known what effect oral contraceptives may have on the infant. Studies have shown oral contraceptives to cause tumors in humans and animals. Use of "high-dose" birth control medicines is not recommended during breast-feeding. It may be necessary for you to use another method of birth control or to stop breast-feeding while taking oral contraceptives. However, your doctor may allow you to begin using one of the "low-dose" oral contraceptives after you have been breast-feeding for a while.

Children—This medicine is frequently used for birth control in teenage females and has not been shown to cause different side effects or problems than it does in adults. However, some teenagers may need extra information on the importance of taking this medication exactly as prescribed in order for it to work.

Other medicines—Although certain medicines should not be used together at all, in other cases two different medicines may be used together even if an interaction might occur. In these cases, your doctor may want to change the dose, or other precautions may be necessary. When you are taking estrogen and progestin birth control pills, it is especially important that your doctor and pharmacist know if you are taking any of the following:

- Acetaminophen (e.g., Tylenol) (with long-term, high-dose use)
- Adrenocorticoids (cortisone-like medicine)
- Amiodarone (e.g., Cordarone)
- Anabolic steroids (dromostanolone [e.g., Drolban], ethylestrenol [e.g., Maxibolin], nandrolone [e.g., Anabolin], oxandrolone [e.g., Anavar], oxymetholone [e.g., Anadrol], stanozolol [e.g., Winstrol])
- Androgens (male hormones)
- Anticoagulants (blood thinners)
- Antithyroid agents (medicine for overactive thyroid)
- Barbiturates
- Bromocriptine (e.g., Parlodel)
- Carbamazepine (e.g., Tegretol)
- Carmustine (e.g., BiCNU)
- Chloroquine (e.g., Aralen)
- Dantrolene (e.g., Dantrium)
- Daunorubicin (e.g., Cerubidine)
- Disulfiram (e.g., Antabuse)
- Divalproex (e.g., Depakote)
- Estrogens (female hormones)
- Etretinate (e.g., Tegison)

- Gold salts
- Griseofulvin (e.g., Fulvicin)
- Hydroxychloroquine (e.g., Plaquenil)
- Medicine for infection
- Mercaptopurine (e.g., Purinethol)
- Methotrexate (e.g., Mexate)
- Methyldopa (e.g., Aldomet)
- Naltrexone (e.g., Trexan) (with long-term, high-dose use)
- Phenothiazines (acetophenazine [e.g., Tindal], chlorproma-zine [e.g., Thorazine], fluphenazine [e.g., Prolixin], meso-ridazine [e.g., Serentil], perphenazine [e.g., Trilafon], pro-chlorperazine [e.g., Compazine], promazine [e.g., Sparine], promethazine [e.g., Phenergan], thioridazine [e.g., Mellaril], trifluoperazine [e.g., Stelazine], triflupromazine [e.g., Ves-prin], trimeprazine [e.g., Temaril])
- Phenylbutazone (e.g., Butazolidin)
- Phenytoin (e.g., Dilantin)
- Plicamycin (e.g., Mithracin)
- Primidone (e.g., Mysoline)
- Rifampin (e.g., Rifadin)
- Tricyclic antidepressants (medicine for depression)
- Valproic acid (e.g., Depakene)

Other medical problems—The presence of other medical problems may affect the use of estrogen and progestin birth control pills. Make sure you tell your doctor if you have any other medical problems, especially:

- Angina pectoris (chest pains on exertion)
- Asthma
- Blood clots (or history of)
- Bone disease
- Breast disease (not cancerous, such as fibrocystic disease [breast cysts], breast lumps, or abnormal mammograms [x-ray pictures of the breast])
- Cancer (or history of or family history of breast cancer)
- Changes in vaginal bleeding
- Diabetes mellitus (sugar diabetes)
- Endometriosis
- Epilepsy
- Fibroid tumors of the uterus

- Gallbladder disease or gallstones (or history of)
- Heart or circulation disease
- High blood cholesterol
- High blood pressure (hypertension)
- Jaundice (or history of, including jaundice during pregnancy)
- Kidney disease
- Liver disease (such as jaundice or porphyria)
- Lumps in breasts
- Mental depression (or history of)
- Migraine headaches
- Scanty or irregular menstrual periods
- Stroke (history of)
- Too much calcium in the blood
- Tuberculosis
- Varicose veins

Before you begin using any new medicine (prescription or nonprescription) or if you develop any new medical problem while you are using this medicine, check with your doctor, nurse, or pharmacist.

Proper Use of This Medicine

Take this medicine only as directed by your doctor. This medicine must be taken exactly on schedule to prevent pregnancy. Try to take the medicine at the same time each day, not more than 24 hours apart, to reduce the possibility of side effects and to provide the best protection.

Nausea may occur during the first few weeks after you start taking this medicine. This effect usually disappears with continued use. If the nausea is bothersome, it can usually be prevented or reduced by taking each dose with food or immediately after food.

Since one of the most important factors in the proper use of oral contraceptives is taking every dose exactly on schedule, you should never let your tablet supply run out. Always keep 1 extra month's supply of tablets on hand. To keep the extra month's supply from becoming too old, use it next, after the pills now being used, and replace the extra supply each month on a regular schedule. The tablets will keep well when kept dry and at room temperature (light will fade some tablet colors but will not change the medicine's effect).

Keep the tablets in the container in which you received them. Most containers aid you in keeping track of your dosage schedule.

Monophasic, biphasic, and triphasic dosing schedules:

- Monophasic cycle dosing schedule: Most available dosing schedules are of the monophasic type. If you are taking tablets of one strength (color) for 20 or 21 days, you are using a monophasic schedule. For the 28-day monophasic cycle you will also take an additional 7 inactive tablets, which are of another color.

- Biphasic cycle dosing schedule:

  —If you are using a biphasic 21-day schedule, you are taking tablets of one strength (color) for 10 days (the 1st phase). You then take tablets of a second strength (color) for the next 11 days (the 2nd phase). For the 28-day biphasic cycle you will also take an additional 7 inactive tablets, which are of a third color.

  —If you are using a biphasic 24-day schedule, you are taking tablets of one strength (color) for 17 days (the 1st phase). You then take tablets of a second strength (color) for the next 7 days (the 2nd phase).

- Triphasic cycle dosing schedule: If you are using a triphasic 21-day schedule, you are taking tablets of one strength (color) for 6 or 7 days depending on the medicine prescribed (the 1st phase). You then take tablets of a second strength (color) for the next 5 to 9 days depending on the medicine prescribed (the 2nd phase). After that, you take tablets of a third strength (color) for the next 5 to 10 days depending on the medicine prescribed (the 3rd phase). At this point, you will have taken a total of 21 tablets. For the 28-day triphasic cycle you will also take an additional 7 inactive tablets, which are of a fourth color.

It is very important that you take the tablets in the same order that they appear in the container. Tablets of different colors in the same package are also different in strength.

Taking the tablets out of order may reduce the effectiveness of the medicine.

Missed dose—If you miss a dose of this medicine:
- For monophasic or biphasic cycles:

   —If you are using a 20-, 21-, or a 24-day schedule and you miss a dose of this medicine for one day, take the missed tablet as soon as you remember. If it is not remembered until the next day, take the missed tablet plus the tablet that is regularly scheduled for that day. This means that you will take 2 tablets on the same day. Then continue on your regular dosing schedule.

   —If you are using a 20-, 21-, or a 24-day schedule and you miss a dose for 2 days in a row, take 2 tablets a day for each of the next 2 days, then continue on your regular dosing schedule. In addition, you should use a second method of birth control to make sure that you are fully protected for the rest of the cycle. Report to your doctor.

   —If you are using a 20-, 21-, or a 24-day schedule and you miss a dose for 3 days or more in a row, stop taking the medicine completely and use another method of birth control until your period begins or until your doctor determines that you are not pregnant. Then restart protection with a new cycle of tablets.

   —If you are using a 28-day schedule and you miss any of the first 21 (active) tablets, follow the instructions for the 21-day schedule depending on how many doses you have missed. If you miss any of the last 7 (inactive) tablets, there is no danger of pregnancy. However, the first tablet (active) of the next month's cycle must be taken on the regularly scheduled day, in spite of any missed doses, if pregnancy is to be avoided. The active and inactive tablets are colored differently for your convenience.

- For triphasic cycles:

   —If you are using a 21-day schedule and you miss a dose of this medicine for one day, take the missed tablet as soon as you remember. If it is not remembered until the next day, take the missed tablet plus the tablet that is regularly scheduled for that day. This means that you will take 2 tablets on the same day. Then continue on your regular dosing schedule. In addition, you should use a second method of birth control to make sure that you are fully protected for the rest of the cycle. Report to your doctor.

—If you are using a 21-day schedule and you miss a dose for 2 days in a row, take 2 tablets a day for each of the next 2 days, then continue on your regular dosing schedule. In addition, you should use a second method of birth control to make sure that you are fully protected for the rest of the cycle. Report to your doctor.

—If you are using a 21-day schedule and you miss a dose for 3 days or more in a row, stop taking the medicine completely and use another method of birth control until your period begins or until your doctor determines that you are not pregnant. Then restart protection with a new cycle of tablets.

—If you are using a 28-day schedule and you miss any of the first 21 (active) tablets, follow the instructions for the 21-day schedule depending on how many doses you have missed. If you miss any of the last 7 (inactive) tablets, there is no danger of pregnancy. However, the first tablet (active) of the next month's cycle must be taken on the regularly scheduled day, in spite of any missed doses, if pregnancy is to be avoided. The active and inactive tablets are colored differently for your convenience.

Storage—To store this medicine:

- Keep out of the reach of children.
- Store away from heat and direct light.
- Do not store in the bathroom, near the kitchen sink, or in other damp places. Heat and moisture may cause the medicine to break down.
- Do not keep outdated medicine or medicine no longer needed. Be sure that any discarded medicine is out of the reach of children.

Precautions While Using This Medicine

It is very important that your doctor check your progress at regular visits to make sure this medicine does not cause unwanted effects. These visits will usually be every 6 to 12 months, but some doctors require them more often.

When you begin to use oral contraceptives, your body will require at least 7 days to adjust before pregnancy will be prevented; therefore, you should *use a second method of birth control for the first cycle (or 3 weeks)* to ensure full protection.

Tell the medical doctor or dentist in charge that you are taking this medicine before any kind of surgery (including dental surgery) or emergency treatment, since this medicine may cause serious blood clots, heart attack, or stroke.

The following medicines may reduce the effectiveness of oral contraceptives. *You should use a second method of birth control during each cycle in which any of the following medicines are used:*

Ampicillin
Adrenocorticoids (cortisone-like medicine)
Bacampicillin
Barbiturates
Carbamazepine (e.g., Tegretol)
Chloramphenicol (e.g., Chloromycetin)
Dihydroergotamine (e.g., D.H.E. 45)
Griseofulvin (e.g., Fulvicin)
Mineral oil
Neomycin, oral
Penicillin V
Phenylbutazone (e.g., Butazolidin)
Phenytoin (e.g., Dilantin)
Primidone (e.g., Mysoline)
Rifampin (e.g., Rifadin)
Sulfonamides (sulfa medicine)
Tetracyclines (medicine for infection)
Tranquilizers
Valproic acid (e.g., Depakene)

Check with your doctor if you have any questions about this.

Vaginal bleeding of various amounts may occur between your regular menstrual periods during the first 3 months of use. This is sometimes called spotting when slight, or break-through bleeding when heavier. If this should occur:

- Continue on your regular dosing schedule.
- The bleeding usually stops within 1 week.
- Check with your doctor if the bleeding continues for more than 1 week.
- After you have been taking oral contraceptives on schedule and for more than 3 months, check with your doctor.

Missed menstrual periods may occur:

- if you have not taken the medicine exactly as scheduled. Pregnancy must be considered a possibility.
- if the medicine is not properly adjusted for your needs.
- if you have taken oral contraceptives for a long time, usually 2 or more years, and stop their use.

Check with your doctor if you miss any menstrual periods so that the cause may be determined.

In some patients using estrogen-containing oral contraceptives, tenderness, swelling, or bleeding of the gums may occur. Brushing and flossing your teeth carefully and regularly and massaging your gums may help prevent this. See your dentist regularly to have your teeth cleaned. Check with your medical doctor or dentist if you have any questions about how to take care of your teeth and gums, or if you notice any tenderness, swelling, or bleeding of your gums. Also, it has been shown that estrogen-containing oral contraceptives may cause a healing problem called dry socket after a tooth has been removed. If you are going to have a tooth removed, tell your dentist or oral surgeon that you are taking oral contraceptives.

Some people who take oral contraceptives may become more sensitive to sunlight than they are normally. When you begin taking this medicine, avoid too much sun and do not use a sunlamp until you see how you react to the sun, especially if you tend to burn easily. If you have a severe reaction, check with your doctor. Some people may develop brown, blotchy spots on exposed areas. These spots usually disappear gradually when the medicine is stopped.

If you wear contact lenses and notice a change in vision or are not able to wear them, check with your doctor.

If you suspect that you may have become pregnant, stop taking this medicine immediately and check with your doctor.

If you are scheduled for any laboratory tests, tell your doctor that you are taking birth control pills.

Do not give this medicine to anyone else. Your doctor has prescribed it only for you after studying your health record and the results of your physical examination. Oral contraceptives may be dangerous for other people because of differences in their health and body make-up.

Check with your doctor before taking any leftover oral contraceptives from an old prescription, especially after a pregnancy. Your old prescription may be dangerous to you now or may allow you to become pregnant if your health has changed since your last physical examination.

Side Effects of This Medicine

Discuss these possible effects with your doctor:

- Along with their needed effects, birth control tablets sometimes cause some unwanted effects such as benign (not cancerous) liver tumors, liver cancer, blood clots, heart attack, and stroke, and problems of the gallbladder, liver, and uterus. Although these effects are rare, they can be very serious and may cause death.
- *Cigarette smoking* during the use of oral contraceptives has been found to increase the risk of serious side effects affecting the heart and/or blood circulation, such as dangerous blood clots, heart attack, or stroke. The risk increases as the age of the patient and the amount of smoking increase. This risk is greater in women age 35 and over. *To reduce the risk of serious side effects, do not smoke cigarettes while using oral contraceptives.*

The following side effects may be caused by blood clots, which could lead to stroke, heart attack, or death. Although these side effects rarely occur, they require immediate medical attention. *Get emergency help immediately* if any of the following side effects occur:

> Abdominal or stomach pain (sudden, severe, or continuing); coughing up blood; headache (severe or sudden); loss of co-ordination (sudden); loss of vision or change in vision (sudden); pains in chest, groin, or leg (especially in calf of leg); shortness of breath (sudden or unexplained); slurring of speech (sudden); weakness, numbness, or pain in arm or leg (unexplained)

Check with your doctor as soon as possible if any of the following side effects occur:

> *Less common or rare*
>
> Bulging eyes; changes in vaginal bleeding (spotting, break-through bleeding, prolonged bleeding, or complete stop-page of bleeding); double vision; fainting; frequent urge to urinate or painful urination; increased blood pressure; loss of vision (gradual, partial, or complete); lumps in, or discharge from, breast; mental depression; pains in stom-ach, side, or abdomen; skin rash, redness, or other skin irritation; swelling, pain, or tenderness in upper abdomen (stomach) area; unusual or dark-colored mole; vaginal discharge (thick, white, or curd-like); vaginal itching or irritation; yellow eyes or skin

Other side effects may occur that usually do not need med-ical attention. These side effects may go away during treat-ment as your body adjusts to the medicine. However, check with your doctor if any of the following side effects continue or are bothersome:

> *More common*
>
> Acne (usually less common after first 3 months); bloating of stomach; cramps of lower stomach; increase or decrease in appetite; nausea; swelling of ankles and feet; swelling and increased tenderness of breasts; unusual tiredness or weakness; unusual weight gain
>
> *Less common or rare*
>
> Brown, blotchy spots on exposed skin;. diarrhea (mild); diz-ziness; headaches or migraine headaches; increased body and facial hair; increased sensitivity to contact lenses; increased skin sensitivity to sun; irritability; some loss of scalp hair; unusual decrease or increase in sexual desire; vomiting; weight loss

Other side effects not listed above may also occur in some patients. If you notice any other effects, check with your doctor.

ETODOLAC Systemic†

A commonly used brand name in the U.S. is Lodine.

Another commonly used name is etodolic acid.

---

†Not commercially available in Canada.

Description

Etodolac (ee-TOE-doe-lac) belongs to the group of medicines called anti-inflammatory analgesics (also called nonsteroidal anti-inflammatory drugs [NSAIDs]). Etodolac is used to relieve some symptoms caused by arthritis (rheumatism), such as inflammation, swelling, stiffness, and joint pain. However, this medicine does not cure arthritis and will help you only as long as you continue to take it.

Etodolac is also used to relieve pain. It is not a narcotic and is not habit-forming. It will not cause physical or mental dependence, as narcotics can. However, etodolac is sometimes used together with a narcotic to provide better pain relief than either medicine used alone.

Etodolac may also be used to treat other conditions as determined by your doctor.

Any anti-inflammatory analgesic can cause side effects, especially when it is used for a long time or in large doses. Some of the side effects are painful or uncomfortable. Others can be more serious, resulting in the need for medical care and sometimes even death. If you will be taking this medicine for more than one or two months or in large amounts, you should discuss with your doctor the good that it can do as well as the risks of taking it. Also, it is a good idea to ask your doctor about other forms of treatment that might

help to reduce the amount of etodolac that you take and/
or the length of treatment.

Etodolac is available only with your medical doctor's or dentist's prescription, in the following dosage form:

Oral
- Capsules (U.S.)

It is very important that you read and understand the following information. If any of it causes you special concern, check with your doctor. Also, *if you have any questions* or if you want more information about this medicine or your medical problem, *ask your doctor, nurse, or pharmacist.*

Before Using This Medicine

In deciding to use a medicine, the risks of taking the medicine must be weighed against the good it will do. This is a decision you and your doctor will make. For etodolac, the following should be considered:

Allergies—Tell your doctor if you have ever had any unusual or allergic reaction to etodolac or to any of the following medicines:

Aspirin or other salicylates
Diclofenac (e.g., Voltaren)
Diflunisal (e.g., Dolobid)
Fenoprofen (e.g., Nalfon)
Floctafenine (e.g., Idarac)
Flurbiprofen, oral (e.g., Ansaid)
Ibuprofen (e.g., Motrin)
Indomethacin (e.g., Indocin)
Ketoprofen (e.g., Orudis)
Ketorolac (e.g., Toradol)
Meclofenamate (e.g., Meclomen)
Mefenamic acid (e.g., Ponstel)
Naproxen (e.g., Naprosyn)
Oxyphenbutazone (e.g., Tandearil)
Phenylbutazone (e.g., Butazolidin)
Piroxicam (e.g., Feldene)
Sulindac (e.g., Clinoril)
Suprofen (e.g., Suprol)
Tiaprofenic acid (e.g., Surgam)
Tolmetin (e.g., Tolectin)
Zomepirac (e.g., Zomax)

Also tell your doctor and pharmacist if you are allergic to any other substances, such as foods, preservatives, or dyes.

Pregnancy—Studies on birth defects with etodolac have not been done in pregnant women. However, etodolac has caused birth defects in animal studies.

There is a chance that regular use of any anti-inflammatory analgesic during the last few months of pregnancy may cause unwanted effects on the heart or blood flow of the fetus or newborn baby. Also, animal studies have shown that, if taken late in pregnancy, etodolac may increase the length of pregnancy, prolong labor, or cause other problems during delivery.

Breast-feeding—It is not known whether etodolac passes into the breast milk. However, it has not been reported to cause problems in nursing babies.

Children—Studies on this medicine have been done only in adult patients, and there is no specific information comparing use of etodolac in children with use in other age groups.

Older adults—This medicine has been tested and has not been shown to cause different side effects or problems in older people than it does in younger adults. However, low doses were used in these studies. Also, experience with other anti-inflammatory analgesics has shown that elderly people are more likely than younger adults to get very sick if the medicine causes stomach problems.

Other medicines—Although certain medicines should not be used together at all, in other cases two different medicines may be used together even if an interaction might occur. In these cases, your doctor may want to change the dose, or other precautions may be necessary. When you are taking etodolac, it is especially important that your doctor and pharmacist know if you are taking any of the following:

- Anticoagulants (blood thinners) or
- Cefamandole (e.g., Mandol) or
- Cefoperazone (e.g., Cefobid) or
- Cefotetan (e.g., Cefotan) or
- Heparin or
- Moxalactam (e.g., Moxam) or

- Plicamycin (e.g., Mithracin) or
- Valproic acid (e.g., Depakene)—Use of any of these medicines together with etodolac may increase the chance of bleeding

- Aspirin or other salicylates or
- Cyclosporine (e.g., Sandimmune) or
- Other inflammation or pain medicine (except narcotics), especially phenylbutazone (e.g., Butazolidin) or
- Tobacco smoking—The chance of serious side effects may be increased

- Lithium (e.g., Lithane) or
- Methotrexate (e.g., Mexate)—Higher blood levels of lithium or methotrexate and an increased chance of side effects may occur

- Probenecid (e.g., Benemid)—Higher blood levels of etodolac and an increased chance of side effects may occur

Other medical problems—The presence of other medical problems may affect the use of etodolac. Make sure you tell your doctor if you have any other medical problems, especially:

- Alcohol abuse or
- Asthma or
- Colitis, stomach ulcer, or other stomach problems, or
- Diabetes mellitus (sugar diabetes) or
- Heart disease or
- High blood pressure or
- Kidney disease or
- Liver disease or
- Systemic lupus erythematosus (SLE)—The chance of serious side effects may be increased
- Hemophilia or other bleeding problems—Etodolac may increase the chance of serious bleeding

Before you begin using any new medicine (prescription or nonprescription) or if you develop any new medical problem while you are using this medicine, check with your doctor, nurse, or pharmacist.

Proper Use of This Medicine

Etodolac may start to relieve pain a little faster if it is taken 30 minutes before meals or 2 hours after meals. However, after the first few doses, take the medicine with food or an antacid to lessen the chance of stomach upset. This is especially important if you will be taking the medicine for a long time, as for arthritis.

Take this medicine with a full glass (8 ounces) of water. Also, do not lie down for about 15 to 30 minutes after taking the medicine. This helps to prevent irritation that may lead to trouble in swallowing.

Do not take more of this medicine, do not take it more often, and do not take it for a longer time than ordered by your medical doctor or dentist. Taking too much of this medicine may increase the chance of unwanted effects, especially in elderly patients.

For patients taking this medicine for *arthritis:*
- This medicine must be taken regularly as ordered by your doctor in order for it to help you. Most anti-inflammatory analgesics usually begin to work within one week, but in severe cases up to two weeks or even longer may pass before you begin to feel better. Also, several weeks may pass before you feel the full effects of the medicine.

Missed dose—If your medical doctor or dentist has ordered you to take this medicine according to a regular schedule, and you miss a dose, take it as soon as you remember. However, if it is almost time for your next dose, skip the missed dose and go back to your regular dosing schedule. Do not double doses.

Storage—To store this medicine:
- Keep out of the reach of children.
- Store away from heat and direct light.
- Do not store this medicine in the bathroom, near the kitchen sink, or in other damp places. Heat or moisture may cause the medicine to break down.
- Do not keep outdated medicine or medicine no longer needed. Be sure that any discarded medicine is out of the reach of children.

Precautions While Using This Medicine

If you will be taking this medicine for a long time, as for arthritis (rheumatism), your doctor should check your progress at regular visits. Your doctor may want to do certain tests to find out if unwanted effects are occurring. The tests are very important because serious side effects, including ulcers or bleeding, can occur without any warning.

Stomach problems may be more likely to occur if you drink alcoholic beverages while being treated with this medicine. Therefore, *do not regularly drink alcoholic beverages while taking this medicine,* unless otherwise directed by your doctor.

Taking certain other medicines together with etodolac may increase the chance of unwanted effects. The risk will depend on how much of each medicine you take every day, and on how long you take the medicines together. Therefore, do not take acetaminophen (e.g., Tylenol) or aspirin or other salicylates together with etodolac for more than a few days, unless otherwise directed by your medical doctor or dentist. Also, *do not take any of the following medicines together with etodolac, unless your medical doctor or dentist has directed you to do so and is following your progress:*

    Diclofenac (e.g., Voltaren)
    Diflunisal (e.g., Dolobid)
    Fenoprofen (e.g., Nalfon)
    Floctafenine (e.g., Idarac)
    Flurbiprofen, oral (e.g., Ansaid)
    Ibuprofen (e.g., Motrin)
    Indomethacin (e.g., Indocin)
    Ketoprofen (e.g., Orudis)
    Ketorolac (e.g., Toradol)
    Meclofenamate (e.g., Meclomen)
    Mefenamic acid (e.g., Ponstel)
    Naproxen (e.g., Naprosyn)
    Phenylbutazone (e.g., Butazolidin)
    Piroxicam (e.g., Feldene)
    Sulindac (e.g., Clinoril)
    Tiaprofenic acid (e.g., Surgam)
    Tolmetin (e.g., Tolectin)

Before having any kind of surgery (including dental surgery), tell the medical doctor or dentist in charge that you are taking this medicine.

This medicine may cause some people to become confused, drowsy, dizzy, or lightheaded. It may also cause blurred vision or other vision problems in some people. *Make sure you know how you react to this medicine before you drive, use machines, or do anything else that could be dangerous if you are dizzy or not able to see well.* If these reactions are especially bothersome, check with your doctor.

Etodolac may interfere with the results of a test that measures the amount of bilirubin (which is normally present in the body) in the urine. Before having any urine tests, be sure to tell the doctor in charge that you are taking etodolac.

For *diabetic patients:*

- Etodolac may cause some urine ketone tests to show higher-than-normal amounts of ketones in your urine. Your doctor may need to find out whether this is a false test result caused by etodolac or whether there is a problem with your diabetes. Therefore, if your test does not show a normal amount of ketones, check with your doctor. Be sure to tell the doctor that you are taking etodolac.

Etodolac may cause your eyes to become more sensitive to light than they are normally. Wearing sunglasses and avoiding too much exposure to bright light may help lessen the discomfort.

Serious side effects, including ulcers or bleeding, can occur during treatment with this medicine. Sometimes serious side effects can occur without any warning. However, possible warning signs often occur, including severe abdominal or stomach cramps, pain, or burning; black, tarry stools; severe, continuing nausea, heartburn, or indigestion; and/or vomiting of blood or material that looks like coffee grounds. *Stop taking this medicine and check with your doctor immediately if you notice any of these warning signs.*

Side Effects of This Medicine

Along with its needed effects, a medicine may cause some unwanted effects. Although not all of these side effects may occur, if they do occur they may need medical attention.

Stop taking this medicine and check with your doctor immediately if any of the following side effects occur:

Less frequent
Bloody or black, tarry stools

Rare
Abdominal or stomach pain, cramping, or burning (severe); blood in urine; fainting; hive-like swellings (large) on face, eyelids, mouth, lips, or tongue; nausea, heartburn, and/or indigestion (severe and continuing); pinpoint red spots on skin; shortness of breath, troubled breathing, wheezing, or tightness in chest; unusual bleeding or bruising; vomiting of blood or material that looks like coffee grounds

Also, check with your doctor as soon as possible if any of the following side effects occur:

Less common
Blurred vision; burning feeling in chest or stomach; fever with or without chills; frequent or painful urination; mental depression; ringing or buzzing in ears; skin rash or itching

Rare
Chest pain; decrease in amount of urine; hives; increased blood pressure; muscle cramps or pain; sores, ulcers, or white spots on mouth or on lips; sore throat (unexplained); swelling and/or tenderness in upper abdominal (stomach) area; swelling of face, fingers, feet, or lower legs; swollen and/or painful glands; unusual tiredness or weakness; weight gain; yellow eyes or skin

Other side effects may occur that usually do not need medical attention. These side effects may go away during treatment as your body adjusts to the medicine. However, check with your doctor if any of the following side effects continue or are bothersome:

More common
Abdominal or stomach cramps, pain, or discomfort (mild to moderate); bloated feeling or gas; diarrhea; dizziness; headache; indigestion or nausea; weakness

Less common or rare

> Constipation; decreased appetite or loss of appetite; drowsiness; flushing; increased sensitivity of eyes to light; increased thirst; nervousness or trouble in sleeping; pounding heartbeat; vomiting

Other side effects not listed above may also occur in some patients. If you notice any other effects, check with your doctor.

FLUCONAZOLE Systemic

A commonly used brand name in the U.S. and Canada is Diflucan.

Description

Fluconazole (floo-KOE-na-zole) is used to help overcome serious fungus infections found throughout the body.

Fluconazole is available only with your doctor's prescription, in the following dosage forms:

Oral
- Tablets (U.S. and Canada)

Parenteral
- Injection (U.S. and Canada)

It is very important that you read and understand the following information. If any of it causes you special concern, check with your doctor. Also, *if you have any questions* or if you want more information about this medicine or your medical problem, *ask your doctor, nurse, or pharmacist.*

Before Using This Medicine

In deciding to use a medicine, the risks of taking the medicine must be weighed against the good it will do. This is a decision you and your doctor will make. For fluconazole, the following should be considered:

Allergies—Tell your doctor if you have ever had any unusual or allergic reaction to fluconazole or other related medicines, such as itraconazole, ketoconazole, or miconazole. Also tell your doctor and pharmacist if you are allergic to any other substances, such as foods, preservatives, or dyes.

Pregnancy—Studies have not been done in pregnant women. However, studies in some animals have shown that fluconazole taken in high doses may cause harm to the fetus. Lower doses have not been shown to cause problems.

Breast-feeding—It is not known whether fluconazole passes into breast milk.

Children—A small number of children have been safely treated with fluconazole. Be sure to discuss with your child's doctor the use of this medicine in children.

Older adults—Many medicines have not been studied specifically in older people. Therefore, it may not be known whether they work exactly the same way they do in younger adults or if they cause different side effects or problems in older people. There is no specific information comparing use of fluconazole in the elderly with use in other age groups.

Other medicines—Although certain medicines should not be used together at all, in other cases 2 different medicines may be used together even if an interaction might occur. In these cases, your doctor may want to change the dose, or other precautions may be necessary. When you are taking fluconazole, it is especially important that your doctor and pharmacist know if you are taking any of the following:

- Chlorpropamide (e.g., Diabinese) or
- Cyclosporine (e.g., Sandimmune) or
- Glipizide (e.g., Glucotrol) or
- Glyburide (e.g., DiaBeta, Micronase) or
- Phenytoin (e.g., Dilantin) or
- Tolbutamide (e.g., Orinase) or
- Warfarin (e.g., Coumadin)—Fluconazole may increase the the effects of these medicines, which may increase the chance of side effects
- Rifampin (e.g., Rifadin)—Rifampin may decrease the effects of fluconazole

Other medical problems—The presence of other medical problems may affect the use of fluconazole. Make sure you

tell your doctor if you have any other medical problems, especially:

- Kidney disease—The effects of fluconazole may be increased in patients with kidney disease
- Liver disease—Patients with liver disease may have an increased chance of side effects

Before you begin using any new medicine (prescription or nonprescription) or if you develop any new medical problem while you are using this medicine, check with your doctor, nurse, or pharmacist.

Proper Use of This Medicine

To help clear up your infection completely, *keep taking this medicine for the full time of treatment,* even if you begin to feel better after a few days. Fungal infections may require many months of treatment even when all your symptoms are gone. *Do not miss any doses.*

Missed dose—If you miss a dose of this medicine, take it as soon as possible. However, if it is almost time for your next dose, skip the missed dose and go back to your regular dosing schedule. Do not double doses.

Storage—To store this medicine:

- Keep out of the reach of children.
- Store away from heat and direct light.
- Do not store in the bathroom, near the kitchen sink, or in other damp places. Heat or moisture may cause the medicine to break down.
- Do not keep outdated medicine or medicine no longer needed. Be sure that any discarded medicine is out of the reach of children.

Precautions While Using This Medicine

It is important that your doctor check your progress at regular visits. This will allow your doctor to check for any unwanted effects.

If your symptoms do not improve within a few weeks, or if they become worse, check with your doctor.

Side Effects of This Medicine

Along with its needed effects, a medicine may cause some unwanted effects. Although not all of these side effects may occur, if they do occur they may need medical attention.

Check with your doctor immediately if any of the following side effects occur:

Rare

> Abdominal pain, especially on the right side under the ribs; dark or amber urine; loss of appetite; reddening, blistering, peeling, or loosening of skin and mucous membranes (insides of mouth); unusual bleeding or bruising; yellow skin or eyes

Other side effects may occur that usually do not need medical attention. These side effects may go away during treatment as your body adjusts to the medicine. However, check with your doctor if any of the following side effects continue or are bothersome:

Less common

> Diarrhea; headache; nausea; stomach pain; vomiting

Other side effects not listed above may also occur in some patients. If you notice any other effects, check with your doctor.

FLUOXETINE   Systemic

A commonly used brand name in the U.S. and Canada is Prozac.

Description

Fluoxetine (floo-OX-uh-teen) is used to treat mental depression.

This medicine is available only with your doctor's prescription, in the following dosage form:

Oral
- Capsules (U.S. and Canada)
- Oral Solution (U.S. and Canada)

It is very important that you read and understand the following information. If any of it causes you special concern, check with your doctor. Also, *if you have any questions* or if you want more information about this medicine or your medical problem, *ask your doctor, nurse, or pharmacist*.

Before Using This Medicine

There have been recent suggestions that the use of fluoxetine may be related to increased thoughts about suicide in a very small number of patients. More study is needed to determine if the medicine caused this effect. Be sure you discuss this, and any possible precautions you should take, with your doctor before taking fluoxetine.

In deciding to use a medicine, the risks of taking the medicine must be weighed against the good it will do. This is a decision you and your doctor will make. For fluoxetine, the following should be considered:

Allergies—Tell your doctor if you have ever had any unusual or allergic reaction to fluoxetine. Also tell your doctor and pharmacist if you are allergic to any other substances, such as foods, preservatives, or dyes.

Pregnancy—Studies have not been done in pregnant women. However, fluoxetine has not been shown to cause birth defects or other problems in animal studies.

Breast-feeding—Fluoxetine may pass into the breast milk. However, this medicine has not been reported to cause problems in nursing babies.

Children—Studies on this medicine have been done only in adult patients, and there is no specific information comparing use of fluoxetine in children with use in other age groups.

Older adults—Many medicines have not been tested in older people. Therefore, it may not be known whether they work exactly the same way they do in younger adults or if they cause different side effects or problems in older people. In studies done to date that included elderly people, fluoxetine did not cause different side effects or problems in older people than it did in younger adults.

Other medicines—Although certain medicines should not be used together at all, in other cases two different medicines may be used together even if an interaction might occur. In these cases, your doctor may want to change the dose, or other precautions may be necessary. When you are taking fluoxetine, it is especially important that your doctor and pharmacist know if you are taking any of the following:

- Anticoagulants (blood thinners) or
- Digitalis glycosides (heart medicine)—Higher or lower blood levels of these medicines or fluoxetine may occur; your doctor may need to change the dose of either medicine

- Central nervous system (CNS) depressants (medicines that cause drowsiness)—The CNS depressant effects may be increased

- Monoamine oxidase (MAO) inhibitors (furazolidone [e.g., Furoxone], isocarboxazid [e.g., Marplan], pargyline [e.g., Eutonyl], phenelzine [e.g., Nardil], procarbazine [e.g., Matulane], tranylcypromine [e.g., Parnate])—Taking fluoxetine while you are taking or within 2 weeks of taking MAO inhibitors may cause confusion, agitation, restlessness, stomach or intestinal symptoms, sudden high body temperature, extremely high blood pressure, and severe convulsions; at least 14 days should be allowed between stopping treatment with an MAO inhibitor and starting treatment with fluoxetine; if you have been taking fluoxetine, at least 5 weeks should be allowed before starting treatment with an MAO inhibitor

- Tryptophan—Taking this medicine with fluoxetine may result in increased agitation or restlessness, and stomach or intestinal problems

Other medical problems—The presence of other medical problems may affect the use of fluoxetine. Make sure you tell your doctor if you have any other medical problems, especially:

- Diabetes—The amount of insulin or oral antidiabetic medicine that you need to take may change

- Kidney disease or
- Liver disease—Higher blood levels of fluoxetine may occur, increasing the chance of side effects
- Seizure disorders (history of)—The risk of seizures may be increased

Before you begin using any new medicine (prescription or nonprescription) or if you develop any new medical problem while you are using this medicine, check with your doctor, nurse, or pharmacist.

Proper Use of This Medicine

Take this medicine only as directed by your doctor, to benefit your condition as much as possible. Do not take more of it, do not take it more often, and do not take it for a longer time than your doctor ordered.

If this medicine upsets your stomach, it may be taken with food.

Sometimes fluoxetine must be taken for up to 4 weeks or longer before you begin to feel better. Your doctor should check your progress at regular visits during this time.

Dosing—The dose of fluoxetine will be different for different patients. *Follow your doctor's orders or the directions on the label.* The following information includes only the average doses of fluoxetine. *If your dose is different, do not change it* unless your doctor tells you to do so:

- Adults: To start, usually 20 mg a day, taken as a single dose in the morning.

Missed dose—If you miss a dose of this medicine, it is not necessary to make up the missed dose. Skip the missed dose and continue with your next scheduled dose. Do not double doses.

Storage—To store this medicine:

- Keep out of the reach of children.
- Store away from heat and direct light.
- Do not store in the bathroom, near the kitchen sink, or in other damp places. Heat or moisture may cause the medicine to break down.

- Do not keep outdated medicine or medicine no longer needed. Be sure that any discarded medicine is out of the reach of children.

Precautions While Using This Medicine

It is important that your doctor check your progress at regular visits, to allow dosage adjustments and help reduce any side effects.

This medicine will add to the effects of alcohol and other CNS depressants (medicines that slow down the nervous system, possibly causing drowsiness). Some examples of CNS depressants are antihistamines or medicine for hay fever, other allergies, or colds; sedatives, tranquilizers, or sleeping medicine; prescription pain medicine or narcotics; barbiturates; medicine for seizures; muscle relaxants; or anesthetics, including some dental anesthetics. *Check with your doctor before taking any of the above while you are using this medicine.*

If you develop a skin rash or hives, stop taking fluoxetine and check with your doctor as soon as possible.

For diabetic patients:
- This medicine may affect blood sugar levels. If you notice a change in the results of your blood or urine sugar tests or if you have any questions, check with your doctor.

This medicine may cause some people to become drowsy. *Make sure you know how you react to fluoxetine before you drive, use machines, or do anything else that could be dangerous if you are not alert.*

Dizziness, lightheadedness, or fainting may occur, especially when you get up from a lying or sitting position. Getting up slowly may help. If this problem continues or gets worse, check with your doctor.

This medicine may cause dryness of the mouth. For temporary relief, use sugarless gum or candy, melt bits of ice in your mouth, or use a saliva substitute. However, if your mouth continues to feel dry for more than 2 weeks, check with your medical doctor or dentist. Continuing dryness of the mouth may increase the chance of dental disease, including tooth decay, gum disease, and fungus infections.

Side Effects of This Medicine

Along with its needed effects, a medicine may cause some unwanted effects. Although not all of these side effects may occur, if they do occur they may need medical attention.

Check with your doctor as soon as possible if any of the following side effects occur:

Less common

Chills or fever; joint or muscle pain; skin rash, hives, or itching; trouble in breathing

Rare

Convulsions (seizures); signs of hypoglycemia (low blood sugar); including anxiety or nervousness, chills, cold sweats, confusion, cool, pale skin, difficulty in concentration, drowsiness, excessive hunger, fast heartbeat, headache, shakiness or unsteady walk, or unusual tiredness or weakness; skin rash or hives that may occur with burning or tingling in fingers, hands, or arms, chills or fever, joint or muscle pain, swelling of feet or lower legs, swollen glands, or trouble in breathing

Symptoms of overdose

Agitation and restlessness; convulsions (seizures); nausea and vomiting (severe); unusual excitement

Other side effects may occur that usually do not need medical attention. These side effects may go away during treatment as your body adjusts to the medicine. However, check with your doctor if any of the following side effects continue or are bothersome:

More common

Anxiety and nervousness; diarrhea; drowsiness; headache; increased sweating; nausea; trouble in sleeping

Less common

Abnormal dreams; change in taste; changes in vision; chest pain; constipation; cough; decreased appetite or weight loss; decreased sexual drive or ability; decrease in concentration; dizziness or lightheadedness; dryness of mouth;

fast or irregular heartbeat; feeling of warmth or heat;
flushing or redness of skin, especially on face and neck;
frequent urination; increased appetite; menstrual pain;
stomach cramps, gas, or pain; stuffy nose; tiredness or
weakness; tremor; vomiting

Other side effects not listed above may also occur in some
patients. If you notice any other effects, check with your
doctor.

Additional Information

Once a medicine has been approved for marketing for a
certain use, experience may show that it is also useful for
other medical problems. Although this use is not included
in product labeling, fluoxetine is used in certain patients
with the following medical condition:
  • Obsessive-compulsive disorder

Other than the above information, there is no additional
information relating to proper use, precautions, or side effects for these uses.

GEMFIBROZIL   Systemic

A commonly used brand name in the U.S. and Canada is Lopid.

Description

Gemfibrozil (gem-FI-broe-zil) is used to lower cholesterol
and triglyceride (fat-like substances) levels in the blood. This
may help prevent medical problems caused by such substances clogging the blood vessels.

Gemfibrozil is available only with your doctor's prescription,
in the following dosage forms:
  Oral
    • Capsules (U.S. and Canada)
    • Tablets (U.S. and Canada)

*It is very important that you read and understand the fol-
lowing information.* If any of it causes you special concern,

check with your doctor. Also, *if you have any questions* or if you want more information about this medicine or your medical problem, *ask your doctor, nurse, or pharmacist.*

Before Using This Medicine

In addition to its helpful effects in treating your medical problem, this type of medicine may have some harmful effects.

Although problems have not been found with gemfibrozil, it is similar in action to another medicine called clofibrate. Studies with clofibrate have suggested that it may increase the patient's risk of cancer, liver disease, pancreatitis (inflammation of the pancreas), gallstones and problems from gallbladder surgery, although it may also decrease the risk of heart attacks. Other studies have not found all of these effects.

Studies with gemfibrozil in rats found an increased risk of liver tumors when doses up to 10 times the human dose were given for a long time.

Be sure you have discussed this with your doctor before taking this medicine.

In deciding to use a medicine, the risks of taking the medicine must be weighed against the good it will do. This is a decision you and your doctor will make. For gemfibrozil, the following should be considered:

Allergies—Tell your doctor if you have ever had any unusual or allergic reaction to gemfibrozil. Also tell your doctor and pharmacist if you are allergic to any other substances, such as foods, preservatives, or dyes.

Diet—Before prescribing medicine for your condition, your doctor will probably try to control your condition by prescribing a personal diet for you. Such a diet may be low in fats, sugars, and/or cholesterol. Many people are able to control their condition by carefully following their doctor's orders for proper diet and exercise. *Medicine is prescribed only when additional help is needed* and is effective only when a schedule of diet and exercise is properly followed.

Also, this medicine is less effective if you are greatly overweight. It may be very important for you to go on a reducing diet. However, check with your doctor before going on any diet.

Make certain your doctor and pharmacist know if you are on a low-sodium, low-sugar, or any other special diet. Most medicines contain more than their active ingredient.

Pregnancy—Gemfibrozil has not been studied in pregnant women. However, studies in animals have shown that high doses of gemfibrozil may increase the number of fetal deaths, although it does not cause birth defects. Make sure your doctor knows if you are pregnant or if you may become pregnant before taking gemfibrozil.

Breast-feeding—Studies in animals have shown that high doses of gemfibrozil may increase the risk of some kinds of tumors. You should consider this when deciding whether to breast-feed your baby while taking this medicine.

Children—There is no specific information about the use of gemfibrozil in children. However, use is not recommended in children under 2 years of age since cholesterol is needed for normal development.

Older adults—Many medicines have not been studied specifically in older people. Therefore, it may not be known whether they work exactly the same way they do in younger adults or if they cause different side effects or problems in older people. There is no specific information comparing use of gemfibrozil in the elderly with use in other age groups.

Other medicines—Although certain medicines should not be used together at all, in other cases two different medicines may be used together even if an interaction might occur. In these cases, your doctor may want to change the dose, or other precautions may be necessary. When you are taking gemfibrozil it is especially important that your doctor and pharmacist know if you are taking any of the following:

- Anticoagulants (blood thinners)—Use with gemfibrozil may increase the effect of the anticoagulant
- Lovastatin—Use with gemfibrozil may cause or worsen muscle or kidney problems

Other medical problems—The presence of other medical problems may affect the use of gemfibrozil. Make sure you tell your doctor if you have any other medical problems, especially:

- Gallbladder disease or
- Gallstones—Gemfibrozil may make these conditions worse
- Kidney disease or
- Liver disease—Higher blood levels of gemfibrozil may result, which may increase the chance of side effects; a decrease in the dose of gemfibrozil may be needed

Before you begin using any new medicine (prescription or nonprescription) or if you develop any new medical problem while you are using this medicine, check with your doctor, nurse, or pharmacist.

Proper Use of This Medicine

Use this medicine only as directed by your doctor. Do not use more or less of it, and do not use it more often or for a longer time than your doctor ordered.

This medicine is usually taken twice a day. If you are taking 2 doses a day, it is best to take the medicine 30 minutes before your breakfast and evening meals.

Follow carefully the special diet your doctor gave you. This is the most important part of controlling your condition and is necessary if the medicine is to work properly.

Missed dose—If you miss a dose of this medicine, take it as soon as possible. However, if it is almost time for your next dose, skip the missed dose and go back to your regular dosing schedule. Do not double doses.

Storage—To store this medicine:

- Keep out of the reach of children.
- Store away from heat and direct light.
- Do not store in the bathroom, near the kitchen sink, or in other damp places. Heat or moisture may cause the medicine to break down.

• Do not keep outdated medicine or medicine no longer needed. Be sure that any discarded medicine is out of the reach of children.

Precautions While Using This Medicine

It is very important that your doctor check your progress at regular visits. This will allow your doctor to see if the medicine is working properly to lower your cholesterol and triglyceride levels and to decide if you should continue to take it.

Do not stop taking this medication without first checking with your doctor. When you stop taking this medicine, your blood cholesterol levels may increase again. Your doctor may want you to follow a special diet to help prevent this from happening.

Side Effects of This Medicine

Along with its needed effects, a medicine may cause some unwanted effects. Although not all of these side effects may occur, if they do occur they may need medical attention.

Check with your doctor immediately if any of the following side effects occur:
   Rare
      Cough or hoarseness; fever or chills; lower back or side pain; painful or difficult urination; stomach pain (severe) with nausea and vomiting

Check with your doctor as soon as possible if either of the following side effects occurs:
   Rare
      Muscle pain; unusual tiredness or weakness

Other side effects may occur that usually do not need medical attention. These side effects may go away during treatment as your body adjusts to the medicine. However, check with your doctor if any of the following side effects continue or are bothersome:
   More common
      Stomach pain, gas, or heartburn

Less common
  Diarrhea; nausea or vomiting; skin rash

Other side effects not listed above may also occur in some patients. If you notice any other effects, check with your doctor.

GUANABENZ   Systemic†

A commonly used brand name in the U.S. is Wytensin.

†Not commercially available in Canada.

Description

Guanabenz (GWAHN-a-benz) belongs to the general class of medicines called antihypertensives. It is used to treat high blood pressure (hypertension).

High blood pressure adds to the workload of the heart and arteries. If it continues for a long time, the heart and arteries may not function properly. This can damage the blood vessels of the brain, heart, and kidneys, resulting in a stroke, heart failure, or kidney failure. High blood pressure may also increase the risk of heart attacks. These problems may be less likely to occur if blood pressure is controlled.

Guanabenz works by controlling nerve impulses along certain nerve pathways. As a result, it relaxes blood vessels so that blood passes through them more easily. This helps to lower blood pressure.

Guanabenz is available only with your doctor's prescription, in the following dosage form:
  Oral
    • Tablets (U.S.)

It is very important that you read and understand the following information. If any of it causes you special concern,

check with your doctor. Also, *if you have any questions* or if you want more information about this medicine or your medical problem, *ask your doctor, nurse, or pharmacist.*

Before Using This Medicine

In deciding to use a medicine, the risks of taking the medicine must be weighed against the good it will do. This is a decision you and your doctor will make. For guanabenz, the following should be considered:

Allergies—Tell your doctor if you have ever had any unusual or allergic reaction to guanabenz. Also tell your doctor and pharmacist if you are allergic to any other substance, such as foods, preservatives, or dyes.

Pregnancy—Studies have not been done in humans. However, studies in rats have shown that guanabenz given in doses 9 to 10 times the maximum human dose caused a decrease in fertility. In addition, 3 to 6 times the maximum human dose caused birth defects (in the skeleton) in mice, and 6 to 9 times the maximum human dose caused death of the fetus in rats.

Breast-feeding—It is not known whether guanabenz passes into breast milk. However, this medicine has not been reported to cause problems in nursing babies.

Children—There is no specific information about the use of guanabenz in children.

Older adults—Dizziness, faintness, or drowsiness may be more likely to occur in the elderly, who are usually more sensitive to the effects of guanabenz.

Other medicines—Although certain medicines should not be used together at all, in other cases two different medicines may be used together even if an interaction might occur. In these cases, your doctor may want to change the dose, or other precautions may be necessary. When you are taking guanabenz, it is especially important that your doctor and pharmacist know if you are taking any of the following:

- Beta-blockers (acebutolol [e.g., Sectral], atenolol [e.g., Tenormin], betaxolol [Kerlone], carteolol [e.g., Cartrol], labetalol [e.g., Normodyne], metoprolol [e.g., Lopressor], nadolol [e.g., Corgard], oxprenolol [e.g., Trasicor], penbutolol [e.g., Levatol], pindolol [e.g., Visken], propranolol [e.g., Inderal], sotalol [e.g., Sotacor], timolol [e.g., Blocadren])—Effects on blood pressure may be increased. Also, the risk of unwanted effects when guanabenz treatment is stopped suddenly may be increased

Other medical problems—The presence of other medical problems may affect the use of guanabenz. Make sure you tell your doctor if you have any other medical problems, especially:

- Heart or blood vessel disease—Lowering blood pressure may make some conditions worse
- Kidney disease or
- Liver disease—Effects may be increased because of slower removal of guanabenz from the body

Before you begin using any new medicine (prescription or nonprescription) or if you develop any new medical problem while you are using this medicine, check with your doctor, nurse, or pharmacist.

Proper Use of This Medicine

Importance of diet:

- When prescribing medicine for your condition, your doctor may also prescribe a personal diet for you. Such a diet may be low in sodium (salt). Most people eat much more sodium than they need and too much sodium in the diet may increase blood pressure. Some foods that contain large amounts of sodium are canned soup, pickles, ketchup, green and ripe olives, relish, frankfurters, soy sauce, and carbonated beverages. Your doctor may want you to limit the amounts of these and other high-sodium foods in your diet. High blood pressure medicine is usually more effective when such a diet is properly followed.
- Also, it may be very important for you to go on a reducing diet. However, check with your doctor before changing your diet.

Many patients who have high blood pressure will not notice any signs of the problem. In fact, many may feel normal. It is very important that you *take your medicine exactly as directed* and that you keep your appointments with your doctor even if you feel well.

Remember that this medicine will not cure your high blood pressure but it does help control it. Therefore, you must continue to take it as directed if you expect to lower your blood pressure and keep it down. *You may have to take high blood pressure medicine for the rest of your life.* If high blood pressure is not treated, it can cause serious problems such as heart failure, blood vessel disease, stroke, or kidney disease.

To help you remember to take your medicine, try to get into the habit of taking it at the same time each day.

Missed dose—If you miss a dose of this medicine, take it as soon as possible. However, if it is almost time for your next dose, skip the missed dose and go back to your regular dosing schedule. Do not double doses. If you miss two or more doses in a row, check with your doctor. If your body suddenly goes without this medicine, some unpleasant effects may occur. If you have any questions about this, check with your doctor.

Storage—To store this medicine:
- Keep out of the reach of children.
- Store away from heat and direct light.
- Do not store in the bathroom, near the kitchen sink, or in other damp places. Heat or moisture may cause the medicine to break down.
- Do not keep outdated medicine or medicine no longer needed. Be sure that any discarded medicine is out of the reach of children.

Precautions While Using This Medicine

It is important that your doctor check your progress at regular visits to make sure that this medicine is working properly.

Check with your doctor before you stop taking guanabenz. Your doctor may want you to reduce gradually the amount you are taking before stopping completely.

Before having any kind of surgery (including dental surgery) or emergency treatment, tell the medical doctor or dentist in charge that you are using this medicine.

Do not take other medicines unless they have been discussed with your doctor. This especially includes over-the-counter (nonprescription) medicines for appetite control, asthma, colds, cough, hay fever, or sinus problems, since they may tend to increase your blood pressure.

Guanabenz will add to the effects of alcohol and other CNS depressants (medicines that slow down the nervous system, possibly causing drowsiness). Some examples of CNS depressants are antihistamines or medicine for hay fever, other allergies, or colds; sedatives, tranquilizers, or sleeping medicine; prescription pain medicine or narcotics; barbiturates; medicine for seizures; muscle relaxants; or anesthetics, including some dental anesthetics. *Check with your doctor before taking any of the above while you are using this medicine.*

Guanabenz may cause some people to become dizzy, drowsy, or less alert than they are normally. *Make sure you know how you react to this medicine before you drive, use machines, or do anything else that could be dangerous if you are dizzy or are not alert.*

Guanabenz may cause dryness of the mouth, nose, and throat. For temporary relief of mouth dryness, use sugarless candy or gum, melt bits of ice in your mouth, or use a saliva substitute. However, if dry mouth continues for more than 2 weeks, check with your medical doctor or dentist. Continuing dryness of the mouth may increase the chance of dental disease, including tooth decay, gum disease, and fungus infections.

Side Effects of This Medicine

Along with its needed effects, a medicine may cause some
unwanted effects. Although not all of these side effects may
occur, if they do occur they may need medical attention.

Check with your doctor as soon as possible if any of the
following side effects occur:

Signs and symptoms of overdose

Dizziness (severe); faintness; irritability; nervousness; pinpoint pupils; slow heartbeat; unusual tiredness or weakness

Other side effects may occur that usually do not need medical attention. These side effects may go away during treatment as your body adjusts to the medicine. However, check
with your doctor if any of the following side effects continue
or are bothersome:

More common

Dizziness; drowsiness; dry mouth; weakness

Less common or rare

Decreased sexual ability; headache; nausea

After you have been using this medicine for a while, unpleasant effects may occur if you stop taking it too suddenly.
After you stop taking this medicine, check with your doctor
if any of the following effects occur:

Anxiety or tenseness; chest pain; fast or irregular heartbeat;
headache; increased salivation; increase in sweating; nausea
or vomiting; nervousness or restlessness; shaking or trembling
of hands or fingers; stomach cramps; trouble in sleeping

Other side effects not listed above may also occur in some
patients. If you notice any other effects, check with your
doctor.

GUANADREL   Systemic†

A commonly used brand name in the U.S. is Hylorel.

---

†Not commercially available in Canada.

Description

Guanadrel (GWAHN-a-drel) belongs to the general class of medicines called antihypertensives. It is used to treat high blood pressure (hypertension).

High blood pressure adds to the workload of the heart and arteries. If it continues for a long time, the heart and arteries may not function properly. This can damage the blood vessels of the brain, heart, and kidneys resulting in a stroke, heart failure, or kidney failure. High blood pressure may also increase the risk of heart attacks. These problems may be less likely to occur if blood pressure is controlled.

Guanadrel works by controlling nerve impulses along certain nerve pathways. As a result, it relaxes the blood vessels so that blood passes through them more easily. This helps to lower blood pressure.

Guanadrel is available only with your doctor's prescription, in the following dosage form:

Oral
 • Tablets (U.S.)

It is very important that you read and understand the following information. If any of it causes you special concern, check with your doctor. Also, *if you have any questions* or if you want more information about this medicine or your medical problem, *ask your doctor, nurse, or pharmacist.*

Before Using This Medicine

In deciding to use a medicine, the risks of taking the medicine must be weighed against the good it will do. This is a decision you and your doctor will make. For guanadrel, the following should be considered:

Allergies—Tell your doctor if you have ever had any unusual or allergic reaction to guanadrel. Also tell your doctor and pharmacist if you are allergic to any other substance, such as foods, preservatives, or dyes.

Pregnancy—Studies have not been done in humans. However, guanadrel has not been shown to cause birth defects or other problems in rats and rabbits given up to 12 times the highest human dose.

Breast-feeding—It is not known whether guanadrel passes into breast milk. However, it has not been reported to cause problems in nursing babies.

Children—There is no specific information about the use of guanadrel in children.

Older adults—Dizziness or faintness may be more likely to occur in the elderly, who are usually more sensitive to the effects of guanadrel.

Other medicines—Although certain medicines should not be used together at all, in other cases two different medicines may be used together even if an interaction might occur. In these cases, your doctor may want to change the dose, or other precautions may be necessary. When you are taking guanadrel, it is especially important that your doctor and pharmacist know if you are taking any of the following:

- Chlorprothixene (e.g., Taractan) or
- Loxapine (e.g., Loxitane) or
- Thiothixene (e.g., Navane) or
- Tricyclic antidepressants (amitriptyline [e.g., Elavil], amoxapine [e.g., Asendin], clomipramine [e.g., Anafranil], desipramine [e.g., Pertofrane], doxepin [e.g., Sinequan], imipramine [e.g., Tofranil], nortriptyline [e.g., Aventyl], protriptyline [e.g., Vivactil], trimipramine [e.g., Surmontil]) or
- Trimeprazine (e.g., Temaril)—May decrease the effects of guanadrel on blood pressure
- Monoamine oxidase (MAO) inhibitors (furazolidone [e.g., Furoxone], isocarboxazid [e.g., Marplan], pargyline [e.g., Eutonyl], phenelzine [e.g., Nardil], procarbazine [e.g., Matulane], tranylcypromine [e.g., Parnate])—Taking guanadrel while you are taking or within 2 weeks of taking MAO inhibitors may cause a severe increase in blood pressure

Other medical problems—The presence of other medical problems may affect the use of guanadrel. Make sure you

tell your doctor if you have any other medical problems, especially:

- Asthma (history of) or
- Diarrhea or
- Pheochromocytoma or
- Stomach ulcer (history of)—May be worsened by guanadrel
- Fever—Effects of guanadrel may be increased
- Heart or blood vessel disease or
- Heart attack or stroke (recent)—Lowering blood pressure may make problems resulting from these conditions worse

Before you begin using any new medicine (prescription or nonprescription) or if you develop any new medical problem while you are using this medicine, check with your doctor, nurse, or pharmacist.

Proper Use of This Medicine

Importance of diet:

- When prescribing medicine for your condition, your doctor may also prescribe a personal diet for you. Such a diet may be low in sodium (salt). Most people eat much more sodium than they need and too much sodium in the diet may increase blood pressure. Some foods that contain large amounts of sodium are canned soup, pickles, ketchup, green and ripe olives, relish, frankfurters, soy sauce, and carbonated beverages. Your doctor may want you to limit the amounts of these and other high-sodium foods in your diet. High blood pressure medicine is usually more effective when such a diet is properly followed.
- Also, it may be very important for you to go on a reducing diet. However, check with your doctor before changing your diet.

Many patients who have high blood pressure will not notice any signs of the problem. In fact, many may feel normal. It is very important that you *take your medicine exactly as directed* and that you keep your appointments with your doctor even if you feel well.

Remember that guanadrel will not cure your high blood pressure but it does help control it. Therefore, you must continue to take it as directed if you expect to lower your blood pressure and keep it down. *You may have to take high blood pressure medicine for the rest of your life.* If high blood pressure is not treated, it can cause serious problems such as heart failure, blood vessel disease, stroke, or kidney disease.

To help you remember to take your medicine, try to get into the habit of taking it at the same time each day.

Missed dose—If you miss a dose of guanadrel, take it as soon as possible. However, if it is almost time for your next dose, skip the missed dose and go back to your regular dosing schedule. Do not double doses.

Storage—To store this medicine:
- Keep out of the reach of children.
- Store away from heat and direct light.
- Do not store in the bathroom, near the kitchen sink, or in other damp places. Heat or moisture may cause the medicine to break down.
- Do not keep outdated medicine or medicine no longer needed. Be sure that any discarded medicine is out of the reach of children.

Precautions While Using This Medicine

It is important that your doctor check your progress at regular visits to make sure that this medicine is working properly.

Dizziness, lightheadedness, or fainting may occur, especially when you get up from a lying or sitting position. This may be more likely to occur in the morning. *Getting up slowly may help.* If you feel dizzy, sit or lie down. When you get up from lying down, sit on the edge of the bed with your feet dangling for 1 or 2 minutes. Then stand up slowly. If the problem continues or gets worse, check with your doctor.

The dizziness, lightheadedness, or fainting is also more likely to occur if you drink alcohol, stand for long periods of time, exercise, or if the weather is hot. *While you are taking guanadrel, be careful in the amount of alcohol you drink. Also, use extra care during exercise or hot weather or if you must stand for long periods of time.*

Do not take other medicines unless they have been discussed with your doctor. This especially includes over-the-counter (nonprescription) medicines for appetite control, asthma, colds, cough, hay fever, or sinus problems, since they may tend to increase your blood pressure.

Before having any kind of surgery (including dental surgery) or emergency treatment, tell the medical doctor or dentist in charge that you are taking guanadrel.

Tell your doctor if you get a fever since that may change the amount of medicine you have to take.

Side Effects of This Medicine

Along with its needed effects, a medicine may cause some unwanted effects. Although not all of these side effects may occur, if they do occur they may need medical attention.

Check with your doctor immediately if either of the following side effects occurs since they may be symptoms of an overdose:

> *Rare*
> > Blurred vision; dizziness or faintness (severe)

Check with your doctor as soon as possible if any of the following side effects occur:

> *More common*
> > Swelling of feet or lower legs
>
> *Less common or rare*
> > Chest pain; shortness of breath

Other side effects may occur that usually do not need medical attention. These side effects may go away during treatment as your body adjusts to the medicine. However, check with your doctor if any of the following side effects continue or are bothersome:

More common
> Difficulty in ejaculating; dizziness, lightheadedness, or faint-
> ing, especially when getting up from a lying or sitting
> position; drowsiness or tiredness

Less common or rare
> Diarrhea or increase in bowel movements; dry mouth; head-
> ache; muscle pain or tremors; nighttime urination

Other side effects not listed above may also occur in some
patients. If you notice any other effects, check with your
doctor.

GUANETHIDINE   Systemic

Some commonly used brand names are:

In the U.S.
> Ismelin
> Generic name product may also be available.

In Canada
> Apo-Guanethidine
> Ismelin

Description

Guanethidine (gwahn-ETH-i-deen) belongs to the general
class of medicines called antihypertensives. It is used to treat
high blood pressure (hypertension).

High blood pressure adds to the workload of the heart and
arteries. If it continues for a long time, the heart and arteries
may not function properly. This can damage the blood vessels of the brain, heart, and kidneys, resulting in a stroke,
heart failure, or kidney failure. High blood pressure may
also increase the risk of heart attacks. These problems may
be less likely to occur if blood pressure is controlled.

Guanethidine works by controlling nerve impulses along certain nerve pathways. As a result, it relaxes the blood vessels
so that blood passes through them more easily. This helps
to lower blood pressure.

Guanethidine is available only with your doctor's prescription, in the following dosage form:

Oral
 • Tablets (U.S. and Canada)

It is very important that you read and understand the following information. If any of it causes you special concern, check with your doctor. Also, *if you have any questions* or if you want more information about this medicine or your medical problem, *ask your doctor, nurse, or pharmacist.*

Before Using This Medicine

In deciding to use a medicine, the risks of taking the medicine must be weighed against the good it will do. This is a decision you and your doctor will make. For guanethidine, the following should be considered:

Allergies—Tell your doctor if you have ever had any unusual or allergic reaction to guanethidine. Also tell your doctor and pharmacist if you are allergic to any other substance, such as foods, preservatives, or dyes.

Pregnancy—Studies on effects in pregnancy have not been done in either humans or animals.

Breast-feeding—Small amounts of guanethidine pass into breast-milk. However, this medicine has not been reported to cause problems in nursing babies.

Children—Although there is no specific information comparing use of guanethidine in children with use in other age groups, this medicine is not expected to cause different side effects or problems in children than it does in adults.

Older adults—Many medicines have not been studied specifically in older people. Therefore, it may not be known whether they work exactly the same way they do in younger adults. Although there is no specific information comparing use of guanethidine in the elderly with use in other age groups, dizziness, lightheadedness, or fainting may be more likely to occur in the elderly, who are more sensitive to the effects of guanethidine.

Other medicines—Although certain medicines should not be used together at all, in other cases two different medicines

may be used together even if an interaction might occur. In these cases, your doctor may want to change the dose, or other precautions may be necessary. When you are taking guanethidine, it is especially important that your doctor and pharmacist know if you are taking any of the following:

- Antidiabetics, oral (diabetes medicine you take by mouth)—Effects may be increased by guanethidine
- Loxapine (e.g., Loxitane) or
- Thioxanthenes (chlorprothixene [e.g., Taractan], thiothixene [e.g., Navane]) or
- Tricyclic antidepressants (amitriptyline [e.g., Elavil], amoxapine [e.g., Asendin], clomipramine [e.g., Anafranil], desipramine [e.g., Pertofrane], doxepin [e.g., Sinequan], imipramine [e.g., Tofranil], nortriptyline [e.g., Aventyl], protriptyline [e.g., Vivactil], trimipramine [e.g., Surmontil]) or
- Trimeprazine (e.g., Temaril)—May decrease the effects of guanethidine on blood pressure
- Minoxidil (e.g., Loniten)—Effects on blood pressure may be greatly increased
- Monoamine oxidase (MAO) inhibitors (furazolidone [e.g., Furoxone], isocarboxazid [e.g., Marplan], phenelzine [e.g., Nardil], procarbazine [e.g., Matulane], selegiline [e.g., Eldepryl], tranylcypromine [e.g., Parnate])—Taking guanethidine while you are taking or within 2 weeks of taking MAO inhibitors may cause a severe increase in blood pressure

Other medical problems—The presence of other medical problems may affect the use of guanethidine. Make sure you tell your doctor if you have any other medical problems, especially:

- Asthma (history of) or
- Diarrhea or
- Pheochromocytoma or
- Stomach ulcer (history of)—May be worsened by guanethidine
- Diabetes mellitus (sugar diabetes)—Effects of medicine used to treat this may be increased by guanethidine
- Fever—Effects of guanethidine may be increased
- Heart or blood vessel disease or
- Heart attack or stroke (recent)—Lowering blood pressure may make problems resulting from these conditions worse

- Kidney disease—May be worsened. Also, effects of guanethidine may be increased because of slower removal of this medicine from the body
- Liver disease—Effects of guanethidine may be increased because of slower removal from the body

Before you begin using any new medicine (prescription or nonprescription) or if you develop any new medical problem while you are using this medicine, check with your doctor, nurse, or pharmacist.

Proper Use of This Medicine

In addition to the use of the medicine your doctor has prescribed, treatment for your high blood pressure may include weight control and care in the types of foods you eat, especially foods high in sodium. Your doctor will tell you which of these are most important for you. You should check with your doctor before changing your diet.

Many patients who have high blood pressure will not notice any signs of the problem. In fact, many may feel normal. It is very important that you *take your medicine exactly as directed* and that you keep your appointments with your doctor even if you feel well.

Remember that guanethidine will not cure your high blood pressure but it does help control it. Therefore, you must continue to take it as directed if you expect to lower your blood pressure and keep it down. *You may have to take high blood pressure medicine for the rest of your life.* If high blood pressure is not treated, it can cause serious problems such as heart failure, blood vessel disease, stroke, or kidney disease.

To help you remember to take your medicine, try to get into the habit of taking it at the same time each day.

Missed dose—If you miss a dose of guanethidine, take it as soon as possible. However, if it is almost time for your next dose, skip the missed dose and go back to your regular dosing schedule. Do not double doses.

Storage—To store this medicine:

- Keep out of the reach of children.
- Store away from heat and direct light.
- Do not store in the bathroom, near the kitchen sink, or in other damp places. Heat or moisture may cause the medicine to break down.
- Do not keep outdated medicine or medicine no longer needed. Be sure that any discarded medicine is out of the reach of children.

Precautions While Using This Medicine

It is important that your doctor check your progress at regular visits to make sure that this medicine is working properly.

Dizziness, lightheadedness, or fainting may occur, especially when you get up from a lying or sitting position. This is more likely to occur in the morning. *Getting up slowly may help.* When you get up from lying down, sit on the edge of the bed with your feet dangling for 1 or 2 minutes. Then stand up slowly. If the problem continues or gets worse, check with your doctor.

The dizziness, lightheadedness, or fainting is also more likely to occur if you drink alcohol, stand for long periods of time, exercise, or if the weather is hot. *While you are taking this medicine, be careful in the amount of alcohol you drink. Also, use extra care during exercise or hot weather or if you must stand for long periods of time.*

Do not take other medicines unless they have been discussed with your doctor. This especially includes over-the-counter (nonprescription) medicines for appetite control, asthma, colds, cough, hay fever, or sinus problems, since they may tend to increase your blood pressure.

Before having any kind of surgery (including dental surgery) or emergency treatment, tell the medical doctor or dentist in charge that you are taking this medicine.

Tell your doctor if you get a fever since that may change the amount of medicine you have to take.

Side Effects of This Medicine

Along with its needed effects, a medicine may cause some unwanted effects. Although not all of these side effects may occur, if they do occur they may need medical attention.

Check with your doctor as soon as possible if any of the following side effects occur:

More common

Swelling of feet or lower legs

Less common or rare

Chest pain; shortness of breath

Other side effects may occur that usually do not need medical attention. These side effects may go away during treatment as your body adjusts to the medicine. However, check with your doctor if any of the following side effects continue or are bothersome:

More common

Diarrhea or increase in bowel movements; dizziness, light-headedness, or fainting, especially when getting up from a lying or sitting position; sexual problems in males; slow heartbeat; stuffy nose; unusual tiredness or weakness

Less common or rare

Blurred vision; drooping eyelids; dryness of mouth; headache; loss of hair on scalp; muscle pain or tremors; nausea or vomiting; nighttime urination; skin rash

Other side effects not listed above may also occur in some patients. If you notice any other effects, check with your doctor.

GUANFACINE Systemic†

A commonly used brand name in the U.S. is Tenex.

---

†Not commercially available in Canada.

Description

Guanfacine (GWAHN-fa-seen) belongs to the general class of medicines called antihypertensives. It is used to treat high blood pressure (hypertension).

High blood pressure adds to the workload of the heart and arteries. If it continues for a long time, the heart and arteries may not function properly. This can damage the blood vessels of the brain, heart, and kidneys, resulting in a stroke, heart failure, or kidney failure. High blood pressure may also increase the risk of heart attacks. These problems may be less likely to occur if blood pressure is controlled.

Guanfacine works by controlling nerve impulses along certain nerve pathways. As a result, it relaxes blood vessels so that blood passes through them more easily. This helps to lower blood pressure.

Guanfacine is available only with your doctor's prescription, in the following dosage form:

Oral
  • Tablets (U.S.)

It is very important that you read and understand the following information. If any of it causes you special concern, check with your doctor. Also, *if you have any questions* or if you want more information about this medicine or your medical problem, *ask your doctor, nurse, or pharmacist.*

Before Using This Medicine

In deciding to use a medicine, the risks of taking the medicine must be weighed against the good it will do. This is a decision you and your doctor will make. For guanfacine, the following should be considered:

Allergies—Tell your doctor if you have ever had any unusual or allergic reaction to guanfacine. Also tell your doctor and pharmacist if you are allergic to any other substance, such as foods, preservatives, or dyes.

Pregnancy—Studies have not been done in humans. However, guanfacine has not been shown to cause birth defects or other problems in rats or rabbits given many times the human dose. In rats and rabbits given extremely high doses (up to 200 times the human dose), there was an increase in deaths of the animal fetus.

Breast-feeding—It is not known whether guanfacine passes into the breast milk. It has not been reported to cause problems in nursing babies.

Children—There is no specific information about the use of guanfacine in children.

Older adults—Dizziness, drowsiness, or faintness may be more likely to occur in the elderly, who are more sensitive to the effects of guanfacine.

Other medicines—Although certain medicines should not be used together at all, in other cases two different medicines may be used together even if an interaction might occur. In these cases, your doctor may want to change the dose, or other precautions may be necessary. When you are taking guanfacine, it is especially important that your doctor and pharmacist know if you are taking any other prescription or nonprescription (over-the-counter [OTC]) medicine.

Other medical problems—The presence of other medical problems may affect the use of guanfacine. Make sure you tell your doctor if you have any other medical problems, especially:
- Heart disease or
- Heart attack or stroke (recent)—Lowering blood pressure may make problems resulting from these conditions worse
- Liver disease—Effects may be increased because of slower removal of guanfacine from the body
- Mental depression—Guanfacine may cause mental depression

Before you begin using any new medicine (prescription or nonprescription) or if you develop any new medical problem while you are using this medicine, check with your doctor, nurse, or pharmacist.

Proper Use of This Medicine

Importance of diet:

- When prescribing medicine for your condition, your doctor may also prescribe a personal diet for you. Such a diet may be low in sodium (salt). Most people eat much more sodium than they need and too much sodium in the diet may increase blood pressure. Some foods that contain large amounts of sodium are canned soup, pickles, ketchup, green and ripe olives, relish, frankfurters, soy sauce, and carbonated beverages. Your doctor may want you to limit the amounts of these and other high-sodium foods in your diet. High blood pressure medicine is usually more effective when such a diet is properly followed.
- Also, it may be very important for you to go on a reducing diet. However, check with your doctor before changing your diet.

Many patients who have high blood pressure will not notice any signs of the problem. In fact, many may feel normal. It is very important that you *take your medicine exactly as directed* and that you keep your appointments with your doctor even if you feel well.

Remember that this medicine will not cure your high blood pressure but it does help control it. Therefore, you must continue to use it as directed if you expect to lower your blood pressure and keep it down. *You may have to take high blood pressure medicine for the rest of your life.* If high blood pressure is not treated, it can cause serious problems such as heart failure, blood vessel disease, stroke, or kidney disease.

Take your daily dose of guanfacine at bedtime. (If you are taking more than one dose a day, take your last dose at bedtime). Taking it this way will help lessen daytime drowsiness.

Missed dose—If you miss a dose of this medicine, take it as soon as possible. However, if it is almost time for your next dose, skip the missed dose and go back to your regular dosing schedule. Do not double doses. *If you miss taking*

*guanfacine for two or more days in a row, check with your
doctor.* If your body suddenly goes without this medicine,
some unwanted effects may occur. If you have any questions
about this, check with your doctor.

Storage—To store this medicine:
- Keep out of the reach of children.
- Store away from heat and direct light.
- Do not store in the bathroom, near the kitchen sink, or
  in other damp places. Heat or moisture may cause the
  medicine to break down.
- Do not keep outdated medicine or medicine no longer
  needed. Be sure any discarded medicine is out of the
  reach of children.

Precautions While Using This Medicine

It is important that your doctor check your progress at regular visits to make sure this medicine is working properly.

Check with your doctor before you stop taking guanfacine.
Your doctor may want you to reduce gradually the amount
you are taking before stopping completely.

Make sure that you have enough guanfacine on hand to last
through weekends, holidays, and vacations. You should not
miss any doses. You may want to ask your doctor for another
written prescription for guanfacine to carry in your wallet
or purse. You can then have it filled if you run out when
you are away from home.

Before having any kind of surgery (including dental surgery)
or emergency treatment, tell the medical doctor or dentist
in charge that you are using this medicine.

*Do not take other medicines unless they have been discussed
with your doctor.* This especially includes over-the-counter
(nonprescription) medicines for appetite control, asthma,
colds, cough, hay fever, or sinus problems, since they may
tend to increase your blood pressure.

Guanfacine will add to the effects of alcohol and other CNS
depressants (medicines that slow down the nervous system,

possibly causing drowsiness). Some examples of CNS depressants are antihistamines or medicine for hay fever, other allergies, or colds; sedatives, tranquilizers, or sleeping medicine; prescription pain medicine or narcotics; barbiturates; medicine for seizures; muscle relaxants; or anesthetics, including some dental anesthetics. *Check with your doctor before taking any of the above while you are using this medicine.*

Guanfacine may cause some people to become dizzy, drowsy, or less alert than they are normally. *Make sure you know how you react to this medicine before you drive, use machines, or do anything else that could be dangerous if you are dizzy or are not alert.*

Guanfacine may cause dryness of the mouth, nose, and throat. For temporary relief of mouth dryness, use sugarless candy or gum, melt bits of ice in your mouth, or use a saliva substitute. However, if dry mouth continues for more than 2 weeks, check with your physician or dentist. Continuing dryness of the mouth may increase the chance of dental disease, including tooth decay, gum disease, and fungus infections.

Side Effects of This Medicine

Along with its needed effects, a medicine may cause some unwanted effects. Although not all of these side effects may occur, if they do occur they may need medical attention.

Check with your doctor as soon as possible if any of the following side effects occur:

Less common

Confusion; mental depression

Signs and symptoms of overdose

Difficulty in breathing; dizziness (extreme) or faintness; slow heartbeat; unusual tiredness or weakness (severe)

Other side effects may occur that usually do not need medical attention. These side effects may go away during treatment as your body adjusts to the medicine. However, check with your doctor if any of the following side effects continue or are bothersome:

More common

Constipation; dizziness; drowsiness; dry mouth

Less common
> Decreased sexual ability; dry, itching, or burning eyes; headache; nausea or vomiting; trouble in sleeping; unusual tiredness or weakness

After you have been using this medicine for a while, unwanted effects may occur if you stop taking it too suddenly. After you stop taking this medicine, check with your doctor if any of the following side effects occur:
> Anxiety or tenseness; chest pain; fast or irregular heartbeat; headache; increased salivation; nausea or vomiting; nervousness or restlessness; shaking or trembling of hands and fingers; stomach cramps; sweating; trouble in sleeping

Other side effects not listed above may also occur in some patients. If you notice any other effects, check with your doctor.

HALOPERIDOL   Systemic

Some commonly used brand names are:
> *In the U.S.*
> > Haldol
> > Haldol Decanoate
> > Generic name product may also be available.
>
> *In Canada*
> > Apo-Haloperidol   Novo-Peridol
> > Haldol   Peridol
> > Haldol LA   PMS Haloperidol
> > Generic name product may also be available.

Description

Haloperidol (ha-loe-PER-i-dole) is used to treat nervous, mental, and emotional conditions. It is also used to control the symptoms of Tourette's disorder. Haloperidol may also be used for other conditions as determined by your doctor.

Haloperidol is available only with your doctor's prescription, in the following dosage forms:

Oral
- Solution (U.S. and Canada)
- Tablets (U.S. and Canada)

Parenteral
- Injection (U.S. and Canada)

It is very important that you read and understand the following information. If any of it causes you special concern, check with your doctor. Also, *if you have any questions* or if you want more information about this medicine or your medical problem, *ask your doctor, nurse, or pharmacist.*

Before Using This Medicine

In deciding to use a medicine, the risks of taking the medicine must be weighed against the good it will do. This is a decision you and your doctor will make. For haloperidol, the following should be considered:

Allergies—Tell your doctor if you have ever had any unusual or allergic reaction to haloperidol. Also tell your doctor and pharmacist if you are allergic to any other substances, such as foods, preservatives, or dyes.

Pregnancy—Haloperidol has not been studied in pregnant women. However, studies in animals given 2 to 20 times the usual maximum human dose of haloperidol have shown reduced fertility, delayed delivery, cleft palate, and an increase in the number of stillbirths and newborn deaths.

Breast-feeding—Haloperidol passes into breast milk. Animal studies have shown that haloperidol in breast milk causes drowsiness and unusual muscle movements in the nursing offspring. Breast-feeding is not recommended during treatment with haloperidol.

Children—Side effects, especially muscle spasms of the neck and back, twisting movements of the body, trembling of fingers and hands, and inability to move the eyes are more likely to occur in children, who usually are more sensitive than adults to the effects of haloperidol.

Older adults—Constipation, dizziness or fainting, drowsiness, dryness of mouth, trembling of the hands and fingers, and symptoms of tardive dyskinesia (such as rapid, worm-like movements of the tongue or any other uncontrolled movements of the mouth, tongue, or jaw, and/or arms and legs) are especially likely to occur in elderly patients, who are usually more sensitive than younger adults to the effects of haloperidol.

Athletes—Haloperidol is banned and, in some cases, tested for in competitors in biathlon and modern pentathlon events by the U.S. Olympic Committee (USOC) .

Other medicines—Although certain medicines should not be used together at all, in other cases 2 different medicines may be used together even if an interaction might occur. In these cases, your doctor may want to change the dose, or other precautions may be necessary. When you are taking haloperidol, it is especially important that your doctor and pharmacist know if you are taking any of the following:

- Amoxapine (e.g., Asendin) or
- Metoclopramide (e.g., Reglan) or
- Metyrosine (e.g., Demser) or
- Other antipsychotics (medicine for mental illness) or
- Pemoline (e.g., Cylert) or
- Pimozide (e.g., Orap) or
- Promethazine (e.g., Phenergan) or
- Rauwolfia alkaloids (alseroxylon [e.g., Rauwiloid], deserpidine [e.g., Harmonyl], rauwolfia serpentina [e.g., Raudixin], reserpine [e.g., Serpasil]) or
- Trimeprazine (e.g., Temaril)—Taking these medicines with haloperidol may increase the frequency and severity of certain side effects
- Central nervous system (CNS) depressants (medicines that cause drowsiness)—Taking these medicines with haloperidol may result in increased CNS and other depressant effects, and in an increased chance of low blood pressure (hypotension)
- Epinephrine (e.g., Adrenalin)—Severe low blood pressure or irregular heartbeat may occur
- Levodopa (e.g., Dopar; Larodopa)—Haloperidol may interfere with the effects of this medicine
- Lithium (e.g., Eskalith; Lithane)—Although lithium and haloperidol are sometimes used together, their use must be closely monitored by your doctor, who may change the amount of medicine you need to take

Other medical problems—The presence of other medical problems may affect the use of haloperidol. Make sure you tell your doctor if you have any other medical problems, especially:

- Alcohol abuse—The risk of heat stroke may be increased
- Difficult urination or
- Glaucoma or
- Heart or blood vessel disease or
- Lung disease or
- Parkinson's disease—Haloperidol may make the condition worse
- Epilepsy—The risk of seizures may be increased
- Kidney disease or
- Liver disease—Higher blood levels of haloperidol may occur, increasing the chance of side effects
- Overactive thyroid—Serious unwanted effects may occur

Before you begin using any new medicine (prescription or nonprescription) or if you develop any new medical problem while you are using this medicine, check with your doctor, nurse, or pharmacist.

Proper Use of This Medicine

If this medicine upsets your stomach, it may be taken with food or milk to lessen stomach irritation.

For patients taking the *liquid form of this medicine*:

- This medicine is to be taken by mouth even if it comes in a dropper bottle. Each dose is to be measured with the specially marked dropper provided with your prescription. Do not use other droppers since they may not deliver the correct amount of medicine.
- This medicine is best taken alone. However, if necessary, it may be mixed with water. If this is done, the mixture should be taken immediately after mixing. Haloperidol should not be taken in tea or coffee, since they cause the medicine to separate out of solution.

Take this medicine only as directed by your doctor. Do not take more of it, do not take it more often, and do not take it for a longer time than your doctor ordered. This is particularly important for children or elderly patients, since they may react very strongly to this medicine.

Continue taking this medicine for the full time of treatment. *Sometimes haloperidol must be taken for several days to several weeks before its full effect is reached.*

Missed dose—If you miss a dose of this medicine, take it as soon as possible. Then take any remaining doses for that day at regularly spaced intervals. Do not double doses.

Storage—To store this medicine:
- Keep out of the reach of children.
- Store away from heat and direct light.
- Do not store the tablet form of this medicine in the bathroom, near the kitchen sink, or in other damp places. Heat or moisture may cause the medicine to break down.
- Keep the liquid form of this medicine from freezing.
- Do not keep outdated medicine or medicine no longer needed. Be sure that any discarded medicine is out of the reach of children.

Precautions While Using This Medicine

Your doctor should check your progress at regular visits, especially during the first few months of treatment with this medicine. The amount of haloperidol you take may be changed often to meet the needs of your condition. This also helps prevent side effects.

Do not stop taking this medicine without first checking with your doctor. Your doctor may want you to reduce gradually the amount you are taking before stopping completely. This will allow your body time to adjust and help avoid a worsening of your medical condition.

This medicine will add to the effects of alcohol and other CNS depressants (medicines that slow down the nervous system, possibly causing drowsiness). Some examples of CNS depressants are antihistamines or medicine for hay fever, other allergies, or colds; sedatives, tranquilizers, or sleeping medicine; prescription pain medicine or narcotics; barbiturates; medicine for seizures; muscle relaxants; or anesthetics, including some dental anesthetics. *Check with your doctor before taking any of the above while you are taking this medicine.*

This medicine may cause some people to become dizzy, drowsy, or less alert than they are normally, especially as the amount of medicine is increased. Even if you take haloperidol at bedtime, you may feel drowsy or less alert on arising. *Make sure you know how you react to this medicine before you drive, use machines, or do anything else that could be dangerous if you are dizzy or are not alert.*

Although not a problem for many patients, dizziness, lightheadedness, or fainting may occur, especially when you get up from a lying or sitting position. Getting up slowly may help. However, if the problem continues or gets worse, check with your doctor.

This medicine will often make you sweat less, causing your body temperature to increase. *Use extra care not to become overheated during exercise or hot weather while you are taking this medicine, since overheating may result in heat stroke.* Also, hot baths or saunas may make you feel dizzy or faint while you are taking this medicine.

Before using any prescription or over-the-counter (OTC) medicine for colds or allergies, check with your doctor. These medicines may increase the chance of heat stroke or other unwanted effects, such as dizziness, dry mouth, blurred vision, and constipation, while you are taking haloperidol.

Before having any kind of surgery, dental treatment, or emergency treatment, tell the medical doctor or dentist in charge that you are using this medicine.

Haloperidol may cause your skin to be more sensitive to sunlight than it is normally. Exposure to sunlight, even for brief periods of time, may cause a skin rash, itching, redness or other discoloration of the skin, or a severe sunburn. When you begin taking this medicine:

- Stay out of direct sunlight, especially between the hours of 10:00 a.m. and 3:00 p.m., if possible.

- Wear protective clothing, including a hat. Also, wear sunglasses.
- Apply a sun block product that has a skin protection factor (SPF) of at least 15. Some patients may require a product with a higher SPF number, especially if they have a fair complexion. If you have any questions about this, check with your doctor or pharmacist.
- Apply a sun block lipstick that has an SPF of at least 15 to protect your lips.
- Do not use a sunlamp or tanning bed or booth.

If you have a severe reaction from the sun, check with your doctor.

Haloperidol may cause dryness of the mouth. For temporary relief, use sugarless candy or gum, melt bits of ice in your mouth, or use a saliva substitute. However, if your mouth continues to feel dry for more than 2 weeks, check with your medical doctor or dentist. Continuing dryness of the mouth may increase the chance of dental disease, including tooth decay, gum disease, and fungus infections.

If you are *receiving this medicine by injection*:
- The effects of the long-acting injection form of this medicine may last for up to 6 weeks. *The precautions and side effects information for this medicine applies during this time.*

Side Effects of This Medicine

Along with its needed effects, haloperidol can sometimes cause serious side effects. Tardive dyskinesia (a movement disorder) may occur and may not go away after you stop using the medicine. Signs of tardive dyskinesia include fine, worm-like movements of the tongue, or other uncontrolled movements of the mouth, tongue, cheeks, jaw, or arms and legs. Other serious but rare side effects may also occur. These include severe muscle stiffness, fever, unusual tiredness or weakness, fast heartbeat, difficult breathing, increased sweating, loss of bladder control, and seizures (neuroleptic malignant syndrome). *You and your doctor should discuss the good this medicine will do as well as the risks of taking it.*

Stop taking haloperidol and get emergency help immediately if any of the following side effects occur:

Rare

Convulsions (seizures); difficult or fast breathing; fast heartbeat or irregular pulse; fever (high); increased sweating; loss of bladder control; muscle stiffness (severe); unusually pale skin; unusual tiredness or weakness

Check with your doctor as soon as possible if any of the following side effects occur:

More common

Difficulty in speaking or swallowing; inability to move eyes; loss of balance control; mask-like face; muscle spasms, especially of the neck and back; restlessness or need to keep moving (severe); shuffling walk; stiffness of arms and legs; trembling and shaking of fingers and hands; twisting movements of body

Less common

Decreased thirst; difficulty in urination; dizziness, lightheadedness, or fainting; hallucinations (seeing or hearing things that are not there); lip smacking or puckering; puffing of cheeks; rapid or worm-like movements of tongue; skin rash; uncontrolled chewing movements; uncontrolled movements of arms and legs

Rare

Hot, dry skin, or lack of sweating; increased blinking or spasms of eyelid; muscle weakness; sore throat and fever; uncontrolled twisting movements of neck, trunk, arms, or legs; unusual bleeding or bruising; unusual facial expressions or body positions; yellow eyes or skin

Symptoms of overdose

Difficulty in breathing (severe); dizziness or lightheadedness (severe); drowsiness (severe); muscle trembling, jerking, stiffness, or uncontrolled movements (severe); unusual tiredness or weakness (severe)

Other side effects may occur that usually do not need medical attention. These side effects may go away during treat-

ment as your body adjusts to the medicine. However, check with your doctor if any of the following side effects continue or are bothersome:

More common

Blurred vision; changes in menstrual period; constipation; dryness of mouth; swelling or pain in breasts (in females); unusual secretion of milk; weight gain

Less common

Decreased sexual ability; drowsiness; increased sensitivity of skin to sun (skin rash, itching, redness or other discoloration of skin, or severe sunburn); nausea or vomiting

Some side effects, such as trembling of fingers and hands, or uncontrolled movements of the mouth, tongue, and jaw, may occur after you have stopped taking this medicine. If you notice any of these effects, check with your doctor as soon as possible.

Other side effects not listed above may also occur in some patients. If you notice any other effects, check with your doctor.

Additional Information

Once a medicine has been approved for marketing for a certain use, experience may show that it is also useful for other medical problems. Although these uses are not included in product labeling, haloperidol is used in certain patients with the following medical conditions:

- Huntington's chorea (an hereditary movement disorder)
- Infantile autism
- Nausea and vomiting caused by cancer chemotherapy

Other than the above information, there is no additional information relating to proper use, precautions, or side effects for these uses.

HEADACHE MEDICINES, ERGOT DERIVATIVE–CONTAINING   Systemic

This information applies to the following medicines:

Dihydroergotamine (dye-hye-droe-er-GOT-a-meen)
Ergotamine (er-GOT-a-meen)
Ergotamine and Caffeine (kaf-EEN)
Ergotamine, Caffeine, and Belladonna Alkaloids (bell-a-DON-a AL-ka-loids)
Ergotamine, Caffeine, Belladonna Alkaloids, and Pentobarbital (pen-toe-BAR-bi-tal)
Ergotamine, Caffeine, and Cyclizine (SYE-kli-zeen)
Ergotamine, Caffeine, and Dimenhydrinate (dye-men-HYE-dri-nate)
Ergotamine, Caffeine, and Diphenhydramine (dye-fen-HYE-dra-mine)

Some commonly used brand names are:

For Dihydroergotamine
In the U.S.
D.H.E. 45

In Canada
Dihydroergotamine-Sandoz

For Ergotamine
In the U.S.
Ergomar   Ergostat

In Canada
Ergomar   Medihaler Ergotamine
Gynergen

For Ergotamine and Caffeine
In the U.S.
Cafergot   Ergo-Caff
Cafertine   Gotamine
Cafetrate   Migergot
Ercaf   Wigraine

Generic name product may also be available.

In Canada
Cafergot

For Ergotamine, Caffeine, and Belladonna Alkaloids*
In Canada
Wigraine

For Ergotamine, Caffeine, Belladonna Alkaloids, and Pentobarbital*
In Canada
Cafergot-PB

For Ergotamine, Caffeine, and Cyclizine*
In Canada
Megral

For Ergotamine, Caffeine, and Dimenhydrinate*
  In Canada
    Gravergol
For Ergotamine, Caffeine, and Diphenhydramine*
  In Canada
    Ergodryl

---

*Not commercially available in the U.S.

Description

Dihydroergotamine and ergotamine belong to the group of medicines known as ergot alkaloids. They are used to treat severe, throbbing headaches, such as migraine and cluster headaches. Dihydroergotamine and ergotamine are not ordinary pain relievers. They will not relieve any kind of pain other than throbbing headaches. Because these medicines can cause serious side effects, they are usually used for patients whose headaches are not relieved by acetaminophen, aspirin, or other pain relievers.

Dihydroergotamine and ergotamine may cause blood vessels in the body to constrict (become narrower). This effect can lead to serious side effects that are caused by a decrease in the flow of blood (blood circulation) to many parts of the body.

The caffeine present in many ergotamine-containing combinations helps ergotamine work better and faster by causing more of it to be quickly absorbed into the body. The belladonna alkaloids, cyclizine, dimenhydrinate, and diphenhydramine in some combinations help to relieve nausea and vomiting, which often occur together with the headaches. Cyclizine, dimenhydinate, diphenhydramine, and pentobarbital also help the patient relax and even sleep. This also helps relieve headaches.

Dihydroergotamine is also used for other conditions, as determined by your doctor.

These medicines are available only with your doctor's prescription, in the following dosage forms:

Oral

Ergotamine
  • Inhalation aerosol (Canada)
  • Sublingual tablets (U.S. and Canada)
  • Tablets (Canada)
Ergotamine and Caffeine
  • Tablets (U.S. and Canada)
Ergotamine, Caffeine, and Belladonna Alkaloids
  • Tablets (Canada)
Ergotamine, Caffeine, Belladonna Alkaloids, and Pentobarbital
  • Tablets (Canada)
Ergotamine, Caffeine, and Cyclizine
  • Tablets (Canada)
Ergotamine, Caffeine, and Dimenhydrinate
  • Capsules (Canada)
Ergotamine, Caffeine, and Diphenhydramine
  • Capsules (Canada)

Parenteral

Dihydroergotamine
  • Injection (U.S. and Canada)

Rectal

Ergotamine and Caffeine
  • Suppositories (U.S. and Canada)
Ergotamine, Caffeine, and Belladonna Alkaloids
  • Suppositories (Canada)
Ergotamine, Caffeine, Belladonna Alkaloids, and Pentobarbital
  • Suppositories (Canada)

It is very important that you read and understand the following information. If any of it causes you special concern, check with your doctor. Also, *if you have any questions* or if you want more information about this medicine or your medical problem, *ask your doctor, nurse, or pharmacist.*

Before Using This Medicine

In deciding to use a medicine, the risks of taking the medicine must be weighed against the good it will do. This is a decision you and your doctor will make. For these headache medicines, the following should be considered:

Allergies—Tell your doctor if you have ever had any unusual or allergic reaction to atropine, belladonna, pentobarbital or other barbiturates, caffeine, cyclizine, dimenhydrinate, diphenhydramine, or an ergot medicine. Also tell your doctor and pharmacist if you are allergic to any other substances, such as foods, preservatives, or dyes.

Pregnancy—Use of dihydroergotamine or ergotamine by pregnant women may cause serious harm, including death of the fetus and miscarriage. Therefore, *these medicines should not be used during pregnancy*.

Breast-feeding—

- *For dihydroergotamine and ergotamine*: These medicines pass into the breast milk and may cause unwanted effects, such as vomiting, diarrhea, weak pulse, changes in blood pressure, or convulsions (seizures) in nursing babies. Large amounts of these medicines may also decrease the flow of breast milk.

- *For caffeine*: Caffeine passes into the breast milk. Large amounts of it may cause the baby to appear jittery or to have trouble in sleeping.

- *For belladonna alkaloids, cyclizine, dimenhydrinate, and diphenhydramine*: These medicines have drying effects. Therefore, it is possible that they may reduce the amount of breast milk in some people. Dimenhydrinate passes into the breast milk. Cylizine may also pass into the breast milk.

- *For pentobarbital*: Pentobarbital passes into the breast milk. Large amounts of it may cause unwanted effects such as drowsiness in nursing babies.

Be sure that you discuss these possible problems with your doctor before taking any of these medicines.

Children—

- *For dihydroergotamine and ergotamine*: These medicines are used to relieve severe, throbbing headaches in children 6 years of age or older. They have not been shown to cause different side effects or problems in children than they do in adults. However, these medicines can cause serious side effects in any patient.

Therefore, it is especially important that you discuss with the child's doctor the good that this medicine may do as well as the risks of using it.

- *For belladonna alkaloids*: Young children, especially children with spastic paralysis or brain damage, may be especially sensitive to the effects of belladonna alkaloids. This may increase the chance of side effects during treatment.

- *For cyclizine, dimenhydrinate, diphenhydramine, and pentobarbital*: Although these medicines often cause drowsiness, some children become excited after taking them.

Older adults—

- *For dihydroergotamine and ergotamine*: The chance of serious side effects caused by decreases in blood flow is increased in elderly people receiving these medicines.

- *For belladonna alkaloids, cyclizine, dimenhydrinate, diphenhydramine, and pentobarbital*: Elderly people are more sensitive than younger adults to the effects of these medicines. This may increase the chance of side effects such as excitement, depression, dizziness, drowsiness, and confusion.

Athletes—

- *For caffeine*: The caffeine in some ergotamine-containing combination medicines is tested for by the International Olympic Committee (IOC), the U.S. Olympic Committee (USOC), and the National Collegiate Athletic Association (NCAA). These groups have set specific limits on the amount of caffeine in the urine they consider to be acceptable. An athlete will be disqualified for competition if the amount of caffeine in the urine is above these limits.

- *For cyclizine, dimenhydrinate, diphenhydramine, and pentobarbital*: These medicines are banned by the USOC for use in competitors in biathlon and modern pentathlon. Use of any of these medicines can lead to disqualification of athletes in these events.

Other medicines—Although certain medicines should not be used together at all, in other cases two different medicines may be used together even if an interaction might occur. In these cases, your doctor may want to change the dose, or other precautions may be necessary. Many medicines can add to or decrease the effects of the belladonna alkaloids, caffeine, cyclizine, dimenhydrinate, diphenhydramine, or pentobarbital present in some of these headache medicines. Therefore, you should tell your doctor and pharmacist if you are taking *any* other prescription or nonprescription (over-the-counter [OTC]) medicine. This is especially important if any medicine you take causes excitement, trouble in sleeping, dryness of the mouth, dizziness, or drowsiness.

When you are taking dihydroergotamine or ergotamine, it is especially important that your doctor and pharmacist know if you are taking any of the following:

- Cocaine or
- Epinephrine by injection [e.g., Epi-Pen] or
- Other ergot medicines (ergoloid mesylates [e.g., Hydergine], ergonovine [e.g., Ergotrate], methylergonovine [e.g., Methergine], methysergide [e.g., Sansert])—The chance of serious side effects caused by dihydroergotamine or ergotamine may be increased

Other medical problems—The presence of other medical problems may affect the use of these headache medicines. Make sure you tell your doctor if you have any other medical problems, especially:

- Agoraphobia (fear of open or public places) or
- Panic attacks or
- Stomach ulcer or
- Trouble in sleeping (insomnia)—Caffeine can make your condition worse
- Diarrhea—Rectal dosage forms (suppositories) will not be effective if you have diarrhea
- Difficult urination or
- Enlarged prostate or
- Glaucoma (not well controlled) or
- Heart or blood vessel disease or
- High blood pressure (not well controlled) or
- Infection or
- Intestinal blockage or other intestinal problems or

- Itching (severe) or
- Kidney disease or
- Liver disease or
- Mental depression or
- Overactive thyroid or
- Urinary tract blockage—The chance of side effects may be increased

Also, tell your doctor if you need, or if you have recently had, an angioplasty (a procedure done to improve the flow of blood in a blocked blood vessel) or surgery on a blood vessel. The chance of serious side effects caused by dihydroergotamine or ergotamine may be increased.

Before you begin using any new medicine (prescription or nonprescription) or if you develop any new medical problem while you are using this medicine, check with your doctor, nurse, or pharmacist.

Proper Use of This Medicine

Use this medicine only as directed by your doctor. Do not use more of it, and do not use it more often, than directed. If the amount you are to use does not relieve your headache, check with your doctor. Taking too much dihydroergotamine or ergotamine, or taking it too often, may cause serious effects, especially in elderly patients. Also, if a headache medicine (especially ergotamine) is used too often for migraines, it may lose its effectiveness or even cause a type of physical dependence. If this occurs, your headaches may actually get worse.

This medicine works best if you:

- *Use it at the first sign of headache or migraine attack. If you get warning signals of a coming migraine, take it before the headache actually starts.*

- *Lie down in a quiet, dark room until you are feeling better.*

Your doctor may direct you to take another medicine to help prevent headaches. *It is important that you follow your doctor's directions, even if your headaches continue to occur.* Headache-preventing medicines may take several weeks to start working. Even after they do start working, your headaches may not go away completely. However, your headaches should occur less often, and they should be less severe and easier to relieve. This can reduce the amount of dihydroergotamine, ergotamine, or pain relievers that you need. If you do not notice any improvement after several weeks of headache-preventing treatment, check with your doctor.

For patients using *dihydroergotamine*:

- Dihydroergotamine is given only by injection. Your doctor or nurse will teach you how to inject yourself with the medicine. Be sure to follow the directions carefully. Check with your doctor or nurse if you have any problems using the medicine.

For patients using *ergotamine inhalation* [e.g., Medihaler Ergotamine]:

- This medicine comes with patient directions. Read them carefully before using the medicine, and check with your doctor or pharmacist if you have any questions.
- To use the inhaler—Remove the cap, then shake the container well. After breathing out, place the mouthpiece of the inhaler in your mouth. Aim it at the back of the throat. Breathe in; at the same time, press the vial down into the adapter. After inhaling the medicine, hold your breath as long as you can.

For patients using the *sublingual (under-the-tongue) tablets of ergotamine*:

- To use—Place the tablet under your tongue and let it remain there until it disappears. The sublingual tablet should not be chewed or swallowed, because it works faster when it is absorbed into the body through the lining of the mouth. Do not eat, drink, or smoke while the tablet is under your tongue.

For patients using *rectal suppository forms of a headache medicine*:

- If the suppository is too soft to use, chill it in the refrigerator for 30 minutes or run cold water over it before removing the foil wrapper.

- If you have been directed to use part of a suppository, you should divide the suppository into pieces that all contain the same amount of medicine. To do this, use a sharp knife and carefully cut the suppository lengthwise (from top to bottom) into pieces that are the same size. The suppository will be easier to cut if it has been kept in the refrigerator.

- To insert the suppository—First remove the foil wrapper and moisten the suppository with cold water. Lie down on your side and use your finger to push the suppository well up into the rectum.

Dosing—The dose of these headache medicines will be different for different patients. *Follow your doctor's orders or the directions on the label.* The following information includes only the average doses of these medicines. *If your dose is different, do not change it* unless your doctor tells you to do so.

For dihydroergotamine

- Adults: For relieving a migraine or cluster headache— 1 mg. If your headache is not better, and no side effects are occurring, a second 1-mg dose may be used at least one hour later.

- Children 6 years of age and older: For relieving a migraine headache—It is not likely that a child will be receiving dihydrogergotamine at home. If a child needs the medicine, the dose will have to be determined by the doctor.

For ergotamine

- Some headache medicines contain only ergotamine. Some of them contain other medicines along with the ergotamine. The number of tablets, capsules, or suppositories that you need for each dose depends on the amount of ergotamine in them. The size of each dose, and the number of doses that you take, also depends on the reason you are taking the medicine and on how you react to the medicine.

- For *oral* (capsule or tablet) and *sublingual* (under-the-tongue tablet) dosage forms:
  —Adults:
  - For relieving a migraine or cluster headache—1 or 2 mg of ergotamine. If your headache is not better, and no side effects are occurring, a second dose and even a third dose may be taken; however the doses should be taken at least 30 minutes apart. People who usually need more than one dose of the medicine, and who do not get side effects from it, may be able to take a larger first dose of not more than 3 mg of ergotamine. This may provide better relief of the headache with only one dose. *The medicine should not be taken more often 2 times a week, at least five days apart.*
  - For preventing cluster headaches—The dose of ergotamine, and the number of doses you need every day, will depend on how many headaches you usually get each day. For some people, 1 or 2 mg of ergotamine once a day may be enough. Other people may need to take 1 or 2 mg of ergotamine 2 or 3 times a day.
  - For all uses—*Do not take more than 6 mg of ergotamine a day in the form of capsules or tablets.*
  —Children 6 years of age and older: For relieving migraine headaches—1 mg of ergotamine. If the headache is not better, and no side effects are occurring, a second dose and even a third dose may be taken; however, the doses should be taken at least 30 minutes apart. *Children should not take more than 3 mg of ergotamine a day in the form of capsules or tablets. Also, this medicine should not be taken more often than 2 times a week, at least five days apart.*

- For *rectal suppository* dosage forms:
  —Adults: For relieving migraine or cluster headaches—Usually 1 mg of ergotamine, but the dose may range from half of this amount to up to 2 mg. If your headache is not better, and no side effects are occurring, a second dose and even a third dose may be used; however the doses should be taken at least 30 minutes

apart. People who usually need more than one dose of the medicine, and who do not get side effects from it, may be able to use a larger first dose of not more than 3 mg. This may provide better relief of the headache with only one dose. *Adults should not use more than 4 mg of ergotamine a day in suppository form. Also, this medicine should not be used more often than 2 times a week, at least five days apart.*

—Children 6 years of age and older: For relieving migraine headaches—One-half or 1 mg of ergotamine. *Children should not receive more than 1 mg a day of ergotamine in suppository form. Also, this medicine should not be used more often than 2 times a week, at least five days apart.*

- For the *oral inhalation* dosage form:

    —Adults: For relieving a migraine or cluster headache—1 spray (1 inhalation). Another inhalation may be used at least 5 minutes later, if needed. Up to a total of 6 inhalations a day may be used, at least 5 minutes apart. *This medicine should not be used more often than 2 times a week, at least five days apart.*

    —Children: To be determined by the doctor.

Storage—To store this medicine:

- Keep out of the reach of children since overdose is especially dangerous in children.
- Store away from heat and direct light.
- Do not store in the bathroom, near the kitchen sink, or in other damp places. Heat or moisture may cause the medicine to break down.
- Suppositories should be stored in a cool place, but not allowed to freeze. Some manufacturers recommend keeping them in a refrigerator; others do not. Follow the directions on the package. However, cutting the suppository into smaller pieces, if you need to do so, will be easier if the suppository is kept in the refrigerator.
- Do not puncture, break, or burn the ergotamine inhalation aerosol container, even after it is empty.

- Do not keep outdated medicine or medicine no longer needed. Be sure that any discarded medicine is out of the reach of children.

Precautions While Using This Medicine

Check with your doctor:

- If your migraine headaches are worse than they were before you started using this medicine, or your headache medicine stops working as well as it did when you first started using it. This may mean that you are in danger of becoming dependent on the headache medicine. *Do not try to get better relief by increasing the dose.*
- If your migraine headaches are occurring more often than they did before you started using this medicine. This is especially important if a new headache occurs within 1 day after you took your last dose of headache medicine, or if you are having headaches every day. This may mean that you are dependent on the headache medicine. *Continuing to take this medicine will cause even more headaches later on.* Your doctor can give you advice on how to relieve the headaches.

Drinking alcoholic beverages can make headaches worse or cause new headaches to occur. People who suffer from severe headaches should probably avoid alcoholic beverages, especially during a headache.

Smoking may increase some of the harmful effects of dihydroergotamine or ergotamine. It is best to avoid smoking for several hours after taking these medicines.

Dihydroergotamine and ergotamine may make you more sensitive to cold temperatures, especially if you have blood circulation problems. They tend to decrease blood flow in the skin, fingers, and toes. Dress warmly during cold weather and be careful during prolonged exposure to cold temperatures. This is especially important for older patients, who are more likely than younger adults to already have problems with their circulation.

If you have a serious infection or illness of any kind, check with your doctor before using this medicine, since you may be more sensitive to its effects.

For patients using *ergotamine inhalation* [e.g., Medihaler Ergotamine]:

- Cough, hoarseness, or throat irritation may occur. Gargling and rinsing your mouth after each dose may help prevent the hoarseness and irritation. However, check with your doctor if these or any other side effects continue or are bothersome.

For patients taking one of the combination medicines that contains *caffeine*:

- Caffeine may interfere with the results of a test that uses dipyridamole (e.g., Persantine) to help find out how well your blood is flowing through certain blood vessels. You should not have any caffeine for at least 12 hours before the test.
- Caffeine may also interfere with some other laboratory tests. Before having any other laboratory tests, tell the person in charge if you have taken a medicine that contains caffeine.

For patients taking one of the combination medicines that contains *belladonna alkaloids, cyclizine, dimenhydrinate, diphenhydramine, or pentobarbital*:

- These medicines may cause some people to have blurred vision or to become drowsy, dizzy, lightheaded, or less alert than they are normally. These effects may be especially severe if you also take CNS depressants (medicines that slow down the nervous system, possibly causing drowsiness) together with one of these combination medicines. Some examples of CNS depressants are antihistamines or medicine for hay fever, other allergies, or colds; sedatives, tranquilizers, or sleeping medicine; prescription pain medicine or narcotics; barbiturates; medicine for seizures; muscle relaxants; and antiemetics (medicines that prevent or relieve nausea or vomiting). If you are not able to lie down for a while, *make sure you know how you react to this medicine*

> *or combination of medicines before you drive, use machines, or do anything else that could be dangerous if you are dizzy or are not alert and able to see well.*

- Belladonna alkaloids, cyclizine, dimenhydrinate, and diphenhydramine may cause dryness of the mouth, nose, and throat. For temporary relief of mouth dryness, use sugarless candy or gum, melt bits of ice in your mouth, or use a saliva substitute.

- Belladonna alkaloids may interfere with certain laboratory tests that check the amount of acid in your stomach. They should not be taken for 24 hours before the test.

- Cyclizine, dimenhydrinate, and diphenhydramine may interfere with skin tests that show whether you are allergic to certain substances. They should not be taken for 3 days before the test.

Side Effects of This Medicine

Along with its needed effects, a medicine may cause some unwanted effects. Although not all of these side effects may occur, if they do occur they may need medical attention.

Check with your doctor immediately if the following side effects occur, because they may mean that you are developing a problem with blood circulation:

Less common or rare

Anxiety or confusion (severe); change in vision; chest pain; increase in blood pressure; pain in arms, legs, or lower back, especially if pain occurs in your calves or heels while you are walking; pale, bluish-colored, or cold hands or feet (not caused by cold temperatures and occurring together with other side effects listed in this section); red or violet-colored blisters on the skin of the hands or feet

Also check with your doctor immediately if any of the following side effects occur, because they may mean that you have taken an overdose of the medicine:

Less common or rare

Convulsions (seizures); diarrhea, nausea, vomiting, or stomach pain or bloating (severe) occurring together with other signs of overdose or of problems with blood circulation;

dizziness, drowsiness, or weakness (severe), occurring together with other signs of overdose or of problems with blood circulation; fast or slow heartbeat; diarrhea; headaches, more often and/or more severe than before; problems with moving bowels, occurring together with pain or discomfort in the rectum (with rectal suppositories only); shortness of breath; unusual excitement

The following side effects may go away after a little while. *Do not take any more medicine while they are present.* If any of them occur together with other signs of problems with blood circulation, *check with your doctor right away.* Even if any of the following side effects occur without other signs of problems with blood circulation, *check with your doctor if any of them continue for more than one hour:*

More common

Itching of skin; coldness, numbness, or tingling in fingers, toes, or face; weakness in legs

Also, check with your doctor as soon as possible if you notice any of the following side effects:

More common

Swelling of face, fingers, feet, or lower legs

Other side effects may occur that usually do not need medical attention. These side effects may go away after a little while. However, check with your doctor if any of the following side effects continue or are bothersome:

More common

Diarrhea, nausea, or vomiting (occurring without other signs of overdose or problems with blood circulation); dizziness or drowsiness (occurring without other signs of overdose or problems with blood circulation, especially with combinations containing cyclizine, dimenhydrinate, diphenhydramine, or pentobarbital); nervousness or restlessness; dryness of mouth (especially with combinations containing belladonna alkaloids, cyclizine, dimenhydrinate, or diphenhydramine)

After you stop taking this medicine, your body may need time to adjust. The length of time this takes depends on the amount of medicine you were taking and how long you took it. During this time check with your doctor if your headaches begin again or worsen.

Other side effects not listed above may also occur in some patients. If you notice any other effects, check with your doctor.

Additional Information

Once a medicine has been approved for marketing for a certain use, experience may show that it is also useful for other medical problems. Although this use is not specifically included in product labeling, dihydroergotamine is sometimes used together with another medicine (heparin) to help prevent blood clots that may occur after certain kinds of surgery. It is also used to prevent or treat low blood pressure in some patients.

For patients receiving this medicine for *preventing blood clots*:

- You may need to receive this medicine two or three times a day for several days in a row. This may increase the chance of problems caused by decreased blood flow. Your doctor or nurse will be following your progress, to make sure that this medicine is not causing problems with blood circulation.

For patients using this medicine to *prevent or treat low blood pressure*:

- Take this medicine every day as directed by your doctor.
- The dose of dihydroergotamine will depend on whether the medicine is going to be injected under the skin or into a muscle, and, sometimes, on the weight of the patient. For these reasons, the dose will have to be determined by your doctor.
- Your doctor will need to check your progress at regular visits, to make sure that the medicine is working properly without causing side effects.
- This medicine is less likely to cause problems with blood circulation in patients with low blood pressure than it is in patients with normal or high blood pressure.

- In patients being treated for low blood pressure, an increase in blood pressure is the wanted effect, not a side effect that may need medical attention.

Other than the above information, there is no additional information relating to proper use, precautions, or side effects for these uses.

HISTAMINE H₂-RECEPTOR ANTAGONISTS   Systemic

This information applies to the following medicines:

    Cimetidine (sye-MET-i-deen)
    Famotidine (fa-MOE-ti-deen)
    Nizatidine (ni-ZA-ti-deen)
    Ranitidine (ra-NIT-ti-deen)

Some commonly used brand names are:

For Cimetidine

In the U.S.

    Tagamet

In Canada

    Apo-Cimetidine   Peptol
    Novocimetine   Tagamet

For Famotidine

In the U.S.

    Pepcid
    Pepcid I.V.

In Canada

    Pepcid
    Pepcid I.V.

For Nizatidine

In the U.S.

    Axid

In Canada

    Axid

For Ranitidine

In the U.S.

    Zantac

In Canada

    Apo-Ranitidine   Zantac-C
    Zantac

Description

Histamine H$_2$-receptor antagonists, also known as H$_2$-blockers, are used to treat duodenal ulcers and prevent their return. They are also used to treat gastric ulcers and in some conditions, such as Zollinger-Ellison disease, in which the stomach produces too much acid. H$_2$-blockers may also be used for other conditions as determined by your doctor.

H$_2$-blockers work by decreasing the amount of acid produced by the stomach.

They are available only with your doctor's prescription, in the following dosage forms:

Oral
Cimetidine
- Oral solution (U.S. and Canada)
- Tablets (U.S. and Canada)
Famotidine
- Oral suspension (U.S.)
- Tablets (U.S. and Canada)
Nizatidine
- Capsules (U.S. and Canada)
Ranitidine
- Capsules (Canada)
- Syrup (U.S. and Canada)
- Tablets (U.S. and Canada)

Parenteral
Cimetidine
- Injection (U.S. and Canada)
Famotidine
- Injection (U.S. and Canada)
Ranitidine
- Injection (U.S. and Canada)

It is very important that you read and understand the following information. If any of it causes you special concern, check with your doctor. Also, *if you have any questions* or if you want more information about this medicine or your medical problem, *ask your doctor, nurse, or pharmacist.*

Before Using This Medicine

In deciding to use a medicine, the risks of taking the medicine must be weighed against the good it will do. This is a decision you and your doctor will make. For H$_2$-blockers, the following should be considered:

Allergies—Tell your doctor if you have ever had any unusual or allergic reaction to cimetidine, famotidine, nizatidine, or ranitidine.

Pregnancy—H$_2$-blockers have not been studied in pregnant women. In animal studies, famotidine and ranitidine have not been shown to cause birth defects or other problems. However, one study in rats suggested that cimetidine may affect male sexual development. More studies are needed to confirm this. Also, studies in rabbits with very high doses have shown that nizatidine causes miscarriages and low birth weights. Make sure your doctor knows if you are pregnant or if you may become pregnant before taking H$_2$-blockers.

Breast-feeding—Cimetidine, famotidine, nizatidine, and ranitidine pass into the breast milk and may cause unwanted effects, such as decreased amount of stomach acid and increased excitement, in the nursing baby. It may be necessary for you to take another medicine or to stop breast-feeding during treatment. Be sure you have discussed the risks and benefits of the medicine with your doctor.

Children—This medicine has been tested in children and, in effective doses, has not been shown to cause different side effects or problems than it does in adults when used for short periods of time.

Older adults—Confusion and dizziness may be especially likely to occur in elderly patients, who are usually more sensitive than younger adults to the effects of H$_2$-blockers.

Other medicines—Although certain medicines should not be used together at all, in other cases two different medicines may be used together even if an interaction might occur. In these cases, your doctor may want to change the dose, or other precautions may be necessary. When you are taking or receiving H$_2$-blockers it is especially important that your doctor and pharmacist know if you are taking any of the following:

- Aminophylline (e.g., Somophyllin) or
- Anticoagulants (blood thinners) or
- Caffeine (e.g., NoDoz) or
- Metoprolol (e.g., Lopressor) or
- Oxtriphylline (e.g., Choledyl) or
- Phenytoin (e.g., Dilantin) or
- Propranolol (e.g., Inderal) or
- Theophylline (e.g., Somophyllin-T) or
- Tricyclic antidepressants (amitriptyline [e.g., Elavil], amoxapine [e.g., Asendin], clomipramine [e.g., Anafranil], desipramine [e.g., Pertofrane], doxepin [e.g., Sinequan], imipramine [e.g., Tofranil], nortriptyline [e.g., Aventyl], protriptyline [e.g., Vivactil], trimipramine [e.g., Surmontil])—Use of these medicines with cimetidine has been shown to increase the effects of cimetidine. This is less of a problem with ranitidine and has not been reported for famotidine or nizatidine. However, all of the H$_2$-blockers are similar, so drug interactions may occur with any of them
- Ketoconazole—H$_2$-blockers may decrease the effects of ketoconazole; H$_2$-blockers should be taken at least 2 hours after ketoconazole

Other medical problems—The presence of other medical problems may affect the use of H$_2$-blockers. Make sure you tell your doctor if you have any other medical problems, especially:

- Kidney disease or
- Liver disease—The H$_2$-blocker may build up in the bloodstream, which may increase the risk of side effects

Before you begin using any new medicine (prescription or nonprescription) or if you develop any new medical problem while you are using this medicine, check with your doctor, nurse, or pharmacist.

Proper Use of This Medicine

For patients taking:

- One dose a day—Take it at bedtime, unless otherwise directed.
- Two doses a day—Take one in the morning and one at bedtime.

- Several doses a day—Take them with meals and at bedtime for best results.

It may take several days before this medicine begins to relieve stomach pain. To help relieve this pain, antacids may be taken with the H$_2$-blocker, unless your doctor has told you not to use them. However, you should wait one-half to one hour between taking the antacid and the H$_2$-blocker.

Take this medicine for the full time of treatment, even if you begin to feel better. Also, it is important that you keep your appointments with your doctor for check-ups so that your doctor will be better able to tell you when to stop taking this medicine.

Missed dose—If you miss a dose of this medicine, take it as soon as possible. However, if it is almost time for your next dose, skip the missed dose and go back to your regular dosing schedule. Do not double doses.

Storage—To store this medicine:
- Keep out of the reach of children.
- Store away from heat and direct light.
- Do not store the tablet form of this medicine in the bathroom, near the kitchen sink, or in other damp places. Heat or moisture may cause the medicine to break down.
- Keep the liquid form of this medicine from freezing.
- Do not keep outdated medicine or medicine no longer needed. Be sure that any discarded medicine is out of the reach of children.

Precautions While Using This Medicine

Some tests may be affected by this medicine. Tell the doctor in charge that you are taking this medicine before:
- You have any skin tests for allergies.
- You have any tests to determine how much acid your stomach produces.

Remember that certain medicines, such as aspirin, and certain foods and drinks (e.g., citrus products, carbonated drinks, etc.) irritate the stomach and may make your problem worse.

Cigarette smoking tends to decrease the effect of H$_2$-blockers by increasing the amount of acid produced by the stomach. This is more likely to affect the stomach's nighttime production of acid. While taking H$_2$-blockers, stop smoking completely, or at least do not smoke after taking the last dose of the day.

Drinking alcoholic beverages while taking cimetidine or ranitidine has been reported to increase the effects of alcohol. Therefore, you should not drink alcoholic beverages while you are taking cimetidine or ranitidine.

Check with your doctor if your ulcer pain continues or gets worse.

Side Effects of This Medicine

Along with its needed effects, a medicine may cause some unwanted effects. Although not all of these side effects may occur, if they do occur they may need medical attention.

Check with your doctor as soon as possible if any of the following side effects occur:

Rare

> Burning, itching, redness, skin rash; confusion; fast, pounding, or irregular heartbeat; fever; slow heartbeat; sore throat and fever; swelling; tightness in chest; unusual bleeding or bruising; unusual tiredness or weakness

Other side effects may occur that usually do not need medical attention. These side effects may go away during treatment as your body adjusts to the medicine. However, check with your doctor if any of the following side effects continue or are bothersome:

Less common or rare

> Blurred vision; constipation; decreased sexual ability (especially in patients with Zollinger-Ellison disease who have received high doses of cimetidine for at least 1 year); decrease in sexual desire; diarrhea; dizziness; drowsiness; dryness of mouth or skin; headache; increased sweating; joint or muscle pain; loss of appetite; loss of hair (temporary); nausea or vomiting; ringing or buzzing in ears; skin rash; swelling of breasts or breast soreness in females and males

Not all of the side effects listed above have been reported for each of these medicines, but they have been reported for at least one of them. All of the H$_2$-blockers are similar, so any of the above side effects may occur with any of these medicines.

Other side effects not listed above may also occur in some patients. If you notice any other effects, check with your doctor.

Additional Information

Once a medicine has been approved for marketing for a certain use, experience may show that it is also useful for other medical problems. Although these uses are not included in product labeling, H$_2$-blockers are used in certain patients with the following medical conditions:

- Damage to the stomach and/or intestines due to stress or trauma
- Hives
- Pancreatic problems
- Stomach or intestinal ulcers (sores) resulting from damage caused by medication used to treat rheumatoid arthritis

Other than the above information, there is no additional information relating to proper use, precautions, or side effects for these uses.

HMG-CoA REDUCTASE INHIBITORS   Systemic

This information applies to the following medicines:

    Lovastatin (LOE-va-sta-tin)
    Pravastatin (PRA-va-stat-in)
    Simvastatin (SIM-va-stat-in)

Some commonly used brand names are:

For Lovastatin
    In the U.S.
        Mevacor
    In Canada
        Mevacor

    Another commonly used name is mevinolin.

For Pravastatin
> *In the U.S.*
>> Pravachol
>
> *In Canada*
>> Pravachol

Another commonly used name is eptastatin.

For Simvastatin
> *In the U.S.*
>> Zocor
>
> *In Canada*
>> Zocor

Other commonly used names are epistatin and synvinolin.

Description

Lovastatin, pravastatin, and simvastatin are used to lower levels of cholesterol and other fats in the blood. This may help prevent medical problems caused by cholesterol clogging the blood vessels.

These medicines belong to the group of medicines called 3-hydroxy-3-methylglutaryl coenzyme A (HMG-CoA) reductase inhibitors. They work by blocking an enzyme that is needed by the body to make cholesterol. Thus, less cholesterol is made.

HMG CoA reductase inhibitors are available only with your doctor's prescription, in the following dosage form:

> *Oral*
>> Lovastatin
>> • Tablets (U.S. and Canada)
>> Pravastatin
>> • Tablets (U.S. and Canada)
>> Simvastatin
>> • Tablets (U.S and Canada)

It is very important that you read and understand the following information. If any of it causes you special concern, check with your doctor. Also, *if you have any questions* or if you want more information about this medicine or your medical problem, *ask your doctor, nurse, or pharmacist.*

Before Using This Medicine

In deciding to use a medicine, the risks of taking the medicine must be weighed against the good it will do. This is a decision you and your doctor will make. For HMG-CoA reductase inhibitors, the following should be considered:

Allergies—Tell your doctor if you have ever had any unusual or allergic reaction to HMG-CoA reductase inhibitors. Also tell your doctor and pharmacist if you are allergic to any other substances, such as foods, preservatives, or dyes.

Diet—Before prescribing medicines to lower your cholesterol, your doctor will probably try to control your condition by prescribing a personal diet for you. Such a diet may be low in fats, sugars, and/or cholesterol. Many people are able to control their condition by carefully following their doctor's orders for proper diet and exercise. *Medicine is prescribed only when additional help is needed* and is effective only when a schedule of diet and exercise is properly followed.

Also, this medicine is less effective if you are greatly overweight. It may be very important for you to go on a reducing diet. However, check with your doctor before going on any diet.

Pregnancy—Use of an HMG-CoA reductase inhibitor is not recommended during pregnancy or in a woman who plans to become pregnant in the near future. These medicines block formation of cholesterol, which is necessary for the fetus to develop properly. In addition, lovastatin has been shown to cause birth defects in animals given very high doses. Be sure you have discussed this with your doctor.

Breast-feeding—These medicines are not recommended for use during breast-feeding because they may cause unwanted effects in nursing babies.

Children—There is no specific information comparing the use of HMG-CoA reductase inhibitors in children with use in other age groups. However, use is not recommended in children under 2 years of age since cholesterol is needed for normal development.

Older adults—Many medicines have not been studied specifically in older people. Therefore, it may not be known whether they work exactly the same way they do in younger adults or if they cause different side effects or problems in older people. There is no specific information comparing the use of HMG-CoA reductase inhibitors in the elderly with use in other age groups.

Other medicines—Although certain medicines should not be used together at all, in other cases two different medicines may be used together even if an interaction might occur. In these cases, your doctor may want to change the dose, or other precautions may be necessary. When you are taking HMG-CoA reductase inhibitors, it is especially important that your doctor and pharmacist know if you are taking any of the following:

- Cyclosporine (e.g., Sandimmune) or
- Gemfibrozil (e.g., Lopid) or
- Niacin—Use of these medicines with an HMG-CoA reductase inhibitor may increase the risk of developing muscle problems and kidney failure

Other medical problems—The presence of other medical problems may affect the use of HMG-CoA reductase inhibitors. Make sure you tell your doctor if you have any other medical problems, especially:

- Alcohol abuse (or history of) or
- Liver disease—Use of this medicine may make liver problems worse
- Convulsions (seizures) or
- Infection (severe) or
- Injury (severe) or
- Low blood pressure or
- Organ transplant with immunosuppressant therapy or major surgery—Increased risk of developing problems that may lead to kidney failure

Before you begin using any new medicine (prescription or nonprescription) or if you develop any new medical problem while you are using this medicine, check with your doctor, nurse, or pharmacist.

Proper Use of This Medicine

Use this medicine only as directed by your doctor. Do not use more or less of it, and do not use it more often or for a longer time than your doctor ordered.

Remember that this medicine will not cure your condition but it does help control it. Therefore, you must continue to take it as directed if you expect to keep your cholesterol levels down.

Follow carefully the special diet your doctor gave you. This is the most important part of controlling your condition, and is necessary if the medicine is to work properly.

For patients taking *lovastatin:*
- This medicine works better when it is taken with food. If you are taking this medicine once a day, take it with the evening meal. If you are taking more than one dose a day, take with meals or snacks.

Missed dose—If you miss a dose of this medicine, take it as soon as possible. However, if it is almost time for your next dose, skip the missed dose and go back to your regular dosing schedule. Do not double doses.

Storage—To store this medicine:
- Keep out of the reach of children.
- Store away from heat and direct light.
- Do not store in the bathroom, near the kitchen sink, or in other damp places. Heat or moisture may cause the medicine to break down.
- Keep the medicine from freezing. Do not refrigerate.
- Do not keep outdated medicine or medicine no longer needed. Be sure that any discarded medicine is out of the reach of children.

Precautions While Using This Medicine

It is very important that your doctor check your progress at regular visits. This will allow your doctor to see if the medicine is working properly to lower your cholesterol levels and that it does not cause unwanted effects.

Do not stop taking this medicine without first checking with your doctor. When you stop taking this medicine, your blood cholesterol levels may increase again. Your doctor may want you to follow a special diet to help prevent this from happening.

Before having any kind of surgery (including dental surgery) or emergency treatment, tell the medical doctor or dentist in charge that you are taking this medicine.

Side Effects of This Medicine

Along with its needed effects, a medicine may cause some unwanted effects. Although not all of these side effects may occur, if they do occur they may need medical attention.

Check with your doctor as soon as possible if any of the following side effects occur:

> *Less common*
>> *For lovastatin, pravastatin, and simvastatin*
>>> Fever; muscle aches or cramps; unusual tiredness or weakness
>>
>> *For lovastatin and pravastatin only (in addition to those listed above)*
>>> Blurred vision

Other side effects may occur that usually do not need medical attention. These side effects may go away during treatment as your body adjusts to the medicine. However, check with your doctor if any of the following side effects continue or are bothersome:

> *Less common*
>> *For lovastatin, pravastatin, and simvastatin*
>>> Constipation; diarrhea; dizziness; gas; heartburn; headache; nausea; skin rash; stomach pain
>>
>> *For lovastatin only (in addition to those listed above)*
>>> Decreased sexual ability; trouble in sleeping

Other side effects not listed above may also occur in some patients. If you notice any other effects, check with your doctor.

HYDRALAZINE   Systemic

Some commonly used brand names are:

In the U.S.
   Apresoline
   Generic name product may also be available.

In Canada
   Apresoline
   Novo-Hylazin

Description

Hydralazine (hye-DRAL-a-zeen) belongs to the general class of medicines called antihypertensives. It is used to treat high blood pressure (hypertension).

High blood pressure adds to the workload of the heart and arteries. If it continues for a long time, the heart and arteries may not function properly. This can damage the blood vessels of the brain, heart, and kidneys, resulting in a stroke, heart failure, or kidney failure. High blood pressure may also increase the risk of heart attacks. These problems may be less likely to occur if blood pressure is controlled.

Hydralazine works by relaxing blood vessels and increasing the supply of blood and oxygen to the heart while reducing its work load.

Hydralazine may also be used for other conditions as determined by your doctor.

Hydralazine is available only with your doctor's prescription, in the following dosage forms:

Oral
   • Tablets (U.S. and Canada)
Parenteral
   • Injection (U.S. and Canada)

It is very important that you read and understand the following information. If any of it causes you special concern, check with your doctor. Also, *if you have any questions* or if you want more information about this medicine or your medical problem, *ask your doctor, nurse, or pharmacist.*

Before Using This Medicine

In deciding to use a medicine, the risks of taking the medicine must be weighed against the good it will do. This is a decision you and your doctor will make. For hydralazine, the following should be considered:

Allergies—Tell your doctor if you have ever had any unusual or allergic reaction to hydralazine. Also tell your doctor and pharmacist if you are allergic to any other substance, such as foods, preservatives, or dyes.

Pregnancy—Hydralazine has not been studied in pregnant women. However, blood problems have been reported in infants of mothers who took hydralazine during pregnancy. In addition, studies in mice have shown that hydralazine causes birth defects (cleft palate, defects in head and face bones). These birth defects may also occur in rabbits, but do not occur in rats. Before taking this medicine, make sure your doctor knows if you are pregnant or if you may become pregnant.

Breast-feeding—It is not known whether hydralazine passes into breast milk.

Children—Although there is no specific information comparing use of hydralazine in children with use in other age groups, this medicine is not expected to cause different side effects or problems in children than it does in adults.

Older adults—Many medicines have not been studied specifically in older people. Therefore, it may not be known whether they work exactly the same way they do in younger adults. Although there is no specific information comparing use of hydralazine in the elderly with use in other age groups, this medicine is not expected to cause different side effects or problems in older people than it does in younger adults. However, dizziness or lightheadedness may be more likely to occur in the elderly, who are more sensitive to the effects of hydralazine.

Other medicines—Although certain medicines should not be used together at all, in other cases two different medicines may be used together even if an interaction might occur. In these cases, your doctor may want to change the dose, or other precautions may be necessary. When you are taking hydralazine, it is especially important that your doctor and pharmacist know if you are taking the following:

- Diazoxide (e.g., Proglycem)—Effect on blood pressure may be increased

Other medical problems—The presence of other medical problems may affect the use of hydralazine. Make sure you tell your doctor if you have any other medical problems, especially:

- Heart or blood vessel disease or
- Stroke—Lowering blood pressure may make problems resulting from these conditions worse
- Kidney disease—Effects may be increased because of slower removal of hydralazine from the body

Before you begin using any new medicine (prescription or nonprescription) or if you develop any new medical problem while you are using this medicine, check with your doctor, nurse, or pharmacist.

Proper Use of This Medicine

For patients taking this medicine *for high blood pressure:*

- In addition to the use of the medicine your doctor has prescribed, treatment for your high blood pressure may include weight control and care in the types of foods you eat, especially foods high in sodium. Your doctor will tell you which of these are most important for you. You should check with your doctor before changing your diet.
- Many patients who have high blood pressure will not notice any signs of the problem. In fact, many may feel normal. It is very important that you *take your medicine exactly as directed* and that you keep your appointments with your doctor even if you feel well.
- Remember that hydralazine will not cure your high blood pressure but it does help control it. Therefore, you must continue to take it as directed if you expect to lower your blood pressure and keep it down. *You may have to take high blood pressure medicine for the*

rest of your life. If high blood pressure is not treated, it can cause serious problems such as heart failure, blood vessel disease, stroke, or kidney disease.

To help you remember to take your medicine, try to get into the habit of taking it at the same time each day.

Missed dose—If you miss a dose of this medicine, take it as soon as possible. However, if it is almost time for your next dose, skip the missed dose and go back to your regular dosing schedule. Do not double doses.

Storage—To store this medicine:

- Keep out of the reach of children.
- Store away from heat and direct light.
- Do not store in the bathroom, near the kitchen sink, or in other damp places. Heat or moisture may cause the medicine to break down.
- Do not keep outdated medicine or medicine no longer needed. Be sure that any discarded medicine is out of the reach of children.

Precautions While Using This Medicine

It is important that your doctor check your progress at regular visits to make sure that this medicine is working properly.

For patients taking this medicine *for high blood pressure:*

- *Do not take other medicines unless they have been discussed with your doctor.* This especially includes over-the-counter (nonprescription) medicines for appetite control, asthma, colds, cough, hay fever, or sinus, since they may tend to increase your blood pressure.

Hydralazine may cause some people to have headaches or to feel dizzy. *Make sure you know how you react to this medicine before you drive, use machines, or do anything else that could be dangerous if you are dizzy or are not alert.*

Side Effects of This Medicine

Along with its needed effects, a medicine may cause some
unwanted effects. Although not all of these side effects may
occur, if they do occur they may need medical attention.

In general, side effects with hydralazine are rare at lower
doses. However, check with your doctor as soon as possible
if any of the following occur:

Less common

> Blisters on skin; chest pain; general feeling of discomfort or
> illness or weakness; joint pain; numbness, tingling, pain,
> or weakness in hands or feet; skin rash or itching; sore
> throat and fever; swelling of feet or lower legs; swelling
> of the lymph glands

Other side effects may occur that usually do not need medical attention. These side effects may go away during treatment as your body adjusts to the medicine. However, check
with your doctor if any of the following side effects continue
or are bothersome:

More common

> Diarrhea; fast or irregular heartbeat; headache; loss of ap-
> petite; nausea or vomiting; pounding heartbeat

Less common

> Constipation; dizziness or lightheadedness; redness or flush-
> ing of face; shortness of breath; stuffy nose; watering or
> irritated eyes

Other side effects not listed above may also occur in some
patients. If you notice any other effects, check with your
doctor.

Additional Information

Once a medicine has been approved for marketing for a
certain use, experience may show that it is also useful for
other medical problems. Although this use is not specifically
included in product labeling, hydralazine is used in certain
patients with the following medical condition:

• Congestive heart failure

Other than the above information, there is no additional information relating to proper use, precautions, or side effects for this use.

INDAPAMIDE   Systemic

Some commonly used brand names are:
In the U.S.
   Lozol
In Canada
   Lozide

Description

Indapamide (in-DAP-a-mide) belongs to the group of medicines known as diuretics. It is commonly used to treat high blood pressure (hypertension).

High blood pressure adds to the workload of the heart and arteries. If it continues for a long time, the heart and arteries may not function properly. This can damage the blood vessels of the brain, heart, and kidneys resulting in a stroke, heart failure, or kidney failure. High blood pressure may also increase the risk of heart attacks. These problems may be less likely to occur if blood pressure is controlled.

Indapamide is also used to help reduce the amount of water in the body by increasing the flow of urine.

Indapamide is available only with your doctor's prescription, in the following dosage form:
   Oral
      • Tablets (U.S. and Canada)

It is very important that you read and understand the following information. If any of it causes you special concern, check with your doctor. Also, *if you have any questions* or if you want more information about this medicine or your medical problem, *ask your doctor, nurse, or pharmacist.*

Before Using This Medicine

In deciding to use a medicine, the risks of taking the medicine must be weighed against the good it will do. This is a decision you and your doctor will make. For indapamide, the following should be considered:

Allergies—Tell your doctor if you have ever had any unusual or allergic reaction to indapamide or other sulfonamide-type medicines. Also tell your doctor and pharmacist if you are allergic to any other substances, such as foods, preservatives, or dyes.

Pregnancy—Studies have not been done in pregnant women. However, indapamide has not been shown to cause birth defects or other problems in animal studies.

In general, diuretics are not useful for normal swelling of feet and hands that occurs during pregnancy. Diuretics should not be taken during pregnancy unless recommended by your doctor.

Breast-feeding—It is not known whether indapamide passes into breast milk. However, this medicine has not been reported to cause problems in nursing babies.

Children—Studies on this medicine have been done only in adult patients, and there is no specific information comparing use of indapamide in children with use in other age groups.

Older adults—Dizziness or lightheadedness and signs and symptoms of too much potassium loss are more likely to occur in the elderly, who are usually more sensitive than younger adults to the effects of indapamide.

Athletes—Diuretics are banned and tested for by the U.S. Olympic Committee (USOC) and the National Collegiate Athletic Association (NCAA). Diuretic use can lead to disqualification in all athletic events.

Other medicines—Although certain medicines should not be used together at all, in other cases two different medicines may be used together even if an interaction might occur. In these cases, your doctor may want to change the dose, or

other precautions may be necessary. When you are taking indapamide, it is especially important that your doctor and pharmacist know if you are taking any of the following:

- Digitalis glycosides (heart medicine)—Use with indapamide may increase the chance of side effects of digitalis glycosides
- Lithium (e.g., Lithane)—Use with indapamide may cause high blood levels of lithium, which may increase the chance of side effects

Other medical problems—The presence of other medical problems may affect the use of indapamide. Make sure you tell your doctor if you have any other medical problems, especially:

- Diabetes mellitus (sugar diabetes) or
- Gout (history of)—Indapamide may make these conditions worse
- Kidney disease—May prevent indapamide from working properly
- Liver disease—Higher blood levels of indapamide may occur, which may increase the chance of side effects

Before you begin using any new medicine (prescription or nonprescription) or if you develop any new medical problem while you are using this medicine, check with your doctor, nurse, or pharmacist.

Proper Use of This Medicine

Indapamide may cause you to have an unusual feeling of tiredness when you begin to take it. You may also notice an increase in the amount of urine or in your frequency of urination. After taking the medicine for a while, these effects should lessen. In general, to keep the increase in urine from affecting your sleep:

- If you are to take a single dose a day, take it in the morning after breakfast.
- If you are to take more than one dose a day, take the last dose no later than 6 p.m., unless otherwise directed by your doctor.

However, it is best to plan your dose or doses according to a schedule that will least affect your personal activities and sleep. Ask your doctor, nurse, or pharmacist to help you plan the best time to take this medicine.

To help you remember to take indapamide, try to get into the habit of taking it at the same time each day.

For patients taking indapamide for *high blood pressure:*

- Importance of diet—When prescribing medicine for your condition your doctor may also prescribe a personal diet for you. Such a diet may be low in sodium (salt). Most people eat much more sodium than they need. Too much sodium in the diet may increase blood pressure. Some foods that contain large amounts of sodium are canned soup, pickles, ketchup, green and ripe olives, relish, frankfurters, soy sauce, and carbonated beverages. Your doctor may want you to limit the amounts of these and other high-sodium foods in your diet. High blood pressure medicine is usually more effective when such a diet is properly followed.

  Also, it may be very important for you to go on a reducing diet. However, check with your doctor before changing your diet.

- Many patients who have high blood pressure will not notice any signs of the problem. In fact, many may feel normal. It is very important that you *take your medicine exactly as directed* and that you keep your appointments with your doctor even if you feel well.

- Remember that this medicine will not cure your high blood pressure but it does help control it. Therefore, you must continue to take it as directed if you expect to lower your blood pressure and keep it down. *You may have to take high blood pressure medicine for the rest of your life.* If high blood pressure is not treated, it can cause serious problems such as heart failure, blood vessel disease, stroke, or kidney disease.

Missed dose—If you miss a dose of this medicine, take it as soon as possible. However, if it is almost time for your next dose, skip the missed dose and go back to your regular dosing schedule. Do not double doses.

Storage—To store this medicine:
- Keep out of the reach of children.
- Store away from heat and direct light.
- Do not store in the bathroom, near the kitchen sink, or in other damp places. Heat or moisture may cause the medicine to break down.
- Do not keep outdated medicine or medicine no longer needed. Be sure that any discarded medicine is out of the reach of children.

Precautions While Using This Medicine

It is important that your doctor check your progress at regular visits to make sure that indapamide is working properly.

This medicine may cause a loss of potassium from your body:
- To help prevent this, your doctor may want you to:
  —eat or drink foods that have a high potassium content (for example, orange or other citrus fruit juices), or
  —take a potassium supplement, or
  —take another medication to help prevent the loss of the potassium in the first place.
- It is very important to follow these directions. Also, it is important not to change your diet on your own. This is more important if you are already on a special diet (as for diabetes), or if you are taking a potassium supplement or a medicine to reduce potassium loss. Extra potassium may not be necessary and, in some cases, too much potassium could be harmful.

Check with your doctor if you become sick and have severe or continuing vomiting or diarrhea. These problems may cause you to lose additional water and potassium.

For patients taking this medicine for *high blood pressure:*
- *Do not take other medicines unless they have been discussed with your doctor.* This especially includes over-the-counter (nonprescription) medicines for ap-

petite control, asthma, colds, hay fever, or sinus problems, since they may tend to increase your blood pressure.

Side Effects of This Medicine

Along with its needed effects, a medicine may cause some unwanted effects. Although not all of these side effects may occur, if they do occur they may need medical attention.

Check with your doctor as soon as possible if any of the following side effects occur:

> Dryness of mouth; increased thirst; irregular heartbeat; mood or mental changes; muscle cramps or pain; nausea or vomiting; unusual tiredness or weakness; weak pulse

> *Rare*

> Skin rash, itching, or hives

Other side effects may occur that usually do not need medical attention. These side effects may go away during treatment as your body adjusts to the medicine. However, check with your doctor if any of the following side effects continue or are bothersome:

> *Less common or rare*

> Diarrhea; dizziness or lightheadedness, especially when getting up from a lying or sitting position; headache; loss of appetite; trouble in sleeping; upset stomach

Other side effects not listed above may also occur in some patients. If you notice any other effects, check with your doctor.

INSULIN   Systemic

This information applies to the following medicines:

> Insulin (IN-su-lin)
> Insulin Human
> Buffered Insulin Human
> Isophane (EYE-so-fayn) Insulin
> Isophane Insulin, Human
> Isophane Insulin and Insulin

Isophane Insulin, Human and Insulin Human
Insulin Zinc
Insulin Zinc, Human
Extended Insulin Zinc
Extended Insulin Zinc, Human
Prompt Insulin Zinc
Protamine (PRO-tah-meen) Zinc Insulin

Some commonly used brand names and other names are:	Generic names:
Regular (Concentrated) Iletin II, U-500 Regular Iletin I Regular Iletin II Regular insulin Regular Insulin Velosulin	Insulin
Humulin R Novolin R Velosulin Human	Insulin Human
Humulin BR	Buffered Insulin Human
Insulatard NPH NPH Iletin I NPH Iletin II NPH insulin NPH Insulin	Isophane Insulin
Humulin N Insulatard NPH Human Novolin N	Isophane Insulin, Human
Mixtard	Isophane Insulin and Insulin
Mixtard Human 70/30 Novolin 70/30	Isophane Insulin, Human and Insulin Human
Lente Iletin I Lente Iletin II Lente insulin Lente Insulin	Insulin Zinc
Humulin L Novolin L	Insulin Zinc, Human
Ultralente Iletin I Ultralente insulin Ultralente Insulin	Extended Insulin Zinc

Humulin U	Extended Insulin Zinc, Human
Semilente Iletin I	Prompt Insulin Zinc
Semilente insulin	
Semilente Insulin	
Protamine Zinc & Iletin I	Protamine Zinc Insulin
Protamine Zinc & Iletin II	
PZI insulin	

Description

Insulin (IN-su-lin) is a hormone that helps the body turn the food we eat into energy. This occurs whether we make our own insulin in the pancreas gland or take it by injection.

Diabetes mellitus (sugar diabetes) is a condition where the body does not make enough insulin to meet its needs or does not properly use the insulin it makes.

Insulin can be obtained from beef or pork pancreas glands or from new processes that produce human insulin. All types of insulin must be injected because, if taken by mouth, insulin is destroyed by chemical reactions in the stomach.

One or more injections of insulin a day may be needed to control your diabetes. Insulin is usually injected before meals or at bedtime. Your doctor will discuss the number of injections you will need, the kind of insulin to use, the correct dose, and the right time to take it.

A prescription is not necessary to purchase most insulin. However, your doctor must first determine your insulin needs and provide you with special instructions for control of your diabetes. Insulin is available in the following dosage forms:

Parenteral

Insulin
  • Injection
Insulin Human
  • Injection
Buffered Insulin Human
  • Injection

Isophane Insulin
  • Injection
Isophane Insulin, Human
  • Injection
Isophane Insulin, Human, and Insulin Human
  • Injection
Insulin Zinc
  • Injection
Insulin Zinc, Human
  • Injection
Extended Insulin Zinc
  • Injection
Extended Insulin Zinc, Human
  • Injection
Prompt Insulin Zinc
  • Injection
Protamine Zinc Insulin
  • Injection

It is very important that you read and understand the following information. If any of it causes you special concern, check with your doctor. Also, *if you have any questions* or if you want more information about this medicine or your medical problem, *ask your doctor, nurse, or pharmacist.*

Before Using This Medicine

In deciding to use a medicine, the risks of taking the medicine must be weighed against the good it will do. This is a decision you and your doctor will make. For insulin, the following should be considered:

Allergies—Tell your doctor if you have ever had any unusual or allergic reaction to insulin. Also tell your doctor and pharmacist if you are allergic to any other substances, such as foods, preservatives, or dyes.

Diet—If you have insulin-dependent diabetes (type I), your doctor will prescribe both insulin and a personalized meal plan for you. Such a diet is low in fat and simple sugars such as table sugar, and sweet foods and beverages. This meal plan is also high in complex carbohydrates (starchy foods) such as cereals, grains, bread, pasta or noodles, starchy vegetables, and dried beans, peas, or lentils. The daily number of calories in this meal plan should be adjusted by your doctor or a registered dietitian to help you reach and maintain a healthy body weight. In addition, meals and snacks are arranged to meet the energy needs of your body at different times of the day. *It is very important that you carefully follow your meal plan.*

Pregnancy—Your requirements for insulin change during pregnancy. Because it is especially important for the health of both you and the baby that your blood sugar be closely controlled, be sure to tell your doctor if you suspect you are pregnant or if you are planning to become pregnant.

Breast-feeding—Insulin does not pass into breast milk and will not affect the nursing infant.

Other medicines—Although certain medicines should not be used together at all, in other cases two different medicines may be used together even if an interaction might occur. In these cases, your doctor may want to change the dose, or other precautions may be necessary. When using insulin, it is especially important that your doctor and pharmacist know if you are taking any of the following:

- Adrenocorticoids (e.g., prednisone or other cortisone-like medicines)—Your dose of either medicine may need to be adjusted because the adrenocorticoids may interfere with insulin and thus increase your blood sugar
- Beta-blockers—Beta-blockers may increase the risk of developing either high or low blood sugar levels. Also, they can mask symptoms of low blood sugar (such as rapid pulse). Because of this, a person with diabetes might not recognize low blood sugar and might not take immediate steps to treat it. Beta-blockers can also cause a low blood sugar level to last longer than it would have normally

Other medical problems—The presence of other medical problems may affect the dose of insulin you need. Be sure to tell your doctor if you have any other medical problems, especially:

- Infections or
- Kidney disease or
- Liver disease or
- Thyroid disease—These conditions may change your daily insulin dose

Before you begin using any new medicine (prescription or nonprescription) or if you develop any new medical problem while you are using this medicine, check with your doctor, nurse, or pharmacist.

Proper Use of This Medicine

Make sure you have the type and strength of insulin that your doctor ordered for you. You may find that keeping an insulin label with you is helpful when buying insulin supplies. The concentration (strength) of insulin is measured by units, and is sometimes expressed in terms such as U-100 insulin.

Insulin doses are measured and given with specially marked insulin syringes. These syringes come in 3 sizes: 30 units, 50 units, and 100 units. Your insulin syringe will allow you to measure the units of insulin that have been prescribed for you, and allow you to easily read the measuring scale.

There are several important steps that will help you successfully prepare your insulin injection. To draw the insulin up into the syringe correctly, you need to follow these steps:

- Wash your hands.
- If your insulin is the intermediate- or long-acting kind (cloudy), be sure that it is completely mixed. Mix the insulin by slowly rolling the bottle between your hands or gently tipping the bottle over a few times.
- Never shake the bottle vigorously (hard).
- Do not use the insulin if it looks lumpy or grainy, seems unusually thick, sticks to the bottle, or seems to be even a little discolored. Do not use the insulin if it contains crystals or if the bottle looks frosted. Regular insulin (short-acting) should be used only if it is clear and colorless.
- Remove the colored protective cap on the bottle. Do *not* remove the rubber stopper.
- Wipe the top of the bottle with an alcohol swab.
- Remove the needle cover of the insulin syringe.
- Draw air into the syringe by pulling back on the plunger. The amount of air should be equal to your insulin dose.

- Gently push the needle through the top of the rubber stopper.
- Push plunger in all the way, to inject air into the bottle.
- Turn the bottle with syringe upside down in one hand. Be sure the tip of the needle is covered by the insulin. With your other hand, draw the plunger back slowly to draw the correct dose of insulin into the syringe.
- Check the insulin in the syringe for air bubbles. To remove air bubbles, push the insulin slowly back into the bottle and draw up your dose again.
- Check your dose again.
- Remove the needle from the bottle and re-cover the needle.

If you are mixing more than 1 type of insulin in the same syringe, you also need to know about the following:

- When mixing regular insulin with another type of insulin, *always* draw the regular insulin into the syringe first. When mixing 2 types of insulins other than regular insulin, it does not matter in what order you draw them.
- After you decide on a certain order for drawing up your insulin, you should use the same order each time.
- Some mixtures of insulins have to be injected immediately. Others may be stable for longer periods of time, which means that you can wait before you inject the mixture. Check with your doctor, nurse, or pharmacist to find out which type you have.
- If your mixture is stable and you mixed it ahead of time, gently turn the filled syringe back and forth to remix the insulins before you inject them. Do not shake the syringe.

After you have your syringe prepared, you are ready to inject the insulin into your body. To do this:

- Clean the site where the injection is to be made with an alcohol swab, and let the area dry.
- Inject the insulin into fatty tissue. Injection sites include your thighs, abdomen (stomach area), upper arms, or buttocks. Generally, insulin is absorbed into the bloodstream most evenly from the abdomen. If you are either

thin or greatly overweight, you may be given special instructions for giving yourself insulin injections.

- Pinch up a large area of skin and hold it firmly. With your other hand, hold the syringe like a pencil. Push the needle straight into the pinched-up skin at a 90-degree angle. Be sure the needle is all the way in. Drawing back on the syringe each time to check for blood (also called routine aspiration) is not necessary.

- Push the plunger all the way down, using less than 5 seconds to inject the dose. Hold an alcohol swab near the needle and pull the needle straight out of the skin.

- Press the swab against the injection site for several seconds. Do not rub.

For patients using *disposable syringes:*

- Manufacturers of disposable syringes recommend that they be used only once, because the sterility of a reused syringe cannot be guaranteed. However, some patients prefer to reuse a syringe until its needle becomes dull. Most insulins have chemicals added that keep them from growing the bacteria that are usually found on the skin. Because of this, some patients may decide to reuse a disposable syringe. However, the syringe should be thrown away when the needle becomes dull, has been bent, or has come into contact with any surface other than the cleaned and swabbed area of skin. Also, if you plan to reuse a syringe, the needle must be recapped after each use. Check with your doctor, nurse, or pharmacist to find out the best way to reuse syringes.

- Laws in some states require that used insulin syringes and needles be destroyed. Be careful when you recap, bend, or break a needle, because these actions increase the chances of a needle-stick injury. It is best to put used syringes and needles in a disposable container that is puncture-resistant or to use a needle-clipping device. The chances of a syringe being reused by someone else is lower if the plunger is taken out of the barrel and broken in half when you dispose of a syringe.

For patients using *a glass syringe and metal needle:*

- This type of syringe and needle may be used repeatedly if it is sterilized each time. You should get an instruction sheet that tells you how to do this. If you need more information on this, ask your doctor, nurse, or pharmacist.

For patients using *an insulin-infusion pump:*

- Regular insulin is the only insulin product that should be used with insulin infusion pumps.
- Do not use the insulin injection if it looks lumpy, cloudy, unusually thick, or even slightly discolored, or if it contains crystals. Use the insulin only if it is clear and colorless.
- Do not mix the buffered regular insulin injection with any other insulin. If you do, crystals may form that will block the pump catheter. Also, the potency of the insulin may change.
- It is important to follow the pump manufacturer's directions on how to load the syringe and/or pump reservoir. Your correct insulin dose may not be given if loading is not done correctly.
- Check the infusion tubing and infusion-site dressing often for improper insulin infusion, as your physician or nurse recommends.

Storage—Storage and expiration date:

- When buying insulin, always check the package expiration date to make sure the insulin will be used before it expires.
- This expiration date applies *only* when the insulin has been stored in the refrigerator. Expiration is much shorter if the insulin is left unrefrigerated. Do not use insulin after the expiration date stated on the label even if the bottle has never been opened. Check with your pharmacist about a possible exchange of bottles.
- An unopened bottle of insulin should be refrigerated until needed. It should never be frozen. Remove the insulin from the refrigerator and allow it to reach room temperature before injecting.

- An insulin bottle in use may be kept at room temperature for up to 1 month. Insulin that has been kept at room temperature for longer than a month should be thrown away.
- Do not expose insulin to extremely hot temperatures or to sunlight. Do not leave insulin in the hot summer sun or in a hot closed car. Extreme heat will cause insulin to become less effective much more quickly.

Precautions While Using This Medicine

It is very important that your doctor check your progress at regular visits, especially during the first few weeks of insulin treatment.

It is very important to follow carefully any instructions from your health care team about:

- Alcohol—Drinking alcohol may cause severe low blood sugar. Discuss this with your health care team.
- Tobacco—If you have been smoking for a long time and suddenly stop, your dosage of insulin may need to be reduced. If you decide to quit, tell your doctor first.
- Meal plan—To be successful in your treatment, you must closely follow the diet your doctor or dietitian prescribed for you. Do not miss or delay your meals.
- Exercise—Ask your doctor what kind of exercise to do, the best time to do it, and how much you should do daily.
- Blood tests—This is the best way to tell whether your diabetes is being controlled properly. Blood sugar testing is a useful guide to help you and your health care team adjust your insulin dose, meal plan, and exercise schedule.
- Urine ketone tests—You will also be asked at certain times to test for acetone, which is an acid that may be released from your bloodstream into your urine when your blood glucose is too high.
- Injection sites—If you carefully select and rotate the sites where you give your insulin injections, you may be able to prevent skin problems. Also, the insulin may be better absorbed into the bloodstream.

- Other medicines—Do not take other medicines unless they have been discussed with your doctor. This especially includes nonprescription medicines such as aspirin, and those for appetite control, asthma, colds, cough, hay fever, or sinus problems.

Insulin can cause low blood sugar (also called insulin reaction or hypoglycemia). Symptoms of low blood sugar are:

Anxious feeling
Cold sweats
Confusion
Cool pale skin
Difficulty in concentration
Drowsiness
Excessive hunger
Headache
Nausea
Nervousness
Rapid pulse
Shakiness
Unusual tiredness or weakness
Vision changes

- Different people may feel different symptoms of low blood sugar (hypoglycemia). It is important that you learn the symptoms of low blood sugar that you usually have so that you can treat it quickly.
- The symptoms of hypoglycemia (low blood sugar) may develop quickly and may result from:

    —delaying or missing a scheduled meal or snack.

    —exercising more than usual.

    —drinking a significant amount of alcohol.

    —taking certain medicines.

    —using too much insulin.

    —sickness (especially with vomiting or diarrhea).

- Eating some form of quick-acting sugar when symptoms of hypoglycemia first appear will usually prevent them from getting worse. Good sources of sugar include:

    Glucose tablets or gel that you can buy
    A restaurant sugar packet
    Fruit juice (4 to 6 ounces or one-half cup)
    Corn syrup (1 tablespoon)

    Honey (1 tablespoon)
    Regular (non-diet) soft drinks (4 to 6 ounces or one-half cup)
    Sugar cubes (6 one-half-inch sized) or table sugar (dissolved in water)

- Do not use chocolate because its fat slows down the sugar entering into the bloodstream.

- If a snack is not scheduled for an hour or more you should also eat some crackers and cheese, or a half a sandwich, or ice cream, or a peanut butter cookie, or drink an 8 ounce glass of milk.

- Symptoms of low blood sugar must be treated before they lead to unconsciousness (passing out). Glucagon is also used in emergency situations such as unconsciousness. Have a glucagon kit available, along with a syringe and needle, and know how to prepare and use it. Members of your household should know how and when to use it, also. Check the expiration date of the glucagon and remind yourself when to buy a new kit. If your kit has expired, ask your pharmacist to exchange it for a new one.

Hyperglycemia (high blood sugar) is another problem related to uncontrolled diabetes. If you have any symptoms of high blood sugar, you need to contact your health care team right away. If it is not treated, severe hyperglycemia can lead to ketoacidosis (diabetic coma) and death. The symptoms of hyperglycemia appear more slowly than those of low blood sugar and usually include:

    Increased urination
    Unusual thirst
    Dry mouth
    Drowsiness
    Flushed, dry skin
    Fruit-like breath odor
    Loss of appetite
    Stomach ache, nausea, or vomiting
    Tiredness
    Troubled breathing (rapid and deep)
    Increased blood sugar level

- Symptoms of ketoacidosis (diabetic coma) that need immediate hospitalization include:

  Flushed, dry skin
  Fruit-like breath odor
  Stomach ache, nausea, or vomiting
  Troubled breathing (rapid and deep)

- Hyperglycemia (high blood sugar) symptoms may occur if you:

  —have a fever, diarrhea, or infection.

  —do not take enough insulin.

  —skip a dose of insulin.

  —do not exercise as much as usual.

  —overeat or do not follow your meal plan.

- Your doctor may recommend changes in your insulin dose or meal plan to avoid hyperglycemia. Symptoms of high blood sugar must be corrected before they progress to more serious conditions. Check with your doctor often to make sure you are controlling your blood sugar.

In case of emergency—There may be a time when you need emergency help for a problem caused by your diabetes. You need to be prepared for these emergencies. It is a good idea to:

- Wear a medical identification (I.D.) bracelet or neck chain at all times. Also, carry an I.D. card in your wallet or purse that says that you have diabetes and lists all of your medicines.

- Keep an extra supply of insulin and syringes with needles on hand.

- Have a glucagon kit and a syringe and needle available and know how to prepare and use it if severe hypoglycemia (low blood sugar) occurs.

- Keep some kind of quick-acting sugar handy to treat hypoglycemia (low blood sugar) symptoms.

In case of illness:

- When you become ill with a cold, fever, or the flu, you need to take your usual insulin dose, even if you feel too sick to eat. This is especially true if you have nausea, vomiting, or diarrhea. Infection usually increases your need for insulin. Call your doctor for specific instructions.

- Continue taking your insulin and try to stay on your regular meal plan. However, if you have trouble eating solid food, drink fruit juices, non-diet soft drinks, or clear soups, or eat small amounts of bland foods. A dietitian or your doctor can give you a list of foods and the amounts to use for sick days.

- Test your blood sugar level at least every 4 hours while you are awake and check your urine for acetone. If acetone is present, call your doctor at once. If you have severe or prolonged vomiting, check with your doctor. Even when you start feeling better, let your doctor know how you are doing.

Travel—If you take a few special precautions when you travel, you are less likely to have problems related to your diabetes during trips away from home. It is a good idea to:

- Carry a recent prescription from your doctor for your diabetes medicine and also for the type of syringe and needles you use.

- Do not make major changes in your meal plan or medicine schedule without advice from your health care team.

- Carry your diabetic supplies on your person or in a purse or briefcase to reduce the possibility of loss.

- Carry snack foods with you in case of delays between meals.

- Make allowances for changing time zones and keep your meal times as close to usual as possible.

- In hot climates, use an insulated container for your insulin.

- When traveling to foreign countries, it is advisable to pack enough diabetic supplies to last until you return home and to have extra or reserve supplies kept separate from your main supplies.

- Carry a letter from your doctor with all the details of your diabetes and medicines you need, including your need for syringes.
- When carrying a large quantity of diabetic supplies, divide them throughout your hand-carried luggage to avoid problems if something is lost, and to avoid possible freezing in airplane storage areas.

ISOTRETINOIN Systemic

Some commonly used brand names are:
> In the U.S.
>> Accutane
> In Canada
>> Accutane Roche

Description

Isotretinoin (eye-soe-TRET-i-noyn) is used to treat severe, disfiguring cystic acne. It should be used only after other acne medicines have been tried and have failed to help the acne. Isotretinoin may also be used to treat other skin diseases as determined by your doctor.

Isotretinoin must not be used to treat women who are able to bear children unless other forms of treatment have been tried first and have failed. Isotretinoin must not be taken during pregnancy, because it causes birth defects in humans. If you are able to bear children, it is very important that you read, understand, and follow the pregnancy warnings for isotretinoin.

This medicine is available only with your doctor's prescription and should be prescribed only by a doctor who has special knowledge in the diagnosis and treatment of severe, uncontrollable cystic acne.

Isotretinoin is available in the following dosage form:
Oral
- Capsules (U.S. and Canada)

It is very important that you read and understand the following information. If any of it causes you special concern, check with your doctor. Also, *if you have any questions* or if you want more information about this medicine or your medical problem, *ask your doctor, nurse, or pharmacist.*

Before Using This Medicine

Isotretinoin comes with patient information. It is very important that you read and understand this information. Be sure to ask your doctor about anything you do not understand.

In deciding to use a medicine, the risks of taking the medicine must be weighed against the good it will do. This is a decision you and your doctor will make. For isotretinoin, the following should be considered:

Allergies—Tell your doctor if you have ever had any unusual or allergic reaction to isotretinoin, etretinate, tretinoin, or vitamin A preparations. Also tell your doctor and pharmacist if you are allergic to any other substances, such as foods, preservatives, or dyes.

Pregnancy—*Isotretinoin must not be taken during pregnancy, because it causes birth defects in humans. In addition, isotretinoin must not be taken if there is a chance that you may become pregnant during treatment or within one month following treatment.* Women who are able to have children must have a pregnancy blood test within 2 weeks before beginning treatment with isotretinoin to make sure they are not pregnant. Treatment with isotretinoin will then be started on the second or third day of the woman's next normal menstrual period. In addition, you must have a pregnancy blood test each month while you are taking this medicine and one month after treatment is completed. Also, *isotretinoin must not be taken unless an effective form of contraception (birth control) has been used for at least 1 month before the beginning of treatment. Contraception must* *be continued during the period of treatment, which is up to 20 weeks, and for 1 month after isotretinoin is stopped. Be sure you have discussed this information with your doctor. In addition, you will be asked to sign an informed consent form stating that you understand the above information.*

Breast-feeding—It is not known whether isotretinoin passes into the breast milk. However, isotretinoin is not recommended during breast-feeding, because it may cause unwanted effects in nursing babies.

Children—Children may be especially sensitive to the effects of isotretinoin. This may increase the chance of side effects during treatment.

Older adults—Many medicines have not been tested in older people. Therefore, it may not be known whether they work exactly the same way they do in younger adults or if they cause different side effects or problems in older people. There is no specific information about the use of isotretinoin in the elderly.

Other medicines—Although certain medicines should not be used together at all, in other cases two different medicines may be used together even if an interaction might occur. In these cases, your doctor may want to change the dose, or other precautions may be necessary. When you are using isotretinoin, it is especially important that your doctor and pharmacist know if you are using any of the following:
- Etretinate (e.g., Tegison) or
- Tretinoin (vitamin A acid) (e.g., Retin-A) or
- Vitamin A or any preparation containing vitamin A—Use of isotretinoin with these medicines will result in an increase in side effects
- Tetracyclines (medicine for infection)—Use of isotretinoin with these medicines may increase the chance of a side effect called pseudotumor cerebri, which is a swelling of the brain

Other medical problems—The presence of other medical problems may affect the use of isotretinoin. Make sure you tell your doctor if you have any other medical problems, especially:
- Alcoholism or excess use of alcohol (or history of) or
- Diabetes mellitus (sugar diabetes) (or a family history of) or

- Family history of high triglyceride (a fat-like substance) levels in the blood or
- Severe weight problems—Use of isotretinoin may increase blood levels of triglyceride (a fat-like substance), which may increase the chance of heart or blood vessel problems in patients who have a family history of high triglycerides, are greatly overweight, are diabetic, or use a lot of alcohol. For persons with diabetes mellitus, use of isotretinoin may also change blood sugar levels

Before you begin using any new medicine (prescription or nonprescription) or if you develop any new medical problem while you are using this medicine, check with your doctor, nurse, or pharmacist.

Proper Use of This Medicine

It is very important that you take isotretinoin only as directed. Do not take more of it, do not take it more often, and do not take it for a longer time than your doctor ordered. To do so may increase the chance of side effects.

Missed dose—If you miss a dose of this medicine, take it as soon as possible. However, if it is almost time for your next dose, skip the missed dose and go back to your regular dosing schedule. Do not double doses.

Storage—To store this medicine:
- Keep out of the reach of children.
- Store away from heat and direct light.
- Do not store in the bathroom, near the kitchen sink, or in other damp places. Heat or moisture may cause the medicine to break down.
- Do not keep outdated medicine or medicine no longer needed. Be sure that any discarded medicine is out of the reach of children.

Precautions While Using This Medicine

Your doctor should check your progress at regular visits to make sure this medicine does not cause unwanted effects.

Isotretinoin causes birth defects in humans if taken during pregnancy. Therefore, if you suspect that you may have become pregnant, stop taking this medicine immediately and check with your doctor.

Do not donate blood to a blood bank while you are taking isotretinoin or for 30 days after you stop taking it. This is to prevent the possibility of a pregnant patient receiving the blood.

Do not take vitamin A or any vitamin supplement containing vitamin A while taking this medicine, unless otherwise directed by your doctor. To do so may increase the chance of side effects.

Drinking too much alcohol while taking this medicine may cause high triglyceride (fat-like substance) levels in the blood and possibly increase the chance of unwanted effects on the heart and blood vessels. Therefore, *while taking this medicine, it is best that you do not drink alcoholic beverages or that you at least reduce the amount you usually drink.* If you have any questions about this, check with your doctor.

For diabetic patients:

• This medicine may affect blood sugar levels. If you notice a change in the results of your blood or urine sugar tests or if you have any questions, check with your doctor.

In some patients, isotretinoin may cause a decrease in night vision. This decrease may occur suddenly. If it does occur, *do not drive, use machines, or do anything else that could be dangerous if you are not able to see well.* Also, check with your doctor.

Isotretinoin may cause dryness of the eyes. Therefore, if you wear contact lenses, your eyes may be more sensitive to them during the time you are taking isotretinoin and for up to about 2 weeks after you stop taking it. To help relieve dryness of the eyes, check with your doctor about using an eye lubricating solution, such as artificial tears. If eye inflammation occurs, check with your doctor.

Some people who take this medicine may become more sensitive to sunlight than they are normally. When you first begin taking this medicine, avoid too much sun and do not use a sunlamp until you see how you react to the sun, especially if you tend to burn easily. If you have a severe reaction, check with your doctor.

Isotretinoin may cause dryness of the mouth and nose. For temporary relief of mouth dryness, use sugarless candy or gum, melt bits of ice in your mouth, or use a saliva substitute. However, if dry mouth continues for more than 2 weeks, check with your medical doctor or dentist. Continuing dryness of the mouth may increase the chance of dental disease, including tooth decay, gum disease, and fungus infections.

For patients taking isotretinoin for acne:
- When you begin taking isotretinoin, your acne may seem to get worse before it gets better. If irritation or other symptoms of your condition become severe, check with your doctor.

Side Effects of This Medicine

Along with its needed effects, a medicine may cause some unwanted effects. Although not all of these side effects may occur, if they do occur they may need medical attention.

Check with your doctor as soon as possible if any of the following side effects occur:

More common

Burning, redness, itching, or other sign of eye inflammation; nosebleeds; scaling, redness, burning, pain, or other sign of inflammation of lips

Less common

Mental depression; skin infection or rash

Rare

Abdominal or stomach pain (severe); bleeding or inflammation of gums; blurred vision or other changes in vision; diarrhea (severe); headache (severe or continuing); mood changes; nausea and vomiting; pain or tenderness of eyes; rectal bleeding; yellow eyes or skin

Other side effects may occur that usually do not need medical attention. These side effects may go away during treat-

ment as your body adjusts to the medicine. However, check
with your doctor if any of the following side effects continue
or are bothersome:

More common

Dryness of mouth or nose; dryness or itching of skin

Less common

Dryness of eyes; headache (mild); increased sensitivity of
skin to sunlight; pain, tenderness, or stiffness in muscles,
bones, or joints; peeling of skin on palms of hands or soles
of feet; stomach upset; thinning of hair; unusual tiredness

Other side effects not listed above may also occur in some
patients. If you notice any other effects, check with your
doctor.

KETOCONAZOLE Systemic

A commonly used brand name in the U.S. and Canada is Nizoral.

Description

Ketoconazole (kee-toe-KON-a-zole) is used to treat fungus
infections. It may be given alone or with other medicines
that are used on the skin for fungus infections. This medicine
may also be used for other problems as determined by your
doctor.

Ketoconazole is available only with your doctor's prescription, in the following dosage forms:

Oral

- Suspension (Canada)
- Tablets (U.S. and Canada)

*It is very important that you read and understand the fol-
lowing information.* If any of it causes you special concern,
check with your doctor. Also, *if you have any questions* or
if you want more information about this medicine or your
medical problem, *ask your doctor, nurse, or pharmacist.*

Before Using This Medicine

In deciding to use a medicine, the risks of taking the medicine must be weighed against the good it will do. This is a decision you and your doctor will make. For ketoconazole, the following should be considered:

Allergies—Tell your doctor if you have ever had any unusual or allergic reaction to ketoconazole, or other related medicines, such as fluconazole, miconazole, or itraconazole. Also tell your doctor and pharmacist if you are allergic to any other substances, such as foods, preservatives, or dyes.

Pregnancy—Studies have not been done in humans. However, studies in rats given doses 10 times the highest recommended human dose have shown that ketoconazole causes webbed toes or fewer toes than normal. When given in higher doses, ketoconazole may also cause other problems in the fetus. Ketoconazole has also been shown to cause difficult labor in rats given doses slightly higher than the highest recommended human dose.

Breast-feeding—Ketoconazole passes into the breast milk and may increase the chance of brain problems in nursing babies. Therefore, you should stop breast-feeding when you begin taking ketoconazole, during treatment, and for 24 to 48 hours after you have finished taking the medicine. During this time the breast milk should be squeezed out or sucked out with a breast pump and thrown away. After the 24 to 48 hours, you may go back to breast-feeding, as directed by your doctor.

Children—This medicine has been tested in a limited number of children 2 years of age and older. In effective doses, the medicine has not been shown to cause different side effects or problems in children than it does in adults.

Older adults—Many medicines have not been studied specifically in older people. Therefore, it may not be known whether they work exactly the same way they do in younger adults or if they cause different side effects or problems in older people. There is no specific information comparing use of ketoconazole in the elderly with use in other age groups.

Other medicines—Although certain medicines should not be used together at all, in other cases two different medicines may be used together even if an interaction might occur. In these cases, your doctor may want to change the dose, or other precautions may be necessary. When you are taking ketoconazole, it is especially important that your doctor and pharmacist know if you are taking any of the following:

- Acetaminophen (e.g., Tylenol) (with long-term, high-dose use) or
- Amiodarone (e.g., Cordarone) or
- Anabolic steroids (nandrolone [e.g., Anabolin], oxandrolone [e.g., Anavar], oxymetholone [e.g., Anadrol], stanozolol [e.g., Winstrol]) or
- Androgens (male hormones) or
- Antithyroid agents (medicine for overactive thyroid) or
- Carmustine (e.g., BiCNU) or
- Chloroquine (e.g., Aralen) or
- Dantrolene (e.g., Dantrium) or
- Daunorubicin (e.g., Cerubidine) or
- Disulfiram (e.g., Antabuse) or
- Divalproex (e.g., Depakote) or
- Estrogens (female hormones) or
- Etretinate (e.g., Tegison) or
- Gold salts (medicine for arthritis) or
- Hydroxychloroquine (e.g., Plaquenil) or
- Mercaptopurine (e.g., Purinethol) or
- Methotrexate (e.g., Mexate) or
- Methyldopa (e.g., Aldomet) or
- Naltrexone (e.g., Trexan) (with long-term, high-dose use) or
- Oral contraceptives (birth control pills) containing estrogen or
- Other anti-infectives by mouth or by injection (medicine for infection) or
- Phenothiazines (acetophenazine [e.g., Tindal], chlorproma-zine [e.g., Thorazine], fluphenazine [e.g., Prolixin], meso-ridazine [e.g., Serentil], perphenazine [e.g., Trilafon], pro-chlorperazine [e.g., Compazine], promazine [e.g., Sparine], promethazine [e.g., Phenergan], thioridazine [e.g., Mellaril], trifluoperazine [e.g., Stelazine], triflupromazine [e.g., Ves-prin], trimeprazine [e.g., Temaril]) or
- Phenytoin (e.g., Dilantin) or
- Plicamycin (e.g., Mithracin) or
- Valproic acid (e.g., Depakene)—Use of these medicines with ketoconazole may increase the chance of side effects af-fecting the liver

- Amantadine (e.g., Symmetrel) or
- Antacids or
- Anticholinergics (medicine for abdominal or stomach spasms or cramps) or
- Antidepressants (medicine for depression) or
- Antidyskinetics (medicine for Parkinson's disease or other conditions affecting control of muscles) or
- Antihistamines or
- Antipsychotics (medicine for mental illness) or
- Buclizine (e.g., Bucladin) or
- Cimetidine (e.g., Tagamet) or
- Cyclizine (e.g., Marezine) or
- Cyclobenzaprine (e.g., Flexeril) or
- Disopyramide (e.g., Norpace) or
- Famotidine (e.g., Pepcid) or
- Flavoxate (e.g., Urispas) or
- Ipratropium (e.g., Atrovent) or
- Meclizine (e.g., Antivert) or
- Methylphenidate (e.g., Ritalin) or
- Nizatidine (e.g., Axid) or
- Omeprazole (e.g., Prilosec) or
- Orphenadrine (e.g., Norflex) or
- Oxybutynin (e.g., Ditropan) or
- Procainamide (e.g., Pronestyl) or
- Promethazine (e.g., Phenergan) or
- Quinidine (e.g., Quinidex) or
- Ranitidine (e.g., Zantac) or
- Trimeprazine (e.g., Temaril)—Use of any of these medicines with ketoconazole may decrease the effects of ketoconazole
- Carbamazepine (e.g., Tegretol)—Use of carbamazepine with ketoconazole may decrease the effects of ketoconazole or increase side effects affecting the liver
- Cyclosporine (e.g., Sandimmune)—Use with ketoconazole may increase the chance of side effects of cyclosporine
- Dideoxyinosine (e.g., ddI, Videx)—Use of dideoxyinosine with ketoconazole may decrease the effects of ketoconazole
- Isoniazid or
- Rifampin—Use of isoniazid or rifampin with ketoconazole may decrease the effects of ketoconazole
- Terfenadine (e.g., Seldane)—Use of terfenadine with ketoconazole may increase the chance for heart problems, such as an irregular heartbeat

Other medical problems—The presence of other medical problems may affect the use of ketoconazole. Make sure you

tell your doctor if you have any other medical problems, especially:

- Achlorhydria (absence of stomach acid) or
- Hypochlorhydria (decreased amount of stomach acid)—Ketoconazole may not be absorbed from the stomach as well in patients who have low or no stomach acid
- Alcohol abuse (or history of) or
- Liver disease—Alcohol abuse or liver disease may increase the chance of side effects caused by ketoconazole

Before you begin using any new medicine (prescription or nonprescription) or if you develop any new medical problem while you are using this medicine, check with your doctor, nurse, or pharmacist.

Proper Use of This Medicine

This medicine may be taken with a meal or snack.

For patients taking the *oral liquid form of ketoconazole:*

- Use a specially marked measuring spoon or other device to measure each dose accurately. The average household teaspoon may not hold the right amount of liquid.

If you have achlorhydria (absence of stomach acid) or hypochlorhydria (decreased amount of stomach acid), your doctor may want you to dissolve each tablet in a teaspoonful of weak hydrochloric acid solution to help you absorb the medicine better. Your doctor or pharmacist can prepare the solution for you. After you dissolve the tablet in the acid solution, add this mixture to a small amount (1 or 2 teaspoonfuls) of water in a glass. Drink the mixture through a plastic or glass drinking straw. Place the straw behind your teeth, as far back in your mouth as you can. This will keep the acid from harming your teeth. Be sure to drink all the liquid to get the full dose of medicine. Then drink about ½ glass of water, swish it around in your mouth, and swallow it.

To help clear up your infection completely, *it is very important that you keep taking this medicine for the full time of treatment,* even if your symptoms begin to clear up or you begin to feel better after a few days. Since fungus infections may be very slow to clear up, you may have to continue taking this medicine every day for as long as 6 months to a year or more. Some fungus infections never clear up completely and require continuous treatment. If you stop taking this medicine too soon, your symptoms may return.

This medicine works best when there is a constant amount in the blood or urine. *To help keep the amount constant, do not miss any doses. Also, it is best to take each dose at the same time every day.* If you need help in planning the best time to take your medicine, check with your doctor, nurse, or pharmacist.

Missed dose—If you do miss a dose of this medicine, take it as soon as possible. This will help to keep a constant amount of medicine in the blood or urine. However, if it is almost time for your next dose, skip the missed dose and go back to your regular dosing schedule. Do not double doses.

Storage—To store this medicine:
- Keep out of the reach of children.
- Store away from heat and direct light.
- Do not store the tablet form of this medicine in the bathroom, near the kitchen sink, or in other damp places. Heat or moisture may cause the medicine to break down.
- Keep the oral liquid form of this medicine from freezing.
- Do not keep outdated medicine or medicine no longer needed. Be sure that any discarded medicine is out of the reach of children.

Precautions While Using This Medicine

It is important that your doctor check your progress at regular visits. This will allow your doctor to check for any unwanted effects.

If your symptoms do not improve within a few weeks, or if they become worse, check with your doctor.

If you are taking antacids, cimetidine (e.g., Tagamet), famotidine (e.g., Pepcid), nizatidine (e.g., Axid), ranitidine (e.g., Zantac), or omeprazole (e.g., Prilosec), while you are taking ketoconazole, take them at least 2 hours after you take ketoconazole. If you take these medicines at the same time that you take ketoconazole, they will keep ketoconazole from working properly.

Liver problems may be more likely to occur if you drink alcoholic beverages while you are taking this medicine. Alcoholic beverages may also cause stomach pain, nausea, vomiting, headache, or flushing or redness of the face. Other alcohol-containing preparations (for example, elixirs, cough syrups, tonics) may also cause problems. These problems may occur for at least a day after you stop taking ketoconazole. Therefore, *you should not drink alcoholic beverages while you are taking this medicine and for at least a day after you stop taking it.*

This medicine may cause your eyes to become more sensitive to light than they are normally. Wearing sunglasses and avoiding too much exposure to bright light may help lessen the discomfort.

This medicine may also cause some people to become dizzy, drowsy, or less alert than they are normally. *Make sure you know how you react to this medicine before you drive, use machines, or do anything else that could be dangerous if you are dizzy or are not alert.* If these reactions are especially bothersome, check with your doctor.

Side Effects of This Medicine

Along with its needed effects, a medicine may cause some unwanted effects. Although not all of these effects may occur, if they do occur they may need medical attention.

Check with your doctor immediately if any of the following side effects occur:

> *Rare*
>> Dark or amber urine; loss of appetite; pale stools; skin rash or itching; stomach pain; unusual tiredness or weakness; yellow eyes or skin

Other side effects may occur that usually do not need medical attention. These side effects may go away during treat-

ment as your body adjusts to the medicine. However, check with your doctor if any of the following side effects continue or are bothersome:

Less common
> Diarrhea; nausea or vomiting

Rare
> Decreased sexual ability in males; dizziness; drowsiness; enlargement of the breasts in males; headache; increased sensitivity of the eyes to light; irregular menstrual periods

Other side effects not listed above may also occur in some patients. If you notice any other effects, check with your doctor.

LEVODOPA   Systemic

This information applies to the following medicines:
> Carbidopa and Levodopa (KAR-bi-doe-pa and LEE-voe-doe-pa)
> Levodopa

Some commonly used brand names are:

For Carbidopa and Levodopa
In the U.S.
> Sinemet   Sinemet CR

In Canada
> Sinemet   Sinemet CR

For Levodopa
In the U.S.
> Dopar   Larodopa

In Canada
> Larodopa

Description

Levodopa is used alone or in combination with carbidopa to treat Parkinson's disease, sometimes referred to as shaking palsy or paralysis agitans. Some patients require the combination of medicine, while others benefit from levodopa alone. By improving muscle control, this medicine allows more normal movements of the body.

Levodopa alone or in combination is available only with your doctor's prescription. It is available in the following dosage forms:

> *Oral*
>> Carbidopa and Levodopa
>> • Tablets (U.S. and Canada)
>> • Extended-release tablets (U.S. and Canada)
>> Levodopa
>> • Capsules (U.S.)
>> • Tablets (U.S. and Canada)

It is very important that you read and understand the following information. If any of it causes you special concern, check with your doctor or pharmacist. Also, *if you have any questions* or if you want more information about this medicine or your medical problem, *ask your doctor, nurse, or pharmacist.*

Before Using This Medicine

In deciding to use a medicine, the risks of taking the medicine must be weighed against the good it will do. This is a decision you and your doctor will make. For levodopa and for carbidopa and levodopa combination, the following should be considered:

Allergies—Tell your doctor if you have ever had any unusual or allergic reaction to levodopa alone or in combination with carbidopa. Also tell your doctor and pharmacist if you are allergic to any other substances, such as foods, preservatives, or dyes.

Diet—Since protein may interfere with the body's response to levodopa, high protein diets should be avoided. Intake of normal amounts of protein should be spaced equally throughout the day.

For patients taking levodopa by itself:

• Pyridoxine (vitamin B_6) has been found to reduce the effects of levodopa when levodopa is taken by itself. This does not happen with the combination of carbidopa and levodopa. *If you are taking levodopa by itself, do not take vitamin products containing vitamin B_6 during treatment, unless prescribed by your doctor.*

- Large amounts of pyridoxine are also contained in some foods such as avocado, bacon, beans, beef liver, dry skim milk, oatmeal, peas, pork, sweet potato, tuna, and certain health foods. Check with your doctor about how much of these foods you may have in your diet while you are taking levodopa. Also, ask your doctor or pharmacist for help when selecting vitamin products.

Pregnancy—Studies have not been done in pregnant women. However, studies in animals have shown that levodopa affects the baby's growth both before and after birth if given during pregnancy in doses many times the human dose. Also, studies in rabbits have shown that levodopa, alone or in combination with carbidopa, causes birth defects.

Breast-feeding—Levodopa and carbidopa pass into the breast milk and may cause unwanted side effects in the nursing baby. Also, levodopa may reduce the flow of breast milk.

Children—Studies on this medicine have been done only in adult patients, and there is no specific information comparing use of levodopa or carbidopa in children with use in other age groups.

Older adults—Elderly people are especially sensitive to the effects of levodopa. This may increase the chance of side effects during treatment.

Other medicines—Although certain medicines should not be used together at all, in other cases 2 different medicines may be used together even if an interaction might occur. In these cases, your doctor may want to change the dose, or other precautions may be necessary. When you are taking levodopa or carbidopa and levodopa combination, it is especially important that your doctor and pharmacist know if you are taking any of the following:

- Cocaine—Cocaine use by individuals taking levodopa, alone or in combination with carbidopa, may cause an irregular heartbeat
- Ethotoin (e.g., Peganone) or
- Haloperidol (e.g., Haldol) or
- Mephenytoin (e.g., Mesantoin) or
- Phenothiazines (acetophenazine [e.g., Tindal], chlorpromazine [e.g., Thorazine], fluphenazine [e.g., Prolixin], meso-

ridazine [e.g., Serentil], perphenazine [e.g., Trilafon], prochlorperazine [e.g., Compazine], promazine [e.g., Sparine], promethazine [e.g., Phenergan], thioridazine [e.g., Mellaril], trifluoperazine [e.g., Stelazine], triflupromazine [e.g., Vesprin], trimeprazine [e.g., Temaril]) or

- Phenytoin (e.g., Dilantin)—Taking these medicines with levodopa may lessen the effects of levodopa
- Monoamine oxidase (MAO) inhibitors (furazolidone [e.g., Furoxone], isocarboxazid [e.g., Marplan], phenelzine [e.g., Nardil], procarbazine [e.g., Matulane], tranylcypromine [e.g., Parnate])—Taking levodopa while you are taking or within 2 weeks of taking monoamine oxidase (MAO) inhibitors may cause sudden extremely high blood pressure; at least 14 days should be allowed between stopping treatment with one medicine and starting treatment with the other medicine
- Pyridoxine (vitamin B_6, e.g., Hexa-Betalin), present in some foods and vitamin formulas (for levodopa used alone)—Pyridoxine reverses the effects of levodopa
- Selegiline—Dosage of levodopa or carbidopa and levodopa combination may need to be decreased

Other medical problems—The presence of other medical problems may affect the use of levodopa. Make sure you tell your doctor if you have any other medical problems, especially:

- Diabetes mellitus (sugar diabetes)—The amount of insulin or antidiabetic medicine that you need to take may change
- Emphysema, asthma, bronchitis, or other chronic lung disease or
- Glaucoma or
- Heart or blood vessel disease or
- Hormone problems or
- Melanoma (a type of skin cancer) (or history of) or
- Mental illness—Levodopa may make the condition worse
- Kidney disease or
- Liver disease—Higher blood levels of levodopa may occur, increasing the chance of side effects
- Seizure disorders, such as epilepsy (history of)—The risk of seizures may be increased
- Stomach ulcer (history of)—The ulcer may occur again

Before you begin using any new medicine (prescription or nonprescription) or if you develop any new medical problem while you are using this medicine, check with your doctor, nurse, or pharmacist.

Proper Use of This Medicine

It is best not to take this medicine with or after food, especially high-protein food, since food may decrease levodopa's effect. However, *to lessen possible stomach upset, your doctor may want you to take food shortly after taking this medicine (about 15 minutes after).* If stomach upset is severe or continues, check with your doctor.

Take this medicine only as directed. Do not take more or less of it, and do not take it more often than your doctor ordered.

For patients taking *carbidopa and levodopa extended-release tablets*:

- Swallow the tablet whole without crushing or chewing, unless your doctor tells you not to. If your doctor tells you to, you may break the tablet in half.

Some people must take this medicine for several weeks or months before full benefit is received. *Do not stop taking it even if you do not think it is working.* Instead, check with your doctor.

Missed dose—If you miss a dose of this medicine, take it as soon as possible. However, if your next scheduled dose is within 2 hours, skip the missed dose and go back to your regular dosing schedule. Do not double doses.

Storage—To store this medicine:

- Keep out of the reach of children.
- Store away from heat and direct light.
- Do not store in the bathroom, near the kitchen sink, or in other damp places. Heat or moisture may cause the medicine to break down.
- Do not keep outdated medicine or medicine no longer needed. Be sure that any discarded medicine is out of the reach of children.

Precautions While Using This Medicine

Before having any kind of surgery (including dental surgery) or emergency treatment, tell the medical doctor or dentist in charge that you are taking this medicine.

For *diabetic patients*:

- This medicine may cause test results for urine sugar or ketones to be wrong. Check with your doctor before depending on home tests using the paper-strip or tablet method.

This medicine may cause some people to become drowsy or less alert than they are normally. *Make sure you know how you react to this medicine before you drive, use machines, or do anything else that could be dangerous if you are not alert.*

Dizziness, lightheadedness, or fainting may occur, especially when you get up from a lying or sitting position. Getting up slowly may help. If the problem continues or gets worse, check with your doctor.

For patients taking levodopa by itself:

- Pyridoxine (vitamin B$_6$) has been found to reduce the effects of levodopa when levodopa is taken by itself. This does not happen with the combination of carbidopa and levodopa. *If you are taking levodopa by itself, do not take vitamin products containing vitamin B$_6$ during treatment, unless prescribed by your doctor.*
- Large amounts of pyridoxine are also contained in some foods such as avocado, bacon, beans, beef liver, dry skim milk, oatmeal, peas, pork, sweet potato, tuna, and certain health foods. Check with your doctor about how much of these foods you may have in your diet while you are taking levodopa. Also, ask your doctor or pharmacist for help when selecting vitamin products.

As your condition improves and your body movements become easier, *be careful not to overdo physical activities. Injuries resulting from falls may occur.* Physical activities must be increased gradually to allow your body to adjust to changing balance, circulation, and coordination. *This is especially important in the elderly.*

After taking this medicine for long periods of time, such as a year or more, some patients suddenly lose the ability to move. Their muscles do not seem to work. This loss of movement may last from a few minutes to several hours. The patient then is able to move as before. This condition may unexpectedly occur again and again. If you should have this problem, sometimes called the "on-off" effect, check with your doctor.

Side Effects of This Medicine

Along with its needed effects, a medicine may cause some unwanted effects. Although not all of these side effects may occur, if they do occur they may need medical attention.

Check with your doctor as soon as possible if any of the following side effects occur:

> *More common*
>> Mental depression; mood or mental changes (such as aggressive behavior); unusual and uncontrolled movements of the body
>
> *Less common—more common when levodopa is used alone*
>> Difficult urination; dizziness or lightheadedness when getting up from a lying or sitting position; irregular heartbeat; nausea or vomiting (severe or continuing); spasm or closing of eyelids (not more common when levodopa is used alone)
>
> *Rare*
>> High blood pressure; stomach pain; unusual tiredness or weakness

Other side effects may occur that usually do not need medical attention. These side effects may go away during treatment as your body adjusts to the medicine. However, check with your doctor if any of the following side effects continue or are bothersome:

> *More common*
>> Anxiety, confusion, or nervousness (especially in elderly patients receiving other medicine for Parkinson's disease)

Less common

Constipation (more common when levodopa is used alone); diarrhea; dryness of mouth; flushing of skin; headache; loss of appetite; muscle twitching; nightmares (more common when levodopa is used alone); trouble in sleeping

This medicine may sometimes cause the urine and sweat to be darker in color than usual. The urine may at first be reddish, then turn to nearly black after being exposed to air. Some bathroom cleaning products will produce a similar effect when in contact with urine containing this medicine. This is to be expected during treatment with this medicine.

Other side effects not listed above may also occur in some patients. If you notice any other effects, check with your doctor.

LITHIUM   Systemic

Some commonly used brand names are:

In the U.S.

Cibalith-S	Lithobid
Eskalith	Lithonate
Eskalith CR	Lithotabs
Lithane	

Generic name product may also be available.

In Canada

Carbolith	Lithane
Duralith	Lithizine

Description

Lithium (LITH-ee-um) is used to treat the manic stage of bipolar disorder (manic-depressive illness). Manic-depressive patients experience severe mood changes, ranging from an excited or manic state (for example, unusual anger or irritability or a false sense of well-being) to depression or sadness. Lithium is used to reduce the frequency and severity of manic states. Lithium may also reduce the frequency and severity of depression in bipolar disorder.

It is not known how lithium works to stabilize a person's mood. However, it does act on the central nervous system. It helps you to have more control over your emotions and helps you cope better with the problems of living.

It is important that you and your family understand all the effects of lithium. These effects depend on your individual condition and response and the amount of lithium you use. You also must know when to contact your doctor if there are problems with the medicine's use. Lithium may also be used for other conditions as determined by your doctor.

This medicine is available only with your doctor's prescription, in the following dosage forms:

Oral

- Capsules (U.S. and Canada)
- Slow-release capsules (Canada)
- Tablets (U.S. and Canada)
- Extended-release tablets (U.S. and Canada)
- Syrup (U.S.).

It is very important that you read and understand the following information. If any of it causes you special concern, check with your doctor. Also, *if you have any questions* or if you want more information about this medicine or your medical problem, *ask your doctor, nurse, or pharmacist.*

Before Using This Medicine

In deciding to use a medicine, the risks of taking the medicine must be weighed against the good it will do. This is a decision you and your doctor will make. For lithium, the following should be considered:

Allergies—Tell your doctor if you have ever had any unusual or allergic reaction to lithium. Also tell your doctor and pharmacist if you are allergic to any other substances, such as foods, preservatives, or dyes.

Diet—Make certain your doctor and pharmacist know if you are on a low-sodium or low-salt diet. Too little salt in your diet could lead to serious side effects.

Pregnancy—Lithium is not recommended for use during pregnancy, especially during the first 3 months. Studies have shown that lithium may rarely cause thyroid problems and heart or blood vessel defects in the baby. It has also been shown to cause muscle weakness and severe drowsiness in newborn babies of mothers taking lithium near time of delivery.

Breast-feeding—Lithium passes into the breast milk. It has been reported to cause unwanted effects such as muscle weakness, lowered body temperature, and heart problems in nursing babies. Before taking this medicine, be sure you have discussed with your doctor the risks and benefits of breast-feeding.

Children—Lithium may cause weakened bones in children during treatment.

Older adults—Unusual thirst, a large volume of urine, diarrhea, drowsiness, loss of appetite, muscle weakness, trembling, slurred speech, nausea or vomiting, goiter, or symptoms of underactive thyroid are especially likely to occur in elderly patients, who are usually more sensitive than younger adults to the effects of lithium.

Other medicines—Although certain medicines should not be used together at all, in other cases 2 different medicines may be used together even if an interaction might occur. In these cases, your doctor may want to change the dose, or other precautions may be necessary. When you are taking lithium, it is especially important that your doctor and pharmacist know if you are taking any of the following:
- Antipsychotics (medicine for mental illness)—Blood levels of both medicines may change, increasing the chance of serious side effects
- Antithyroid agents (medicine for overactive thyroid) or
- Medicine for asthma, bronchitis, emphysema, sinusitis, or cystic fibrosis that contains the following:
    Calcium iodide or
    Iodinated glycerol or
    Potassium iodide—Unwanted effects on the thyroid gland may occur

- Diuretics (water pills) or
- Medicine for inflammation or pain, except narcotics—Higher blood levels of lithium may occur, increasing the chance of serious side effects

Other medical problems—The presence of other medical problems may affect the use of lithium. Make sure you tell your doctor if you have any other medical problems, especially:

- Brain disease or
- Schizophrenia—You may be especially sensitive to lithium and mental effects (such as increased confusion) may occur
- Diabetes mellitus (sugar diabetes)—Lithium may increase the blood levels of insulin; the dose of insulin you need to take may change
- Difficult urination or
- Infection (severe) or
- Kidney disease—Higher blood levels of lithium may occur, increasing the chance of serious side effects
- Epilepsy or
- Heart disease or
- Parkinson's disease or
- Psoriasis or
- Thyroid disease—Lithium may make the condition worse
- Leukemia (history of)—Lithium may cause the leukemia to occur again

Before you begin using any new medicine (prescription or nonprescription) or if you develop any new medical problem while you are using this medicine, check with your doctor, nurse, or pharmacist.

Proper Use of This Medicine

Take this medicine after a meal or snack. Doing so will reduce stomach upset, tremors, or weakness and may also prevent a laxative effect.

For patients taking the *long-acting or slow-release form* of lithium:

- Swallow the tablet or capsule whole.
- Do not break, crush, or chew before swallowing.

For patients taking the *syrup form* of lithium:
- Dilute the syrup in fruit juice or another flavored beverage before taking.

During treatment with lithium, drink 2 or 3 quarts of water or other fluids each day, and use a normal amount of salt in your food, unless otherwise directed by your doctor.

Take this medicine exactly as directed. Do not take more or less of it, do not take it more or less often, and do not take it for a longer time than your doctor ordered. To do so may increase the chance of unwanted effects.

Sometimes lithium must be taken for 1 to several weeks before you begin to feel better.

In order for lithium to work properly, it must be taken every day in regularly spaced doses as ordered by your doctor. This is necessary to keep a constant amount of lithium in your blood. To help keep the amount constant, do not miss any doses and *do not stop taking the medicine even if you feel better.*

Missed dose—If you do miss a dose of this medicine, take it as soon as possible. However, if it is within 2 hours (about 6 hours for extended-release tablets or slow-release capsules) of your next dose, skip the missed dose and go back to your regular dosing schedule. Do not double doses.

Storage—To store this medicine:
- Keep out of the reach of children.
- Store away from heat and direct light.
- Do not store in the bathroom, near the kitchen sink, or in other damp places. Heat or moisture may cause the medicine to break down.
- Keep the syrup form of this medicine from freezing.
- Do not keep outdated medicine or medicine no longer needed. Be sure that any discarded medicine is out of the reach of children.

Precautions While Using This Medicine

Your doctor should check your progress at regular visits to make sure that the medicine is working properly and that possible side effects are avoided. Laboratory tests may be necessary.

Lithium may not work properly as it should if you drink large amounts of caffeine-containing coffee, tea, or colas.

This medicine may cause some people to become dizzy, drowsy, or less alert than they are normally. *Make sure you know how you react to this medicine before you drive, use machines, or do anything else that could be dangerous if you are dizzy or are not alert.*

Use extra care in hot weather and during activities that cause you to sweat heavily, such as hot baths, saunas, or exercising. The loss of too much water and salt from your body could lead to serious side effects from this medicine.

If you have an infection or illness that causes heavy sweating, vomiting, or diarrhea, check with your doctor. The loss of too much water and salt from your body could lead to serious side effects from lithium.

Do not go on a diet to lose weight and do not make a major change in your diet without first checking with your doctor. Improper dieting could cause the loss of too much water and salt from your body and could lead to serious side effects from this medicine.

For patients taking the *slow-release capsules or the extended-release tablets*:
- Do not use this medicine interchangeably with other lithium products.

It is important that you and your family know the early symptoms of lithium overdose or toxicity and when to call the doctor.

Side Effects of This Medicine

Along with its needed effects, a medicine may cause some unwanted effects. Although not all of these side effects may occur, if they do occur they may need medical attention.

Check with your doctor immediately if any of the following side effects occur:

Early symptoms of overdose or toxicity

Diarrhea; drowsiness; loss of appetite; muscle weakness; nausea or vomiting; slurred speech; trembling

Late symptoms of overdose or toxicity

Blurred vision; clumsiness or unsteadiness; confusion; convulsions (seizures); dizziness; increase in amount of urine; trembling (severe)

Check with your doctor as soon as possible if any of the following side effects occur:

Less common

Fainting; fast or slow heartbeat; irregular pulse; troubled breathing (especially during hard work or exercise); unusual tiredness or weakness; weight gain

Rare

Blue color and pain in fingers and toes; coldness of arms and legs; dizziness; eye pain; headache; noises in the ears; vision problems

Signs of low thyroid function

Dry, rough skin; hair loss; hoarseness; mental depression; sensitivity to cold; swelling of feet or lower legs; swelling of neck; unusual excitement

Other side effects may occur that usually do not need medical attention. These side effects may go away during treatment as your body adjusts to the medicine. However, check with your doctor if any of the following side effects continue or are bothersome:

More common

Increased frequency of urination or loss of bladder control—more common in women than in men, usually beginning two to seven years after start of treatment; increased thirst; nausea (mild); trembling of hands (slight)

Less common

Acne or skin rash; bloated feeling or pressure in the stomach; muscle twitching (slight)

Other side effects not listed above may also occur in some patients. If you notice any other effects, check with your doctor.

Additional Information

Once a medicine has been approved for marketing for a certain use, experience may show that it is also useful for other medical problems. Although these uses are not specifically included in product labeling, lithium is used in certain patients with the following medical conditions:

- Cluster headaches
- Mental depression
- Neutropenia (a blood condition in which there is a decreased number of a certain type of white blood cells)

Other than the above information, there is no additional information relating to proper use, precautions, or side effects for these uses.

LOXAPINE Systemic

Some commonly used brand names are:

In the U.S.

Loxitane	Loxitane IM
Loxitane C	

Generic name product may also be available.

In Canada

Loxapac

Description

Loxapine (LOX-a-peen) is used to treat nervous, mental, and emotional conditions.

Loxapine is available only with your doctor's prescription, in the following dosage forms:

Oral
- Solution (U.S. and Canada)
- Capsules (U.S.)
- Tablets (Canada)

Parenteral
- Injection (U.S. and Canada)

It is very important that you read and understand the following information. If any of it causes you special concern, check with your doctor. Also, *if you have any questions* or if you want more information about this medicine or your medical problem, *ask your doctor, nurse, or pharmacist.*

Before Using This Medicine

In deciding to use a medicine, the risks of taking the medicine must be weighed against the good it will do. This is a decision you and your doctor will make. For loxapine, the following should be considered:

Allergies—Tell your doctor if you have ever had any unusual or allergic reaction to loxapine or amoxapine. Also tell your doctor and pharmacist if you are allergic to any other substances, such as foods, preservatives, or dyes.

Pregnancy— Loxapine has not been shown to cause birth defects or other problems in humans. However, animal studies have shown unwanted effects in the fetus.

Breast-feeding—It is not known if loxapine passes into breast milk. This medicine has not been reported to cause problems in nursing babies.

Children—Studies on this medicine have been done only in adult patients, and there is no specific information about its use in children.

Older adults—Elderly patients are usually more sensitive than younger adults to the effects of loxapine. Constipation, dizziness or fainting, drowsiness, dry mouth, trembling of the hands and fingers, and symptoms of tardive dyskinesia (such as rapid, worm-like movements of the tongue or any other uncontrolled movements of the mouth, tongue, or jaw, and/or arms and legs) are especially likely to occur in elderly patients.

Athletes—Loxapine is banned and, in some cases, tested for in competitors in certain events by the U.S. Olympic Committee (USOC) and the National Collegiate Athletic Association (NCAA).

Other medicines—Although certain medicines should not be used together at all, in other cases 2 different medicines may be used together even if an interaction might occur. In these cases, your doctor may want to change the dose, or other precautions may be necessary. When you are taking loxapine, it is especially important that your doctor and pharmacist know if you are taking any of the following:

- Amoxapine (e.g., Asendin) or
- Methyldopa (e.g., Aldomet) or
- Metoclopramide (e.g., Reglan) or
- Metyrosine (e.g., Demser) or
- Other antipsychotics (medicine for mental illness) or
- Pemoline (e.g., Cylert) or
- Pimozide (e.g., Orap) or
- Promethazine (e.g., Phenergan) or
- Rauwolfia alkaloids (alseroxylon [e.g., Rauwiloid], deserpidine [e.g., Harmonyl], rauwolfia serpentina [e.g., Raudixin], reserpine [e.g., Serpasil]) or
- Trimeprazine (e.g., Temaril)—Taking these medicines with loxapine may increase the chance and seriousness of some side effects
- Central nervous system (CNS) depressants—Taking these medicines with loxapine may increase the CNS depressant effects
- Guanadrel (e.g., Hylorel) or
- Guanethidine (e.g., Ismelin)—Loxapine may decrease the effects of these medicines

Other medical problems—The presence of other medical problems may affect the use of loxapine. Make sure you tell your doctor if you have any other medical problems, especially:

- Alcohol abuse—CNS depressant effects may be increased
- Enlarged prostate or
- Glaucoma (or predisposition to) or

- Parkinson's disease or
- Difficult urination—Loxapine may make the condition worse
- Heart or blood vessel disease—An increased risk of low blood pressure (hypotension) or changes in the rhythm of your heart may occur
- Liver disease—Higher blood levels of loxapine may occur, increasing the chance of side effects
- Seizure disorders—Loxapine may increase the risk of seizures

Before you begin using any new medicine (prescription or nonprescription) or if you develop any new medical problem while you are using this medicine, check with your doctor, nurse, or pharmacist.

Proper Use of This Medicine

This medicine may be taken with food or a full glass (8 ounces) of water or milk to reduce stomach irritation.

For patients taking the *oral solution*:

- Measure the solution only with the dropper provided by the manufacturer. This will give a more accurate dose.

The liquid medicine must be mixed with orange juice or grapefruit juice just before you take it to make it easier to take.

Do not take more of this medicine, do not take it more often, and do not take it for a longer time than your doctor ordered. To do so may increase the chance of unwanted effects.

Missed dose—If you miss a dose of this medicine, take it as soon as possible. However, if it is within one hour of your next dose, skip the missed dose and go back to your regular dosing schedule. Do not double doses.

Storage—To store this medicine:

- Keep out of the reach of children.
- Store away from heat and direct light.
- Do not store the capsule or tablet form of this medicine in the bathroom, near the kitchen sink, or in other damp

places. Heat or moisture may cause the medicine to break down.

- Keep the liquid form of this medicine from freezing.
- Do not keep outdated medicine or medicine no longer needed. Be sure that any discarded medicine is out of the reach of children.

Precautions While Using This Medicine

Your doctor should check your progress at regular visits, especially during the first few months of treatment with this medicine. The amount of loxapine you take may be changed often to meet the needs of your condition and to help avoid side effects.

Do not stop taking this medicine without first checking with your doctor. Your doctor may want you to reduce gradually the amount you are taking before stopping completely. This will allow your body time to adjust and to keep your condition from becoming worse.

This medicine will add to the effects of alcohol and other CNS depressants (medicines that slow down the nervous system, possibly causing drowsiness). Some examples of CNS depressants are antihistamines or medicine for hay fever, other allergies, or colds; sedatives, tranquilizers, or sleeping medicine; prescription pain medicine or narcotics; barbiturates; medicine for seizures; or anesthetics, including some dental anesthetics. *Check with your doctor before taking any of the above while you are taking this medicine.*

Do not take this medicine within an hour or two of taking antacids or medicine for diarrhea. Taking them too close together may make this medicine less effective.

This medicine may cause some people to become drowsy or less alert than they are normally, especially as the amount of medicine is increased. Even if you take this medicine at bedtime, you may feel drowsy or less alert on arising. *Make sure you know how you react to this medicine before you drive, use machines, or do anything else that could be dangerous if you are not alert.*

Although not a problem for most patients, dizziness, light-headedness, or fainting may occur, especially when you get up from a lying or sitting position. Getting up slowly may help. However, if the problem continues or gets worse, check with your doctor.

Loxapine may cause your skin to be more sensitive to sunlight than it is normally. Exposure to sunlight, even for brief periods of time, may cause a skin rash, itching, redness or other discoloration of the skin, or a severe sunburn. When you begin taking this medicine:

- Stay out of direct sunlight, especially between the hours of 10:00 a.m. and 3:00 p.m., if possible.
- Wear protective clothing, including a hat. Also, wear sunglasses.
- Apply a sun block product that has a skin protection factor (SPF) of at least 15. Some patients may require a product with a higher SPF number, especially if they have a fair complexion. If you have any questions about this, check with your doctor or pharmacist.
- Apply a sun block lipstick that has an SPF of at least 15 to protect your lips.
- Do not use a sunlamp or tanning bed or booth.

If you have a severe reaction from the sun, check with your doctor.

Loxapine may cause dryness of the mouth. For temporary relief, use sugarless candy or gum, melt bits of ice in your mouth, or use a saliva substitute. However, if your mouth continues to feel dry for more than 2 weeks, check with your medical doctor or dentist. Continuing dryness of the mouth may increase the chance of dental disease, including tooth decay, gum disease, and fungus infections.

Before having any kind of surgery, dental treatment, or emergency treatment, tell the medical doctor or dentist in charge that you are taking this medicine.

Side Effects of This Medicine

Along with its needed effects, loxapine can sometimes cause serious side effects. Tardive dyskinesia (a movement disorder) may occur and may not go away after you stop using the medicine. Signs of tardive dyskinesia include fine, worm-like movements of the tongue, or other uncontrolled movements of the mouth, tongue, cheeks, jaw, or arms and legs. Other serious but rare side effects may also occur. These include severe muscle stiffness, fever, unusual tiredness or weakness, fast heartbeat, difficult breathing, increased sweating, loss of bladder control, and seizures (neuroleptic malignant syndrome). *You and your doctor should discuss the good this medicine will do as well as the risks of taking it.*

Stop taking loxapine and get emergency help immediately if any of the following side effects occur:

> *Rare*
>> Convulsions (seizures); difficult or fast breathing; fast heartbeat or irregular pulse; fever (high); high or low blood pressure; increased sweating; loss of bladder control; muscle stiffness (severe); unusually pale skin; unusual tiredness or weakness

Check with your doctor immediately if any of the following side effects occur:

> *More common*
>> Lip smacking or puckering; puffing of cheeks; rapid or fine, worm-like movements of tongue; uncontrolled chewing movements; uncontrolled movements of arms or legs

Also, check with your doctor as soon as possible if any of the following side effects occur:

> *More common (occurring with increase of dosage)*
>> Difficulty in speaking or swallowing; loss of balance control; mask-like face; restlessness or desire to keep moving; shuffling walk; slowed movements; stiffness of arms and legs; trembling and shaking of fingers and hands

> *Less common*
>> Constipation (severe); difficult urination; inability to move eyes; muscle spasms, especially of the neck and back; skin rash; twisting movements of the body

> *Rare*
>> Sore throat and fever; unusual bleeding or bruising; yellow eyes or skin

Symptoms of overdose

Dizziness (severe); drowsiness (severe); muscle trembling, jerking, stiffness, or uncontrolled movements (severe); troubled breathing (severe); unusual tiredness or weakness (severe)

Other side effects may occur that usually do not need medical attention. These side effects may go away during treatment as your body adjusts to the medicine. However, check with your doctor if any of the following side effects continue or are bothersome:

More common

Blurred vision; confusion; dizziness, lightheadedness, or fainting; drowsiness; dryness of mouth

Less common

Constipation (mild); decreased sexual ability; enlargement of breasts (males and females); headache; increased sensitivity of skin to sun; missing menstrual periods; nausea or vomiting; trouble in sleeping; unusual secretion of milk; weight gain

Certain side effects of this medicine may occur after you have stopped taking it. Check with your doctor as soon as possible if you notice any of the following effects after you have stopped taking loxapine:

Dizziness; nausea and vomiting; puffing of cheeks; rapid or wormlike movements of the tongue; stomach upset or pain; trembling of fingers and hands; uncontrolled chewing movements

Other side effects not listed above may also occur in some patients. If you notice any other effects, check with your doctor.

Additional Information

Once a medicine has been approved for marketing for a certain use, experience may show that it is also useful for other medical problems. Although this use is not included in product labeling, loxapine is used in certain patients with the following medical condition:

• Anxiety associated with mental depression

Other than the above information, there is no additional information relating to proper use, precautions, or side effects for this use.

MAPROTILINE   Systemic

A commonly used brand name in the U.S. and Canada is Ludiomil.
   Generic name product may also be available in the U.S.

Description

Maprotiline (ma-PROE-ti-leen) belongs to the group of medicines known as tetracyclic antidepressants or "mood elevators." It is used to relieve mental depression, including anxiety that sometimes occurs with depression.

Maprotiline is available only with your doctor's prescription, in the following dosage form:

Oral
   • Tablets (U.S. and Canada)

It is very important that you read and understand the following information. If any of it causes you special concern, check with your doctor. Also, *if you have any questions* or if you want more information about this medicine or your medical problem, *ask your doctor, nurse, or pharmacist.*

Before Using This Medicine

In deciding to use a medicine, the risks of taking the medicine must be weighed against the good it will do. This is a decision you and your doctor will make. For maprotiline, the following should be considered:

Allergies—Tell your doctor if you have ever had any unusual or allergic reaction to maprotiline or tricyclic antidepressants. Also tell your doctor and pharmacist if you are allergic to any other substances, such as foods, preservatives, or dyes.

Pregnancy—Maprotiline has not been studied in pregnant women. However, this medicine has not been shown to cause birth defects or other problems in animal studies.

Breast-feeding—Maprotiline passes into the breast milk. However, this medicine has not been reported to cause problems in nursing babies.

Children—Studies on this medicine have been done only in adult patients, and there is no specific information comparing use of maprotiline in children with use in other age groups.

Older adults—Drowsiness, dizziness or lightheadedness; confusion; vision problems; dryness of mouth; constipation; and difficulty in urinating may be especially likely to occur in elderly patients, who are usually more sensitive than younger adults to the effects of maprotiline.

Athletes—Maprotiline is banned and, in some cases, tested for in competitors in biathlon and modern pentathlon events by the U.S. Olympic Committee (USOC).

Other medicines—Although certain medicines should not be used together at all, in other cases 2 different medicines may be used together even if an interaction might occur. In these cases, your doctor may want to change the dose, or other precautions may be necessary. When you are taking maprotiline, it is especially important that your doctor and pharmacist know if you are taking any of the following:

- Amphetamines or
- Appetite suppressants (diet pills) or
- Medicine for asthma or other breathing problems or
- Medicine for colds, sinus problems, or hay fever or other allergies (including nose drops or sprays)—Using these medicines with maprotiline may cause serious unwanted effects on your heart and blood pressure
- Central nervous system (CNS) depressants—Taking these medicines with maprotiline may increase the CNS depressant effects
- Monoamine oxidase (MAO) inhibitors (furazolidone [e.g., Furoxone], isocarboxazid [e.g., Marplan], phenelzine [e.g., Nardil], procarbazine [e.g., Matulane], selegiline [e.g., Eldepryl], tranylcypromine [e.g., Parnate])—Taking mapro-

anything else that could be dangerous if you are not alert or able to see well.

Dizziness, lightheadedness, or fainting may occur, especially when you get up from a lying or sitting position. Getting up slowly may help. If this problem continues or gets worse, check with your doctor.

Maprotiline may cause dryness of the mouth. For temporary relief, use sugarless gum or candy, melt bits of ice in your mouth, or use a saliva substitute. However, if your mouth continues to feel dry for more than 2 weeks, check with your medical doctor or dentist. Continuing dryness of the mouth may increase the chance of dental disease, including tooth decay, gum disease, and fungus infections.

Before having any kind of surgery, dental treatment, or emergency treatment, tell the medical doctor or dentist in charge that you are using this medicine.

Do not stop taking this medicine without first checking with your doctor. Your doctor may want you to reduce gradually the amount you are taking before stopping completely. This will allow your body to adjust properly and will reduce the possibility of unwanted effects.

Side Effects of This Medicine

Along with its needed effects, a medicine may cause some unwanted effects. Although not all of these side effects may occur, if they do occur they may need medical attention.

Check with your doctor as soon as possible if any of the following side effects occur:

More common
> Skin rash, redness, swelling, or itching

Less common
> Constipation (severe); convulsions (seizures); nausea or vomiting; shakiness or trembling; unusual excitement

Rare
> Breast enlargement—in males and females; confusion (especially in the elderly); difficulty in urinating; fainting; hallucinations (seeing, hearing, or feeling things that are

not there); inappropriate secretion of milk—in females; irregular heartbeat (pounding, racing, skipping); sore throat and fever; swelling of testicles; yellow eyes or skin

Symptoms of overdose

Convulsions (seizures); dizziness (severe); drowsiness (severe); fast or irregular heartbeat; fever; muscle stiffness or weakness (severe); restlessness or agitation; trouble in breathing; vomiting

Other side effects may occur that usually do not need medical attention. These side effects may go away during treatment as your body adjusts to the medicine. However, check with your doctor if any of the following side effects continue or are bothersome:

More common

Blurred vision; decreased sexual ability; dizziness or light-headedness (especially in the elderly); drowsiness; dryness of mouth; headache; increased or decreased sexual drive; tiredness or weakness

Less common

Constipation (mild); diarrhea; heartburn; increased appetite and weight gain; increased sensitivity of skin to sunlight; increased sweating; trouble in sleeping; weight loss

After you stop taking this medicine, your body will need time to adjust. This usually takes about 3 to 10 days. Continue to follow the precautions listed above during this period of time.

Other side effects not listed above may also occur in some patients. If you notice any other effects, check with your doctor.

Additional Information

Once a medicine has been approved for marketing for a certain use, experience may show that it is also useful for other medical problems. Although this use in not included in product labeling, maprotiline is used in certain patients with the following medical condition:

• Chronic neurogenic pain (a certain type of pain that is continuing)

Other than the above information, there is no additional information relating to proper use, precautions, or side effects for these uses.

METHOTREXATE—For Noncancerous Conditions   Systemic

Some commonly used brand names in the U.S. are:

Folex   Mexate-AQ
Folex PFS   Rheumatrex
Mexate

Generic name product may also be available in the U.S. and Canada.

Another commonly used name is amethopterin.

Description

Methotrexate (meth-o-TREX-ate) belongs to the group of medicines known as antimetabolites. It is used to treat psoriasis and rheumatoid arthritis. It may also be used for other conditions as determined by your doctor.

Methotrexate blocks an enzyme needed by the cell to live. This interferes with the growth of certain cells, such as skin cells in psoriasis that are growing rapidly. Since the growth of normal body cells may also be affected by methotrexate, other effects will also occur. Some of these may be serious and must be reported to your doctor. Other effects, like hair loss, may not be serious but may cause concern. Some effects may not occur for months or years after the medicine is used.

Before you begin treatment with methotrexate, you and your doctor should talk about the good this medicine will do as well as the risks of using it.

Methotrexate is available only with your doctor's prescription, in the following dosage forms:

Oral
- Tablets (U.S. and Canada)

Parenteral
- Injection (U.S. and Canada)

It is very important that you read and understand the following information. If any of it causes you special concern,

check with your doctor. Also, *if you have any questions* or if you want more information about this medicine or your medical problem, *ask your doctor, nurse, or pharmacist*.

Before Using This Medicine

In deciding to use a medicine, the risks of taking the medicine must be weighed against the good it will do. This is a decision you and your doctor will make. For methotrexate, the following should be considered:

Allergies—Tell your doctor if you have ever had any unusual or allergic reaction to methotrexate.

Pregnancy—There is a good chance that this medicine may cause birth defects if either the male or female is taking it at the time of conception or if it is taken during pregnancy. Methotrexate may cause harm or even death of the fetus. In addition, this medicine may rarely cause temporary sterility.

Methotrexate is not recommended during pregnancy. Be sure that you have discussed this with your doctor before taking this medicine. It is best to use some kind of birth control while you are taking methotrexate. Tell your doctor right away if you think you have become pregnant while taking methotrexate.

Breast-feeding—Tell your doctor if you are breast-feeding or if you intend to breast-feed during treatment with this medicine. Because methotrexate may cause serious side effects, breast-feeding is generally not recommended while you are taking it.

Children—Newborns and other infants may be more sensitive to the effects of methotrexate. However, in other children it is not expected to cause different side effects or problems than it does in adults.

Older adults—Side effects may be more likely to occur in the elderly, who are usually more sensitive to the effects of methotrexate.

Other medicines—Although certain medicines should not be used together at all, in other cases two different medicines

may be used together even if an interaction might occur. In these cases, your doctor may want to change the dose, or other precautions may be necessary. When you are taking methotrexate, it is especially important that your doctor and pharmacist know if you are taking any other prescription or nonprescription (over-the-counter [OTC]) medicine. They should also be told if you have ever been treated with x-rays or cancer medicines or if you drink alcohol.

Other medical problems—The presence of other medical problems may affect the use of methotrexate. Make sure you tell your doctor if you have any other medical problems, especially:

- Alcohol abuse (or history of)—Increased risk of unwanted effects on the liver
- Chickenpox (including recent exposure) or
- Herpes zoster (shingles)—Risk of severe disease affecting other parts of the body
- Colitis
- Disease of the immune system
- Infection—Methotrexate can reduce immunity to infection
- Intestine blockage or
- Kidney disease or
- Liver disease—Effects may be increased because of slower removal of methotrexate from the body
- Mouth sores or inflammation or
- Stomach ulcer—May be worsened

Before you begin using any new medicine (prescription or nonprescription) or if you develop any new medical problem while you are using this medicine, check with your doctor, nurse, or pharmacist.

Proper Use of This Medicine

Take this medicine only as directed by your doctor. Do not take more or less of it, and do not take it more often than your doctor ordered. The exact amount of medicine you need has been carefully worked out. Taking too much may increase the chance of side effects, while taking too little may not improve your condition.

Methotrexate may cause nausea. Even if you begin to feel ill, *do not stop using this medicine without first checking with your doctor*. Ask your doctor, nurse, or pharmacist for ways to lessen these effects. If you begin vomiting, check with your doctor.

If you vomit shortly after taking a dose of methotrexate, check with your doctor. You will be told whether to take the dose again or to wait until the next scheduled dose.

Missed dose—If you miss a dose of this medicine, do not take the missed dose at all and do not double the next one. Instead, go back to your regular dosing schedule and check with your doctor.

Storage—To store this medicine:
- Keep out of the reach of children.
- Store away from heat and direct light.
- Do not store in the bathroom, near the kitchen sink, or in other damp places. Heat or moisture may cause the medicine to break down.
- Do not keep outdated medicine or medicine no longer needed. Be sure that any discarded medicine is out of the reach of children.

Precautions While Using This Medicine

It is very important that your doctor check your progress at regular visits to make sure that this medicine is working properly and to check for unwanted effects.

Do not drink alcohol while using this medicine. Alcohol can increase the chance of liver problems.

Some patients who take methotrexate may become more sensitive to sunlight than they are normally. When you first begin taking methotrexate, avoid too much sun and do not use a sunlamp until you see how you react to the sun, especially if you tend to burn easily. In case of a severe burn, check with your doctor. This is especially important if you are taking this medicine for psoriasis because sunlight can make the psoriasis worse.

Do not take medicine for inflammation or pain (aspirin or other salicylates, diclofenac, diflunisal, fenoprofen, ibuprofen, indomethacin, ketoprofen, meclofenamate, mefenamic acid, naproxen, phenylbutazone, piroxicam, sulindac, suprofen, tolmetin) without first checking with your doctor. These medicines may increase the effects of methotrexate, which could be harmful.

While you are being treated with methotrexate, and after you stop treatment with it, *do not have any immunizations (vaccinations) without your doctor's approval.* Methotrexate may lower your body's resistance and there is a chance you might get the infection the immunization is meant to prevent. In addition, other persons living in your household should not take or should not have recently taken oral polio vaccine since there is a chance they could pass the polio virus on to you. Also, avoid other persons who have taken oral polio vaccine. Do not get close to them, and do not stay in the same room with them for very long. If you cannot take these precautions, you should consider wearing a protective face mask that covers the nose and mouth.

Methotrexate can lower the number of white blood cells in your blood temporarily, increasing the chance of getting an infection. It can also lower the number of platelets, which are necessary for proper blood clotting. If this occurs, there are certain precautions you can take, especially when your blood count is low, to reduce the risk of infection or bleeding:

- If you can, avoid people with infections. *Check with your doctor immediately* if you think you are getting an infection or if you get a fever or chills, cough or hoarseness, lower back or side pain, or painful or difficult urination.
- *Check with your doctor immediately* if you notice any unusual bleeding or bruising; black, tarry stools; blood in urine or stools; or pinpoint red spots on your skin.
- Be careful when using a regular toothbrush, dental floss, or toothpick. Your medical doctor, dentist, or nurse may recommend other ways to clean your teeth and gums. Check with your medical doctor before having any dental work done.

- Do not touch your eyes or the inside of your nose unless you have just washed your hands and have not touched anything else in the meantime.
- Be careful not to cut yourself when you are using sharp objects such as a safety razor or fingernail or toenail cutters.
- Avoid contact sports or other situations where bruising or injury could occur.

Side Effects of This Medicine

Along with their needed effects, medicines like methotrexate can sometimes cause unwanted effects such as blood problems, kidney problems, stomach or liver problems, loss of hair, and other side effects. These and others are described below. Also, because of the way these medicines act on the body, there is a chance that they might cause other unwanted effects that may not occur until months or years after the medicine is used. These delayed effects may include certain types of cancer, such as leukemia. Discuss these possible effects with your doctor.

Although not all of these side effects may occur, if they do occur they may need medical attention.

Check with your doctor immediately if any of the following side effects occur:

Less common

Diarrhea; reddening of skin; sores in mouth and on lips; stomach pain

Rare

Black, tarry stools; blood in urine or stools; blurred vision; convulsions (seizures); cough or hoarseness; fever or chills; lower back or side pain; painful or difficult urination; pinpoint red spots on skin; shortness of breath; unusual bleeding or bruising

Check with your doctor as soon as possible if any of the following side effects occur:

Rare

Back pain; dark urine; dizziness; drowsiness; headache; unusual tiredness or weakness; yellow eyes or skin

Other side effects may occur that usually do not need medical attention. These side effects may go away during treatment as your body adjusts to the medicine. Also, your doctor or nurse may be able to tell you about ways to prevent or reduce some of these side effects. Check with your doctor or nurse if any of the following side effects continue or are bothersome or if you have any questions about them:

Less common or rare

Acne; boils; loss of appetite; nausea or vomiting; pale skin; skin rash or itching

This medicine may cause a temporary loss of hair in some people. After treatment with methotrexate has ended, normal hair growth should return.

Other side effects not listed above may also occur in some patients. If you notice any other effects, check with your doctor.

Additional Information

Once a medicine has been approved for marketing for a certain use, experience may show that it is also useful for other medical problems. Although these uses are not included in product labeling, methotrexate is used in certain patients with the following medical conditions:

- Psoriatic arthritis
- Systemic dermatomyositis

Other than the above information, there is no additional information relating to proper use, precautions, or side effects for these uses.

METHYLDOPA   Systemic

Some commonly used brand names are:

In the U.S.

Aldomet

Generic name product may also be available.

In Canada
    Aldomet   Dopamet
    Apo-Methyldopa   Novomedopa
    Generic name product may also be available.

Description

Methyldopa (meth-ill-DOE-pa) belongs to the general class of medicines called antihypertensives. It is used to treat high blood pressure (hypertension).

High blood pressure adds to the workload of the heart and arteries. If it continues for a long time, the heart and arteries may not function properly. This can damage the blood vessels of the brain, heart, and kidneys, resulting in a stroke, heart failure, or kidney failure. High blood pressure may also increase the risk of heart attacks. These problems may be less likely to occur if blood pressure is controlled.

Methyldopa works by controlling impulses along certain nerve pathways. As a result, it relaxes blood vessels so that blood passes through them more easily. This helps to lower blood pressure.

Methyldopa is available only with your doctor's prescription, in the following dosage forms:

Oral
  • Oral suspension (U.S.)
  • Tablets (U.S. and Canada)

Parenteral
  • Injection (U.S. and Canada)

It is very important that you read and understand the following information. If any of it causes you special concern, check with your doctor. Also, *if you have any questions* or if you want more information about this medicine or your medical problem, *ask your doctor, nurse, or pharmacist.*

Before Using This Medicine

In deciding to use a medicine, the risks of taking the medicine must be weighed against the good it will do. This is a decision you and your doctor will make. For methyldopa, the following should be considered:

Allergies—Tell your doctor if you have ever had any unusual or allergic reaction to methyldopa. Also tell your doctor and pharmacist if you are allergic to any other substances, such as foods, sulfites or other preservatives, or dyes. Some methyldopa products may contain sulfites. Your doctor, nurse, or pharmacist can help you avoid products that may cause a problem.

Pregnancy—Methyldopa has not been studied in pregnant women in the first and second trimesters (the first 6 months of pregnancy). However, studies in pregnant women during the third trimester (the last 3 months of pregnancy) have not shown that methyldopa causes birth defects or other problems.

Breast-feeding—Although methyldopa passes into breast milk, it has not been reported to cause problems in nursing babies.

Children—Although there is no specific information comparing use of methyldopa in children with use in other age groups, this medicine is not expected to cause different side effects or problems in children than it does in adults.

Older adults—Dizziness or lightheadedness and drowsiness may be more likely to occur in the elderly, who are more sensitive to the effects of methyldopa.

Other medicines—Although certain medicines should not be used together at all, in other cases two different medicines may be used together even if an interaction might occur. In these cases, your doctor may want to change the dose, or other precautions may be necessary. When taking methyldopa, it is especially important that your doctor and pharmacist know if you are taking any of the following:

- Monoamine oxidase (MAO) inhibitors (furazolidone [e.g., Furoxone], isocarboxazid [e.g., Marplan], phenelzine [e.g., Nardil], procarbazine [e.g., Matulane], selegiline [e.g., Eldepryl], tranylcypromine [e.g., Parnate])—Taking methyldopa while you are taking or within 2 weeks of taking MAO inhibitors may cause nervousness in patients receiving MAO inhibitors; headache, severe high blood pressure, and hallucinations have been reported

Other medical problems—The presence of other medical problems may affect the use of methyldopa. Make sure you tell your doctor if you have any other medical problems, especially:

- Angina (chest pain)—Methyldopa may worsen the condition
- Kidney disease or
- Liver disease—Effects of methyldopa may be increased because of slower removal from the body
- Mental depression (history of)—Methyldopa can cause mental depression
- Parkinson's disease—Methyldopa may worsen condition
- Pheochromocytoma—Methyldopa may interfere with tests for the condition; in addition, there have been reports of increased blood pressure
- If you have taken methyldopa in the past and developed liver problems

Before you begin using any new medicine (prescription or nonprescription) or if you develop any new medical problem while you are using this medicine, check with your doctor, nurse, or pharmacist.

Proper Use of This Medicine

In addition to the use of the medicine your doctor has prescribed, treatment for your high blood pressure may include weight control and care in the types of foods you eat, especially foods high in sodium. Your doctor will tell you which of these are most important for you. You should check with your doctor before changing your diet.

Many patients who have high blood pressure will not notice any signs of the problem. In fact, many may feel normal. It is very important that you *take your medicine exactly as directed* and that you keep your appointments with your doctor even if you feel well.

Remember that methyldopa will not cure your high blood pressure but it does help control it. Therefore, you must continue to take it as directed if you expect to lower your blood pressure and keep it down. *You may have to take high blood pressure medicine for the rest of your life.* If high blood pressure is not treated, it can cause serious problems such as heart failure, blood vessel disease, stroke, or kidney disease.

To help you remember to take your medicine, try to get into the habit of taking it at the same time each day.

Missed dose—If you miss a dose of this medicine, take it as soon as possible. However, if it is almost time for your next dose, skip the missed dose and go back to your regular dosing schedule. Do not double doses.

Storage—To store this medicine:
- Keep out of the reach of children.
- Store away from heat and direct light.
- Do not store in the bathroom, near the kitchen sink, or in other damp places. Heat or moisture may cause the medicine to break down.
- Keep the oral liquid form of this medicine from freezing.
- Do not keep outdated medicine or medicine no longer needed. Be sure that any discarded medicine is out of the reach of children.

Precautions While Using This Medicine

It is important that your doctor check your progress at regular visits to make sure that this medicine is working properly.

Do not take other medicines unless they have been discussed with your doctor. This especially includes over-the-counter (nonprescription) medicines for appetite control, asthma, colds, cough, hay fever, or sinus problems, since they may tend to increase your blood pressure.

If you have a fever and there seems to be no reason for it, check with your doctor. This is especially important during the first few weeks you take methyldopa, since fever may be a sign of a serious reaction to this medicine.

Before having any kind of surgery (including dental surgery) or emergency treatment, make sure the medical doctor or dentist in charge knows that you are taking this medicine.

Methyldopa may cause some people to become drowsy or less alert than they are normally. This is more likely to happen when you begin to take it or when you increase the amount of medicine you are taking. *Make sure you know how you react to this medicine before you drive, use machines, or do anything else that could be dangerous if you are not alert.*

Dizziness, lightheadedness, or fainting may occur, especially when you get up from a lying or sitting position. Getting up slowly may help, but if the problem continues or gets worse, check with your doctor.

Methyldopa may cause dryness of the mouth. For temporary relief, use sugarless candy or gum, melt bits of ice in your mouth, or use a saliva substitute. However, if your mouth continues to feel dry for more than 2 weeks, check with your medical doctor or dentist. Continuing dryness of the mouth may increase the chance of dental disease, including tooth decay, gum disease, and fungus infections.

Tell the doctor in charge that you are taking this medicine before you have any medical tests. The results of some tests may be affected by this medicine.

Side Effects of This Medicine

Along with its needed effects, a medicine may cause some unwanted effects. Although not all of these side effects may occur, if they do occur they may need medical attention.

Check with your doctor immediately if the following side effect occurs:

> *Less common*
> Fever, shortly after starting to take this medicine

Check with your doctor as soon as possible if any of the following side effects occur:

> *More common*
> Swelling of feet or lower legs
>
> *Less common*
> Mental depression or anxiety; nightmares or unusually vivid dreams

Rare

Dark or amber urine; diarrhea or stomach cramps (severe or continuing); fever, chills, troubled breathing, and fast heartbeat; general feeling of discomfort or illness or weakness; joint pain; pale stools; skin rash or itching; stomach pain (severe) with nausea and vomiting; tiredness or weakness after having taken this medicine for several weeks (continuing); yellow eyes or skin

Other side effects may occur that usually do not need medical attention. These side effects may go away during treatment as your body adjusts to the medicine. However, check with your doctor if any of the following side effects continue or are bothersome:

More common

Drowsiness; dryness of mouth; headache

Less common

Decreased sexual ability or interest in sex; diarrhea; dizziness or lightheadedness when getting up from a lying or sitting position; nausea or vomiting; numbness, tingling, pain, or weakness in hands or feet; slow heartbeat; stuffy nose; swelling of breasts or unusual milk production

Other side effects not listed above may also occur in some patients. If you notice any other effects, check with your doctor.

METOCLOPRAMIDE   Systemic

Some commonly used brand names are:

In the U.S.

Clopra	Reclomide
Octamide	Reglan
Octamide PFS	

Generic name product may also be available.

In Canada

Apo-Metoclop	Maxeran
Emex	Reglan

Description

Metoclopramide (met-oh-KLOE-pra-mide) is a medicine that increases the movements or contractions of the stomach and intestines. When given by injection it is used to help diagnose certain problems of the stomach and/or intestines. It is also used by injection to prevent the nausea and vomiting that may occur after treatment with anticancer medicines. Another medicine may be used with metoclopramide to prevent side effects that may occur when metoclopramide is used with anticancer medicines.

When taken by mouth, metoclopramide is used to treat the symptoms of a certain type of stomach problem called diabetic gastroparesis. It relieves symptoms such as nausea, vomiting, continued feeling of fullness after meals, and loss of appetite. Metoclopramide is also used, for a short time, to treat symptoms such as heartburn in patients who suffer esophageal injury from a backward flow of gastric acid into the esophagus.

Metoclopramide may also be used for other conditions as determined by your doctor.

Metoclopramide is available only with your doctor's prescription. It is available in the following dosage forms:

Oral
- Tablets (U.S. and Canada)
- Syrup (U.S. and Canada)

Parenteral
- Injection (U.S. and Canada)

It is very important that you read and understand the following information. If any of it causes you special concern, check with your doctor. Also, *if you have any questions* or if you want more information about this medicine or your medical problem, *ask your doctor, nurse, or pharmacist.*

Before Using This Medicine

In deciding to use a medicine, the risks of taking the medicine must be weighed against the good it will do. This is a decision you and your doctor will make. For metoclopramide, the following should be considered:

Allergies—Tell your doctor if you have ever had any unusual or allergic reaction to metoclopramide, procaine, or procainamide. Also tell your doctor and pharmacist if you are allergic to any other substances, such as foods, preservatives, or dyes.

Pregnancy—Not enough studies have been done in humans to determine metoclopramide's safety during pregnancy. However, metoclopramide has not been shown to cause birth defects or other problems in animal studies.

Breast-feeding—Although metoclopramide passes into the breast milk, it has not been shown to cause problems in nursing babies.

Children—Muscle spasms, especially of jaw, neck, and back, and tic-like (jerky) movements of head and face may be especially likely to occur in children, who are usually more sensitive than adults to the effects of metoclopramide. Premature and full-term infants may develop blood problems if given high doses of metoclopramide.

Older adults—Shuffling walk and trembling and shaking of hands may be especially likely to occur in elderly patients after they have taken metoclopramide over a long time.

Athletes— Metoclopramide is banned and, in some cases, tested for in competitors in biathlon and modern pentathlon events by the U.S. Olympic Committee (USOC).

Other medicines—Although certain medicines should not be used together at all, in other cases 2 different medicines may be used together even if an interaction might occur. In these cases, your doctor may want to change the dose, or other precautions may be necessary. When you are taking metoclopramide, it is especially important that your doctor and pharmacist know if you are taking the following:

- Central nervous system (CNS) depressants (medicine that causes drowsiness)—Use with metoclopramide may cause severe drowsiness

Other medical problems—The presence of other medical problems may affect the use of metoclopramide. Make sure you tell your doctor if you have any other medical problems, especially:

- Abdominal or stomach bleeding or
- Asthma or
- High blood pressure or
- Intestinal blockage or
- Parkinson's disease—Metoclopramide may make these conditions worse
- Epilepsy—Metoclopramide may increase the risk of having a seizure
- Kidney disease (severe) or
- Liver disease (severe)—Higher blood levels of metoclopramide may result, possibly increasing the chance of side effects

Before you begin using any new medicine (prescription or nonprescription) or if you develop any new medical problem while you are using this medicine, check with your doctor, nurse, or pharmacist.

Proper Use of This Medicine

Take this medicine 30 minutes before meals and at bedtime, unless otherwise directed by your doctor.

Take metoclopramide only as directed. Do not take more of it, do not take it more often, and do not take it for a longer time than your doctor ordered. To do so may increase the chance of side effects.

Missed dose—If you miss a dose of this medicine, take it as soon as possible. However, if it is almost time for your next dose, skip the missed dose and go back to your regular dosing schedule. Do not double doses.

Storage—To store this medicine:

- Keep out of the reach of children.
- Store away from heat and direct light.
- Do not store the tablet form of this medicine in the bathroom, near the kitchen sink, or in other damp places. Heat or moisture may cause the medicine to break down.
- Keep the syrup form of this medicine from freezing.

- Do not keep outdated medicine or medicine no longer needed. Be sure that any discarded medicine is out of the reach of children.

Precautions While Using This Medicine

This medicine will add to the effects of alcohol and other CNS depressants (medicines that slow down the nervous system, possibly causing drowsiness). Some examples of CNS depressants are antihistamines or medicine for hay fever, other allergies, or colds; sedatives, tranquilizers, or sleeping medicine; prescription pain medicine or narcotics; barbiturates; medicine for seizures; muscle relaxants; or anesthetics, including some dental anesthetics. *Check with your doctor before taking any of the above while you are using this medicine.*

This medicine may cause some people to become dizzy, light-headed, drowsy, or less alert than they are normally. *Make sure you know how you react to this medicine before you drive, use machines, or do anything else that could be dangerous if you are dizzy or are not alert.*

Side Effects of This Medicine

Along with its needed effects, a medicine may cause some unwanted effects. Although not all of these side effects may occur, if they do occur they may need medical attention.

Check with your doctor as soon as possible if any of the following side effects occur:

Rare

Chills; difficulty in speaking or swallowing; dizziness or fainting; fast or irregular heartbeat; fever; general feeling of tiredness or weakness; headache (severe or continuing); increase in blood pressure; lip smacking or puckering; loss of balance control; mask-like face; rapid or worm-like movements of tongue; shuffling walk; sore throat; stiffness of arms or legs; trembling and shaking of hands and fingers; uncontrolled chewing movements; uncontrolled movements of arms and legs

*With high doses—may occur within minutes of receiving
a dose of metoclopramide and last for 2 to 24 hours*
>   Aching or discomfort in lower legs; panic-like sensation; sensation of crawling in legs; unusual nervousness, restlessness, or irritability

*Symptoms of overdose—may also occur rarely with usual
doses, especially in children and young adults, and with
high doses used to treat the nausea and vomiting caused
by anticancer medicines*
>   Confusion; drowsiness (severe)

Other side effects may occur that usually do not need medical attention. These side effects may go away during treatment as your body adjusts to the medicine. However, check with your doctor if any of the following side effects continue or are bothersome:

More common
>   Diarrhea—with high doses; drowsiness; restlessness

Less common or rare
>   Breast tenderness and swelling; changes in menstruation; constipation; depression; increased flow of breast milk; nausea; skin rash; trouble in sleeping; unusual dryness of mouth; unusual irritability

Other side effects not listed above may also occur in some patients. If you notice any other effects, check with your doctor.

Additional Information

Once a medicine has been approved for marketing for a certain use, experience may show that it is also useful for other medical problems. Although these uses are not included in product labeling, metoclopramide is used in certain patients with the following medical conditions:

- Failure of the stomach to empty its contents
- Nausea and vomiting caused by other medicines
- Persistent hiccups
- Prevention of aspirating fluid into the lungs during surgery
- Vascular headaches

Other than the above information, there is no additional information relating to proper use, precautions, or side effects for these uses.

METRONIDAZOLE   Systemic

Some commonly used brand names are:

In the U.S.

Flagyl	Metric 21
Flagyl I.V.	Metro I.V.
Flagyl I.V. RTU	Protostat
Metizol	

Generic name product may also be available.

In Canada

Apo-Metronidazole	Novonidazol
Flagyl	PMS Metronidazole
Neo-Metric	Trikacide

Generic name product may also be available.

Description

Metronidazole (me-troe-NI-da-zole) is used to treat infections. It may also be used for other problems as determined by your doctor. It will not work for colds, flu, or other virus infections.

Metronidazole is available only with your doctor's prescription, in the following dosage forms:

Oral
- Capsules (Canada)
- Tablets (U.S. and Canada)

Parenteral
- Injection (U.S. and Canada)

It is very important that you read and understand the following information. If any of it causes you special concern, check with your doctor. Also, *if you have any questions* or if you want more information about this medicine or your medical problem, *ask your doctor, nurse, or pharmacist.*

Before Using This Medicine

In deciding to use a medicine, the risks of taking the medicine must be weighed against the good it will do. This is a decision you and your doctor will make. For metronidazole, the following should be considered:

Allergies—Tell your doctor if you have ever had any unusual or allergic reaction to metronidazole. Also tell your doctor and pharmacist if you are allergic to any other substances, such as foods, preservatives, or dyes.

Pregnancy—Studies have not been done in humans. Metronidazole has not been shown to cause birth defects in animal studies; however, use is not recommended during the first trimester of pregnancy.

Breast-feeding—Use is not recommended in nursing mothers since metronidazole passes into the breast milk and may cause unwanted effects in the baby. However, in some infections your doctor may want you to stop breast-feeding and take this medicine for a short time. During this time the breast milk should be squeezed out or sucked out with a breast pump and thrown away. One or two days after you finish taking this medicine, you may go back to breast-feeding.

Children—Metronidazole has been used in children and, in effective doses, has not been shown to cause different side effects or problems in children than it does in adults.

Older adults—Many medicines have not been studied specifically in older people. Therefore, it may not be known whether they work exactly the same way they do in younger adults or if they cause different side effects or problems in older people. There is no specific information comparing use of metronidazole in the elderly with use in other age groups.

Other medicines—Although certain medicines should not be used together at all, in other cases two different medicines may be used together even if an interaction might occur. In these cases, your doctor may want to change the dose, or other precautions may be necessary. When you are taking metronidazole, it is especially important that your doctor and pharmacist know if you are taking any of the following:

- Anticoagulants (blood thinners)—Patients taking anticoagulants with metronidazole may have an increased chance of bleeding

- Disulfiram (e.g., Antabuse)—Patients taking disulfiram with metronidazole may have an increase in side effects affecting the central nervous system

Other medical problems—The presence of other medical problems may affect the use of metronidazole. Make sure you tell your doctor if you have any other medical problems, especially:

- Blood disease or a history of blood disease—Metronidazole may make the condition worse
- Central nervous system (CNS) disease, including epilepsy—Metronidazole may increase the chance of seizures (convulsions) or other CNS side effects
- Heart disease—Patients receiving metronidazole by injection may have a worsening of heart disease
- Liver disease, severe—Patients with severe liver disease may have an increase in side effects

Before you begin using any new medicine (prescription or nonprescription) or if you develop any new medical problem while you are using this medicine, check with your doctor, nurse, or pharmacist.

Proper Use of This Medicine

If this medicine upsets your stomach, it may be taken with meals or a snack. If stomach upset (nausea, vomiting, stomach pain, or diarrhea) continues, check with your doctor.

To help clear up your infection completely, *keep taking this medicine for the full time of treatment,* even if you begin to feel better after a few days. If you stop taking this medicine too soon, your symptoms may return.

In some kinds of infections, this medicine works best when there is a constant amount in the blood. *To help keep the amount constant, do not miss any doses. Also, it is best to take the doses at evenly spaced times, day and night.* For example, if you are to take 4 doses a day, the doses should be spaced about 6 hours apart. If this interferes with your sleep or other daily activities, or if you need help in planning the best times to take your medicine, check with your doctor, nurse, or pharmacist.

Missed dose—If you do miss a dose of this medicine, take it as soon as possible. This will help to keep a constant amount of medicine in the blood. However, if it is almost time for your next dose, skip the missed dose and go back to your regular dosing schedule. Do not double doses.

Storage—To store this medicine:

- Keep out of the reach of children.
- Store away from heat and direct light.
- Do not store the capsule or tablet form of this medicine in the bathroom, near the kitchen sink, or in other damp places. Heat or moisture may cause the medicine to break down.
- Do not keep outdated medicine or medicine no longer needed. Be sure that any discarded medicine is out of the reach of children.

Precautions While Using This Medicine

If your symptoms do not improve within a few days, or if they become worse, check with your doctor.

Drinking alcoholic beverages while taking this medicine may cause stomach pain, nausea, vomiting, headache, or flushing or redness of the face. Other alcohol-containing preparations (for example, elixirs, cough syrups, tonics) may also cause problems. These problems may last for at least a day after you stop taking metronidazole. Also, this medicine may cause alcoholic beverages to taste different. Therefore, *you should not drink alcoholic beverages or take other alcohol-containing preparations while you are taking this medicine and for at least a day after stopping it*.

Metronidazole may cause dryness of the mouth, an unpleasant or sharp metallic taste, and a change in taste sensation. For temporary relief of dry mouth, use sugarless candy or gum, melt bits of ice in your mouth, or use a saliva substitute. However, if your mouth continues to feel dry for more than 2 weeks, check with your medical doctor or dentist. Continuing dryness of the mouth may increase the chance of dental disease, including tooth decay, gum disease, and fungus infections.

This medicine may also cause some people to become dizzy or lightheaded. *Make sure you know how you react to this medicine before you drive, use machines, or do anything else that could be dangerous if you are dizzy or are not alert.* If these reactions are especially bothersome, check with your doctor.

If you are taking this medicine for trichomoniasis (an infection of the sex organs in males and females), your doctor may want to treat your sexual partner at the same time you are being treated, even if he or she has no symptoms. Also, it may be desirable to use a condom (prophylactic) during intercourse. These measures will help keep you from getting the infection back again from your partner. If you have any questions about this, check with your doctor.

Side Effects of This Medicine

Along with its needed effects, a medicine may cause some unwanted effects. Although not all of these side effects may occur, if they do occur they may need medical attention.

Check with your doctor immediately if any of the following side effects occur:

   Less common
   Numbness, tingling, pain, or weakness in hands or feet
   Rare
   Convulsions (seizures)

Also, check with your doctor as soon as possible if any of the following side effects occur:

   Less common
   Any vaginal irritation, discharge, or dryness not present before use of this medicine; clumsiness or unsteadiness; mood or other mental changes; skin rash, hives, redness, or itching; sore throat and fever; stomach and back pain (severe)

   For injection form
   Pain, tenderness, redness, or swelling over vein in which the medicine is given

Other side effects may occur that usually do not need medical attention. These side effects may go away during treat-

ment as your body adjusts to the medicine. However, check with your doctor if any of the following side effects continue or are bothersome:

More common

   Diarrhea; dizziness or lightheadedness; headache; loss of appetite; nausea or vomiting; stomach pain or cramps

Less common or rare

   Change in taste sensation; dryness of mouth; unpleasant or sharp metallic taste

In some patients metronidazole may cause dark urine. This is only temporary and will go away when you stop taking this medicine.

Other side effects not listed above may also occur in some patients. If you notice any other effects, check with your doctor.

Additional Information

Once a medicine has been approved for marketing for a certain use, experience may show that it is also useful for other medical problems. Although these uses are not included in product labeling, metronidazole is used in certain patients with the following medical conditions:

- Antibiotic-associated colitis
- Bacterial vaginosis
- Balantidiasis
- Dental infections
- Gastritis or ulcer due to *Helicobacter pylori*
- Giardiasis
- Inflammatory bowel disease

For patients taking this medicine for *giardiasis*:

- After treatment, it is important that your doctor check whether or not the infection in your intestinal tract has been cleared up completely.

Other than the above information, there is no additional information relating to proper use, precautions, or side effects for this use.

MISOPROSTOL Systemic

A commonly used brand name in the U.S. and Canada is Cytotec.

Description

Misoprostol (mye-soe-PROST-ole) is taken to prevent stomach ulcers in patients taking anti-inflammatory drugs, including aspirin. Misoprostol may also be used for other conditions as determined by your doctor.

Misoprostol helps the stomach protect itself against acid damage. It also decreases the amount of acid produced by the stomach.

This medicine is available only with your doctor's prescription, in the following dosage form:

Oral
- Tablets (U.S. and Canada)

It is very important that you read and understand the following information. If any of it causes you special concern, check with your doctor. Also, *if you have any questions* or if you want more information about this medicine or your medical problem, *ask your doctor, nurse, or pharmacist.*

Before Using This Medicine

In deciding to use a medicine, the risks of taking the medicine must be weighed against the good it will do. This is a decision you and your doctor will make. For misoprostol, the following should be considered:

Allergies—Tell your doctor if you have ever had any unusual or allergic reaction to misoprostol. Also tell your doctor and pharmacist if you are allergic to any other substances, such as foods, preservatives, or dyes.

Pregnancy—*Misoprostol must not be used during pregnancy.* It has been shown to cause contractions and bleeding of the uterus. Misoprostol may also cause miscarriage.

Before starting to take this medicine you must have had a negative pregnancy test within the previous 2 weeks. Also, you must start taking misoprostol only on the second or third day of your next normal menstrual period. In addition, it will be necessary that you use an effective form of birth control while taking this medicine. Be sure that you have discussed this with your doctor before taking this medicine.

Breast-feeding—It is not known whether misoprostol passes into breast milk. However, misoprostol is not recommended for use during breast-feeding because it may cause diarrhea in nursing babies.

Children—Studies on this medicine have been done only in adult patients, and there is no specific information comparing use of misoprostol in children with use in other age groups.

Older adults—This medicine has been tested and has not been shown to cause different side effects or problems in older people than it does in younger adults.

Other medicines—Although certain medicines should not be used together at all, in other cases two different medicines may be used together even if an interaction might occur. In these cases, your doctor may want to change the dose, or other precautions may be necessary. Tell your doctor and pharmacist if you are taking any other prescription or non-prescription (over-the-counter [OTC]) medicine.

Other medical problems—The presence of other medical problems may affect the use of misoprostol. Make sure you tell your doctor if you have any other medical problems, especially:

- Blood vessel disease—Medicines similar to misoprostol have been shown to make this condition worse
- Epilepsy (uncontrolled)—Medicines similar to misoprostol have been shown to cause convulsions (seizures)

Before you begin using any new medicine (prescription or nonprescription) or if you develop any new medical problem while you are using this medicine, check with your doctor, nurse, or pharmacist.

Proper Use of This Medicine

Misoprostol is best taken with or after meals and at bedtime, unless otherwise directed by your doctor.

Missed dose—If you miss a dose of this medicine, take it as soon as possible. However, if it is almost time for your next dose, skip the missed dose and go back to your regular dosing schedule. Do not double doses.

Storage—To store this medicine:
- Keep out of the reach of children.
- Store away from heat and direct light.
- Do not store in the bathroom, near the kitchen sink, or in other damp places. Heat or moisture may cause the medicine to break down.
- Do not keep outdated medicine or medicine no longer needed. Be sure that any discarded medicine is out of the reach of children.

Precautions While Using This Medicine

Misoprostol may cause miscarriage if taken during pregnancy. Therefore, if you suspect that you may have become pregnant, stop taking this medicine immediately and check with your doctor.

This medicine may cause diarrhea in some people. The diarrhea will usually disappear within a few days as your body adjusts to the medicine. However, check with your doctor if the diarrhea is severe and/or does not stop after a week. Your doctor may have to lower the dose of misoprostol you are taking.

Side Effects of This Medicine

Along with its needed effects, a medicine may cause some unwanted effects. Some side effects may occur that usually do not need medical attention. These side effects may go away during treatment as your body adjusts to the medicine. However, check with your doctor if any of the following side effects continue or are bothersome:

More common
    Abdominal or stomach pain (mild); diarrhea

Less common or rare

> Bleeding from vagina; constipation; cramps in lower abdo-
> men or stomach area; gas; headache; nausea and/or vom-
> iting

Other side effects not listed above may also occur in some
patients. If you notice any other effects, check with your
doctor.

Additional Information

Once a medicine has been approved for marketing for a
certain use, experience may show that it is also useful for
other medical problems. Although this use is not included
in product labeling, misoprostol is used in certain patients
with the following medical condition:

- Duodenal ulcers

For patients taking this medicine for *duodenal ulcers*:

- Antacids may be taken with misoprostol, if needed, to
  help relieve stomach pain, unless you are otherwise directed by your doctor. However, do not take magnesium-containing antacids, since they may cause diarrhea or worsen the diarrhea that is sometimes caused
  by misoprostol.

- Take this medicine for the full time of treatment, even
  if you begin to feel better. Also, it is important that
  you keep your appointments with your doctor so that
  your doctor will be better able to tell you when to stop
  taking this medicine.

- *Misoprostol is not normally taken for more than 4
  weeks when used to treat duodenal ulcers.* However,
  your doctor may order treatment for a second 4-week
  period if needed.

Other than the above information, there is no additional
information relating to proper use, precautions, or side effects for these uses.

NARCOTIC ANALGESICS—For Pain Relief   Systemic

This information applies to the following medicines:

    Buprenorphine (byoo-pre-NOR-feen)
    Butorphanol (byoo-TOR-fa-nole)
    Codeine (KOE-deen)
    Hydrocodone (hye-droe-KOE-done)
    Hydromorphone (hye-droe-MOR-fone)
    Levorphanol (lee-VOR-fa-nole)
    Meperidine (me-PER-i-deen)
    Methadone (METH-a-done)
    Morphine (MOR-feen)
    Nalbuphine (NAL-byoo-feen)
    Opium Injection (OH-pee-um)
    Oxycodone (ox-i-KOE-done)
    Oxymorphone (ox-i-MOR-fone)
    Pentazocine (pen-TAZ-oh-seen)
    Propoxyphene (proe-POX-i-feen)

This information does *not* apply to Opium Tincture or Paregoric.

Some commonly used brand names are:

For Buprenorphine
    In the U.S.
        Buprenex

For Butorphanol
    In the U.S.
        Stadol
    In Canada
        Stadol

For Codeine
    In the U.S.
        Available by generic name.
    In Canada
        Paveral
        Generic name product may also be available.

For Hydrocodone*
    In Canada
        Hycodan‡
        Robidone

For Hydromorphone
    In the U.S.
        Dilaudid
        Dilaudid-HP
        Generic name product may also be available.

In Canada
> Dilaudid
> Dilaudid-HP

Another commonly used name is dihydromorphinone.

For Levorphanol
In the U.S.
> Levo-Dromoran
>
> Generic name product may also be available.

In Canada
> Levo-Dromoran

Another commonly used name is levorphan.

For Meperidine
In the U.S.
> Demerol
>
> Generic name product may also be available.

In Canada
> Demerol
>
> Generic name product may also be available.

Another commonly used name is pethidine.

For Methadone§
In the U.S.
> Dolophine
> Methadose
>
> Generic name product may also be available.

For Morphine
In the U.S.

Astramorph	RMS Uniserts
Astramorph PF	Roxanol
Duramorph	Roxanol 100
M S Contin	Roxanol SR
MSIR	

Generic name product may also be available.

In Canada

Epimorph	M.O.S.-S.R.
Morphine H.P.	M S Contin
Morphitec	Roxanol
M.O.S.	Statex

Generic name product may also be available.

For Nalbuphine
In the U.S.
> Nubain
>
> Generic name product may also be available.

In Canada
    Nubain

For Opium
  In the U.S.
    Pantopon

  In Canada
    Pantopon

Another commonly used name is papaveretum.

For Oxycodone
  In the U.S.
    Roxicodone

  In Canada
    Supeudol

For Oxymorphone
  In the U.S.
    Numorphan

  In Canada
    Numorphan

For Pentazocine
  In the U.S.
    Talwin
    Talwin-Nx

  In Canada
    Talwin

For Propoxyphene
  In the U.S.

Darvon	Doxaphene
Darvon-N	Profene
Dolene	Pro Pox
Doraphen	Propoxycon

    Generic name product may also be available.

  In Canada

Darvon-N	642
Novopropoxyn	

Another commonly used name is dextropropoxyphene.

---

*Not commercially available in the U.S.
‡For Canadian product only. In the U.S., *Hycodan* also contains homatropine; in Canada, *Hycodan* contains only hydrocodone.
§In Canada, methadone is available only through doctors who have received special approval to prescribe it.

Description

Narcotic (nar-KOT-ik) analgesics (an-al-JEE-zicks) are used to relieve pain. Some of these medicines are also used just before or during an operation to help the anesthetic work better. Codeine and hydrocodone are also used to relieve coughing. Methadone is also used to help some people control their dependence on heroin or other narcotics. Narcotic analgesics may also be used for other conditions as determined by your doctor.

Narcotic analgesics act in the central nervous system (CNS) to relieve pain. Some of their side effects are also caused by actions in the CNS.

If a narcotic is used for a long time, it may become habit-forming (causing mental or physical dependence). Physical dependence may lead to withdrawal side effects when you stop taking the medicine.

These medicines are available only with your medical doctor's or dentist's prescription. For some of them, prescriptions cannot be refilled and you must obtain a new prescription from your medical doctor or dentist each time you need the medicine. In addition, other rules and regulations may apply when methadone is used to treat narcotic dependence.

These medicines are available in the following dosage forms:

Oral

Codeine
- Oral solution (U.S. and Canada)
- Tablets (U.S. and Canada)

Hydrocodone
- Syrup (Canada)
- Tablets (Canada)

Hydromorphone
- Tablets (U.S. and Canada)

Levorphanol
- Tablets (U.S. and Canada)

Meperidine
- Syrup (U.S.)
- Tablets (U.S. and Canada)

Methadone
- Oral concentrate (U.S.)
- Oral solution (U.S.)
- Tablets (U.S.)
- Dispersible tablets (U.S.)

Morphine
- Oral solution (U.S. and Canada)
- Syrup (Canada)
- Tablets (U.S. and Canada)
- Extended-release tablets (U.S. and Canada)

Oxycodone
- Oral solution (U.S.)
- Tablets (U.S. and Canada)

Pentazocine
- Tablets (Canada)

Pentazocine and Naloxone
- Tablets (U.S.)

Propoxyphene
- Capsules (U.S. and Canada)
- Oral suspension (U.S.)
- Tablets (U.S. and Canada)

Parenteral

Buprenorphine
- Injection (U.S.)

Butorphanol
- Injection (U.S. and Canada)

Codeine
- Injection (U.S. and Canada)

Hydromorphone
- Injection (U.S. and Canada)

Levorphanol
- Injection (U.S. and Canada)

Meperidine
- Injection (U.S. and Canada)

Methadone
- Injection (U.S.)

Morphine
- Injection (U.S. and Canada)

Nalbuphine
- Injection (U.S. and Canada)

Opium
- Injection (U.S. and Canada)

Oxymorphone
- Injection (U.S. and Canada)

Pentazocine
- Injection (U.S. and Canada)

Rectal

Hydromorphone
- Suppositories (U.S. and Canada)

Morphine
- Suppositories (U.S. and Canada)

Oxycodone
- Suppositories (Canada)

Oxymorphone
- Suppositories (U.S. and Canada)

It is very important that you read and understand the following information. If any of it causes you special concern, check with your doctor. Also, *if you have any questions* or if you want more information about this medicine or your medical problem, *ask your doctor, nurse, or pharmacist.*

Before Using This Medicine

In deciding to use a medicine, the risks of taking the medicine must be weighed against the good it will do. This is a decision you and your doctor will make. For narcotic analgesics, the following should be considered:

Allergies—Tell your doctor if you have ever had any unusual or allergic reaction to any of the narcotic analgesics. Also tell your doctor and pharmacist if you are allergic to any other substances, such as foods, preservatives, or dyes.

Pregnancy—Although studies on birth defects with narcotic analgesics have not been done in pregnant women, these medicines have not been reported to cause birth defects. However, hydrocodone, hydromorphone, and morphine caused birth defects in animals when given in very large doses. Buprenorphine and codeine did not cause birth defects in animal studies, but they caused other unwanted effects. Butorphanol, nalbuphine, pentazocine, and propoxyphene did not cause birth defects in animals. There is no information about whether other narcotic analgesics cause birth defects in animals.

Too much use of a narcotic during pregnancy may cause the baby to become dependent on the medicine. This may lead to withdrawal side effects after birth. Also, some of these medicines may cause breathing problems in the newborn infant if taken just before delivery.

Breast-feeding—Most narcotic analgesics have not been reported to cause problems in nursing babies. However, when the mother is taking large amounts of methadone (in a methadone maintenance program), the nursing baby may become dependent on the medicine. Also, butorphanol, codeine, meperidine, morphine, opium, and propoxyphene pass into the breast milk.

Children—Breathing problems may be especially likely to occur in children younger than 2 years of age. These children are usually more sensitive than adults to the effects of narcotic analgesics. Also, unusual excitement or restlessness may be more likely to occur in children receiving these medicines.

Older adults—Elderly people are especially sensitive to the effects of narcotic analgesics. This may increase the chance of side effects, especially breathing problems, during treatment.

Athletes—Narcotic analgesics are banned and tested for by the U.S. Olympic Committee (USOC). Narcotic use can lead to disqualification of athletes in USOC-sponsored events.

Other medicines—Although certain medicines should not be used together at all, in other cases two different medicines may be used together even if an interaction might occur. In these cases, your doctor may want to change the dose, or other precautions may be necessary. When you are taking a narcotic analgesic, it is especially important that your doctor and pharmacist know if you are taking any of the following:

- Carbamazepine (e.g., Tegretol)—Propoxyphene may increase the blood levels of carbamazepine, which increases the chance of serious side effects
- Central nervous system (CNS) depressants or
- Monoamine oxidase (MAO) inhibitors (furazolidone [e.g., Furoxone], isocarboxazid [e.g., Marplan], pargyline [e.g., Eutonyl], phenelzine [e.g., Nardil], procarbazine [e.g., Matulane], tranylcypromine [e.g., Parnate] (taken currently or within the past 2 weeks) or

- Tricyclic antidepressants (amitriptyline [e.g., Elavil], amoxapine [e.g., Asendin], clomipramine [e.g., Anafranil], desipramine [e.g., Pertofrane], doxepin [e.g., Sinequan], imipramine [e.g., Tofranil], nortriptyline [e.g., Aventyl], protriptyline [e.g., Vivactil], trimipramine [e.g., Surmontil])—The chance of side effects may be increased; the combination of meperidine (e.g., Demerol) and MAO inhibitors is especially dangerous
- Naltrexone (e.g., Trexan)—Narcotics will not be effective in people taking naltrexone
- Rifampin (e.g., Rifadin)—Rifampin decreases the effects of methadone and may cause withdrawal symptoms in people who are dependent on methadone
- Zidovudine (e.g., AZT, Retrovir)—Morphine may increase the blood levels of zidovudine and increase the chance of serious side effects

Other medical problems—The presence of other medical problems may affect the use of narcotic analgesics. Make sure you tell your doctor if you have any other medical problems, especially:

- Alcohol abuse, or history of, or
- Drug dependence, especially narcotic abuse, or history of, or
- Emotional problems—The chance of side effects may be increased; also, withdrawal symptoms may occur if a narcotic you are dependent on is replaced by buprenorphine, butorphanol, nalbuphine, or pentazocine
- Brain disease or head injury or
- Emphysema, asthma, or other chronic lung disease or
- Enlarged prostate or problems with urination or
- Gallbladder disease or gallstones—Some of the side effects of narcotic analgesics can be dangerous if these conditions are present
- Colitis or
- Heart disease or
- Kidney disease or
- Liver disease or
- Underactive thyroid—The chance of side effects may be increased
- Convulsions (seizures), history of—Some of the narcotic analgesics can cause convulsions

Before you begin using any new medicine (prescription or nonprescription) or if you develop any new medical problem while you are using this medicine, check with your doctor, nurse, or pharmacist.

Proper Use of This Medicine

Some narcotic analgesics given by injection may be given at home to patients who do not need to be in the hospital. If you are using an injection form of this medicine at home, *make sure you clearly understand and carefully follow your doctor's instructions.*

To take the *syrup form of meperidine:*
- Unless otherwise directed by your medical doctor or dentist, *take this medicine mixed with a half glass (4 ounces) of water* to lessen the numbing effect of the medicine on your mouth and throat.

To take the *oral liquid forms of methadone:*
- *This medicine may have to be mixed with water or another liquid before you take it.* Read the label carefully for directions. If you have any questions about this, check with your doctor, nurse, or pharmacist.

To take the *dispersible tablet form of methadone:*
- *These tablets must be stirred into water or fruit juice just before each dose is taken. Read the label carefully for directions.* If you have any questions about this, check with your doctor, nurse, or pharmacist.

To take *oral liquid forms of morphine:*
- This medicine may be mixed with a glass of fruit juice just before you take it, if desired, to improve the taste.

To take *long-acting morphine tablets:*
- *These tablets must be swallowed whole.* Do not break, crush, or chew them before swallowing.

To use *suppositories:*
- If the suppository is too soft to insert, chill it in the refrigerator for 30 minutes or run cold water over it before removing the foil wrapper.

- To insert the suppository: First remove the foil wrapper and moisten the suppository with cold water. Lie down on your side and use your finger to push the suppository well up into the rectum.

Take this medicine only as directed by your medical doctor or dentist. Do not take more of it, do not take it more often, and do not take it for a longer time than your medical doctor or dentist ordered. This is especially important for young children and elderly patients, who are especially sensitive to the effects of narcotic analgesics. If too much is taken, the medicine may become habit-forming (causing mental or physical dependence) or lead to medical problems because of an overdose.

If you think this medicine is not working properly after you have been taking it for a few weeks, *do not increase the dose.* Instead, check with your doctor.

Missed dose—If your medical doctor or dentist has ordered you to take this medicine according to a regular schedule and you miss a dose, take it as soon as you remember. However, if it is almost time for your next dose, skip the missed dose and go back to your regular dosing schedule. *Do not double doses.*

Storage—To store this medicine:

- Keep out of the reach of children. Overdose is very dangerous in young children.
- Store away from heat and direct light.
- Do not store tablets or capsules in the bathroom, near the kitchen sink, or in other damp places. Heat or moisture may cause the medicine to break down.
- Store hydromorphone, oxycodone, or oxymorphone suppositories in the refrigerator.
- Keep liquid (including injections) and suppository forms of the medicine from freezing.
- Do not keep outdated medicine or medicine no longer needed. Be sure that any discarded medicine is out of the reach of children.

Precautions While Using This Medicine

If you will be taking this medicine for a long time (for example, for several months at a time), your doctor should check your progress at regular visits.

Narcotic analgesics will add to the effects of alcohol and other CNS depressants (medicines that slow down the nervous system, possibly causing drowsiness). Some examples of CNS depressants are antihistamines or medicine for hay fever, other allergies, or colds; sedatives, tranquilizers, or sleeping medicine; other prescription pain medicines including other narcotics; barbiturates; medicine for seizures; muscle relaxants; or anesthetics, including some dental anesthetics. *Do not drink alcoholic beverages, and check with your medical doctor or dentist before taking any of the medicines listed above, while you are using this medicine.*

This medicine may cause some people to become drowsy, dizzy, or lightheaded, or to feel a false sense of well-being. *Make sure you know how you react to this medicine before you drive, use machines, or do anything else that could be dangerous if you are dizzy or are not alert and clearheaded.*

Dizziness, lightheadedness, or fainting may occur, especially when you get up suddenly from a lying or sitting position. Getting up slowly may help lessen this problem.

Nausea or vomiting may occur, especially after the first couple of doses. This effect may go away if you lie down for a while. However, if nausea or vomiting continues, check with your medical doctor or dentist. Lying down for a while may also help relieve some other side effects, such as dizziness or lightheadedness, that may occur.

Before having any kind of surgery (including dental surgery) or emergency treatment, tell the medical doctor or dentist in charge that you are taking this medicine.

Narcotic analgesics may cause dryness of the mouth. For temporary relief, use sugarless candy or gum, melt bits of ice in your mouth, or use a saliva substitute. However, if dry mouth continues for more than 2 weeks, check with your dentist. Continuing dryness of the mouth may increase the chance of dental disease, including tooth decay, gum disease, and fungus infections.

If you have been taking this medicine regularly for several weeks or more, *do not suddenly stop using it without first checking with your doctor*. Your doctor may want you to reduce gradually the amount you are taking before stopping completely, in order to lessen the chance of withdrawal side effects.

If you think you or someone else may have taken an overdose, get emergency help at once. Taking an overdose of this medicine or taking alcohol or CNS depressants with this medicine may lead to unconsciousness or death. Signs of overdose include convulsions (seizures), confusion, severe nervousness or restlessness, severe dizziness, severe drowsiness, slow or troubled breathing, and severe weakness.

Side Effects of This Medicine

Along with its needed effects, a medicine may cause some unwanted effects. Although not all of these side effects may occur, if they do occur they may need medical attention.

Get emergency help immediately if any of the following symptoms of overdose occur:

  Cold, clammy skin; confusion; convulsions (seizures); dizziness (severe); drowsiness (severe); low blood pressure; nervousness or restlessness (severe); pinpoint pupils of eyes; slow heartbeat; slow or troubled breathing; weakness (severe)

Also, check with your doctor as soon as possible if any of the following side effects occur:

Less common or rare

  Dark urine (for propoxyphene only); fast, slow, or pounding heartbeat; feelings of unreality; hallucinations (seeing, hearing, or feeling things that are not there); hives, itching, or skin rash; increased sweating (more common with hydrocodone, meperidine, and methadone); irregular breathing; mental depression or other mood or mental changes; pale stools (for propoxyphene only); redness or flushing of face (more common with hydrocodone, meperidine, and methadone); ringing or buzzing in the ears; shortness of breath, wheezing, or troubled breathing;

swelling of face; trembling or uncontrolled muscle movements; unusual excitement or restlessness (especially in
children); yellow eyes or skin (for propoxyphene only)

Other side effects may occur that usually do not need medical attention. These side effects may go away during treatment as your body adjusts to the medicine. However, check
with your doctor if any of the following side effects continue
or are bothersome:

More common

Dizziness, lightheadedness, or feeling faint; drowsiness; nausea or vomiting

Less common or rare

Blurred or double vision or other changes in vision; constipation (more common with long-term use and with codeine); decrease in amount of urine; difficult or painful
urination; dry mouth; false sense of well-being; frequent
urge to urinate; general feeling of discomfort or illness;
headache; loss of appetite; nervousness or restlessness;
nightmares or unusual dreams; redness, swelling, pain, or
burning at place of injection; stomach cramps or pain;
trouble in sleeping; unusual tiredness or weakness

After you stop using this medicine, your body may need
time to adjust. The length of time this takes depends on the
amount of medicine you were using and how long you used
it. During this period of time check with your doctor if you
notice any of the following side effects:

Body aches; diarrhea; fast heartbeat; fever, runny nose, or sneezing; gooseflesh; increased sweating; increased yawning; loss
of appetite; nausea or vomiting; nervousness, restlessness, or
irritability; shivering or trembling; stomach cramps; trouble
in sleeping; unusually large pupils of eyes; weakness

Other side effects not listed above may also occur in some
patients. If you notice any other effects, check with your
doctor.

NARCOTIC ANALGESICS AND ACETAMINOPHEN   Systemic

This information applies to the following medicines:

Acetaminophen (a-seat-a-MIN-oh-fen) and Codeine (KOE-deen)
Acetaminophen, Codeine, and Caffeine (kaf-EEN)
Dihydrocodeine (dye-hye-droe-KOE-deen), Acetaminophen, and Caffeine
Hydrocodone (hye-droe-KOE-done) and Acetaminophen
Meperidine (me-PER-i-deen) and Acetaminophen
Oxycodone (ox-i-KOE-done) and Acetaminophen
Pentazocine (pen-TAZ-oh-seen) and Acetaminophen
Propoxyphene (proe-POX-i-feen) and Acetaminophen

Some commonly used brand names are:

For Acetaminophen and Codeine
In the U.S.

Acetaco	Proval
Aceta with Codeine	Pyregesic-C
Capital with Codeine	Tylaprin with Codeine
M-Gesic	Tylenol with Codeine
Myapap with Codeine	Tylenol with Codeine No.1
Phenaphen with Codeine	Tylenol with Codeine No.2
No.2‡	Tylenol with Codeine No.3
Phenaphen with Codeine	Tylenol with Codeine No.4
No.3‡	Ty-Pap with Codeine
Phenaphen with Codeine	Ty-Tab with Codeine No.2
No.4‡	Ty-Tab with Codeine No.3
Phenaphen-650 with Codeine	Ty-Tab with Codeine No.4

Generic name product may also be available.

In Canada

Empracet-30	Rounox and Codeine 15
Empracet-60	Rounox and Codeine 30
Emtec-30	Rounox and Codeine 60
Lenoltec with Codeine No.4	Tylenol with Codeine No.4

Another commonly used name is APAP with codeine.

For Acetaminophen, Codeine, and Caffeine
In the U.S.

Codalan No.1	Codalan No.3
Codalan No.2	

In Canada

Atasol-8
Atasol-15
Atasol-30
Codamin #2
Codamin #3
Codaminophen
Exdol-8
Exdol-15
Exdol-30
Lenoltec with Codeine No.1
Lenoltec with Codeine No.2

Lenoltec with Codeine No.3
Novogesic C8
Novogesic C15
Novogesic C30
Tylenol No.1
Tylenol No.1 Forte
Tylenol with Codeine
Tylenol with Codeine No.2
Tylenol with Codeine No.3
Veganin

Generic name product may also be available.

For Dihydrocodeine, Acetaminophen, and Caffeine†
In the U.S.
Compal

Another commonly used name is drocode, acetaminophen, and caffeine.

For Hydrocodone and Acetaminophen†
In the U.S.

Allay
Amacodone
Anexsia
Anexsia 7.5
Anodynos DHC
Anolor DH 5
Bancap-HC
Co-Gesic
Dolacet
Duocet
Duradyne DHC
HY-5
Hycomed
Hycopap
Hyco-Pap
Hydrocet
Hydrogesic
HY-PHEN

Lorcet-HD
Lorcet Plus
Lortab
Lortab 5
Lortab 7
Megagesic
Norcet
Norcet 7.5
Polygesic
Propain-HC
Rogesic No.3
Senefen III
Ultragesic
Vapocet
Vicodin
Vicodin ES
Zydone

Generic name product may also be available.

Another commonly used name is hydrocodone with APAP.

For Meperidine and Acetaminophen†
In the U.S.
Demerol-APAP

For Oxycodone and Acetaminophen
In the U.S.

Percocet
Roxicet

Roxicet 5/500
Tylox

Generic name product may also be available.

In Canada
    Endocet   Percocet
    Oxycocet   Percocet-Demi

Another commonly used name is oxycodone with APAP.

For Pentazocine and Acetaminophen†
In the U.S.
    Talacen

For Propoxyphene and Acetaminophen†
In the U.S.

Darvocet-N 50	E-Lor
Darvocet-N 100	Genagesic
Dolene-AP-65	Propacet 100
Doxapap-N	Pro Pox with APAP
D-Rex 65	Wygesic

Generic name product may also be available.

Another commonly used name is propoxyphene with APAP.

---

†Not commercially available in Canada.

‡In Canada, *Phenaphen with Codeine* is different from the product with that name in the U.S. The Canadian product contains phenobarbital, ASA, and codeine.

Description

Combination medicines containing narcotic (nar-KOT-ik) analgesics (an-al-JEE-zicks) and acetaminophen are used to relieve pain. A narcotic analgesic and acetaminophen used together may provide better pain relief than either medicine used alone. In some cases, relief of pain may come at lower doses of each medicine.

Narcotic analgesics act in the central nervous system (CNS) to relieve pain. Many of their side effects are also caused by actions in the CNS. When narcotics are used for a long time, your body may get used to them so that larger amounts are needed to relieve pain. This is called tolerance to the medicine. Also, when narcotics are used for a long time or in large doses, they may become habit-forming (causing mental or physical dependence). Physical dependence may lead to withdrawal symptoms when you stop taking the medicine.

Acetaminophen does not become habit-forming when taken for a long time or in large doses, but it may cause other unwanted effects, including liver damage, if too much is taken.

In the U.S., these medicines are available only with your medical doctor's or dentist's prescription. In Canada, some acetaminophen, codeine, and caffeine combinations are available without a prescription.

These medicines are available in the following dosage forms:

Oral

Acetaminophen and Codeine
- Capsules (U.S.)
- Elixir (U.S. and Canada)
- Oral suspension (U.S.)
- Tablets (U.S. and Canada)

Acetaminophen, Codeine, and Caffeine
- Capsules (Canada)
- Tablets (U.S. and Canada)

Dihydrocodeine, Acetaminophen, and Caffeine
- Capsules (U.S.)

Hydrocodone and Acetaminophen
- Capsules (U.S.)
- Oral solution (U.S.)
- Tablets (U.S.)

Meperidine and Acetaminophen
- Tablets (U.S.)

Oxycodone and Acetaminophen
- Capsules (U.S.)
- Oral solution (U.S.)
- Tablets (U.S. and Canada)

Pentazocine and Acetaminophen
- Tablets (U.S.)

Propoxyphene and Acetaminophen
- Capsules (U.S.)
- Tablets (U.S.)

It is very important that you read and understand the following information. If any of it causes you special concern, check with your doctor. Also, *if you have any questions* or if you want more information about this medicine or your medical problem, *ask your doctor, nurse, or pharmacist.*

Before Using This Medicine

In deciding to use a medicine, the risks of taking the medicine must be weighed against the good it will do. This is a decision you and your doctor will make. For narcotic analgesic and acetaminophen combinations, the following should be considered:

Allergies—Tell your doctor if you have ever had any unusual or allergic reaction to acetaminophen or to a narcotic analgesic. Also tell your doctor and pharmacist if you are allergic to any other substances, such as foods, preservatives, or dyes.

Pregnancy—

- *For acetaminophen*: Although studies on birth defects with acetaminophen have not been done in pregnant women, it has not been reported to cause birth defects or other problems.

- *For narcotic analgesics*: Although studies on birth defects with narcotic analgesics have not been done in pregnant women, they have not been reported to cause birth defects. However, hydrocodone caused birth defects in animal studies when very large doses were used. Codeine did not cause birth defects in animals, but it caused slower development of bones and other toxic or harmful effects in the fetus. Pentazocine and propoxyphene did not cause birth defects in animals. There is no information about whether dihydrocodeine, meperidine, or oxycodone cause birth defects in animals.

  Too much use of a narcotic during pregnancy may cause the fetus to become dependent on the medicine. This may lead to withdrawal side effects in the newborn baby. Also, some of these medicines may cause breathing problems in the newborn baby if taken just before or during delivery.

- *For caffeine:* Studies in humans have not shown that caffeine (contained in some of these combination medicines) causes birth defects. However, studies in animals have shown that caffeine causes birth defects when given in very large doses (amounts equal to those present in 12 to 24 cups of coffee a day).

Breast-feeding—Acetaminophen, codeine, meperidine, and propoxyphene pass into the breast milk. It is not known whether other narcotic analgesics pass into the breast milk. However, these medicines have not been reported to cause problems in nursing babies.

Children—Breathing problems may be especially likely to occur when narcotic analgesics are given to children younger than 2 years of age. These children are usually more sensitive than adults to the effects of narcotic analgesics. Also, unusual excitement or restlessness may be more likely to occur in children receiving these medicines.

Acetaminophen has been tested in children and has not been shown to cause different side effects or problems in children than it does in adults.

Older adults—Elderly people are especially sensitive to the effects of narcotic analgesics. This may increase the chance of side effects, especially breathing problems, during treatment.

Acetaminophen has been tested and has not been shown to cause different side effects or problems in older people than it does in younger adults.

Athletes—Narcotic analgesics are banned and tested for by the U.S. Olympic Committee (USOC). Narcotic use can lead to disqualification of athletes in USOC-sponsored events. Also, some of these combination medicines contain caffeine, which is tested for by the USOC and the National Collegiate Athletic Association (NCAA). These 2 groups have set specific limits on the amount of caffeine in the urine that they consider to be acceptable. An athlete will be disqualified for competition if the amount of caffeine in the urine is above these limits.

Other medicines—Although certain medicines should not be used together at all, in other cases two different medicines may be used together even if an interaction might occur. In these cases, your doctor may want to change the dose, or

other precautions may be necessary. When you are taking a narcotic analgesic and acetaminophen combination, it is especially important that your doctor and pharmacist know if you are taking any of the following:

- Carbamazepine (e.g., Tegretol)—Propoxyphene may increase the blood levels of carbamazepine, which increases the chance of serious side effects
- Central nervous system (CNS) depressants or
- Monoamine oxidase (MAO) inhibitors (furazolidone [e.g., Furoxone], isocarboxazid [e.g., Marplan], pargyline [e.g., Eutonyl], phenelzine [e.g., Nardil], procarbazine [e.g., Matulane], tranylcypromine [e.g., Parnate]) (taken currently or within the past 2 weeks) or
- Tricyclic antidepressants (amitriptyline [e.g., Elavil], amoxapine [e.g., Asendin], clomipramine [e.g., Anafranil], desipramine [e.g., Pertofrane], doxepin [e.g., Sinequan], imipramine [e.g., Tofranil], nortriptyline [e.g., Aventyl], protriptyline [e.g., Vivactil], trimipramine [e.g., Surmontil])—Taking these medicines together with a narcotic analgesic may increase the chance of serious side effects
- Naltrexone (e.g., Trexan)—Naltrexone keeps narcotic analgesics from working to relieve pain; people taking naltrexone should take pain relievers that do not contain a narcotic
- Zidovudine (e.g., AZT, Retrovir)—Acetaminophen may increase the blood levels of zidovudine, which increases the chance of serious side effects

Other medical problems—The presence of other medical problems may affect the use of narcotic analgesic and acetaminophen combinations. Make sure you tell your doctor if you have any other medical problems, especially:

- Alcohol and/or other drug abuse, or history of, or
- Brain disease or head injury or
- Colitis or
- Convulsions (seizures), history of, or
- Emotional problems or mental illness or
- Emphysema, asthma, or other chronic lung disease or
- Hepatitis or other liver disease or
- Kidney disease or
- Underactive thyroid—The chance of serious side effects may be increased

- Enlarged prostate or problems with urination or
- Gallbladder disease or gallstones—Some of the effects of narcotic analgesics may be especially serious in people with these medical problems
- Heart disease—Caffeine (present in some of these combination medicines) can make some kinds of heart disease worse

Before you begin using any new medicine (prescription or nonprescription) or if you develop any new medical problem while you are using this medicine, check with your doctor, nurse, or pharmacist.

Proper Use of This Medicine

Take this medicine only as directed by your medical doctor or dentist. Do not take more of it, do not take it more often, and do not take it for a longer time than your medical doctor or dentist ordered. This is especially important for young children and elderly patients, who may be more sensitive than other people to the effects of narcotic analgesics. If too much of a narcotic analgesic is taken, it may become habit-forming (causing mental or physical dependence) or lead to medical problems because of an overdose. Taking too much acetaminophen may cause liver damage.

If you think that this medicine is not working properly after you have been taking it for a few weeks, *do not increase the dose*. Instead, check with your medical doctor or dentist.

Missed dose—If your medical doctor or dentist has ordered you to take this medicine according to a regular schedule and you miss a dose, take it as soon as you remember. However, if it is almost time for your next dose, skip the missed dose and go back to your regular dosing schedule. *Do not double doses.*

Storage—To store this medicine:
- Keep out of the reach of children. Overdose is very dangerous in young children.
- Store away from heat and direct light.
- Do not store tablets or capsules in the bathroom, near the kitchen sink, or in other damp places. Heat or moisture may cause the medicine to break down.

- Keep the liquid forms of this medicine from freezing.
- Do not keep outdated medicine or medicine no longer needed. Be sure that any discarded medicine is out of the reach of children.

Precautions While Using This Medicine

If you will be taking this medicine for a long time (for example, for several months at a time), or in high doses, your doctor should check your progress at regular visits.

Check the labels of all nonprescription (over-the-counter [OTC]) and prescription medicines you now take. If any contain acetaminophen or a narcotic be especially careful, since taking them while taking this medicine may lead to overdose. If you have any questions about this, check with your medical doctor, dentist, or pharmacist.

The narcotic analgesic in this medicine will add to the effects of alcohol and other CNS depressants (medicines that slow down the nervous system, possibly causing drowsiness). Some examples of CNS depressants are antihistamines or medicine for hay fever, other allergies, or colds; sedatives, tranquilizers, or sleeping medicine; other prescription pain medicine or narcotics; barbiturates; medicine for seizures; muscle relaxants; or anesthetics, including some dental anesthetics. Also, there may be a greater risk of liver damage if large amounts of alcoholic beverages are used while you are taking acetaminophen. *Do not drink alcoholic beverages, and check with your medical doctor or dentist before taking any of the medicines listed above, while you are using this medicine.*

Too much use of the acetaminophen in this combination medicine together with certain other medicines may increase the chance of unwanted effects. The risk will depend on how much of each medicine you take every day, and on how long you take the medicines together. If your doctor directs you to take these medicines together on a regular basis, follow his or her directions carefully. However, do not take this medicine together with any of the following medicines for more than a few days, unless your doctor has directed you to do so and is following your progress:

Aspirin or other salicylates
Diclofenac (e.g., Voltaren)
Diflunisal (e.g., Dolobid)
Fenoprofen (e.g., Nalfon)
Floctafenine (e.g., Idarac)
Flurbiprofen, oral (e.g., Ansaid)
Ibuprofen (e.g., Motrin)
Indomethacin (e.g., Indocin)
Ketoprofen (e.g., Orudis)
Ketorolac (e.g., Toradol)
Meclofenamate (e.g., Meclomen)
Mefenamic acid (e.g., Ponstel)
Naproxen (e.g., Naprosyn)
Phenylbutazone (e.g., Butazolidin)
Piroxicam (e.g., Feldene)
Sulindac (e.g., Clinoril)
Tiaprofenic acid (e.g., Surgam)
Tolmetin (e.g., Tolectin)

This medicine may cause some people to become drowsy, dizzy, or lightheaded, or to feel a false sense of well-being. *Make sure you know how you react to this medicine before you drive, use machines, or do anything else that could be dangerous if you are dizzy or are not alert and clearheaded.*

Dizziness, lightheadedness, or fainting may occur, especially when you get up suddenly from a lying or sitting position. Getting up slowly may help lessen this problem.

Nausea or vomiting may occur, especially after the first couple of doses. This effect may go away if you lie down for a while. However, if nausea or vomiting continues, check with your medical doctor or dentist. Lying down for a while may also help relieve some other side effects, such as dizziness or lightheadedness, that may occur.

Before having any kind of surgery (including dental surgery) or emergency treatment, tell the medical doctor or dentist in charge that you are taking this medicine.

Narcotic analgesics may cause dryness of the mouth. For temporary relief, use sugarless candy or gum, melt bits of ice in your mouth, or use a saliva substitute. However, if dry mouth continues for more than 2 weeks, check with your dentist. Continuing dryness of the mouth may increase the chance of dental disease, including tooth decay, gum disease, and fungus infections.

If you have been taking this medicine regularly for several weeks or more, *do not suddenly stop taking it without first checking with your doctor.* Your doctor may want you to reduce gradually the amount you are taking before stopping completely, to lessen the chance of withdrawal side effects. This will depend on which of these medicines you have been taking, and the amount you have been taking every day.

If you think you or someone else may have taken an over-dose of this medicine, get emergency help at once. Taking an overdose of this medicine or taking alcohol or CNS depressants with this medicine may lead to unconsciousness or death. Signs of overdose of narcotics include convulsions (seizures), confusion, severe nervousness or restlessness, severe dizziness, severe drowsiness, shortness of breath or troubled breathing, and severe weakness. Signs of severe acetaminophen overdose may not occur until several days after the overdose is taken.

Side Effects of This Medicine

Along with its needed effects, a medicine may cause some unwanted effects. Although not all of these side effects may occur, if they do occur they may need medical attention.

Get emergency help immediately if any of the following symptoms of overdose occur:
> Cold, clammy skin; confusion (severe); convulsions (seizures); diarrhea; dizziness (severe); drowsiness (severe); increased sweating; low blood pressure; nausea or vomiting (continuing); nervousness or restlessness (severe); pinpoint pupils of eyes; shortness of breath or unusually slow or troubled breathing; slow heartbeat; stomach cramps or pain; weakness (severe)

Also, check with your doctor as soon as possible if any of the following side effects occur:

Less common or rare

Black, tarry stools; bloody or cloudy urine; confusion; dark urine; difficult or painful urination; fast, slow, or pounding heartbeat; frequent urge to urinate; hallucinations (seeing, hearing, or feeling things that are not there); increased sweating; irregular breathing or wheezing; mental depression; pain in lower back and/or side (severe and/or sharp); pale stools; pinpoint red spots on skin; redness or flushing of face; ringing or buzzing in ears; skin rash, hives, or itching; sore throat and fever; sudden decrease in amount of urine; swelling of face; trembling or uncontrolled muscle movements; unusual bleeding or bruising; unusual excitement (especially in children); yellow eyes or skin

Other side effects may occur that usually do not need medical attention. These side effects may go away during treatment as your body adjusts to the medicine. However, check with your medical doctor or dentist if any of the following side effects continue or are bothersome:

More common

Dizziness, lightheadedness, or feeling faint; drowsiness; nausea or vomiting; unusual tiredness or weakness

Less common or rare

Blurred or double vision or other changes in vision; constipation (more common with long-term use and with codeine or meperidine); dry mouth; false sense of well-being; general feeling of discomfort or illness; headache; loss of appetite; nervousness or restlessness; nightmares or unusual dreams; trouble in sleeping

Although not all of the side effects listed above have been reported for all of these combination medicines, they have been reported for at least one of them. However, since all of the narcotic analgesics are very similar, any of the above side effects may occur with any of these medicines.

After you stop using this medicine, your body may need time to adjust. The length of time this takes depends on which of these medicines you were taking, the amount of medicine you were using, and how long you used it. During this time check with your doctor if you notice any of the following side effects:

Body aches; diarrhea; fast heartbeat; fever, runny nose, or sneezing; gooseflesh; increased sweating; increased yawning; loss of appetite; nausea or vomiting; nervousness, restlessness, or irritability; shivering or trembling; stomach cramps; trouble in sleeping; weakness

Other side effects not listed above may also occur in some patients. If you notice any other effects, check with your doctor.

NARCOTIC ANALGESICS AND ASPIRIN   Systemic

This information applies to the following medicines:
  Aspirin, Caffeine, and Dihydrocodeine (dye-hye-droe-KOE-deen)
  Aspirin (AS-pir-in) and Codeine (KOE-deen)
  Aspirin, Codeine, and Caffeine (kaf-EEN)
  Aspirin, Codeine, and Caffeine, Buffered
  Hydrocodone (hye-droe-KOE-done) and Aspirin
  Hydrocodone, Aspirin, and Caffeine
  Oxycodone (ox-i-KOE-done) and Aspirin
  Pentazocine (pen-TAZ-oh-seen) and Aspirin
  Propoxyphene (proe-POX-i-feen) and Aspirin
  Propoxyphene, Aspirin, and Caffeine
Some commonly used brand names are:

For Aspirin, Caffeine, and Dihydrocodeine†
  In the U.S.
    Synalgos-DC
    Generic name product may also be available.
Other commonly used names are dihydrocodeine compound and drocode and aspirin.

For Aspirin and Codeine
  In the U.S.

Emcodeine No.2	Empirin with Codeine No.2
Emcodeine No.3	Empirin with Codeine No.3
Emcodeine No.4	Empirin with Codeine No.4

    Generic name product may also be available.

  In Canada‡
    Coryphen with Codeine

For Aspirin, Codeine, and Caffeine*
  In Canada‡

A.C.&C.	222 Forte
Anacin with Codeine	222
Ancasal 8	282
Ancasal 15	292
Ancasal 30	293
C2 with Codeine	

For Aspirin, Codeine, and Caffeine, Buffered*
  In Canada‡
    C2 Buffered with Codeine

For Hydrocodone and Aspirin†
  In the U.S.

Azdone	Lortab ASA

For Hydrocodone, Aspirin, and Caffeine†
  In the U.S.
    Damason-P

For Oxycodone and Aspirin
  In the U.S.

Percodan	Roxiprin
Percodan-Demi	

Generic name product may also be available.

  In Canada‡

Endodan	Percodan
Oxycodan	Percodan-Demi

For Pentazocine and Aspirin†
  In the U.S.
    Talwin Compound

For Propoxyphene and Aspirin
  In the U.S.

Darvon with A.S.A.	Darvon-N with A.S.A.

  In Canada‡
    Darvon-N with A.S.A.

For Propoxyphene, Aspirin, and Caffeine
  In the U.S.

Bexophene	Doraphen Compound-65
Cotanal-65	Doxaphene Compound
Darvon Compound	Margesic A-C
Darvon Compound-65	Pro Pox Plus

Generic name product may also be available.

Another commonly used name is propoxyphene hydrochloride compound.

---

   *Not commercially available in the U.S.
   †Not commercially available in Canada.
   ‡In Canada, *Aspirin* is a brand name. Acetylsalicylic acid is the generic name in Canada. ASA, a synonym for acetylsalicylic acid, is the term that commonly appears on Canadian product labels.

Description

Combination medicines containing narcotic (nar-KOT-ik) analgesics (an-al-JEE-zicks) and aspirin are used to relieve pain. A narcotic analgesic and aspirin used together may provide better pain relief than either medicine used alone. In some cases, relief of pain may come at lower doses of each medicine.

Narcotic analgesics act in the central nervous system (CNS) to relieve pain. Many of their side effects are also caused by actions in the CNS. When narcotics are used for a long time, your body may get used to them so that larger amounts are needed to relieve pain. This is called tolerance to the medicine. Also, when narcotics are used for a long time or in large doses, they may become habit-forming (causing mental or physical dependence). Physical dependence may lead to withdrawal symptoms when you stop taking the medicine.

Aspirin does not become habit-forming when taken for a long time or in large doses, but it may cause other unwanted effects if too much is taken.

In the U.S., these medicines are available only with your medical doctor's or dentist's prescription. In Canada, some strengths of aspirin, codeine, and caffeine combination are available without a prescription.

These medicines are available in the following dosage forms:
   Oral
      Aspirin, Caffeine, and Dihydrocodeine
         • Capsules (U.S.)

Aspirin and Codeine
- Tablets (U.S. and Canada)

Aspirin, Codeine, and Caffeine
- Tablets (Canada)

Aspirin, Codeine, and Caffeine, Buffered
- Tablets (Canada)

Hydrocodone and Aspirin
- Tablets (U.S.)

Hydrocodone, Aspirin, and Caffeine
- Tablets (U.S.)

Oxycodone and Aspirin
- Tablets (U.S. and Canada)

Pentazocine and Aspirin
- Tablets (U.S.)

Propoxyphene and Aspirin
- Capsules (U.S. and Canada)
- Tablets (U.S.)

Propoxyphene, Aspirin, and Caffeine
- Capsules (U.S. and Canada)
- Tablets (Canada)

It is very important that you read and understand the following information. If any of it causes you special concern, check with your doctor. Also, *if you have any questions* or if you want more information about this medicine or your medical problem, *ask your doctor, nurse, or pharmacist.*

Before Using This Medicine

In deciding to use a medicine, the risks of taking the medicine must be weighed against the good it will do. This is a decision you and your doctor will make. For narcotic analgesic and aspirin combinations, the following should be considered:

Allergies—Tell your doctor if you have ever had any unusual or allergic reaction to a narcotic analgesic, aspirin or other salicylates, including methyl salicylate (oil of wintergreen), or any of the following medicines:

Diclofenac (e.g., Voltaren)
Diflunisal (e.g., Dolobid)
Fenoprofen (e.g., Nalfon)
Floctafenine (e.g., Idarac)
Flurbiprofen, oral (e.g., Ansaid)
Ibuprofen (e.g., Motrin)

Indomethacin (e.g., Indocin)
Ketoprofen (e.g., Orudis)
Ketorolac (e.g., Toradol)
Meclofenamate (e.g., Meclomen)
Mefenamic acid (e.g., Ponstel)
Naproxen (e.g., Naprosyn)
Oxyphenbutazone (e.g., Tandearil)
Phenylbutazone (e.g., Butazolidin)
Piroxicam (e.g., Feldene)
Sulindac (e.g., Clinoril)
Suprofen (e.g., Suprol)
Tiaprofenic acid (e.g., Surgam)
Tolmetin (e.g., Tolectin)
Zomepirac (e.g., Zomax)

Also tell your doctor and pharmacist if you are allergic to any other substances, such as foods, preservatives, or dyes.

Pregnancy—

- *For aspirin*: Studies in humans have not shown that aspirin causes birth defects. However, studies in animals have shown that aspirin causes birth defects.

  Some reports have suggested that too much use of aspirin late in pregnancy may cause a decrease in the newborn's weight and possible death of the fetus or newborn baby. However, the mothers in these reports had been taking much larger amounts of aspirin than are usually recommended. Studies of mothers taking aspirin in the doses that are usually recommended did not show these effects. However, regular use of aspirin late in pregnancy may cause unwanted effects on the heart or blood flow in the fetus or in the newborn baby. Also, use of aspirin during the last 2 weeks of pregnancy may cause bleeding problems in the fetus before or during delivery or in the newborn baby.

  Too much use of aspirin during the last 3 months of pregnancy may increase the length of pregnancy, prolong labor, cause other problems during delivery, or cause severe bleeding in the mother before, during, or after delivery. *Do not take aspirin during the last 3 months of pregnancy unless it has been ordered by your doctor.*

- *For narcotic analgesics*: Although studies on birth defects with narcotic analgesics have not been done in pregnant women, they have not been reported to cause birth defects. However, hydrocodone caused birth defects in animal studies when given in very large doses. Codeine did not cause birth defects in animals, but it caused slower development of bones and other toxic or harmful effects on the fetus. Pentazocine and propoxyphene did not cause birth defects in animals. There is no information about whether dihydrocodeine or oxycodone causes birth defects in animals.

  Too much use of a narcotic during pregnancy may cause the fetus to become dependent on the medicine. This may lead to withdrawal side effects in the newborn baby. Also, some of these medicines may cause breathing problems in the newborn baby if taken just before or during delivery.

- *For caffeine*: Studies in humans have not shown that caffeine (contained in some of these combination medicines) causes birth defects. However, studies in animals have shown that caffeine causes birth defects when given in very large doses (amounts equal to those present in 12 to 24 cups of coffee a day).

Breast-feeding—These combination medicines have not been reported to cause problems in nursing babies. However, aspirin, caffeine, codeine, and propoxyphene pass into the breast milk. It is not known whether dihydrocodeine, hydrocodone, oxycodone, or pentazocine passes into the breast milk.

Children—*Do not give a medicine containing aspirin to a child or a teenager with a fever or other symptoms of a virus infection, especially flu or chickenpox, without first discussing its use with your child's doctor*. This is very important because aspirin may cause a serious illness called Reye's syndrome in children with fever caused by a virus infection, especially flu or chickenpox. Children who do not have a virus infection may also be more sensitive to the effects of aspirin, especially if they have a fever or have lost large amounts of body fluid because of vomiting, diarrhea, or sweating. This may increase the chance of side effects during treatment.

The narcotic analgesic in this combination medicine can cause breathing problems, especially in children younger than 2 years of age. These children are usually more sensitive than adults to the effects of narcotic analgesics. Also, unusual excitement or restlessness may be more likely to occur in children receiving these medicines.

Older adults—Elderly people are especially sensitive to the effects of aspirin and of narcotic analgesics. This may increase the chance of side effects, especially breathing problems caused by narcotic analgesics, during treatment.

Athletes—Narcotic analgesics are banned and tested for by the U.S. Olympic Committee (USOC). Narcotic use can lead to disqualification of athletes in most USOC-sponsored athletic events. Also, some of these combination medicines contain caffeine, which is tested for by the USOC and the National Collegiate Athletic Association (NCAA). These two groups have set specific limits on the amount of caffeine in the urine they consider to be acceptable. An athlete will be disqualified for competition if the amount of caffeine in the urine is above these limits.

Other medicines—Although certain medicines should not be used together at all, in other cases two different medicines may be used together even if an interaction might occur. In these cases, your doctor may want to change the dose, or other precautions may be necessary. When you are taking a narcotic analgesic and aspirin combination, it is especially important that your doctor and pharmacist know if you are taking any of the following:
  • Anticoagulants (blood thinners) or
  • Carbenicillin by injection (e.g., Geopen) or
  • Cefamandole (e.g., Mandol) or
  • Cefoperazone (e.g., Cefobid) or
  • Cefotetan (e.g., Cefotan) or
  • Dipyridamole (e.g., Persantine) or
  • Divalproex (e.g., Depakote) or
  • Heparin or
  • Medicine for inflammation or pain, except narcotics, or

- Moxalactam (e.g., Moxam) or
- Pentoxifylline (e.g., Trental) or
- Plicamycin (e.g., Mithracin) or
- Ticarcillin (e.g., Ticar) or
- Valproic acid (e.g., Depakene)—Taking these medicines together with aspirin may increase the chance of bleeding
- Antidiabetics, oral (diabetes medicine you take by mouth)— Aspirin may increase the effects of the antidiabetic medicine; a change in the dose of the antidiabetic medicine may be needed if aspirin is taken regularly
- Carbamazepine (e.g., Tegretol)—Propoxyphene can increase the blood levels of carbamazepine, which increases the chance of serious side effects
- Central nervous system (CNS) depressants or
- Diarrhea medicine or
- Methotrexate (e.g., Mexate) or
- Tricyclic antidepressants (amitriptyline [e.g., Elavil], amoxapine [e.g., Asendin], clomipramine [e.g., Anafranil], desipramine [e.g., Pertofrane], doxepin [e.g., Sinequan], imipramine [e.g., Tofranil], nortriptyline [e.g., Aventyl], protriptyline [e.g., Vivactil], trimipramine [e.g., Surmontil]) or
- Vancomycin (e.g., Vancocin)—The chance of side effects may be increased
- Naltrexone (e.g., Trexan)—Naltrexone keeps narcotic analgesics from working to relieve pain; people taking naltrexone should use pain relievers that do not contain a narcotic
- Probenecid (e.g., Benemid) or
- Sulfinpyrazone (e.g., Anturane)—Aspirin can keep these medicines from working as well for treating gout; also, use of sulfinpyrazone and aspirin together may increase the chance of bleeding
- Urinary alkalizers (medicine that makes the urine less acid, such as acetazolamide [e.g., Diamox], calcium- and/or magnesium-containing antacids, dichlorphenamide [e.g., Daranide], methazolamide [e.g., Neptazane], potassium or sodium citrate and/or citric acid, sodium bicarbonate [baking soda])—These medicines may make aspirin less effective by causing it to be removed from the body more quickly
- Zidovudine (e.g., AZT, Retrovir)—Higher blood levels of zidovudine and an increased chance of serious side effects may occur

Other medical problems—The presence of other medical problems may affect the use of narcotic analgesic and aspirin combinations. Make sure you tell your doctor if you have any other medical problems, especially:

- Alcohol and/or other drug abuse, or history of, or
- Asthma, allergies, and nasal polyps (history of) or
- Brain disease or head injury or
- Colitis or
- Convulsions (seizures), history of, or
- Emotional problems or mental illness or
- Emphysema or other chronic lung disease or
- Kidney disease or
- Liver disease or
- Underactive thyroid—The chance of serious side effects may be increased

- Anemia or
- Overactive thyroid or
- Stomach ulcer or other stomach problems—Aspirin may make these conditions worse

- Enlarged prostate or problems with urination or
- Gallbladder disease or gallstones—Narcotic analgesics have side effects that may be dangerous if these medical problems are present

- Gout—Aspirin can make this condition worse and can also lessen the effects of some medicines used to treat gout

- Heart disease—Large amounts of aspirin and caffeine (present in some of these combination medicines) can make some kinds of heart disease worse

- Hemophilia or other bleeding problems or
- Vitamin K deficiency—Aspirin increases the chance of serious bleeding

Before you begin using any new medicine (prescription or nonprescription) or if you develop any new medical problem while you are using this medicine, check with your doctor, nurse, or pharmacist.

Proper Use of This Medicine

Take this medicine with food or a full glass (8 ounces) of water to lessen stomach irritation.

Do not take this medicine if it has a strong vinegar-like odor. This odor means the aspirin in it is breaking down. If you have any questions about this, check with your doctor or pharmacist.

Take this medicine only as directed by your medical doctor or dentist. Do not take more of it, do not take it more often, and do not take it for a longer time than your medical doctor or dentist ordered. This is especially important for children and elderly patients, who are usually more sensitive to the effects of these medicines. If too much of a narcotic analgesic is taken, it may become habit-forming (causing mental or physical dependence) or lead to medical problems because of an overdose. Also, taking too much aspirin may cause stomach problems or lead to medical problems because of an overdose.

If you think that this medicine is not working as well after you have been taking it for a few weeks, *do not increase the dose.* Instead, check with your medical doctor or dentist.

Missed dose—If your medical doctor or dentist has ordered you to take this medicine according to a regular schedule and you miss a dose, take it as soon as you remember. However, if it is almost time for your next dose, skip the missed dose and go back to your regular dosing schedule. *Do not double doses.*

Storage—To store this medicine:
- Keep out of the reach of children. Overdose is very dangerous in young children.
- Store away from heat and direct light.
- Do not store this medicine in the bathroom, near the kitchen sink, or in other damp places. Heat or moisture may cause the medicine to break down.
- Do not keep outdated medicine or medicine no longer needed. Be sure that any discarded medicine is out of the reach of children.

Precautions While Using This Medicine

If you will be taking this medicine for a long time (for example, for several months at a time), your doctor should check your progress at regular visits.

Check the labels of all nonprescription (over-the-counter [OTC]) and prescription medicines you now take. If any contain a narcotic, aspirin, or other salicylates, be especially careful, since taking them while taking this medicine may lead to overdose. If you have any questions about this, check with your physician, dentist, or pharmacist.

This medicine will add to the effects of alcohol and other CNS depressants (medicines that slow down the nervous system, possibly causing drowsiness). Some examples of CNS depressants are antihistamines or medicine for hay fever, other allergies, or colds; sedatives, tranquilizers, or sleeping medicine; other prescription pain medicine or narcotics; barbiturates; medicine for seizures; muscle relaxants; or anesthetics, including some dental anesthetics. Also, stomach problems may be more likely to occur if you drink alcoholic beverages while you are taking aspirin. *Do not drink alcoholic beverages, and check with your medical doctor or dentist before taking any of the medicines listed above, while you are using this medicine.*

Taking acetaminophen or certain other medicines together with the aspirin in this combination medicine may increase the chance of unwanted effects. The risk will depend on how much of each medicine you take every day, and on how long you take the medicines together. If your doctor directs you to take these medicines together on a regular basis, follow his or her directions carefully. However, do not take acetaminophen or any of the following medicines together with this combination medicine for more than a few days, unless your doctor has directed you to do so and is following your progress:

    Diclofenac (e.g., Voltaren)
    Diflunisal (e.g., Dolobid)
    Fenoprofen (e.g., Nalfon)
    Floctafenine (e.g., Idarac)
    Flurbiprofen, oral (e.g., Ansaid)
    Ibuprofen (e.g., Motrin)
    Indomethacin (e.g., Indocin)
    Ketoprofen (e.g., Orudis)
    Ketorolac (e.g., Toradol)
    Meclofenamate (e.g., Meclomen)
    Mefenamic acid (e.g., Ponstel)

Naproxen (e.g., Naprosyn)
Phenylbutazone (e.g., Butazolidin)
Piroxicam (e.g., Feldene)
Sulindac (e.g., Clinoril)
Tiaprofenic acid (e.g., Surgam)
Tolmetin (e.g., Tolectin)

This medicine may cause some people to become drowsy, dizzy, or lightheaded, or to feel a false sense of well-being. *Make sure you know how you react to this medicine before you drive, use machines, or do anything else that could be dangerous if you are dizzy or are not alert and clearheaded.*

Dizziness, lightheadedness, or fainting may occur, especially when you get up suddenly from a lying or sitting position. Getting up slowly may help lessen this problem.

Nausea or vomiting may occur, especially after the first couple of doses. This effect may go away if you lie down for a while. However, if nausea or vomiting continues, check with your doctor. Lying down for a while may also help some other side effects, such as dizziness or lightheadedness.

Before having any kind of surgery (including dental surgery) or emergency treatment, tell the medical doctor or dentist in charge that you are taking this medicine.

Do not take this medicine for 5 days before any surgery, including dental surgery, unless otherwise directed by your medical doctor or dentist. Taking aspirin during this time may cause bleeding problems.

If you are taking one of the combination medicines containing buffered aspirin, and you are also taking a tetracycline antibiotic, do not take the two medicines within 3 to 4 hours of each other. Taking them too close together may prevent the tetracycline from being absorbed by your body. If you have any questions about this, check with your doctor or pharmacist.

For *diabetic patients:*

- False urine sugar test results may occur if you are regularly taking 8 or more 325-mg (5-grain) or 5 or more 500-mg doses of aspirin a day. Smaller amounts or occasional use of aspirin usually will not affect urine sugar tests. If you have any questions about this, check with your doctor, nurse, or pharmacist, especially if your diabetes is not well controlled.

Narcotic analgesics may cause dryness of the mouth. For temporary relief, use sugarless candy or gum, melt bits of ice in your mouth, or use a saliva substitute. However, if dry mouth continues for more than 2 weeks, check with your dentist. Continuing dryness of the mouth may increase the chance of dental disease, including tooth decay, gum disease, and fungus infections.

If you have been taking this medicine regularly for several weeks or more, *do not suddenly stop using it without first checking with your doctor*. Depending on which of these medicines you have been taking, and the amount you have been taking every day, your doctor may want you to reduce gradually the amount you are taking before stopping completely, to lessen the chance of withdrawal side effects.

If you think you or someone else may have taken an overdose of this medicine, get emergency help at once. Taking an overdose of this medicine or taking alcohol or CNS depressants with this medicine may lead to unconsciousness or death. Signs of overdose of this medicine include convulsions (seizures); hearing loss; confusion; ringing or buzzing in the ears; severe excitement, nervousness, or restlessness; severe dizziness, severe drowsiness, shortness of breath or troubled breathing, and severe weakness.

Side Effects of This Medicine

Along with its needed effects, a medicine may cause some unwanted effects. Although not all of these side effects may occur, if they do occur they may need medical attention.

Get emergency help immediately if any of the following symptoms of overdose occur:

Any loss of hearing; bloody urine; cold, clammy skin; confusion (severe); convulsions (seizures); diarrhea (severe or continuing); dizziness or lightheadedness (severe); drowsiness (severe); excitement, nervousness, or restlessness (severe); fever;

hallucinations (seeing, hearing, or feeling things that are not there); headache (severe or continuing); increased sweating; increased thirst; low blood pressure; nausea or vomiting (severe or continuing); pinpoint pupils of eyes; ringing or buzzing in the ears; shortness of breath or unusually slow or troubled breathing; slow heartbeat; stomach pain (severe or continuing); uncontrollable flapping movements of the hands (especially in elderly patients); vision problems; weakness (severe)

Also, check with your doctor as soon as possible if any of the following side effects occur:

Less common or rare

Bloody or black, tarry stools; confusion; dark urine; fast, slow, or pounding heartbeat; increased sweating (more common with hydrocodone); irregular breathing; mental depression; pale stools; redness or flushing of face (more common with hydrocodone); skin rash, hives, or itching; stomach pain (severe); swelling of face; tightness in chest or wheezing; trembling or uncontrolled muscle movements; unusual excitement (especially in children); unusual tiredness or weakness; vomiting of blood or material that looks like coffee grounds; yellow eyes or skin

Other side effects may occur that usually do not need medical attention. These side effects may go away during treatment as your body adjusts to the medicine. However, check with your doctor if any of the following side effects continue or are bothersome:

More common

Dizziness, lightheadedness, or feeling faint; drowsiness; heartburn or indigestion; nausea or vomiting; stomach pain (mild)

Less common or rare

Blurred or double vision or other changes in vision; constipation (more common with long-term use and with codeine); difficult, painful, or decreased urination; dryness of mouth; false sense of well-being; frequent urge to urinate; general feeling of discomfort or illness; headache; loss of appetite; nervousness or restlessness; nightmares or unusual dreams; trouble in sleeping; unusual tiredness; unusual weakness

Although not all of the side effects listed above have been reported for all of these medicines, they have been reported for at least one of them. However, since all of the narcotic analgesics are very similar, any of the above side effects may occur with any of these medicines.

After you stop using this medicine, your body may need time to adjust. The length of time this takes depends on which of these medicines you were taking, the amount of medicine you were using, and how long you used it. During this period of time check with your doctor if you notice any of the following side effects:

Body aches; diarrhea; fever, runny nose, or sneezing; gooseflesh; increased sweating; increased yawning; loss of appetite; nausea or vomiting; nervousness, restlessness, or irritability; shivering or trembling; stomach cramps; trouble in sleeping; weakness

Other side effects not listed above may also occur in some patients. If you notice any other effects, check with your medical doctor or dentist.

NICOTINE   Systemic

Some commonly used brand names are:
In the U.S.
    Habitrol   Nicotrol
    Nicoderm   ProStep
    Nicorette

In Canada
    Habitrol   Nicorette
    Nicoderm

Description

Nicotine (NIK-o-teen), in a flavored chewing gum or a skin patch, is used to help you stop smoking. It is used for up to 12 to 20 weeks as part of a supervised stop-smoking program. These programs may include education, counseling, and psychological support. Using nicotine replacement products without taking part in a supervised stop-smoking program has not been shown to be effective.

- As you chew nicotine gum, nicotine passes through the lining of your mouth and into your body.
- When you wear a nicotine patch, nicotine passes through your skin into your bloodstream.

This nicotine takes the place of nicotine that you would otherwise get from smoking. In this way, the withdrawal effects of not smoking are less severe. Then, as your body adjusts to not smoking, the use of the nicotine gum is decreased gradually, or the strength of the patches is decreased over a few weeks. Finally, use is stopped altogether.

Children, pregnant women, and nonsmokers should not use nicotine gum or patches because of unwanted effects.

Nicotine gum and patches are available only with your doctor's prescription, in the following dosage forms:

Oral
- Chewing gum tablets (U.S. and Canada)

Topical
- Transdermal (stick-on) skin patch (U.S. and Canada)

It is very important that you read and understand the following information. If any of it causes you special concern, check with your doctor or pharmacist. Also, *if you have any questions* or if you want more information about this medicine or your medical problem, *ask your doctor, nurse, or pharmacist.*

Before Using This Medicine

In deciding to use a medicine, the risks of taking the medicine must be weighed against the good it will do. This is a decision you and your doctor will make. For nicotine gum, the following should be considered:

Allergies—Tell your doctor if you have ever had any unusual or allergic reaction to nicotine. Also tell your doctor and pharmacist if you are allergic to any other substances, such as foods, preservatives, or dyes. If you plan to use the nic-

otine patches, tell your doctor if you have ever had a rash
or irritation from adhesive tape or bandages.

Pregnancy—Nicotine, whether from smoking or from the
gum or patches, is not recommended during pregnancy.
Studies in humans show that miscarriages have occurred in
pregnant women using nicotine replacement products. In
addition, studies in animals have shown that nicotine can
cause harmful effects in the fetus.

Breast-feeding—Nicotine passes into breast milk and may
cause unwanted effects in the baby. It may be necessary for
you to stop breast-feeding during treatment.

Children—Small amounts of nicotine can cause serious harm
in children. Even used nicotine patches contain enough nicotine to cause problems in children.

Older adults—Nicotine gum and patches have been used in
a limited number of patients 60 years of age or older, and
have not been shown to cause different side effects or problems in older people than in younger adults.

Other medicines—Although certain medicines should not be
used together at all, in other cases 2 different medicines may
be used together even if an interaction might occur. In these
cases, your doctor may want to change the dose, or other
precautions may be necessary. When you are using nicotine
gum or patches, it is especially important that your doctor
and pharmacist know if you are taking any of the following:
- Aminophylline (e.g., Somophyllin) or
- Insulin or
- Oxtriphylline (e.g., Choledyl) or
- Propoxyphene (e.g., Darvon) or
- Propranolol (e.g., Inderal) or
- Theophylline (e.g., Somophyllin-T)—Stopping smoking may
  increase the effects of these medicines; the amount of med-
  icine you need to take may change

Other medical problems—The presence of other medical
problems may affect the use of nicotine gum or patches.
Make sure you tell your doctor if you have any other medical
problems, especially:
- Dental problems (with gum only) or
- Diabetes mellitus (sugar diabetes) or

- Heart or blood vessel disease or
- High blood pressure or
- Inflammation of mouth or throat (with gum only) or
- Irritated skin (with patches only) or
- Overactive thyroid or
- Pheochromocytoma (PCC) or
- Stomach ulcer or
- Temporomandibular (jaw) joint disorder (TMJ) (with gum only)—Nicotine gum or patches may make the condition worse

Before you begin using any new medicine (prescription or nonprescription) or if you develop any new medical problem while you are using this medicine, check with your doctor, nurse, or pharmacist.

Proper Use of This Medicine

For patients using the *chewing gum tablets:*

- Nicotine gum usually comes with patient directions. *Read the directions carefully before using this medicine.*
- *When you feel the urge to smoke, chew one piece of gum very slowly* until you taste it or feel a slight tingling in your mouth. Stop chewing, and place ("park") the chewing gum tablet between your cheek and gum until the taste or tingling is almost gone. Then chew slowly until you taste it again. Continue chewing and stopping ("parking") in this way for about 30 minutes in order to get the full dose of nicotine.
- *Do not chew too fast*, do not chew more than one piece at a time, and do not chew a piece of gum too soon after another. To do so may cause unwanted side effects or an overdose. Also, slower chewing will reduce the possibility of belching.
- *Use nicotine gum exactly as directed by your doctor.* Remember that it is also important to participate in a stop-smoking program during treatment. This may make it easier for you to stop smoking.
- As your urge to smoke becomes less frequent, *gradually reduce the number of pieces of gum you chew each day*

until you are chewing one or two pieces a day. This
may be possible within 2 to 3 months.

- *Remember to carry nicotine gum with you at all times*
  in case you feel the sudden urge to smoke. One cigarette
  may be enough to start you on the smoking habit again.

- Using hard sugarless candy between doses of gum may
  help to relieve the discomfort in your mouth.

For patients using the *transdermal system (skin patch):*

- *Use this medicine exactly as directed by your doctor.*
  It will work only if applied correctly. *This medicine
  usually comes with patient instructions. Read them
  carefully before using this product.* Remember that it
  is also important to participate in a stop-smoking program during treatment. This may make it easier for you
  to stop smoking.

- Do not remove the patch from its sealed pouch until
  you are ready to put it on your skin. The patch may
  not work as well if it is unwrapped too soon.

- Do not try to trim or cut the adhesive patch to adjust
  the dosage. Check with your doctor if you think the
  medicine is not working as it should.

- Apply the patch to a clean, dry area of skin on your
  upper arm, chest, or back. Choose an area that is not
  very oily, has little or no hair, and is free of scars, cuts,
  burns, or any other skin irritations.

- Press the patch firmly in place with the palm of your
  hand for about 10 seconds. Make sure there is good
  contact with your skin, especially around the edges of
  the patch.

- The patch should stay in place even when you are showering, bathing, or swimming. Apply a new patch if one
  falls off.

- Rinse your hands with plain water after you have finished applying the patch to your skin. Nicotine on your
  hands could get into your eyes and nose and cause stinging, redness, or more serious problems. Using soap to
  wash your hands will increase the amount of nicotine
  that passes through your skin.

- After 16 or 24 hours, depending on which product you are using, remove the patch. Choose a different place on your skin to apply the next patch. Do not put a new patch in the same place for at least one week. Do not leave the patch on for more than 24 hours. It will not work as well after that time and it may irritate your skin.

- After removing a used patch, fold the patch in half with the sticky sides together. Place the folded, used patch in its protective pouch or in aluminum foil. Make sure to dispose of it out of the reach of children and pets.

- Try to change the patch at the same time each day. If you want to change the time when you put on your patch, just remove the patch you are wearing and put on a new patch. After that, apply a fresh patch at the new time each day.

Storage—To store this medicine:

- Keep out of the reach of children because even small doses of nicotine can cause serious harm in children.

- Store away from heat and direct light.

- Do not store in the bathroom, near the kitchen sink, or in other damp places. Heat or moisture may cause the medicine to break down.

- Do not keep outdated medicine or medicine no longer needed. Be sure that any discarded medicine is out of the reach of children and pets.

Precautions While Using This Medicine

Your doctor should check your progress at regular visits to make sure that the nicotine gum or patches are working properly and that possible side effects are avoided.

Do not smoke during treatment with nicotine gum or patches because of the risk of nicotine overdose.

Nicotine should not be used in pregnancy. If there is a possibility you might become pregnant, you may want to use some type of birth control. If you think you may have become pregnant, stop taking this medicine immediately and check with your doctor.

Nicotine products must be kept out of the reach of children and pets. Even used nicotine patches contain enough nicotine to cause problems in children. If a child chews or swallows one or more pieces of nicotine gum, contact your doctor or poison control center at once. If a child puts on a nicotine patch or plays with a patch that is out of the sealed pouch, take it away from the child and contact your doctor or poison control center at once.

For patients using the *chewing gum tablets:*

- *Do not chew more than 30 pieces of gum a day.* Chewing too many pieces may be harmful because of the risk of overdose.
- *Do not use nicotine gum for longer than 6 months.* To do so may result in physical dependence on the nicotine.
- *If the gum sticks to your dental work, stop using it and check with your medical doctor or dentist.* Dentures or other dental work may be damaged because nicotine gum is stickier and harder to chew than ordinary gum.

For patients using the *transdermal system (skin patch):*

- Mild itching, burning, or tingling may occur when the patch is first applied, and should go away within an hour. After a patch is removed, the skin underneath it may be somewhat red. It should not remain red for more than a day. *If you get a skin rash from the patch, or if the skin becomes swollen or very red, call your doctor.* Do not put on a new patch. If you become allergic to the nicotine in the patch, you could get sick from using cigarettes or other products that contain nicotine.
- *Do not use nicotine patches for longer than 12 to 20 weeks* (depending on the product) if you have stopped smoking, because continuing use of nicotine in any form can be harmful and addictive.

Side Effects of This Medicine

Along with its needed effects, a medicine may cause some unwanted effects. Although not all of these side effects may occur, if they do occur they may need medical attention.

Check with your doctor as soon as possible if any of the following side effects occur:

More common

Injury to mouth, teeth, or dental work—with chewing gum only

Rare

Irregular heartbeat; rash or hives; redness, swelling, and itching at the site of application of the patch that lasts longer than 1 day

Symptoms of overdose (may occur in the following order)

Nausea and/or vomiting; increased watering of mouth (severe); abdominal or stomach pain (severe); diarrhea (severe); cold sweat; headache (severe); dizziness (severe); drooling; disturbed hearing and vision; confusion; weakness (severe); fainting; low blood pressure; difficulty in breathing (severe); fast, weak, or irregular heartbeat; convulsions (seizures)

Other side effects may occur that usually do not need medical attention. These side effects may go away during treatment as your body adjusts to the medicine. However, check with your doctor if any of the following side effects continue or are bothersome:

More common

Belching—with chewing gum only; fast heartbeat; headache (mild); increased appetite; increased watering of mouth (mild)—with chewing gum only; jaw muscle ache—with chewing gum only; redness, itching, and/or burning at site of application of patch—usually stops within an hour; sore mouth or throat—with chewing gum only

Less common or rare

Constipation; coughing (increased); diarrhea; dizziness or lightheadedness (mild); drowsiness; dryness of mouth; hiccups—with chewing gum only; hoarseness—with chewing gum only; irritability or nervousness; loss of appetite; menstrual pain; muscle or joint pain; stomach upset or indigestion (mild); sweating (increased); trouble in sleeping or unusual dreams

Other side effects not listed above may also occur in some patients. If you notice any other effects, check with your doctor.

NITRATES—Lingual Aerosol   Systemic

This information applies to nitroglycerin oral spray.
A commonly used brand name in the U.S. and Canada is Nitrolingual.
Another commonly used name is glyceryl trinitrate.

Description

Nitrates (NYE-trates) are used to treat the symptoms of angina (chest pain). Depending on the type of dosage form and how it is taken, nitrates are used to treat angina in three ways:

- to relieve an attack that is occurring by using the medicine when the attack begins;
- to prevent attacks from occurring by using the medicine just before an attack is expected to occur; or
- to reduce the number of attacks that occur by using the medicine regularly on a long-term basis.

When used as a lingual (in the mouth) spray, nitroglycerin is used either to relieve the pain of angina attacks or to prevent an expected angina attack.

Nitroglycerin works by relaxing blood vessels and increasing the supply of blood and oxygen to the heart while reducing its work load.

Nitroglycerin as discussed here is available only with your doctor's prescription, in the following dosage form:

Oral
- Lingual aerosol (U.S. and Canada)

It is very important that you read and understand the following information. If any of it causes you special concern,

check with your doctor. Also, *if you have any questions* or
if you want more information about this medicine or your
medical problem, *ask your doctor, nurse, or pharmacist.*

Before Using This Medicine

In deciding to use a medicine, the risks of taking the medicine must be weighed against the good it will do. This is a
decision you and your doctor will make. For nitroglycerin
lingual aerosol, the following should be considered:

Allergies—Tell your doctor if you have ever had any unusual
or allergic reaction to nitrates or nitrites. Also tell your doctor and pharmacist if you are allergic to any other substance,
such as certain foods, preservatives, or dyes.

Pregnancy—Studies have not been done in humans. However, nitroglycerin has not been shown to cause problems.

Breast-feeding—It is not known whether this medicine passes
into breast milk. However, nitroglycerin has not been reported to cause problems in nursing babies.

Children—There is no specific information about the use of
nitrates in children.

Older adults—Dizziness or lightheadedness may be more
likely to occur in the elderly, who may be more sensitive to
the effects of nitrates.

Other medicines—Although certain medicines should not be
used together at all, in other cases two different medicines
may be used together even if an interaction might occur. In
these cases, your doctor may want to change the dose, or
other precautions may be necessary. When you are taking
nitroglycerin, it is especially important that your doctor and
pharmacist know if you are taking any of the following:

- Antihypertensives (high blood pressure medicine) or
- Other heart medicine—May increase the effects of nitroglycerin on blood pressure

Other medical problems—The presence of other medical
problems may affect the use of nitroglycerin. Make sure you
tell your doctor if you have any other medical problems,
especially:

- Anemia (severe)
- Glaucoma—May be worsened by nitroglycerin
- Head injury (recent) or
- Stroke (recent)—Nitroglycerin may increase pressure in the brain, which can make problems worse
- Heart attack (recent)—Nitroglycerin may lower blood pressure, which can aggravate problems associated with heart attack
- Kidney disease or
- Liver disease—Effects may be increased because of slower removal of nitroglycerin from the body
- Overactive thyroid

Before you begin using any new medicine (prescription or nonprescription) or if you develop any new medical problem while you are using this medicine, check with your doctor, nurse, or pharmacist.

Proper Use of This Medicine

Use nitroglycerin spray exactly as directed by your doctor. It will work only if used correctly.

This medicine usually comes with patient instructions. Read them carefully before you actually need to use it. Then, if you need the medicine quickly, you will know how to use it.

To use nitroglycerin lingual spray:
- Remove the plastic cover. *Do not shake the container.*
- Hold the container upright. With the container held close to your mouth, press the button to spray onto or under your tongue. *Do not inhale the spray.*
- Release the button and close your mouth. Avoid swallowing immediately after using the spray.

For patients using nitroglycerin oral spray *to relieve the pain of an angina attack*:
- *When you begin to feel an attack of angina starting (chest pains or a tightness or squeezing in the chest), sit down. Then use 1 or 2 sprays as directed by your doctor.* This medicine works best when you are standing

or sitting. However, since you may become dizzy, light-headed, or faint soon after using a spray, it is safer to sit rather than stand while the medicine is working. If you become dizzy or faint while sitting, take several deep breaths and bend forward with your head between your knees.

- Remain calm and you should feel better in a few minutes.

- *This medicine usually gives relief in less than 5 minutes.* However, if the pain is not relieved, use a second spray. If the pain continues for another 5 minutes, a third spray may be used. *If you still have the chest pains after a total of 3 sprays in a 15-minute period, contact your doctor or go to a hospital emergency room immediately.*

For patients using nitroglycerin oral spray *to prevent an expected angina attack*:

- You may prevent anginal chest pains for up to 1 hour by using a spray 5 to 10 minutes before expected emotional stress or physical exertion that in the past seemed to bring on an attack.

Storage—To store this medicine:

- Keep out of the reach of children.
- Store away from heat and direct light.
- Keep the medicine from freezing.
- Do not puncture, break, or burn the aerosol container, even after it is empty.
- Do not keep outdated medicine or medicine no longer needed. Be sure that any discarded medicine is out of the reach of children.

Precautions While Using This Medicine

If you have been using this medicine regularly for several weeks, do not suddenly stop using it. Stopping suddenly may bring on attacks of angina. Check with your doctor for the best way to reduce gradually the amount you are using before stopping completely.

Dizziness, lightheadedness, or faintness may occur, especially when you get up quickly from a lying or sitting position. Getting up slowly may help. If you feel dizzy, sit or lie down.

The dizziness, lightheadedness, or fainting is also more likely to occur if you drink alcohol, stand for long periods of time, exercise, or if the weather is hot. *While you are taking this medicine, be careful in the amount of alcohol you drink. Also, use extra care during exercise or hot weather or if you must stand for long periods of time.*

After using a dose of this medicine you may get a headache that lasts for a short time. This is a common side effect, which should become less noticeable after you have used the medicine for a while. If this effect continues or if the headaches are severe, check with your doctor.

Side Effects of This Medicine

Along with its needed effects, a medicine may cause some unwanted effects. Although not all of these side effects may occur, if they do occur they may need medical attention.

Check with your doctor as soon as possible if any of the following side effects occur:

> *Rare*
>> Blurred vision; dry mouth; headache (severe or prolonged); skin rash
>
> *Signs and symptoms of overdose (in the order in which they may occur)*
>> Bluish-colored lips, fingernails, or palms of hands; dizziness (extreme) or fainting; feeling of extreme pressure in head; shortness of breath; unusual tiredness or weakness; weak and fast heartbeat; fever; convulsions (seizures)

Other side effects may occur that usually do not need medical attention. These side effects may go away during treatment as your body adjusts to the medicine. However, check with your doctor if any of the following side effects continue or are bothersome:

More common

Dizziness or lightheadedness, especially when getting up from a lying or sitting position; fast pulse; flushing of face and neck; headache; nausea or vomiting; restlessness

Other side effects not listed above may also occur in some patients. If you notice any other effects, check with your doctor.

NITRATES—Sublingual, Chewable, or Buccal Systemic

This information applies to the following medicines:

Erythrityl Tetranitrate (e-RI-thri-till tet-ra-NYE-trate)
Isosorbide Dinitrate (eye-soe-SOR-bide dye-NYE-trate)
Nitroglycerin (nye-troe-GLI-ser-in)

Note: This information does *not* apply to amyl nitrite or pentaerythritol tetranitrate.

Some commonly used brand names are:

For Erythrityl Tetranitrate
In the U.S. and Canada
Cardilate

Some other commonly used names are eritrityl tetranitrate and erythritol tetranitrate.

For Isosorbide Dinitrate
In the U.S.

Isonate	Isordil
Isorbid	Sorbitrate

Generic name product may also be available.

In Canada

Apo-ISDN	Isordil
Coronex	

For Nitroglycerin
In the U.S.
Nitrogard
Nitrostat

Generic name product may also be available.

In Canada
Nitrogard SR
Nitrostat

Generic name product may also be available.

Another commonly used name is glyceryl trinitrate.

Description

Nitrates (NYE-trates) are used to treat the symptoms of angina (chest pain). Depending on the type of dosage form and how it is taken, nitrates are used to treat angina in three ways:

- to relieve an attack that is occurring by using the medicine when the attack begins;
- to prevent attacks from occurring by using the medicine just before an attack is expected to occur; or
- to reduce the number of attacks that occur by using the medicine regularly on a long-term basis.

Nitrates are available in different forms. Sublingual nitrates are generally placed under the tongue where they dissolve and are absorbed through the lining of the mouth. Some can also be used buccally, being placed under the lip or in the cheek. The chewable dosage forms, after being chewed and held in the mouth before swallowing, are absorbed in the same way. *It is important to remember that each dosage form is different and that the specific directions for each type must be followed if the medicine is to work properly.*

Nitrates that are used *to relieve the pain* of an angina attack include:

- sublingual nitroglycerin;
- buccal nitroglycerin;
- sublingual isosorbide dinitrate; and
- chewable isosorbide dinitrate.

Those that can be used *to prevent expected attacks* of angina include:

- sublingual nitroglycerin;
- buccal nitroglycerin;
- sublingual erythrityl tetranitrate;
- sublingual isosorbide dinitrate; and
- chewable isosorbide dinitrate.

Products that are used regularly on a long-term basis *to reduce the number of attacks* that occur include:

- buccal nitroglycerin;
- oral/sublingual erythrityl tetranitrate; and

- chewable isosorbide dinitrate; and
- sublingual isosorbide dinitrate.

Nitrates work by relaxing blood vessels and increasing the supply of blood and oxygen to the heart while reducing its work load.

Nitrates may also be used for other conditions as determined by your doctor.

The nitrates discussed here are available only with your doctor's prescription, in the following dosage forms:

Buccal

Nitroglycerin
- Tablets (U.S. and Canada)

Chewable

Isosorbide dinitrate
- Tablets (U.S.)

Sublingual

Erythrityl tetranitrate
- Tablets (U.S. and Canada)
Isosorbide dinitrate
- Tablets (U.S. and Canada)
Nitroglycerin
- Tablets (U.S. and Canada)

It is very important that you read and understand the following information. If any of it causes you special concern, check with your doctor. Also, *if you have any questions* or if you want more information about this medicine or your medical problem, *ask your doctor, nurse, or pharmacist.*

Before Using This Medicine

In deciding to use a medicine, the risks of taking the medicine must be weighed against the good it will do. This is a decision you and your doctor will make. For nitrates, the following should be considered:

Allergies—Tell your doctor if you have ever had any unusual or allergic reaction to nitrates or nitrites. Also tell your doctor and pharmacist if you are allergic to any other substance, such as certain foods, preservatives, or dyes.

Pregnancy—Although nitrates have not been shown to cause problems in humans, studies in rabbits given large doses of isosorbide dinitrate have shown adverse effects on the fetus. Studies have not been done with erythrityl tetranitrate, nitroglycerin, or pentaerythrityl tetranitrate.

Breast-feeding—It is not known whether this medicine passes into breast milk. However, nitrates have not been reported to cause problems in nursing babies.

Children—There is no specific information about the use of nitrates in children.

Older adults—Dizziness or lightheadedness may be more likely to occur in the elderly, who may be more sensitive to the effects of nitrates.

Other medicines—Although certain medicines should not be used together at all, in other cases two different medicines may be used together even if an interaction might occur. In these cases, your doctor may want to change the dose, or other precautions may be necessary. When you are taking nitrates, it is especially important that your doctor and pharmacist know if you are taking any of the following:
- Antihypertensives (high blood pressure medicine) or
- Other heart medicine—May increase the effects of nitrates on blood pressure

Other medical problems—The presence of other medical problems may affect the use of nitroglycerin. Make sure you tell your doctor if you have any other medical problems, especially:
- Anemia (severe)
- Glaucoma—May be worsened by nitrates
- Head injury (recent) or
- Stroke (recent)—Nitrates may increase pressure in the brain, which can make problems worse
- Heart attack (recent)—Nitrates may lower blood pressure, which can aggravate problems associated with heart attack
- Kidney disease or
- Liver disease—Effects may be increased because of slower removal of nitroglycerin from the body
- Overactive thyroid

Before you begin using any new medicine (prescription or nonprescription) or if you develop any new medical problem while you are using this medicine, check with your doctor, nurse, or pharmacist.

Proper Use of This Medicine

Take this medicine exactly as directed by your doctor. It will work only if taken correctly.

Sublingual tablets should not be chewed, crushed, or swallowed. They work much faster when absorbed through the lining of the mouth. Place the tablet under the tongue, between the lip and gum, or between the cheek and gum and let it dissolve there. Do not eat, drink, smoke, or use chewing tobacco while a tablet is dissolving.

Buccal extended-release tablets should not be chewed, crushed, or swallowed. They are designed to release a dose of nitroglycerin over a period of hours, not all at once.

- Allow the tablet to dissolve slowly in place between the upper lip and gum (above the front teeth), or between the cheek and upper gum. If food or drink is to be taken during the 3 to 5 hours when the tablet is dissolving, place the tablet between the *upper* lip and gum, above the front teeth. If you have dentures, you may place the tablet anywhere between the cheek and gum.
- Touching the tablet with your tongue or drinking hot liquids may cause the tablet to dissolve faster.
- Do not go to sleep while a tablet is dissolving because it could slip down your throat and cause choking.
- If you accidentally swallow the tablet, replace it with another one.
- Do not use chewing tobacco while a tablet is in place.

Chewable tablets must be chewed well and held in the mouth for about 2 minutes before you swallow them. This will allow the medicine to be absorbed through the lining of the mouth.

For patients using *nitroglycerin or isosorbide dinitrate to relieve the pain of an angina attack*:

- *When you begin to feel an attack of angina starting (chest pains or a tightness or squeezing in the chest), sit down. Then place a tablet in your mouth, either sublingually or buccally, or chew a chewable tablet.* This medicine works best when you are standing or sitting. However, since you may become dizzy, light-headed, or faint soon after using a tablet, it is safer to sit rather than stand while the medicine is working. If you become dizzy or faint while sitting, take several deep breaths and bend forward with your head between your knees.

- Remain calm and you should feel better in a few minutes.

- *This medicine usually gives relief in 1 to 5 minutes.* However, if the pain is not relieved, and you are using:

  —Sublingual tablets, either sublingually or buccally: Use a second tablet. If the pain continues for another 5 minutes, a third tablet may be used. *If you still have the chest pains after a total of 3 tablets in a 15-minute period, contact your doctor or go to a hospital emergency room immediately.*

  —Buccal extended-release tablets: *Use a sublingual (under the tongue) nitroglycerin tablet and check with your doctor.* Do not use another buccal tablet since the effects of a buccal tablet last for several hours.

For patients using *nitroglycerin, erythrityl tetranitrate, or isosorbide dinitrate to prevent an expected angina attack:*

- You may prevent anginal chest pains for up to 1 hour (6 hours for the extended-release nitroglycerin tablet) by using a buccal or sublingual tablet or chewing a chewable tablet 5 to 10 minutes before expected emotional stress or physical exertion that in the past seemed to bring on an attack.

For patients using *isosorbide dinitrate or extended-release buccal nitroglycerin regularly on a long-term basis to reduce the number of angina attacks that occur:*

- Chewable or sublingual isosorbide dinitrate and buccal extended-release nitroglycerin tablets can be used either to prevent angina attacks or to help relieve an attack that has already started.

Missed dose—For patients using isosorbide dinitrate or extended-release buccal nitroglycerin regularly on a long-term basis to reduce the number of angina attacks that occur:

- If you miss a dose of this medicine, use it as soon as possible. However, if the next scheduled dose is within 2 hours, skip the missed dose and go back to your regular dosing schedule. Do not double doses.

Stability and storage—

For sublingual nitroglycerin

- When properly stored, sublingual nitroglycerin tablets retain their strength until the expiration date printed on the original label. However, because of patient usage, changing temperature and moisture, shaking, and repeated bottle opening, the tablets may be good for only 3 to 6 months. The "stabilized" sublingual tablets may stay good for a longer period of time but require the same care in storage and use.

- Some people think they should test the strength of their sublingual nitroglycerin tablets by looking for a tingling or burning sensation, a feeling of warmth or flushing, or a headache, after a tablet has been dissolved under the tongue. This kind of testing is not completely reliable since some patients may be unable to detect these effects. In addition, newer, stabilized sublingual nitroglycerin tablets are less likely to produce these detectable effects.

- To help keep the nitroglycerin tablets at full strength:
  —keep the medicine in the original glass, screw-cap bottle. For patients who wish to carry a small number of tablets with them for emergency use, a specially designed container is available. However, only containers specifically labeled as suitable for use with nitroglycerin sublingual tablets should be used.

  —remove the cotton plug that comes in the bottle and *do not* put it back.

—*put the cap on the bottle quickly and tightly after each use.*

—to select a tablet for use, pour several into the bottle cap, take one, and pour the others back into the bottle. Try not to hold them in the palm of your hand because they may pick up moisture and crumble.

—do not keep other medicines in the same bottle with the nitroglycerin since they will weaken the nitroglycerin effect.

—keep the medicine handy at all times but try not to carry the bottle close to the body. Medicine may lose strength because of body warmth. Instead, carry the tightly closed bottle in your purse or the pocket of a jacket or other loose-fitting clothing whenever possible.

—store the bottle of nitroglycerin tablets in a cool, dry place. Storage at average room temperature away from direct heat or direct sunlight is best. Do not store in the refrigerator or in a bathroom medicine cabinet because the moisture usually present in these areas may cause the tablets to crumble if the container is not tightly closed. Do not keep the tablets in your automobile glove compartment.

• Keep out of the reach of children.
• Do not keep outdated medicine or medicine no longer needed. Be sure that any discarded medicine is out of the reach of children.

For erythrityl tetranitrate, isosorbide dinitrate, and buccal extended-release nitroglycerin

• These forms of nitrates are more stable than sublingual nitroglycerin.
• Keep out of the reach of children.
• Store away from heat and direct light.
• Do not store in the bathroom, near the kitchen sink, or in other damp places. Heat or moisture may cause the medicine to break down.
• Do not keep outdated medicine or medicine no longer needed. Be sure that any discarded medicine is out of the reach of children.

Precautions While Using This Medicine

If you have been taking this medicine regularly for several weeks, do not suddenly stop using it. Stopping suddenly may bring on attacks of angina. Check with your doctor for the best way to reduce gradually the amount you are taking before stopping completely.

Dizziness, lightheadedness, or faintness may occur, especially when you get up quickly from a lying or sitting position. Getting up slowly may help. If you feel dizzy, sit or lie down.

The dizziness, lightheadedness, or fainting is also more likely to occur if you drink alcohol, stand for long periods of time, exercise, or if the weather is hot. *While you are taking this medicine, be careful in the amount of alcohol you drink. Also, use extra care during exercise or hot weather or if you must stand for long periods of time.*

After taking a dose of this medicine you may get a headache that lasts for a short time. This is a common side effect, which should become less noticeable after you have taken the medicine for a while. If this effect continues or if the headaches are severe, check with your doctor.

Side Effects of This Medicine

Along with its needed effects, a medicine may cause some unwanted effects. Although not all of these side effects may occur, if they do occur they may need medical attention.

Check with your doctor as soon as possible if any of the following side effects occur:

Rare

   Blurred vision; dry mouth; headache (severe or prolonged); skin rash

Signs and symptoms of overdose (in the order in which they may occur)

   Bluish-colored lips, fingernails, or palms of hands; dizziness (extreme) or fainting; feeling of extreme pressure in head; shortness of breath; unusual tiredness or weakness; weak and fast heartbeat; fever; convulsions (seizures)

Other side effects may occur that usually do not need medical attention. These side effects may go away during treatment as your body adjusts to the medicine. However, check with your doctor if any of the following side effects continue or are bothersome:

> *More common*
>> Dizziness or lightheadedness, especially when getting up from a lying or sitting position; fast pulse; flushing of face and neck; headache; nausea or vomiting; restlessness

Other side effects not listed above may also occur in some patients. If you notice any other effects, check with your doctor.

NITRATES—Topical   Systemic

This information applies to nitroglycerin ointment and transdermal patches.

Some commonly used brand names are:

For nitroglycerin ointment

In the U.S.

Nitro-Bid	Nitrong
Nitrol	Nitrostat

Generic name product may also be available.

In Canada

Nitro-Bid	Nitrong
Nitrol	

Another commonly used name is glyceryl trinitrate.

For nitroglycerin transdermal patches

In the U.S.

Deponit	Nitro-Dur II
Nitrocine	NTS
Nitrodisc	Transderm-Nitro
Nitro-Dur	

Generic name product may also be available.

In Canada

Transderm-Nitro

Another commonly used name is glyceryl trinitrate.

Description

Nitrates (NYE-trates) are used to treat the symptoms of angina (chest pain). Depending on the type of dosage form and how it is taken, nitrates are used to treat angina in three ways:

- to relieve an attack that is occurring by using the medicine when the attack begins;
- to prevent attacks from occurring by using the medicine just before an attack is expected to occur; or
- to reduce the number of attacks that occur by using the medicine regularly on a long-term basis.

When applied to the skin, nitrates are used to reduce the number of angina attacks that occur. The only nitrate available for this purpose is topical nitroglycerin (nye-troe-GLI-ser-in).

Topical nitroglycerin is absorbed through the skin. It works by relaxing blood vessels and increasing the supply of blood and oxygen to the heart while reducing its work load. This helps prevent future angina attacks from occurring.

Topical nitroglycerin may also be used for other conditions as determined by your doctor.

Nitroglycerin as discussed here is available only with your doctor's prescription, in the following dosage forms:

Topical
- Ointment (U.S. and Canada)
- Transdermal (stick-on) patch (U.S. and Canada)

It is very important that you read and understand the following information. If any of it causes you special concern, check with your doctor. Also, *if you have any questions* or if you want more information about this medicine or your medical problem, *ask your doctor, nurse, or pharmacist.*

Before Using This Medicine

In deciding to use a medicine, the risks of taking the medicine must be weighed against the good it will do. This is a decision you and your doctor will make. For nitroglycerin applied to the skin, the following should be considered:

Allergies—Tell your doctor if you have ever had any unusual or allergic reaction to nitrates or nitrites. Also tell your doctor and pharmacist if you are allergic to any other substance, such as certain foods, preservatives, or dyes.

Pregnancy—Studies have not been done in humans. However, nitroglycerin has not been shown to cause problems.

Breast-feeding—It is not known whether this medicine passes into breast milk. However, nitroglycerin has not been reported to cause problems in nursing babies.

Children—There is no specific information about the use of nitrates in children.

Older adults—Dizziness or lightheadedness may be more likely to occur in the elderly, who may be more sensitive to the effects of nitrates.

Other medicines—Although certain medicines should not be used together at all, in other cases two different medicines may be used together even if an interaction might occur. In these cases, your doctor may want to change the dose, or other precautions may be necessary. When you are using nitroglycerin, it is especially important that your doctor and pharmacist know if you are taking any of the following:
- Antihypertensives (high blood pressure medicine) or
- Other heart medicine—May increase the effects of nitroglycerin on blood pressure

Other medical problems—The presence of other medical problems may affect the use of nitroglycerin. Make sure you tell your doctor if you have any other medical problems, especially:
- Anemia (severe)
- Glaucoma—May be worsened by nitroglycerin
- Head injury (recent) or
- Stroke (recent)—Nitroglycerin may increase pressure in the brain, which can make problems worse
- Heart attack (recent)—Nitroglycerin may lower blood pressure, which can aggravate problems associated with heart attack

- Kidney disease or
- Liver disease—Effects may be increased because of slower removal of nitroglycerin from the body
- Overactive thyroid

Before you begin using any new medicine (prescription or nonprescription) or if you develop any new medical problem while you are using this medicine, check with your doctor, nurse, or pharmacist.

Proper Use of This Medicine

Use nitroglycerin exactly as directed by your doctor. It will work only if applied correctly.

The ointment and transdermal forms of nitroglycerin are used to reduce the number of angina attacks. They will not relieve an attack that has already started because they work too slowly. Check with your doctor if you need a fast-acting medicine to relieve the pain of an angina attack.

This medicine usually comes with patient instructions. Read them carefully before using.

For patients using the *ointment* form of this medicine:

- Before applying a new dose of ointment, remove any ointment remaining on the skin from a previous dose. This will allow the fresh ointment to release the nitroglycerin properly.
- This medicine comes with dose-measuring papers. Use them to measure the length of ointment squeezed from the tube and to apply the ointment to the skin. *Do not rub or massage the ointment into the skin; just spread in a thin, even layer, covering an area of the same size each time it is applied.*
- Apply the ointment to skin that has little or no hair.
- Apply each dose of ointment to a different area of skin to prevent irritation or other skin problems.
- If your doctor has ordered an occlusive dressing (airtight covering, such as kitchen plastic wrap) to be applied over this medicine, make sure you know how to apply it. Since occlusive dressings increase the amount

of medicine absorbed through the skin and the possibility of side effects, use them only as directed. If you have any questions about this, check with your doctor, nurse, or pharmacist.

For patients using the *transdermal (stick-on patch) system*:

- Do not try to trim or cut the adhesive patch to adjust the dosage. Check with your doctor if you think the medicine is not working as it should.
- Apply the patch to a clean, dry skin area with little or no hair and free of scars, cuts, or irritation. Remove the previous patch before applying a new one.
- Apply a new patch if the first one becomes loose or falls off.
- Apply each dose to a different area of skin to prevent skin irritation or other problems.

Missed dose—

- For patients using the *ointment* form of this medicine: If you miss a dose of this medicine, apply it as soon as possible unless the next scheduled dose is within 2 hours. Then go back to your regular dosing schedule. Do not increase the amount used.
- For patients using the *transdermal (stick-on patch) system*: If you miss a dose of this medicine, apply it as soon as possible. Then go back to your regular dosing schedule.

Storage—

- To store the *ointment* form of this medicine:

    —Keep out of the reach of children.

    —Store the tube of nitroglycerin ointment in a cool place and keep it tightly closed.

    —Do not keep outdated medicine or medicine no longer needed. Be sure that any discarded medicine is out of the reach of children.

- To store the *transdermal (stick-on patch) system*:

    —Keep out of the reach of children.

    —Store away from heat and direct light.

—Do not store in the bathroom, near the kitchen sink, or in other damp places. Heat or moisture may cause the medicine to break down.

—Do not keep outdated medicine or medicine no longer needed. Be sure that any discarded medicine is out of the reach of children.

Precautions While Using This Medicine

If you have been using nitroglycerin regularly for several weeks or more, do not suddenly stop using it. Stopping suddenly may bring on attacks of angina. Check with your doctor for the best way to reduce gradually the amount you are using before stopping completely.

Dizziness, lightheadedness, or faintness may occur, especially when you get up quickly from a lying or sitting position. Getting up slowly may help. If you feel dizzy, sit or lie down.

The dizziness, lightheadedness, or fainting is also more likely to occur if you drink alcohol, stand for long periods of time, exercise, or if the weather is hot. *While you are taking this medicine, be careful in the amount of alcohol you drink. Also, use extra care during exercise or hot weather or if you must stand for long periods of time.*

After using a dose of this medicine you may get a headache that lasts for a short time. This is a common side effect, which should become less noticeable after you have used the medicine for a while. If this effect continues, or if the headaches are severe, check with your doctor.

Side Effects of This Medicine

Along with its needed effects, a medicine may cause some unwanted effects. Although not all of these side effects may occur, if they do occur they may need medical attention.

Check with your doctor as soon as possible if any of the following side effects occur:

Rare

Blurred vision; dry mouth; headache (severe or prolonged)

Signs and symptoms of overdose (in the order in which they may occur)
> Bluish-colored lips, fingernails, or palms of hands; dizziness (extreme) or fainting; feeling of extreme pressure in head; shortness of breath; unusual tiredness or weakness; weak and fast heartbeat; fever; convulsions (seizures)

Other side effects may occur that usually do not need medical attention. These side effects may go away during treatment as your body adjusts to the medicine. However, check with your doctor if any of the following side effects continue or are bothersome:

More common
> Dizziness or lightheadedness, especially when getting up from a lying or sitting position; fast pulse; flushing of face and neck; headache; nausea or vomiting; restlessness

Less common
> Sore, reddened skin

Other side effects not listed above may also occur in some patients. If you notice any other effects, check with your doctor.

NITROFURANTOIN   Systemic

Some commonly used brand names are:
> *In the U.S.*

Furadantin	Macrodantin
Furalan	Nitrofuracot
Furatoin	

> Generic name product may also be available.

> *In Canada*

Apo-Nitrofurantoin	Nephronex
Macrodantin	Novofuran

Description

Nitrofurantoin (nye-troe-fyoor-AN-toyn) belongs to the family of medicines called anti-infectives. It is used to treat infections of the urinary tract. It may also be used for other conditions as determined by your doctor.

Nitrofurantoin is available only with your doctor's prescription, in the following dosage forms:

Oral
- Capsules (U.S. and Canada)
- Oral Suspension (U.S. and Canada)
- Tablets (U.S. and Canada)

It is very important that you read and understand the following information. If any of it causes you special concern, check with your doctor. Also, *if you have any questions* or if you want more information about this medicine or your medical problem, *ask your doctor, nurse, or pharmacist*.

Before Using This Medicine

In deciding to use a medicine, the risks of taking the medicine must be weighed against the good it will do. This is a decision you and your doctor will make. For nitrofurantoin, the following should be considered:

Allergies—Tell your doctor if you have ever had any unusual or allergic reaction to nitrofurantoin or to any related medicines such as furazolidone (e.g., Furoxone) or nitrofurazone (e.g., Furacin). Also tell your doctor and pharmacist if you are allergic to any other substances, such as foods, preservatives, or dyes.

Pregnancy—Nitrofurantoin should not be used if you are within a week or 2 of your delivery date or during labor and delivery. It may cause problems in the infant.

Breast-feeding—Nitrofurantoin passes into the breast milk in small amounts and may cause problems in nursing babies with glucose-6-phosphate dehydrogenase (G6PD) deficiency.

Children—Infants under the age of 1 month should not be given this medicine because they are especially sensitive to the effects of nitrofurantoin.

Older adults—Elderly people may be more sensitive to the effects of nitrofurantoin. This may increase the chance of side effects during treatment.

Other medicines—Although certain medicines should not be used together at all, in other cases two different medicines

may be used together even if an interaction might occur. In these cases, your doctor may want to change the dose, or other precautions may be necessary. When you are taking nitrofurantoin, it is especially important that your doctor and pharmacist know if you are taking any of the following:

- Acetohydroxamic acid (e.g., Lithostat) or
- Antidiabetics, oral (diabetes medicine you take by mouth) or
- Dapsone or
- Furazolidone (e.g., Furoxone) or
- Methyldopa (e.g., Aldomet) or
- Primaquine or
- Procainamide (e.g., Pronestyl) or
- Quinidine (e.g., Quinidex) or
- Sulfonamides (sulfa medicine) or
- Sulfoxone (e.g., Diasone) or
- Vitamin K (e.g., AquaMEPHYTON, Synkayvite)—Patients who take nitrofurantoin with any of these medicines may have an increase in side effects affecting the blood

- Carbamazepine (e.g., Tegretol) or
- Chloroquine (e.g., Aralen) or
- Cisplatin (e.g., Platinol) or
- Cytarabine (e.g., Cytosar-U) or
- Disulfiram (e.g., Antabuse) or
- Ethotoin (e.g., Peganone) or
- Hydroxychloroquine (e.g., Plaquenil) or
- Lindane, topical (e.g., Kwell) or
- Lithium (e.g., Lithane) or
- Mephenytoin (e.g., Mesantoin) or
- Mexiletine (e.g., Mexitil) or
- Other anti-infectives by mouth or by injection (medicine for infection) or
- Pemoline (e.g., Cylert) or
- Phenytoin (e.g., Dilantin) or
- Pyridoxine (e.g., Hexa-Betalin) (with long-term, high-dose use) or
- Quinine (e.g., Quinamm) or
- Vincristine (e.g., Oncovin) or
- Diphtheria, tetanus, and pertussis (DTP) vaccine—Patients who take nitrofurantoin with any of these medicines, or who have received a DTP vaccine within the last 30 days or are going to receive a DTP may have an increase in side effects affecting the nervous system

- Probenecid (e.g., Benemid) or
- Sulfinpyrazone (e.g., Anturane)—Patients who take nitrofurantoin with any of these medicines may have an increase in side effects

Other medical problems—The presence of other medical problems may affect the use of nitrofurantoin. Make sure you tell your doctor if you have any other medical problems, especially:

- Glucose-6-phosphate dehydrogenase (G6PD) deficiency—Nitrofurantoin may cause anemia in patients with G6PD deficiency
- Kidney disease (other than infection)—Nitrofurantoin may cause an increased chance of side effects and be less effective in patients with kidney disease
- Lung disease or
- Nerve damage—Patients with lung disease or nerve damage may have an increase in side effects when they take nitrofurantoin

Before you begin using any new medicine (prescription or nonprescription) or if you develop any new medical problem while you are using this medicine, check with your doctor, nurse, or pharmacist.

Proper Use of This Medicine

Do not give this medicine to infants up to 1 month of age.

Nitrofurantoin is best taken with food or milk. This may lessen stomach upset and help your body absorb the medicine better.

For patients taking the *oral liquid form of this medicine:*

- Shake the oral liquid forcefully before each dose to help make it pour more smoothly and to be sure the medicine is evenly mixed.
- Use a specially marked measuring spoon or other device to measure each dose accurately. The average household teaspoon may not hold the right amount of liquid.
- May be mixed with water, milk, fruit juices, or infants' formulas. If mixed with other liquids, take immediately after mixing. Be sure to drink all the liquid in order to get the full dose of medicine.

To help clear up your infection completely, *keep taking this medicine for the full time of treatment,* even if you begin to feel better after a few days. *Do not miss any doses.*

Missed dose—If you do miss a dose of this medicine, take it as soon as possible. However, if it is almost time for your next dose and your dosing schedule is:

- Three or more doses a day—Space the missed dose and the next dose 2 to 4 hours apart.

Then go back to your regular dosing schedule.

Storage—To store this medicine:

- Keep out of the reach of children.
- Store away from heat and direct light.
- Do not store the capsule or tablet form of this medicine in the bathroom, near the kitchen sink, or in other damp places. Heat or moisture may cause the medicine to break down.
- Keep the oral liquid form of this medicine from freezing.
- Do not keep outdated medicine or medicine no longer needed. Be sure that any discarded medicine is out of the reach of children.

Precautions While Using This Medicine

It is important that your doctor check your progress at regular visits if you will be taking this medicine for a long time.

If your symptoms do not improve within a few days, or if they become worse, check with your doctor.

For *diabetic patients:*

- *This medicine may cause false test results with some urine sugar tests.* Check with your doctor before changing your diet or the dosage of your diabetes medicine.

Side Effects of This Medicine

Along with its needed effects, a medicine may cause some unwanted effects. Although not all of these side effects may occur, if they do occur they may need medical attention.

Check with your doctor immediately if any of the following side effects occur:

More common

Chest pain; chills; cough; fever; troubled breathing

Less common

Dizziness; drowsiness; headache; numbness, tingling, or burning of face or mouth; sore throat and fever

Rare

Itching; joint pain; pale skin; skin rash; unusual tiredness or weakness; yellow eyes or skin

Other side effects may occur that usually do not need medical attention. These side effects may go away during treatment as your body adjusts to the medicine. However, check with your doctor if any of the following side effects continue or are bothersome:

More common

Abdominal or stomach pain or upset; diarrhea; loss of appetite; nausea or vomiting

This medicine may cause the urine to become rust-yellow to brown. This side effect does not require medical attention.

Other side effects not listed above may also occur in some patients. If you notice any other effects, check with your doctor.

NORFLOXACIN   Systemic

A commonly used brand name in the U.S. and Canada is Noroxin.

Description

Norfloxacin (nor-FLOX-a-sin) is used in the treatment of infections caused by bacteria. They work by killing bacteria or preventing their growth. This medicine will not work for colds, flu, or other virus infections.

Norfloxacin is used to treat infections of the urinary tract. It may also be used for other problems as determined by your doctor.

This medicine is available only with your doctor's prescription, in the following dosage form:

    Oral
      • Tablets (U.S. and Canada)

It is very important that you read and understand the following information. If any of it causes you special concern, check with your doctor. Also, *if you have any questions* or if you want more information about this medicine or your medical problem, *ask your doctor, nurse, or pharmacist.*

Before Using This Medicine

In deciding to use a medicine, the risks of taking the medicine must be weighed against the good it will do. This is a decision you and your doctor will make. For norfloxacin, the following should be considered:

Allergies—Tell your doctor if you have ever had any unusual or allergic reaction to norfloxacin or to any related medicines such as cinoxacin (e.g., Cinobac), ciprofloxacin (e.g., Cipro), ofloxacin (e.g., Floxin), or nalidixic acid (e.g., NegGram). Also tell your doctor and pharmacist if you are allergic to any other substances, such as foods, preservatives, or dyes.

Pregnancy—Studies have not been done in humans. However, use is not recommended during pregnancy since norfloxacin has been shown to cause bone problems in young animals. Studies in some monkeys have shown that norfloxacin causes a decrease in successful pregnancies and may kill the fetus when given in doses of 10 to 15 times the highest human dose. Studies in rats, rabbits, and mice, and other studies in monkeys have not shown that norfloxacin causes birth defects when given in doses 6 to 50 times the usual human dose.

Breast-feeding—It is not known whether norfloxacin passes into the breast milk. Norfloxacin has not been shown to pass into breast milk when it was given in low doses. However, other related medicines do pass into the breast milk. Also, norfloxacin has been shown to cause bone problems in young animals. Therefore, use is not recommended in nursing mothers.

Children—Use is not recommended for infants, children, or adolescents since norfloxacin has been shown to cause bone problems in young animals.

Older adults—Many medicines have not been studied specifically in older people. Therefore, it may not be known whether they work exactly the same way they do in younger adults. Although there is no specific information comparing use of norfloxacin in the elderly with use in other age groups, this medicine is not expected to cause different side effects or problems in older people than it does in younger adults.

Other medicines—Although certain medicines should not be used together at all, in other cases two different medicines may be used together even if an interaction might occur. In these cases, your doctor may want to change the dose, or other precautions may be necessary. When you are taking norfloxacin, it is especially important that your doctor and pharmacist know if you are taking any of the following:

- Antacids or
- Sucralfate—Antacids or sucralfate may decrease the effectiveness of norfloxacin
- Theophylline (e.g., Somophyllin-T, Theodur, Elixophyllin)—Norfloxacin may increase the chance of side effects from theophylline

- Warfarin (e.g., Coumadin)—Norfloxacin may increase the chance of side effects from warfarin

Other medical problems—The presence of other medical problems may affect the use of norfloxacin. Make sure you tell your doctor if you have any other medical problems, especially:

- Kidney disease, severe—Patients with kidney disease may have an increased chance of side effects
- Seizures or a history of seizures—Patients with a history of seizures may have an increased chance of seizures when taking this medicine

Before you begin using any new medicine (prescription or nonprescription) or if you develop any new medical problem while you are using this medicine, check with your doctor, nurse, or pharmacist.

Proper Use of This Medicine

Do not give this medicine to infants or children unless otherwise directed by your doctor. It has been shown to cause bone problems in young animals.

Norfloxacin is best taken with a full glass (8 ounces) of water on an empty stomach (either 1 hour before or 2 hours after meals). *Several additional glasses of water should be taken every day,* unless otherwise directed by your doctor. Drinking extra water will help to prevent unwanted effects of norfloxacin, especially if you are taking high doses.

To help clear up your infection completely, *keep taking norfloxacin for the full time of treatment,* even if you begin to feel better after a few days. If you stop taking this medicine too soon, your symptoms may return.

This medicine works best when there is a constant amount in the blood or urine. *To help keep the amount constant, do not miss any doses. Also, it is best to take the doses at evenly spaced times day and night.* For example, if you are to take 2 doses a day, the doses should be spaced about 12 hours apart. If this interferes with your sleep or other daily activities, or if you need help in planning the best times to take your medicine, check with your doctor, nurse, or pharmacist.

Missed dose—If you do miss a dose of this medicine, take it as soon as possible. This will help to keep a constant amount of medicine in the blood or urine. However, if it is almost time for your next dose, skip the missed dose and go back to your regular dosing schedule. Do not double doses.

Storage—To store this medicine:
* Keep out of the reach of children.
* Store away from heat and direct light.
* Do not store in the bathroom, near the kitchen sink, or in other damp places. Heat or moisture may cause the medicine to break down.
* Do not keep outdated medicine or medicine no longer needed. Be sure that any discarded medicine is out of the reach of children.

Precautions While Using This Medicine

If your symptoms do not improve within a few days, or if they become worse, check with your doctor.

If you are taking antacids or sucralfate, do not take them at the same time that you take norfloxacin. Antacids and sucralfate may keep norfloxacin from working properly. Take antacids and sucralfate *at least* 2 to 3 hours after you take this medicine.

This medicine may cause your eyes to become more sensitive to light than they are normally. Wearing sunglasses and avoiding too much exposure to bright light may help lessen the discomfort.

Norfloxacin may cause your skin to be more sensitive to sunlight than it is normally. Exposure to sunlight, even for brief periods of time, may cause a skin rash, itching, redness or other discoloration of the skin, or a severe sunburn. When you begin taking this medicine:
* Stay out of direct sunlight, especially between the hours of 10:00 a.m. and 3:00 p.m., if possible.

- Wear protective clothing, including a hat. Also, wear sunglasses.
- Apply a sun block product that has a skin protection factor (SPF) of at least 15. Some patients may require a product with a higher SPF number, especially if they have a fair complexion. If you have any questions about this, check with your doctor or pharmacist.
- Apply a sun block lipstick that has an SPF of at least 15 to protect your lips.
- Do not use a sunlamp or tanning bed or booth.

If you have a severe reaction from the sun, check with your doctor.

This medicine may cause some people to become dizzy, light-headed, drowsy, or less alert than they are normally. *Make sure you know how you react to this medicine before you drive, use machines, or do anything else that could be dangerous if you are dizzy or are not alert.* If these reactions occur, check with your doctor.

Side Effects of This Medicine

Along with its needed effects, a medicine may cause some unwanted effects. Although not all of these side effects may occur, if they do occur they may need medical attention.

Check with your doctor as soon as possible if any of the following side effects occur:

Rare

Confusion; convulsions (seizures); mental depression; muscle tremors; skin rash, itching, or redness; swelling of neck or face; swollen or inflamed joints or tendons

Other side effects may occur that usually do not need medical attention. These side effects may go away during treatment as your body adjusts to the medicine. However, check with your doctor if any of the following side effects continue or are bothersome:

More common

Abdominal or stomach pain or upset; constipation; diarrhea; dizziness; drowsiness; headache; lightheadedness; loss of appetite; nausea or vomiting; trouble in sleeping

Less common or rare
Increased sensitivity to sunlight

Other side effects not listed above may also occur in some patients. If you notice any other effects, check with your doctor.

Additional Information

Once a medicine has been approved for marketing for a certain use, experience may show that it is also useful for other medical problems. Although these uses are not included in product labeling, norfloxacin is used in certain patients with the following medical conditions:

- Bacterial gastroenteritis
- Gonorrhea—not treatable with penicillin

Other than the above information, there is no additional information relating to proper use, precautions, or side effects for these uses.

OFLOXACIN   Systemic

Some commonly used brand names are:
In the U.S.
Floxin
Floxin IV
In Canada
Floxin

Description

Ofloxacin (oe-FLOX-a-sin) is used to treat bacterial infections in many different parts of the body. It works by killing bacteria or preventing their growth. However, this medicine will not work for colds, flu, or other virus infections.

Ofloxacin is available only with your doctor's prescription, in the following dosage forms:
Oral
- Tablets (U.S. and Canada)

Parenteral
- Injection (U.S.)

It is very important that you read and understand the following information. If any of it causes you special concern, check with your doctor. Also, *if you have any questions* or if you want more information about this medicine or your medical problem, *ask your doctor, nurse, or pharmacist.*

Before Using This Medicine

In deciding to use a medicine, the risks of taking the medicine must be weighed against the good it will do. This is a decision you and your doctor will make. For ofloxacin, the following should be considered:

Allergies—Tell your doctor if you have ever had any unusual or allergic reaction to ofloxacin or to any related medicines such as cinoxacin (e.g., Cinobac), ciprofloxacin (e.g., Cipro), nalidixic acid (e.g., NegGram), or norfloxacin (e.g., Noroxin). Also tell your doctor and pharmacist if you are allergic to any other substances, such as foods, preservatives, or dyes.

Pregnancy—Studies have not been done in humans. However, use is not recommended during pregnancy since ofloxacin has been reported to cause bone development problems in young animals.

Breast-feeding—Ofloxacin passes into human breast milk. Since ofloxacin has been reported to cause bone development problems in young animals, breast-feeding is not recommended during treatment with this medicine.

Children—Use is not recommended in infants, children, or adolescents since ofloxacin has been shown to cause bone development problems in young animals.

Older adults—This medicine has been tested and has not been shown to cause different side effects or problems in older people than it does in younger adults.

Other medicines—Although certain medicines should not be used together at all, in other cases two different medicines

may be used together even if an interaction might occur. In these cases, your doctor may want to change the dose, or other precautions may be necessary. When you are using ofloxacin, it is especially important that your doctor and pharmacist know if you are taking any of the following:

- Antacids, aluminum- or magnesium-containing—Aluminum- or magnesium-containing antacids may keep ofloxacin from working properly

Other medical problems—The presence of other medical problems may affect the use of ofloxacin. Make sure you tell your doctor if you have any other medical problems, especially:

- Kidney disease or
- Liver disease—Patients with kidney or liver disease may have an increased chance of side effects

Before you begin using any new medicine (prescription or nonprescription) or if you develop any new medical problem while you are using this medicine, check with your doctor, nurse, or pharmacist.

Proper Use of This Medicine

Do not give ofloxacin to infants, children, or adolescents unless otherwise directed by your doctor. Also, *do not take ofloxacin if you are pregnant or breast-feeding*. This medicine has been shown to cause bone development problems in young animals.

Ofloxacin is best taken on an empty stomach with a full glass (8 ounces) of water. Several additional glasses of water should be taken every day, unless you are otherwise directed by your doctor.

To help clear up your infection completely, *keep taking ofloxacin for the full time of treatment,* even if you begin to feel better after a few days. If you stop taking this medicine too soon, your symptoms may return.

This medicine works best when there is a constant amount in the blood or urine. *To help keep the amount constant, do not miss any doses. Also, it is best to take the doses at evenly spaced times, day and night.* For example, if you are to take 2 doses a day, the doses should be spaced about 12 hours apart. If this interferes with your sleep or other daily activities, or if you need help in planning the best times to take your medicine, check with your doctor, nurse, or pharmacist.

Missed dose—If you do miss a dose of this medicine, take it as soon as possible. This will help to keep a constant amount of medicine in the blood or urine. However, if it is almost time for your next dose, skip the missed dose and go back to your regular dosing schedule. Do not double doses.

Storage—To store this medicine:
- Keep out of the reach of children.
- Store away from heat and direct light.
- Do not store in the bathroom, near the kitchen sink, or in other damp places. Heat or moisture may cause the medicine to break down.
- Do not keep outdated medicine or medicine no longer needed. Be sure that any discarded medicine is out of the reach of children.

Precautions While Using This Medicine

If your symptoms do not improve within a few days, or if they become worse, check with your doctor.

If you are taking aluminum- or magnesium-containing antacids, do not take them at the same time that you take ofloxacin. It is best to take these medicines at least 2 hours before or at least 2 hours after you take ofloxacin. These medicines may keep ofloxacin from working properly.

Ofloxacin may cause some people to become dizzy or less alert than they are normally. *Make sure you know how you react to this medicine before you drive, use machines, or do anything else that could be dangerous if you are dizzy or are not alert.* If these reactions are especially bothersome, check with your doctor.

Side Effects of This Medicine

Along with its needed effects, a medicine may cause some unwanted effects. Although not all of these side effects may occur, if they do occur they may need medical attention.

Check with your doctor immediately if any of the following side effects occur:

Rare

Agitation; confusion; hallucinations (seeing, hearing, or feeling things that are not there); mood changes; pain or redness at place of injection; shortness of breath; skin rash, itching, or redness

Other side effects may occur that usually do not need medical attention. These side effects may go away during treatment as your body adjusts to the medicine. However, check with your doctor if any of the following side effects continue or are bothersome:

More common

Abdominal or stomach pain or discomfort; diarrhea; dizziness; headache; nausea or vomiting; trouble in sleeping

Other side effects not listed above may also occur in some patients. If you notice any other effects, check with your doctor.

OLSALAZINE   Oral

A commonly used brand name in the U.S. and Canada is Dipentum.

Other commonly used names are sodium azodisalicylate and azodisal sodium.

Description

Olsalazine (ole-SAL-a-zeen) is used in patients who have had ulcerative colitis to prevent the condition from occurring again. It works inside the bowel by helping to reduce the inflammation and other symptoms of the disease.

Olsalazine is available only with your doctor's prescription, in the following dosage form:

Oral
- Capsules (U.S. and Canada)

It is very important that you read and understand the following information. If any of it causes you special concern, check with your doctor. Also, *if you have any questions* or if you want more information about this medicine or your medical problem, *ask your doctor, nurse, or pharmacist.*

Before Using This Medicine

In deciding to use a medicine, the risks of taking the medicine must be weighed against the good it will do. This is a decision you and your doctor will make. For olsalazine, the following should be considered:

Allergies—Tell your doctor if you have ever had any unusual or allergic reaction to olsalazine, mesalamine, or any salicylates (for example, aspirin). Also tell your doctor and pharmacist if you are allergic to any other substances, such as foods, preservatives, or dyes.

Pregnancy—Studies have not been done in humans. However, studies in rats have shown that olsalazine causes birth defects and other problems at doses 5 to 20 times the human dose. Before taking this medicine, make sure your doctor knows if you are pregnant or if you may become pregnant.

Breast-feeding—It is not known whether olsalazine passes into the breast milk.

Children—Studies on this medicine have been done only in adult patients, and there is no specific information comparing use of olsalazine in children with use in other age groups.

Older adults—Many medicines have not been studied specifically in older people. Therefore, it may not be known whether they work exactly the same way they do in younger adults. Although there is no specific information comparing use of olsalazine in the elderly with use in other age groups, this medicine is not expected to cause different side effects or problems in older people than it does in younger adults.

Other medicines—Although certain medicines should not be used together at all, in other cases two different medicines

may be used together even if an interaction might occur. In these cases, your doctor may want to change the dose, or other precautions may be necessary. When you are using olsalazine, it is especially important that your doctor and pharmacist know if you are taking any other medicines.

Other medical problems—The presence of other medical problems may affect the use of olsalazine. Make sure you tell your doctor if you have any other medical problems, especially:

- Kidney disease—The use of olsalazine may cause further damage to the kidneys

Before you begin using any new medicine (prescription or nonprescription) or if you develop any new medical problem while you are using this medicine, check with your doctor, nurse, or pharmacist.

Proper Use of This Medicine

Olsalazine is best taken with food, to lessen stomach upset and diarrhea. If stomach or intestinal problems continue or are bothersome, check with your doctor.

Keep taking this medicine for the full time of treatment, even if you begin to feel better after a few days. *Do not miss any doses.*

Missed dose—If you do miss a dose of this medicine, take it as soon as possible. However, if it is almost time for your next dose, skip the missed dose and go back to your regular dosing schedule. Do not double doses.

Storage—To store this medicine:

- Keep out of the reach of children.
- Store away from heat and direct light.
- Do not store this medicine in the bathroom, near the kitchen sink, or in other damp places. Heat or moisture may cause the medicine to break down.
- Do not keep outdated medicine or medicine no longer needed. Be sure that any discarded medicine is out of the reach of children.

Precautions While Using This Medicine

It is very important that your doctor check your progress at regular visits, especially if you will be taking it for a long time. Olsalazine may cause blood problems.

Side Effects of This Medicine

Along with its needed effects, a medicine may cause some unwanted effects. Although not all of these side effects may occur, if they do occur they may need medical attention.

Check with your doctor as soon as possible if any of the following side effects occur:

Rare

Bloody diarrhea; fever; pale skin; skin rash; sore throat; unusual bleeding or bruising; unusual tiredness or weakness; yellow eyes or skin

Other side effects may occur that usually do not need medical attention. These side effects may go away during treatment as your body adjusts to the medicine. However, check with your doctor if any of the following side effects continue or are bothersome:

More common

Abdominal or stomach pain or upset; diarrhea; loss of appetite; nausea or vomiting

Less common

Aching joints and muscles; acne; anxiety or depression, drowsiness or dizziness; headache; insomnia

Other side effects not listed above may also occur in some patients. If you notice any other effects, check with your doctor.

OMEPRAZOLE   Systemic

Some commonly used brand names are:

In the U.S.
Prilosec

In Canada
Losec

Description

Omeprazole (o-MEP-ra-zole) is used to treat certain conditions in which there is too much acid in the stomach. It is used to treat duodenal ulcers and gastroesophageal reflux disease, a condition in which the acid in the stomach washes back up into the esophagus. Omeprazole is also used to treat Zollinger-Ellison disease, a condition in which the stomach produces too much acid. It may also be used for other conditions as determined by your doctor.

Omeprazole works by decreasing the amount of acid produced by the stomach.

This medicine is available only with your doctor's prescription.

Oral

- Delayed-release capsules (U.S. and Canada)

It is very important that you read and understand the following information. If any of it causes you special concern, check with your doctor. Also, *if you have any questions* or if you want more information about this medicine or your medical problem, *ask your doctor, nurse, or pharmacist.*

Before Using This Medicine

In deciding to use a medicine, the risks of taking the medicine must be weighed against the good it will do. This is a decision you and your doctor will make. For omeprazole, the following should be considered:

Allergies—Tell your doctor if you have ever had any unusual or allergic reaction to omeprazole. Also tell your doctor and pharmacist if you are allergic to any other substances, such as foods, preservatives, or dyes.

Pregnancy—Studies have not been done in humans. However, studies in animals have shown that omeprazole may cause harm to the fetus.

Breast-feeding—Omeprazole may pass into the breast milk. Since this medicine has been shown to cause unwanted effects, such as tumors and cancer in animals, it may be necessary for you to take another medicine or to stop breast-feeding during treatment. Be sure you have discussed the risks and benefits of the medicine with your doctor.

Children—There is no specific information comparing the use of omeprazole in children with use in other age groups.

Older adults—Many medicines have not been studied specifically in older people. Therefore, it may not be known whether they work exactly the same way they do in younger adults or if they cause different side effects or problems in older people. There is no specific information comparing use of omeprazole in the elderly with use in other age groups.

Other medicines—Although certain medicines should not be used together at all, in other cases two different medicines may be used together even if an interaction might occur. In these cases, your doctor may want to change the dose, or other precautions may be necessary. When you are taking omeprazole, it is especially important that your doctor and pharmacist know if you are taking any of the following:

- Anticoagulants (blood thinners) or
- Diazepam (e.g., Valium) or
- Phenytoin (e.g., Dilantin)—Use with omeprazole may cause high blood levels of these medicines, which may increase the chance of side effects

Other medical problems—The presence of other medical problems may affect the use of omeprazole. Make sure you tell your doctor if you have any other medical problems, especially:

- Liver disease or a history of liver disease—This condition may cause omeprazole to build up in the body

Before you begin using any new medicine (prescription or nonprescription) or if you develop any new medical problem while you are using this medicine, check with your doctor, nurse, or pharmacist.

Proper Use of This Medicine

Take omeprazole immediately before a meal, preferably in the morning.

It may take several days before this medicine begins to relieve stomach pain. To help relieve this pain, antacids may be taken with omeprazole, unless your doctor has told you not to use them.

Swallow the capsule whole. Do not crush, break, chew, or open the capsule.

Take this medicine for the full time of treatment, even if you begin to feel better. Also, keep your appointments with your doctor for check-ups so that your doctor will be better able to tell you when to stop taking this medicine.

Missed dose—If you miss a dose of this medicine, take it as soon as possible. However, if it is almost time for your next dose, skip the missed dose and go back to your regular dosing schedule. Do not double doses.

Storage—To store this medicine:
- Keep out of the reach of children.
- Store away from heat and direct light.
- Do not store in the bathroom, near the kitchen sink, or in other damp places. Heat or moisture may cause the medicine to break down.
- Do not keep outdated medicine or medicine no longer needed. Be sure that any discarded medicine is out of the reach of children.

Precautions While Using This Medicine

If your condition does not improve, or if it becomes worse, check with your doctor.

Side Effects of This Medicine

Along with its needed effects, a medicine may cause some unwanted effects. Although not all of these side effects may occur, if they do occur they may need medical attention.

Check with your doctor as soon as possible if any of the following side effects occur:

Rare

Bloody or cloudy urine; continuing ulcers or sores in mouth; difficult, burning, or painful urination; frequent urge to urinate; sore throat and fever; unusual bleeding or bruising; unusual tiredness or weakness

Other side effects may occur that usually do not need medical attention. These side effects may go away during treatment as your body adjusts to the medicine. However, check with your doctor if any of the following side effects continue or are bothersome:

More common

Abdominal or stomach pain

Less common

Chest pain; constipation; diarrhea or loose stools; dizziness; gas; headache; heartburn; muscle pain; nausea and vomiting; skin rash or itching; unusual drowsiness; unusual tiredness

Other side effects not listed above may also occur in some patients. If you notice any other effects, check with your doctor.

Additional Information

Once a medicine has been approved for marketing for a certain use, experience may show that it is also useful for other medical problems. Although this use is not included in product labeling, omeprazole is used in certain patients with the following medical condition:

• Gastric ulcer

Other than the above information, there is no additional information relating to proper use, precautions, or side effects for these uses.

ORPHENADRINE AND ASPIRIN   Systemic

Some commonly used brand names are:

In the U.S.

Norgesic   N3 Gesic
Norgesic Forte   N3 Gesic Forte
Norphadrine   Orphenagesic
Norphadrine Forte   Orphenagesic Forte

In Canada‡
   Norgesic   Norgesic Forte

   ‡In Canada, *Aspirin* is a brand name. Acetylsalicylic acid is the generic
name in Canada. ASA, a synonym for acetylsalicylic acid, is the term that
commonly appears on Canadian product labels.

Description

Orphenadrine (or-FEN-a-dreen) and aspirin (AS-pir-in) combination is used to help relax certain muscles in your body and relieve the pain and discomfort caused by strains, sprains, or other injury to your muscles. However, this medicine does not take the place of rest, exercise, or other treatment that your doctor may recommend for your medical problem.

Orphenadrine acts in the central nervous system (CNS) to produce its muscle relaxant effects. Actions in the CNS may also be responsible for some of its side effects. Orphenadrine also has other actions (antimuscarinic) that may be responsible for some of its side effects.

This combination medicine also contains caffeine (kaf-EEN).

In the U.S., this combination medicine is available only with your doctor's prescription. In Canada, it is available without a prescription.

These medicines are available in the following dosage forms:
   Oral
      • Tablets (U.S. and Canada)

It is very important that you read and understand the following information. If any of it causes you special concern, check with your doctor. Also, *if you have any questions* or if you want more information about this medicine or your medical problem, *ask your doctor, nurse, or pharmacist.*

Before Using This Medicine

In deciding to use a medicine, the risks of taking the medicine must be weighed against the good it will do. This is a decision you and your doctor will make. For orphenadrine and aspirin combination, the following should be considered:

Allergies—Tell your doctor if you have ever had any unusual or allergic reaction to orphenadrine, caffeine, aspirin or other salicylates including methyl salicylate (oil of wintergreen), or to any of the following medicines:

    Diclofenac (e.g., Voltaren)
    Diflunisal (e.g., Dolobid)
    Fenoprofen (e.g., Nalfon)
    Floctafenine (e.g., Idarac)
    Flurbiprofen, oral (e.g., Ansaid)
    Ibuprofen (e.g., Motrin)
    Indomethacin (e.g., Indocin)
    Ketoprofen (e.g., Orudis)
    Ketorolac (e.g., Toradol)
    Meclofenamate (e.g., Meclomen)
    Mefenamic acid (e.g., Ponstel)
    Naproxen (e.g., Naprosyn)
    Oxyphenbutazone (e.g., Tandearil)
    Phenylbutazone (e.g., Butazolidin)
    Piroxicam (e.g., Feldene)
    Sulindac (e.g., Clinoril)
    Suprofen (e.g., Suprol)
    Tiaprofenic acid (e.g., Surgam)
    Tolmetin (e.g., Tolectin)
    Zomepirac (e.g., Zomax)

Also tell your doctor and pharmacist if you are allergic to any other substances, such as foods, preservatives, or dyes.

Pregnancy—

- *For aspirin:* Studies in humans have not shown that aspirin causes birth defects. However, aspirin has caused birth defects in animal studies.

  Some reports have suggested that too much use of aspirin late in pregnancy may cause a decrease in the newborn's weight and possible death of the fetus or newborn baby. However, the mothers in these reports had been taking much larger amounts of aspirin than are usually recommended. Studies of mothers taking aspirin in the doses that are usually recommended did not show these unwanted effects.

  Regular use of aspirin late in pregnancy may cause unwanted effects on the heart or blood flow in the fetus or in the newborn baby. Also, use of aspirin during the last 2 weeks of pregnancy may cause bleeding problems in the fetus before or during delivery or in the newborn baby. In addition, too much use of aspirin during the last 3 months of pregnancy may increase the length of pregnancy, prolong labor, cause other problems during delivery, or cause severe bleeding in the mother before, during, or after delivery. *Do not take aspirin during the last 3 months of pregnancy unless it has been ordered by your doctor.*

- *For orphenadrine:* Orphenadrine has not been reported to cause birth defects or other problems in humans.

Breast-feeding—This medicine has not been shown to cause problems in nursing babies. However, aspirin passes into the breast milk. Also, caffeine passes into the breast milk in small amounts. It is not known whether orphenadrine passes into the breast milk.

Children—*Do not give a medicine containing aspirin to a child or a teenager with a fever or other symptoms of a virus infection, especially flu or chickenpox, without first discussing its use with your child's doctor.* This is very important because aspirin may cause a serious illness called Reye's syndrome in children with fever caused by a virus infection, especially flu or chickenpox. Children who do not have a virus infection may also be more sensitive to the effects of aspirin, especially if they have a fever or have lost large amounts of body fluid because of vomiting, diarrhea, or sweating. This may increase the chance of side effects during treatment.

There is no specific information about the use of orphenadrine in children.

Older adults—Elderly people are especially sensitive to the effects of aspirin. This may increase the chance of side effects during treatment.

There is no specific information about the use of orphenadrine in the elderly.

Athletes—Muscle relaxants such as orphenadrine are banned and tested for in shooters by the U.S. Olympic Committee

(USOC) and National Collegiate Athletic Association
(NCAA). Orphenadrine use can lead to disqualification of
shooters in most events. Also, the caffeine in this combination medicine is tested for by the USOC and the NCAA.
These two groups have set specific limits on the amount of
caffeine in the urine they consider to be acceptable. An
athlete will be disqualified for competition if the amount of
caffeine in the urine is above these limits.

Other medicines—Although certain medicines should not be
used together at all, in other cases two different medicines
may be used together even if an interaction might occur. In
these cases, your doctor may want to change the dose, or
other precautions may be necessary. When you are taking
orphenadrine and aspirin combination, it is especially important that your doctor and pharmacist know if you are
taking any of the following:

- Anticoagulants (blood thinners) or
- Carbenicillin by injection (e.g., Geopen) or
- Cefamandole (e.g., Mandol) or
- Cefoperazone (e.g., Cefobid) or
- Cefotetan (e.g., Cefotan) or
- Dipyridamole (e.g., Persantine) or
- Divalproex (e.g., Depakote) or
- Heparin or
- Medicine for inflammation or pain, except narcotics, or
- Moxalactam (e.g., Moxam) or
- Pentoxifylline (e.g., Trental) or
- Plicamycin (e.g., Mithracin) or
- Ticarcillin (e.g., Ticar) or
- Valproic acid (e.g., Depakene)—Taking these medicines to-
  gether with aspirin may increase the chance of bleeding
- Anticholinergics (medicine for abdominal or stomach spasms
  or cramps) or
- Central nervous system (CNS) depressants or
- Methotrexate (e.g., Mexate) or
- Tricyclic antidepressants (amitriptyline [e.g., Elavil], amox-
  apine [e.g., Asendin], clomipramine [e.g., Anafranil], desipramine [e.g., Pertofrane], doxepin [e.g., Sinequan], imipramine [e.g., Tofranil], nortriptyline [e.g., Aventyl],
  protriptyline [e.g., Vivactil], trimipramine [e.g., Surmontil])
  or
- Vancomycin (e.g., Vancocin)—The chance of side effects may
  be increased

- Antidiabetics, oral (diabetes medicine you take by mouth)—Aspirin may increase the effects of the antidiabetic medicine; a change in dose may be needed if aspirin is taken regularly
- Probenecid (e.g., Benemid) or
- Sulfinpyrazone (e.g., Anturane)—Aspirin can keep these medicines from working properly for treating gout; also, taking aspirin together with sulfinpyrazone may increase the chance of bleeding
- Urinary alkalizers (medicine that makes the urine less acid, such as acetazolamide [e.g., Diamox], dichlorphenamide [e.g., Daranide], methazolamide [e.g., Neptazane], potassium or sodium citrate and/or citric acid)—These medicines may make aspirin less effective by causing it to be removed from the body more quickly
- Zidovudine (e.g., AZT; Retrovir)—Aspirin may increase the blood levels of zidovudine, which increases the chance of serious side effects

Other medical problems—The presence of other medical problems may affect the use of orphenadrine and aspirin combination. Make sure you tell your doctor if you have any other medical problems, especially:

- Anemia or
- Overactive thyroid or
- Stomach ulcer or other stomach problems—Aspirin may make your condition worse
- Asthma, allergies, and nasal polyps, history of or
- Glucose-6-phosphate dehydrogenase (G6PD) deficiency or
- Kidney disease or
- Liver disease—The chance of side effects may be increased
- Disease of the digestive tract, especially esophagus disease or intestinal blockage, or
- Enlarged prostate or
- Fast or irregular heartbeat or
- Glaucoma or
- Myasthenia gravis or
- Urinary tract blockage—Orphenadrine has side effects that may be harmful to people with these conditions
- Gout—Aspirin can make this condition worse and can also lessen the effects of some medicines used to treat gout
- Heart disease—The chance of some side effects may be increased. Also, the caffeine present in this combination medicine can make your condition worse

- Hemophilia or other bleeding problems or
- Vitamin K deficiency—Aspirin may increase the chance of
  bleeding

Before you begin using any new medicine (prescription or nonprescription) or if you develop any new medical problem while you are using this medicine, check with your doctor, nurse, or pharmacist.

Proper Use of This Medicine

Take this medicine with food or a full glass (8 ounces) of water to lessen stomach irritation.

Do not take this medicine if it has a strong vinegar-like odor. This odor means the aspirin in it is breaking down. If you have any questions about this, check with your doctor or pharmacist.

Do not take more of this medicine than your doctor ordered to lessen the chance of side effects or overdose.

Missed dose—If you miss a dose of this medicine and remember within an hour or so of the missed dose, take it right away. But if you do not remember until later, skip the missed dose and go back to your regular dosing schedule. Do not double doses.

Storage—To store this medicine:
- Keep out of the reach of children. Overdose of aspirin is especially dangerous in young children.
- Store away from heat and direct light.
- Do not store this medicine in the bathroom, near the kitchen sink, or in other damp places. Heat or moisture may cause the medicine to break down.
- Do not keep outdated medicine or medicine no longer needed. Be sure that any discarded medicine is out of the reach of children.

Precautions While Using This Medicine

If you will be taking this medicine for a long time (for example, more than a few weeks), your doctor should check your progress at regular visits.

Check the labels of all nonprescription (over-the-counter [OTC]) and prescription medicines you now take. If any contain orphenadrine or aspirin or other salicylates be especially careful, since taking them while taking this medicine may lead to overdose. If you have any questions about this, check with your doctor or pharmacist.

Too much use of acetaminophen or certain other medicines together with the aspirin in this combination medicine may increase the chance of unwanted effects. The risk depends on how much of each medicine you take every day, and on how long you take the medicines together. If your doctor directs you to take these medicines together on a regular basis, follow his or her directions carefully. However, do not take acetaminophen or any of the following medicines together with this combination medicine for more than a few days, unless your doctor has directed you to do so and is following your progress:

    Diclofenac (e.g., Voltaren)
    Diflunisal (e.g., Dolobid)
    Fenoprofen (e.g., Nalfon)
    Floctafenine (e.g., Idarac)
    Flurbiprofen, oral (e.g., Ansaid)
    Ibuprofen (e.g., Motrin)
    Indomethacin (e.g., Indocin)
    Ketoprofen (e.g., Orudis)
    Ketorolac (e.g., Toradol)
    Meclofenamate (e.g., Meclomen)
    Mefenamic acid (e.g., Ponstel)
    Naproxen (e.g., Naprosyn)
    Phenylbutazone (e.g., Butazolidin)
    Piroxicam (e.g., Feldene)
    Sulindac (e.g., Clinoril)
    Tiaprofenic acid (e.g., Surgam)
    Tolmetin (e.g., Tolectin)

For *diabetic patients:*

- The aspirin in this combination medicine may cause false urine sugar test results if you are regularly taking 6 or more of the regular-strength tablets or 3 or more of the double-strength tablets of this medicine a day. Smaller doses or occasional use of aspirin usually will not affect urine sugar tests. If you have any questions about this, check with your doctor, nurse, or pharmacist, especially if your diabetes is not well controlled.

Do not take this medicine for 5 days before any surgery, including dental surgery, unless otherwise directed by your medical doctor or dentist. Taking aspirin during this time may cause bleeding problems.

The orphenadrine in this combination medicine may add to the effects of alcohol and other CNS depressants (medicines that slow down the nervous system, possibly causing drowsiness). Some examples of CNS depressants are antihistamines or medicine for hay fever, other allergies, or colds; sedatives, tranquilizers, or sleeping medicine; prescription pain medicine or narcotics; barbiturates; medicine for seizures; other muscle relaxants; or anesthetics, including some dental anesthetics. Also, stomach problems may be more likely to occur if you drink alcoholic beverages while you are taking aspirin. *Do not drink alcoholic beverages, and check with your doctor before taking any of the medicines listed above, while you are using this medicine.*

This medicine may cause some people to have blurred vision or to become drowsy, dizzy, lightheaded, faint, or less alert than they are normally. *Make sure you know how you react to this medicine before you drive, use machines, or do anything else that could be dangerous if you are dizzy or are not alert.*

Dryness of the mouth may occur while you are taking this medicine. For temporary relief, use sugarless candy or gum, melt bits of ice in your mouth, or use a saliva substitute. However, if dry mouth continues for more than 2 weeks, check with your dentist. Continuing dryness of the mouth may increase the chance of dental disease, including tooth decay, gum disease, and fungus infections.

If you think that you or someone else may have taken an overdose of this medicine, get emergency help at once. Taking an overdose of this medicine may cause unconsciousness or death. Signs of overdose include convulsions (seizures), hearing loss, confusion, ringing or buzzing in the ears, severe drowsiness or tiredness, severe excitement or nervousness, and fast or deep breathing.

Side Effects of This Medicine

Along with its needed effects, a medicine may cause some unwanted effects. Although not all of these side effects may occur, if they do occur they may need medical attention.

Get emergency help immediately if any of the following symptoms of overdose occur:

Any loss of hearing; bloody urine; confusion; convulsions (seizures); diarrhea; dizziness or lightheadedness (severe); drowsiness (severe); excitement or nervousness (severe); fast or deep breathing; hallucinations (seeing, hearing, or feeling things that are not there); headache (severe or continuing); increased sweating; nausea or vomiting (severe or continuing); ringing or buzzing in the ears (continuing); uncontrollable flapping movements of the hands, especially in elderly patients; unexplained fever; unusual thirst; vision problems

Symptoms of overdose in children

Changes in behavior; drowsiness or tiredness (severe); fast or deep breathing

Also, check with your doctor as soon as possible if any of the following side effects occur:

Less common or rare

Abdominal or stomach pain, cramping, or burning (severe); bloody or black, tarry stools; decreased urination; eye pain; fainting; fast or pounding heartbeat; shortness of breath, troubled breathing, tightness in chest, or wheezing; skin rash, hives, itching, or redness; sores, ulcers, or white spots on lips or in mouth; swollen and/or painful glands; unusual bleeding or bruising; unusual tiredness or weakness; vomiting of blood or material that looks like coffee grounds

Other side effects may occur that usually do not need medical attention. These side effects may go away during treatment as your body adjusts to the medicine. However, check with your doctor if any of the following side effects continue or are bothersome:

More common

Abdominal or stomach cramps, pain, or discomfort (mild to moderate); dryness of mouth; heartburn or indigestion; nausea or vomiting (mild)

Less common

Blurred or double vision or other vision problems; confusion; constipation; difficult urination; dizziness or lightheadedness; drowsiness; excitement, nervousness, or restlessness; headache; muscle weakness; trembling; unusually large pupils of eyes

Other side effects not listed above may also occur in some patients. If you notice any other effects, check with your doctor.

PENICILLINS Systemic

This information applies to the following medicines:

Amoxicillin (a-mox-i-SILL-in)
Amoxicillin and Clavulanate (klav-yoo-LAN-ate)
Ampicillin (am-pi-SILL-in)
Ampicillin and Sulbactam (sul-BAK-tam)
Azlocillin (az-loe-SILL-in)
Bacampicillin (ba-kam-pi-SILL-in)
Carbenicillin (kar-ben-i-SILL-in)
Cloxacillin (klox-a-SILL-in)
Cyclacillin (sye-kla-SILL-in)
Dicloxacillin (dye-klox-a-SILL-in)
Methicillin (meth-i-SILL-in)
Mezlocillin (mez-loe-SILL-in)
Nafcillin (naf-SILL-in)
Oxacillin (ox-a-SILL-in)
Penicillin G (pen-i-SILL-in)
Penicillin V
Piperacillin (pi-PER-a-sill-in)
Ticarcillin (tye-kar-SILL-in)
Ticarcillin and Clavulanate

Some commonly used brand names and other names are:

For Amoxicillin
In the U.S.

Amoxil	Trimox
Larotid	Wymox
Polymox	

Generic name product may also be available.

In Canada
    Amoxil   Novamoxin
    Apo-Amoxi   Nu-Amoxi

Another commonly used name for amoxicillin is amoxicilline.

For Amoxicillin and Clavulanate
   In the U.S.
    Augmentin

   In Canada
    Clavulin

For Ampicillin
   In the U.S.
    Omnipen   Polycillin-N
    Omnipen-N   Principen
    Polycillin

   Generic name product may also be available.

   In Canada
    Ampicin   Nu-Ampi
    Apo-Ampi   Penbritin
    Novo Ampicillin

For Ampicillin and Sulbactam†
   In the U.S.
    Unasyn

For Azlocillin†
   In the U.S.
    Azlin

For Bacampicillin
   In the U.S.
    Spectrobid

   In Canada
    Penglobe

For Carbenicillin
   In the U.S.
    Geocillin   Geopen

   In Canada
    Geopen Oral   Pyopen

Another commonly used name for carbenicillin indanyl sodium is carindacillin.

For Cloxacillin
   In the U.S.
    Cloxapen   Tegopen

   Generic name product may also be available.

   In Canada
    Apo-Cloxi   Nu-Cloxi
    Novocloxin   Orbenin
                                   Tegopen

For Cyclacillin†
In the U.S.
Generic name product may also be available.
Another commonly used name for cyclacillin is ciclacillin.

For Dicloxacillin†
In the U.S.
Dycill   Pathocil
Dynapen
Generic name product may also be available.

For Methicillin†
In the U.S.
Staphcillin
Another commonly used name for methicillin is meticillin.

For Mezlocillin†
In the U.S.
Mezlin

For Nafcillin
In the U.S.
Nafcil   Unipen
Nallpen
Generic name product may also be available.
In Canada
Unipen

For Oxacillin†
In the U.S.
Bactocill   Prostaphlin
Generic name product may also be available.

For Penicillin G
In the U.S.
Bicillin L-A   Pfizerpen
Crysticillin 300 AS   Pfizerpen-AS
Pentids   Wycillin
Generic name product may also be available.
In Canada
Ayercillin   Megacillin
Bicillin L-A   Wycillin
Crystapen
Generic name product may also be available.
Another commonly used name for penicillin G benzathine is benzathine benzylpenicillin.

For Penicillin V
In the U.S.

Beepen-VK	Robicillin VK
Betapen-VK	V-Cillin K
Ledercillin VK	Veetids
Pen Vee K	

Generic name product may also be available.

In Canada

Apo-Pen-VK	Nu-Pen-VK
Ledercillin	Pen Vee
Nadopen-V 200	PVF
Nadopen-V 400	PVF K
Nadopen-VK	V-Cillin K
Novopen-VK	VC-K

Another commonly used name for penicillin V is phenoxymethylpenicillin.

For Piperacillin
In the U.S.
Pipracil

In Canada
Pipracil

For Ticarcillin
In the U.S.
Ticar

In Canada
Ticar

For Ticarcillin and Clavulanate
In the U.S.
Timentin

In Canada
Timentin

---

†Not commercially available in Canada.

Description

Penicillins are used in the treatment of bacterial infections. They work by killing bacteria or preventing their growth.

There are several different kinds of penicillins. Each is used to treat different kinds of bacterial infections. One kind of penicillin usually may not be used in place of another.

Penicillins are used to treat bacterial infections in many different parts of the body. They are sometimes given with other antibacterial medicines. Carbenicillin taken by mouth is used only to treat bacterial infections of the urinary tract and prostate gland. Penicillin G and penicillin V are also used to prevent "strep" infections in patients with a history of rheumatic heart disease. Piperacillin is given by injection to prevent bacterial infections before, during, and after surgery also. Some of the penicillins may also be used for other problems as determined by your doctor. However, none of the penicillins will work for colds, flu, or other virus infections.

Penicillins are available only with your doctor's prescription, in the following dosage forms:

Oral

Amoxicillin
- Capsules (U.S. and Canada)
- Oral suspension (U.S. and Canada)
- Chewable tablets (U.S. and Canada)

Amoxicillin and Clavulanate
- Oral suspension (U.S. and Canada)
- Tablets (U.S. and Canada)
- Chewable tablets (U.S.)

Ampicillin
- Capsules (U.S. and Canada)
- Oral suspension (U.S. and Canada)

Bacampicillin
- Oral suspension (U.S.)
- Tablets (U.S. and Canada)

Carbenicillin
- Tablets (U.S. and Canada)

Cloxacillin
- Capsules (U.S. and Canada)
- Oral solution (U.S. and Canada)

Cyclacillin
- Tablets (U.S.)

Dicloxacillin
- Capsules (U.S.)
- Oral suspension (U.S.)

Nafcillin
- Capsules (U.S.)
- Oral solution (U.S.)
- Tablets (U.S.)

Oxacillin
- Capsules (U.S.)
- Oral solution (U.S.)

Penicillin G Benzathine
- Oral suspension (Canada)

Penicillin G Potassium
- Oral solution (U.S.)
- Tablets (U.S. and Canada)

Penicillin V Benzathine
- Oral suspension (Canada)

Penicillin V Potassium
- Oral solution (U.S. and Canada)
- Tablets (U.S. and Canada)

Parenteral

Ampicillin
- Injection (U.S. and Canada)

Ampicillin and Sulbactam
- Injection (U.S.)

Azlocillin
- Injection (U.S.)

Carbenicillin
- Injection (U.S. and Canada)

Cloxacillin
- Injection (Canada)

Methicillin
- Injection (U.S.)

Mezlocillin
- Injection (U.S.)

Nafcillin
- Injection (U.S. and Canada)

Oxacillin
- Injection (U.S.)

Penicillin G Benzathine
- Injection (U.S. and Canada)

Penicillin G Potassium
- Injection (U.S. and Canada)

Penicillin G Procaine
- Injection (U.S. and Canada)

Penicillin G Sodium
- Injection (U.S. and Canada)

Piperacillin
- Injection (U.S. and Canada)

Ticarcillin
- Injection (U.S. and Canada)

Ticarcillin and Clavulanate
- Injection (U.S. and Canada)

It is very important that you read and understand the following information. If any of it causes you special concern, check with your doctor. Also, *if you have any questions* or if you want more information about this medicine or your medical problem, *ask your doctor, nurse, or pharmacist.*

Before Using This Medicine

In deciding to use a medicine, the risks of taking the medicine must be weighed against the good it will do. This is a decision you and your doctor will make. For penicillins, the following should be considered:

Allergies—Tell your doctor if you have ever had any unusual or allergic reaction to any of the penicillins, cephalosporins, griseofulvin (e.g., Fulvicin), or penicillamine (e.g., Cuprimine). Also tell your doctor and pharmacist if you are allergic to any other substances, such as foods, preservatives, or dyes, or procaine (e.g., Novocain) or other ester-type anesthetics (medicines that cause numbing) if you are receiving penicillin G procaine.

Pregnancy—Studies have not been done in pregnant women. However, penicillins have not been shown to cause birth defects or other problems in animals given more than 25 times the usual human dose.

Breast-feeding—Most penicillins pass into the breast milk. Even though only small amounts may pass into breast milk, allergic reactions, diarrhea, fungus infections, and skin rash may occur in nursing babies.

Children—Many penicillins have been used in children and, in effective doses, are not expected to cause different side effects or problems in children than they do in adults.

Older adults—Penicillins have been used in the elderly and have not been shown to cause different side effects or problems in older people than they do in younger adults.

Other medicines—Although certain medicines should not be used together at all, in other cases two different medicines may be used together even if an interaction might occur. In these cases, your doctor may want to change the dose, or

other precautions may be necessary. When you are taking a penicillin, it is especially important that your doctor and pharmacist know if you are taking any of the following:

- Amiloride (e.g., Midamor) or
- Captopril (e.g., Capoten) or
- Enalapril (e.g., Vasotec) or
- Lisinopril (e.g., Prinivil, Zestril) or
- Potassium-containing medicine or
- Spironolactone (e.g., Aldactone) or
- Triamterene (e.g., Dyrenium)—Use of these medicines with penicillin G by injection may cause an increase in side effects

- Anticoagulants (blood thinners) or
- Dipyridamole (e.g., Persantine) or
- Divalproex (e.g., Depakote) or
- Heparin (e.g., Panheprin) or
- Inflammation or pain medicine (except narcotics) or
- Moxalactam (e.g., Moxam) or
- Pentoxifylline (e.g., Trental) or
- Plicamycin (e.g., Mithracin) or
- Sulfinpyrazone (e.g., Anturane) or
- Valproic acid (e.g., Depakene)—Use of these medicines with carbenicillin or ticarcillin may increase the chance of bleeding

- Cholestyramine (e.g., Questran) or
- Colestipol (e.g., Colestid)—Use of these medicines with oral penicillin G may prevent penicillin G from working properly

- Oral contraceptives (birth control pills) containing estrogen— Use of ampicillin, bacampicillin, or penicillin V with estrogen-containing oral contraceptives may prevent oral contraceptives from working properly, increasing the chance of pregnancy

- Probenecid (e.g., Benemid)—Probenecid increases the blood level of many penicillins. Although your doctor may give you probenecid with a penicillin to treat some infections, in other cases, this effect may be unwanted and may increase the chance of side effects

Other medical problems—The presence of other medical problems may affect the use of penicillins. Make sure you tell your doctor if you have any other medical problems, especially:

- Allergy, general (such as asthma, eczema, hay fever, hives), history of—Patients with a history of general allergies may be more likely to have a severe reaction to penicillins if an allergy develops

- Bleeding problems, history of—Patients with a history of bleeding problems may have an increased chance of bleeding when receiving carbenicillin or ticarcillin
- Kidney disease—Patients with kidney disease may have an increased chance of side effects
- Mononucleosis, infectious ("mono")—Patients with infectious mononucleosis may have an increased chance of skin rash
- Stomach or intestinal disease, history of (especially colitis, including colitis caused by antibiotics, or enteritis)—Patients with a history of stomach or intestinal disease may be more likely to develop colitis while taking penicillins

Before you begin using any new medicine (prescription or nonprescription) or if you develop any new medical problem while you are using this medicine, check with your doctor, nurse, or pharmacist.

Proper Use of This Medicine

Penicillins (except bacampicillin tablets, amoxicillin, amoxicillin and clavulanate combination, and penicillin V) are best taken with a full glass (8 ounces) of water on an empty stomach (either 1 hour before or 2 hours after meals) unless otherwise directed by your doctor.

For patients taking *amoxicillin, amoxicillin and clavulanate combination, and penicillin V:*

- Amoxicillin, amoxicillin and clavulanate combination, and penicillin V may be taken on a full or empty stomach.
- The *liquid form of amoxicillin* may also be taken straight or mixed with formulas, milk, fruit juice, water, ginger ale, or other cold drinks. If mixed with other liquids, take immediately after mixing. Be sure to drink all the liquid to get the full dose of medicine.

For patients taking *bacampicillin:*

- The liquid form of this medicine is best taken with a full glass (8 ounces) of water on an empty stomach (either 1 hour before or 2 hours after meals) unless otherwise directed by your doctor.

- The tablet form of this medicine may be taken on a full or empty stomach.

For patients taking *penicillin G by mouth:*

- Do not drink acidic fruit juices (for example, orange or grapefruit juice) or other acidic beverages within 1 hour of taking penicillin G since this may keep the medicine from working properly.

For patients taking the *oral liquid form of penicillins:*

- This medicine is to be taken by mouth even if it comes in a dropper bottle. If this medicine does not come in a dropper bottle, use a specially marked measuring spoon or other device to measure each dose accurately. The average household teaspoon may not hold the right amount of liquid.

- Do not use after the expiration date on the label. The medicine may not work properly after that date. If you have any questions about this, check with your pharmacist.

For patients taking the *chewable tablet form of penicillins:*

- Tablets should be chewed or crushed before they are swallowed.

To help clear up your infection completely, *keep taking this medicine for the full time of treatment*, even if you begin to feel better after a few days. *If you have a "strep" infection, you should keep taking this medicine for at least 10 days. This is especially important in "strep" infections. Serious heart problems could develop later* if your infection is not cleared up completely. Also, if you stop taking this medicine too soon, your symptoms may return.

This medicine works best when there is a constant amount in the blood or urine. *To help keep the amount constant, do not miss any doses. Also, it is best to take the doses at evenly spaced times, day and night*. For example, if you are to take 4 doses a day, the doses should be spaced about 6 hours apart. If this interferes with your sleep or other daily activities, or if you need help in planning the best times to take your medicine, check with your doctor, nurse, or pharmacist.

Missed dose—If you do miss a dose of this medicine, take it as soon as possible. This will help to keep a constant amount of medicine in the blood or urine. However, if it is almost time for your next dose, skip the missed dose and go back to your regular dosing schedule. Do not double doses.

Storage—To store this medicine:
- Keep out of the reach of children.
- Store away from heat and direct light.
- Do not store the capsule or tablet form of penicillins in the bathroom, near the kitchen sink, or in other damp places. Heat or moisture may cause the medicine to break down.
- Store the oral liquid form of penicillins in the refrigerator because heat will cause this medicine to break down. However, keep the medicine from freezing. Follow the directions on the label.
- Do not keep outdated medicine or medicine no longer needed. Be sure that any discarded medicine is out of the reach of children.

Precautions While Using This Medicine

If your symptoms do not improve within a few days, or if they become worse, check with your doctor.

If you have ever had an allergic reaction to any of the penicillins, your doctor may want you to carry a medical identification (ID) card or wear a medical ID bracelet stating this.

In some patients, penicillins may cause diarrhea.
- Severe diarrhea may be a sign of a serious side effect. *Do not take any diarrhea medicine without first checking with your doctor.* Diarrhea medicines may make your diarrhea worse or make it last longer.
- For mild diarrhea, diarrhea medicine containing kaolin or attapulgite (e.g., Kaopectate tablets, Diasorb) may be taken. However, other kinds of diarrhea medicine

should not be taken. They may make your diarrhea worse or make it last longer.
- If you have any questions about this or if mild diarrhea continues or gets worse, check with your doctor or pharmacist.

Oral contraceptives (birth control pills) containing estrogen may not work properly if you take them while you are taking ampicillin, bacampicillin, or penicillin V. Unplanned pregnancies may occur. You should use a different or additional means of birth control while you are taking any of these penicillins. If you have any questions about this, check with your doctor or pharmacist.

For *diabetic patients:*
- *Amoxicillin, amoxicillin and clavulanate combination, ampicillin, ampicillin and sulbactam combination, bacampicillin, and penicillin G may cause false test results with some urine sugar tests.* Check with your doctor before changing your diet or the dosage of your diabetes medicine.

Tell the doctor in charge that you are taking this medicine before you have any medical tests. The results of some tests may be affected by this medicine.

Side Effects of This Medicine

Along with its needed effects, a medicine may cause some unwanted effects. Although not all of these side effects may occur, if they do occur they may need medical attention.

Stop taking this medicine and get emergency help immediately if any of the following side effects occur:

Rare *(may be less common with some penicillins)*

Difficulty in breathing; lightheadedness; skin rash, hives, itching, or wheezing

In addition to the side effects mentioned above, *check with your doctor immediately* if any of the following side effects occur:

Rare (may be more common with some penicillins)

> Abdominal or stomach cramps and pain (severe); abdominal bloating; blood in urine; convulsions (seizures); decreased amount of urine; diarrhea (watery and severe), which may also be bloody; fever; joint pain; sore throat and fever; unusual bleeding or bruising
>
> (some of the above side effects may also occur up to several weeks after you stop taking any of these medicines)

Other side effects may occur that usually do not need medical attention. These side effects may go away during treatment as your body adjusts to the medicine. However, check with your doctor if any of the following side effects continue or are bothersome:

> *More common (may be less common with some penicillins)*
>
> Diarrhea (mild); nausea or vomiting; sore mouth or tongue

Overdose is very unlikely to occur with penicillins. However, if you think that you or someone else, especially a child, has taken too much, check with your doctor. Severe diarrhea, nausea, or vomiting may need to be treated.

Other side effects not listed above may also occur in some patients. If you notice any other effects, check with your doctor.

PENTOXIFYLLINE Systemic

A commonly used brand name in the U.S. and Canada is Trental.

Description

Pentoxifylline (pen-tox-IF-i-lin) is a medicine that improves the flow of blood through blood vessels. It is used to reduce leg pain caused by poor blood circulation. Pentoxifylline makes it possible to walk farther before having to rest because of leg cramps.

Pentoxifylline is available only with your doctor's prescription, in the following dosage form:

Oral
- Extended-release tablets (U.S. and Canada)

It is very important that you read and understand the following information. If any of it causes you special concern, check with your doctor. Also, *if you have any questions* or if you want more information about this medicine or your medical problem, *ask your doctor, nurse, or pharmacist.*

Before Using This Medicine

In deciding to use a medicine, the risks of taking the medicine must be weighed against the good it will do. This is a decision you and your doctor will make. For pentoxifylline, the following should be considered:

Allergies—Tell your doctor if you have ever had any unusual or allergic reaction to pentoxifylline or to other xanthines such as aminophylline, caffeine, dyphylline, ethylenediamine (contained in aminophylline), oxtriphylline, theobromine, or theophylline. Also tell your doctor and pharmacist if you are allergic to any other substances, such as foods, preservatives, or dyes.

Pregnancy—Studies have not been done in humans. Although pentoxifylline has not been shown to cause birth defects in animals, it has caused other harmful effects in rats given doses 25 times the maximum human dose.

Breast-feeding—Pentoxifylline passes into the breast milk. The medicine has not been reported to cause problems in nursing babies. However, pentoxifylline has caused noncancerous tumors in animals when given for a long time in doses much larger than are used in humans. Therefore, your doctor may not want you to breast-feed while taking it. Be sure that you discuss the risks and benefits of this medicine with your doctor.

Older adults—Side effects may be more likely to occur in the elderly, who are usually more sensitive than younger adults to the effects of pentoxifylline.

Other medicines—Although certain medicines should not be used together at all, in other cases two different medicines

may be used together even if an interaction might occur. In these cases, your doctor may want to change the dose, or other precautions may be necessary. When you are taking pentoxifylline, it is important that your doctor and pharmacist know if you are taking *any* other prescription or non-prescription (over-the-counter [OTC]) medicine, or if you smoke tobacco.

Other medical problems—The presence of other medical problems may affect the use of pentoxifylline. Make sure you tell your doctor if you have any other medical problems, especially:

- Kidney disease or
- Liver disease—The chance of side effects may be increased

Before you begin using any new medicine (prescription or nonprescription) or if you develop any new medical problem while you are using this medicine, check with your doctor, nurse, or pharmacist.

Proper Use of This Medicine

Swallow the tablet whole. Do not crush, break, or chew it before swallowing.

Pentoxifylline should be taken with meals to lessen the chance of stomach upset. Taking an antacid with the medicine may also help.

Missed dose—If you miss a dose of this medicine, take it as soon as possible. However, if it is almost time for your next dose, skip the missed dose and go back to your regular dosing schedule. Do not double doses.

Storage—To store this medicine:

- Keep out of the reach of children.
- Store away from heat and direct light.
- Do not store in the bathroom, near the kitchen sink, or in other damp places. Heat or moisture may cause the medicine to break down.
- Do not keep outdated medicine or medicine no longer needed. Be sure that any discarded medicine is out of the reach of children.

Precautions While Using This Medicine

It may take several weeks for this medicine to work. If you feel that pentoxifylline is not working, do not stop taking it on your own. Instead, check with your doctor.

Smoking tobacco may worsen your condition since nicotine may further narrow your blood vessels. Therefore, it is best to avoid smoking.

Side Effects of This Medicine

Along with its needed effects, a medicine may cause some unwanted effects. Although not all of these side effects may occur, if they do occur they may need medical attention.

Check with your doctor as soon as possible if any of the following side effects occur:

Rare

Chest pain; irregular heartbeat

Signs and symptoms of overdose (in the order in which they may occur)

Drowsiness; flushing; faintness; unusual excitement; convulsions (seizures)

Other side effects may occur that usually do not need medical attention. These side effects may go away during treatment as your body adjusts to the medicine. However, check with your doctor if any of the following side effects continue or are bothersome:

Less common

Dizziness; headache; nausea or vomiting; stomach discomfort

Other side effects not listed above may also occur in some patients. If you notice any other effects, check with your doctor.

PERGOLIDE Systemic

A commonly used brand name in the U.S. and Canada is Permax.

Description

Pergolide (PER-go-lide) belongs to the group of medicines known as ergot alkaloids. It is used with levodopa or with carbidopa and levodopa combination to treat people who have Parkinson's disease. It works by stimulating certain parts of the central nervous system (CNS) that are involved in this disease.

Pergolide is available only with your doctor's prescription, in the following dosage form:

Oral
- Tablets (U.S. and Canada)

It is very important that you read and understand the following information. If any of it causes you special concern, check with your doctor. Also, *if you have any questions* or if you want more information about this medicine or your medical problem, *ask your doctor, nurse, or pharmacist.*

Before Using This Medicine

In deciding to use a medicine, the risks of taking the medicine must be weighed against the good it will do. This is a decision you and your doctor will make. For pergolide, the following should be considered:

Allergies—Tell your doctor if you have ever had any unusual or allergic reaction to pergolide or other ergot medicines such as ergotamine. Also tell your doctor and pharmacist if you are allergic to any other substances, such as foods, preservatives, or dyes.

Pregnancy—Studies have not been done in pregnant women. However, pergolide has not been shown to cause birth defects or other problems in animal studies.

Breast-feeding—This medicine may stop milk from being produced.

Children—Studies on this medicine have been done only in adult patients, and there is no specific information about its use in children.

Older adults—This medicine has been tested and has not been shown to cause different side effects or problems in older people than it does in younger adults.

Other medicines—Although certain medicines should not be used together at all, in other cases 2 different medicines may be used together even if an interaction might occur. In these cases, your doctor may want to change the dose, or other precautions may be necessary. When you are taking pergolide, it is especially important that your doctor and pharmacist know if you are taking any other prescription or nonprescription (over-the-counter [OTC]) medicine.

Other medical problems—The presence of other medical problems may affect the use of pergolide. Make sure you tell your doctor if you have any other medical problems, especially:

- Heart disease or
- Mental problems (history of)—Pergolide may make the condition worse

Before you begin using any new medicine (prescription or nonprescription) or if you develop any new medical problem while you are using this medicine, check with your doctor, nurse, or pharmacist.

Proper Use of This Medicine

If pergolide upsets your stomach, it may be taken with meals. If stomach upset continues, check with your doctor.

Missed dose—If you miss a dose of this medicine, take it as soon as you remember it. However, if it is almost time for your next dose, skip the missed dose and go back to your regular dosing schedule. Do not double doses.

Storage—To store this medicine:

- Keep out of the reach of children.
- Store away from heat and direct light.

- Do not store in the bathroom, near the kitchen sink, or in other damp places. Heat or moisture may cause the medicine to break down.
- Do not keep outdated medicine or medicine no longer needed. Be sure that any discarded medicine is out of the reach of children.

Precautions While Using This Medicine

It is important that your doctor check your progress at regular visits, to make sure that this medicine is working and to check for unwanted effects.

This medicine may cause some people to become drowsy, dizzy, or less alert than they are normally. *Make sure you know how you react to this medicine before you drive, use machines, or do anything else that could be dangerous if you are dizzy or are not alert.*

Dizziness, lightheadedness, or fainting may occur after the first doses of pergolide, especially when you get up from a lying or sitting position. Getting up slowly may help. Taking the first dose at bedtime or when you are able to lie down may also lessen problems. If the problem continues or gets worse, check with your doctor.

Pergolide may cause dryness of the mouth. For temporary relief, use sugarless candy or gum, melt bits of ice in your mouth, or use a saliva substitute. However, if your mouth continues to feel dry for more than 2 weeks, check with your medical doctor or dentist. Continuing dryness of the mouth may increase the chance of dental disease, including tooth decay, gum disease, and fungus infections.

It may take several weeks for pergolide to work. Do not stop taking this medicine or reduce the amount you are taking without first checking with your doctor.

Side Effects of This Medicine

Along with its needed effects, a medicine may cause some unwanted effects. Although not all of these side effects may occur, if they do occur they may need medical attention.

Check with your doctor immediately if any of the following side effects occur:

Rare

Chest pain (severe); convulsions (seizures); fainting; fast heartbeat; headache (severe or continuing); increased sweating; nausea and vomiting (continuing or severe); nervousness; unexplained shortness of breath; vision changes, such as blurred vision or temporary blindness; weakness (sudden)

Also, check with your doctor as soon as possible if any of the following side effects occur:

More common

Confusion; hallucinations (seeing, hearing, or feeling things that are not there); pain or burning while urinating; uncontrolled movements of the body, such as the face, tongue, arms, hands, head, and upper body

Less common

High blood pressure

Other side effects may occur that usually do not need medical attention. These side effects may go away during treatment as your body adjusts to the medicine. However, check with your doctor if any of the following side effects continue or are bothersome:

More common

Abdominal or stomach pain; constipation; dizziness or lightheadedness, especially when getting up from a lying or sitting position; drowsiness; lower back pain; nausea; runny nose; weakness

Less common

Chills; diarrhea; dryness of mouth; loss of appetite; swelling of the face; vomiting

Other side effects not listed above may also occur in some patients. If you notice any other effects, check with your doctor.

PHENOTHIAZINES   Systemic

This information applies to the following medicines:

Acetophenazine (a-set-oh-FEN-a-zeen)
Chlorpromazine (klor-PROE-ma-zeen)

Fluphenazine (floo-FEN-a-zeen)
Mesoridazine (mez-oh-RID-a-zeen)
Methotrimeprazine (meth-oh-trim-EP-ra-zeen)
Pericyazine (pair-ee-SYE-a-zeen)
Perphenazine (per-FEN-a-zeen)
Pipotiazine (pip-oh-TYE-a-zeen)
Prochlorperazine (proe-klor-PAIR-a-zeen)
Promazine (PROE-ma-zeen)
Thiopropazate (thye-oh-PROE-pa-zayt)
Thioproperazine (thye-oh-proe-PAIR-a-zeen)
Thioridazine (thye-oh-RID-a-zeen)
Trifluoperazine (trye-floo-oh-PAIR-a-zeen)
Triflupromazine (trye-floo-PROE-ma-zeen)

Note: This information does *not* apply to Ethopropazine, Promethazine, Propiomazine, and Trimeprazine.

Some commonly used brand names are:

For Acetophenazine†
In the U.S.
Tindal

For Chlorpromazine
In the U.S.
Ormazine   Thorazine Spansule
Thorazine   Thor-Prom
Thorazine Concentrate

Generic name product may also be available.

In Canada
Chlorpromanyl-5   Largactil Liquid
Chlorpromanyl-20   Largactil Oral Drops
Chlorpromanyl-40   Novo-Chlorpromazine
Largactil

Generic name product may also be available.

For Fluphenazine
In the U.S.
Permitil   Prolixin Concentrate
Permitil Concentrate   Prolixin Decanoate
Prolixin   Prolixin Enanthate

Generic name product may also be available.

In Canada
Apo-Fluphenazine   Moditen HCl
Modecate   Moditen HCl-H.P.
Modecate Concentrate   Permitil
Moditen Enanthate

For Mesoridazine
In the U.S.
Serentil
Serentil Concentrate

In Canada
    Serentil

For Methotrimeprazine
In the U.S.
    Levoprome

In Canada
    Nozinan   Nozinan Oral Drops
    Nozinan Liquid

For Pericyazine*
In Canada
    Neuleptil

For Perphenazine
In the U.S.
    Trilafon
    Trilafon Concentrate

    Generic name product may also be available.

In Canada
    Apo-Perphenazine   Trilafon
    PMS Perphenazine   Trilafon Concentrate

    Generic name product may also be available.

For Pipotiazine*
In Canada
    Piportil L_4

For Prochlorperazine
In the U.S.
    Compa-Z   Cotranzine
    Compazine   Ultrazine-10
    Compazine Spansule

    Generic name product may also be available.

In Canada
    PMS Prochlorperazine   Stemetil
    Prorazin   Stemetil Liquid

    Generic name product may also be available.

For Promazine
In the U.S.
    Primazine   Sparine
    Prozine-50

    Generic name product may also be available.

In Canada

    Generic name product may be available.

For Thiopropazate*
In Canada
    Dartal

For Thioproperazine*
  In Canada
    Majeptil

For Thioridazine
  In the U.S.
    Mellaril   Mellaril-S
    Mellaril Concentrate

    Generic name product may also be available.

  In Canada
    Apo-Thioridazine   Novo-Ridazine
    Mellaril   PMS Thioridazine

For Trifluoperazine
  In the U.S.
    Stelazine
    Stelazine Concentrate

    Generic name product may also be available.

  In Canada
    Apo-Trifluoperazine   Stelazine
    Novo-Flurazine   Stelazine Concentrate
    PMS Trifluoperazine   Terfluzine
    Solazine   Terfluzine Concentrate

For Triflupromazine†
  In the U.S.
    Vesprin

---

*Not commercially available in the U.S.
†Not commercially available in Canada.

Description

Phenothiazines (FEE-noe-THYE-a-zeens) are used to treat nervous, mental, and emotional disorders. Some are used also to control anxiety or agitation in certain patients, severe nausea and vomiting, severe hiccups, and moderate to severe pain in some hospitalized patients. Chlorpromazine is also used in the treatment of certain types of porphyria, and with other medicines in the treatment of tetanus. Phenothiazines may also be used for other conditions as determined by your doctor.

Phenothiazines are available only with your doctor's prescription in the following dosage forms:

  Oral
    Acetophenazine
      • Tablets (U.S.)

Chlorpromazine
- Extended-release capsules (U.S.)
- Oral concentrate (U.S. and Canada)
- Syrup (U.S. and Canada)
- Tablets (U.S. and Canada)

Fluphenazine
- Elixir (U.S. and Canada)
- Oral solution (U.S.)
- Tablets (U.S. and Canada)

Mesoridazine
- Oral solution (U.S.)
- Tablets (U.S. and Canada)

Methotrimeprazine
- Oral solution (Canada)
- Syrup (Canada)
- Tablets (Canada)

Pericyazine
- Capsules (Canada)
- Oral solution (Canada)

Perphenazine
- Oral solution (U.S. and Canada)
- Syrup (Canada)
- Tablets (U.S. and Canada)

Prochlorperazine
- Extended-release capsules (U.S.)
- Syrup (U.S. and Canada)
- Tablets (U.S. and Canada)

Promazine
- Tablets (U.S.)

Thiopropazate
- Tablets (Canada)

Thioproperazine
- Tablets (Canada)

Thioridazine
- Oral solution (U.S. and Canada)
- Oral suspension (U.S. and Canada)
- Tablets (U.S. and Canada)

Trifluoperazine
- Oral solution (U.S. and Canada)
- Syrup (Canada)
- Tablets (U.S. and Canada)

Parenteral

Chlorpromazine
- Injection (U.S. and Canada)

Fluphenazine
- Injection (U.S. and Canada)

Mesoridazine
- Injection (U.S.)

Methotrimeprazine
- Injection (U.S. and Canada)

Perphenazine
- Injection (U.S. and Canada)

Pipotiazine
- Injection (Canada)

Prochlorperazine
- Injection (U.S. and Canada)

Promazine
- Injection (U.S. and Canada)

Trifluoperazine
- Injection (U.S. and Canada)

Triflupromazine
- Injection (U.S.)

Rectal

Chlorpromazine
- Suppositories (U.S. and Canada)

Prochlorperazine
- Suppositories (U.S. and Canada)

It is very important that you read and understand the following information. If any of it causes you special concern, check with your doctor. Also, *if you have any questions* or if you want more information about this medicine or your medical problem, *ask your doctor, nurse, or pharmacist.*

Before Using This Medicine

In deciding to use a medicine, the risks of taking the medicine must be weighed against the good it will do. This is a decision you and your doctor will make. For phenothiazines, the following should be considered:

Allergies—Tell your doctor if you have ever had any unusual or allergic reaction to phenothiazines. Also tell your doctor and pharmacist if you are allergic to any other substances, such as foods, preservatives, or dyes.

Pregnancy—Although studies have not been done in pregnant women, some side effects, such as jaundice and muscle tremors and other movement disorders, have occurred in a few newborns whose mothers received phenothiazines close to the time of delivery. Studies in animals have shown that chlorpromazine and trifluoperazine, given in doses many times the usual human dose, may cause birth defects.

Breast-feeding—Phenothiazines pass into the breast milk and may cause drowsiness and a greater chance of unusual muscle movement in the nursing baby.

Children—Certain side effects, such as muscle spasms of the face, neck, and back, tic-like or twitching movements, inability to move the eyes, twisting of the body, or weakness of the arms and legs, are more likely to occur in children, especially those with severe illness or dehydration. Children are usually more sensitive than adults to some of the side effects of phenothiazines.

Older adults—Constipation, dizziness or fainting, drowsiness, dryness of mouth, trembling of the hands and fingers, and symptoms of tardive dyskinesia (such as rapid, worm-like movements of the tongue or any other uncontrolled movements of the mouth, tongue, or jaw, and/or arms and legs) are especially likely to occur in elderly patients, who are usually more sensitive than younger adults to the effects of phenothiazines.

Athletes—Phenothiazines are banned and, in some cases, tested for in competitors in biathlon and modern pentathlon events by the U.S. Olympic Committee (USOC). Use of phenothiazines can lead to the disqualification of athletes in these events.

Other medicines—Although certain medicines should not be used together at all, in other cases 2 different medicines may be used together even if an interaction might occur. In these cases, your doctor may want to change the dose, or other precautions may be necessary. When you are taking phenothiazines, it is especially important that your doctor and pharmacist know if you are taking any of the following:

- Amantadine (e.g., Symmetrel) or
- Antihypertensives (high blood pressure medicine) or
- Bromocriptine (e.g., Parlodel) or

- Deferoxamine (e.g., Desferal) or
- Diuretics (water pills) or
- Levobunolol (e.g., Betagan) or
- Medicine for heart disease or
- Metipranolol (e.g., OptiPranolol)
- Nabilone (e.g., Cesamet) (with high doses) or
- Narcotic pain medicine or
- Nimodipine (e.g., Nimotop) or
- Other antipsychotics (medicine for mental illness) or
- Pentamidine (e.g., Pentam) or
- Pimozide (e.g., Orap)
- Promethazine (e.g., Phenergan) or
- Trimeprazine (e.g., Temaril)—Severe low blood pressure may occur
- Antidepressants (medicine for depression)—The risk of serious side effects may be increased
- Antithyroid agents (medicine for overactive thyroid) or
- Central nervous system (CNS) depressants (medicines that cause drowsiness)—There may be an increased chance of blood problems
- Epinephrine (e.g., Adrenalin)—Severe low blood pressure and fast heartbeat may occur
- Levodopa (e.g., Dopar)—Phenothiazines may prevent levodopa from working properly in the treatment of Parkinson's disease
- Lithium (e.g., Lithane, Lithizine)—The amount of medicine you need to take may change
- Methyldopa (e.g., Aldomet) or
- Metoclopramide (e.g., Reglan) or
- Metyrosine (e.g. Demser) or
- Pemoline (e.g., Cylert) or
- Rauwolfia alkaloids (alseroxylon [e.g., Rauwiloid], deserpidine [e.g., Harmonyl], rauwolfia serpentina [e.g., Raudixin], reserpine [e.g., Serpasil])—Taking these medicines with phenothiazines may increase the chance and severity of certain side effects
- Metrizamide—When this dye is used for myelograms, the risk of seizures may be increased

Other medical problems—The presence of other medical problems may affect the use of phenothiazines. Make sure you tell your doctor if you have any other medical problems, especially:

- Alcohol abuse—Certain side effects such as heat stroke may be more likely to occur
- Blood disease or
- Breast cancer or
- Difficult urination or
- Enlarged prostate or
- Glaucoma or
- Heart or blood vessel disease or
- Lung disease or
- Parkinson's disease or
- Seizure disorders or
- Stomach ulcers—Phenothiazines may make the condition worse
- Liver disease—Higher blood levels of phenothiazines may occur, increasing the chance of side effects
- Reye's syndrome—There may be an increased chance of unwanted effects on the liver

Before you begin using any new medicine (prescription or nonprescription) or if you develop any new medical problem while you are using this medicine, check with your doctor, nurse, or pharmacist.

Proper Use of This Medicine

For patients taking this medicine *by mouth:*

- This medicine may be taken with food or a full glass (8 ounces) of water or milk to reduce stomach irritation.

- *If your medicine comes in a dropper bottle,* measure each dose with the special dropper provided with your prescription and dilute it in ½ a glass (4 ounces) of orange or grapefruit juice or water.

- If you are taking the *extended-release capsule form* of this medicine, each dose should be swallowed whole. Do not break, crush, or chew before swallowing.

For patients using the *suppository form* of this medicine:

- If the suppository is too soft to insert, chill it in the refrigerator for 30 minutes or run cold water over it before removing the foil wrapper.

- To insert the suppository: First remove the foil wrapper and moisten the suppository with cold water. Lie down on your side and use your finger to push the suppository well up into the rectum.

Do not take more of this medicine and do not take it more often than your doctor ordered. This is particularly important for children or elderly patients, since they may react very strongly to this medicine.

Sometimes this medicine must be taken for several weeks before its full effect is reached when it is used to treat mental and emotional conditions.

Missed dose—If you miss a dose of this medicine and your dosing schedule is:

- One dose a day: Take the missed dose as soon as possible. Then go back to your regular dosing schedule. However, if you do not remember the missed dose until the next day, skip it and go back to your regular dosing schedule. Do not double doses.

- More than one dose a day: If you remember within an hour or so of the missed dose, take it right away. However, if you do not remember until later, skip the missed dose and go back to your regular dosing schedule. Do not double doses.

If you have any questions about this, check with your doctor.

Storage—To store this medicine:

- Keep out of the reach of children.
- Store away from heat and direct light.
- Do not store the capsule or tablet form of this medicine in the bathroom, near the kitchen sink, or in other damp places. Heat or moisture may cause the medicine to break down.
- Keep the liquid form of this medicine from freezing.
- Do not keep outdated medicine or medicine no longer needed. Be sure that any discarded medicine is out of the reach of children.

Precautions While Using This Medicine

Your doctor should check your progress at regular visits, especially during the first few months of treatment with this medicine. This will allow your dosage to be changed if necessary to meet your needs.

Do not stop taking this medicine without first checking with your doctor. Your doctor may want you to reduce gradually the amount you are taking before stopping completely. This is to prevent side effects and to keep your condition from becoming worse.

Do not take this medicine within two hours of taking antacids or medicine for diarrhea. Taking these products too close together may make this medicine less effective.

This medicine will add to the effects of alcohol and other CNS depressants (medicines that slow down the nervous system, possibly causing drowsiness). Some examples of CNS depressants are antihistamines or medicine for hay fever, other allergies, or colds; sedatives, tranquilizers, or sleeping medicine; prescription pain medicine or narcotics; barbiturates; medicine for seizures; muscle relaxants; or anesthetics, including some dental anesthetics. *Check with your doctor before taking any of the above while you are using this medicine.*

Before using any prescription or over-the-counter (OTC) medicine for colds or allergies, check with your doctor. These medicines may increase the chance of heat stroke or other unwanted effects, such as dizziness, dry mouth, blurred vision, and constipation, while you are taking a phenothiazine.

Before you have any medical tests, tell the medical doctor in charge that you are taking this medicine. The results of some tests (such as electrocardiogram [ECG] readings, certain pregnancy tests, the metyrapone test, and urine bilirubin tests) may be affected by this medicine.

Before having any kind of surgery, dental treatment, or emergency treatment, tell the medical doctor or dentist in charge that you are using this medicine.

This medicine may cause some people to become drowsy or less alert than they are normally. Even if this medicine is taken only at bedtime, it may cause some people to feel drowsy or less alert on arising. *Make sure you know how you react to this medicine before you drive, use machines, or do anything else that could be dangerous if you are not alert.*

Phenothiazines may cause blurred vision, difficulty in reading, or other changes in vision, especially during the first few weeks of treatment. Do not drive, use machines, or do anything else that could be dangerous if you are not able to see well. *If the problem continues or gets worse, check with your doctor.*

Dizziness, lightheadedness, or fainting may occur, especially when you get up from a lying or sitting position. Getting up slowly may help. If the problem continues or gets worse, check with your doctor.

This medicine may make you sweat less, causing your body temperature to increase. *Use extra care not to become overheated during exercise or hot weather while you are taking this medicine,* since overheating may result in heat stroke. Also, hot baths or saunas may make you feel dizzy or faint while you are taking this medicine.

This medicine may also make you more sensitive to cold temperatures. Dress warmly during cold weather. Be careful during prolonged exposure to cold, such as in winter sports or swimming in cold water.

Phenothiazines may cause dryness of the mouth. For temporary relief, use sugarless candy or gum, melt bits of ice in your mouth, or use a saliva substitute. However, if your mouth continues to feel dry for more than 2 weeks, check with your medical doctor or dentist. Continuing dryness of the mouth may increase the chance of dental disease, including tooth decay, gum disease, and fungus infections.

Phenothiazines may cause your skin to be more sensitive to sunlight than it is normally. Exposure to sunlight, even for brief periods of time, may cause a skin rash, itching, redness

or other discoloration of the skin, or a severe sunburn. When
you begin taking this medicine:

- Stay out of direct sunlight, especially between the hours
  of 10:00 a.m. and 3:00 p.m., if possible.
- Wear protective clothing, including a hat. Also, wear
  sunglasses.
- Apply a sun block product that has a skin protection
  factor (SPF) of at least 15. Some patients may require
  a product with a higher SPF number, especially if they
  have a fair complexion. If you have any questions about
  this, check with your doctor or pharmacist.
- Apply a sun block lipstick that has an SPF of at least
  15 to protect your lips.
- Do not use a sunlamp or tanning bed or booth.

*If you have a severe reaction from the sun, check with your
doctor.*

Phenothiazines may cause your eyes to be more sensitive to
sunlight than they are normally. Exposure to sunlight over
a period of time (several months to years) may cause blurred
vision, change in color vision, or difficulty in seeing at night.
When you go out during the daylight hours, even on cloudy
days, wear sunglasses that block ultraviolet (UV) light. Ordinary sunglasses may not protect your eyes. If you have
any questions about the kind of sunglasses to wear, check
with your medical doctor or eye doctor.

If you are taking a liquid form of this medicine, avoid
getting it on your skin or clothing because it may cause a
skin rash or other irritation.

If you are receiving this medicine by injection:

- The effects of the long-acting injection form of this
  medicine may last for up to 12 weeks. *The precautions
  and side effects information for this medicine applies
  during this time.*

Side Effects of This Medicine

Along with their needed effects, phenothiazines can sometimes cause serious side effects. Tardive dyskinesia (a movement disorder) may occur and may not go away after you

stop using the medicine. Signs of tardive dyskinesia include fine, worm-like movements of the tongue, or other uncontrolled movements of the mouth, tongue, cheeks, jaw, or arms and legs. Other serious but rare side effects may also occur. These include severe muscle stiffness, fever, unusual tiredness or weakness, fast heartbeat, difficult breathing, increased sweating, loss of bladder control, and seizures (neuroleptic malignant syndrome). *You and your doctor should discuss the good this medicine will do as well as the risks of taking it.*

Stop taking this medicine and check with your doctor immediately if any of the following side effects occur:
> *Rare*
>> Convulsions (seizures); difficult or fast breathing; fast heartbeat or irregular pulse; fever; high or low blood pressure; increased sweating; loss of bladder control; muscle stiffness (severe); unusually pale skin; unusual tiredness or weakness

Check with your doctor immediately if any of the following side effects occur:
> *More common*
>> Lip smacking or puckering; puffing of cheeks; rapid or fine, worm-like movements of tongue; uncontrolled chewing movements; uncontrolled movements of arms or legs

Also, check with your doctor as soon as possible if any of the following side effects occur:
> *More common*
>> Blurred vision, change in color vision, or difficulty in seeing at night; difficulty in speaking or swallowing; fainting; inability to move eyes; loss of balance control; mask-like face; muscle spasms (especially of face, neck, and back); restlessness or need to keep moving; shuffling walk; stiffness of arms or legs; tic-like or twitching movements; trembling and shaking of hands and fingers; twisting movements of body; weakness of arms and legs

> *Less common*
>> Difficulty in urinating; skin rash; sunburn (severe)

Rare

Abdominal or stomach pains; aching muscles and joints; confusion; fever and chills; hot, dry skin or lack of sweating; muscle weakness; nausea, vomiting, or diarrhea; painful, inappropriate penile erection (continuing); skin discoloration (tan or blue-gray); skin itching (severe); sore throat and fever; unusual bleeding or bruising; yellow eyes or skin

Other side effects may occur that usually do not need medical attention. These side effects may go away during treatment as your body adjusts to the medicine. However, check with your doctor if any of the following side effects continue or are bothersome:

More common

Constipation; decreased sweating; dizziness; drowsiness; dryness of mouth; nasal congestion

Less common

Changes in menstrual period; decreased sexual ability; increased sensitivity of skin to sunlight (skin rash, itching, redness or other discoloration of skin, or severe sunburn); swelling or pain in breasts; unusual secretion of milk; weight gain (unusual)

After you stop using this medicine, your body may need time to adjust. The length of time this takes depends on the amount of medicine you are using and how long you used it. During this time, check with your doctor if you notice dizziness, nausea and vomiting, stomach pain, trembling of the fingers and hands, or any of the following symptoms of tardive dyskinesia:

Lip smacking or puckering; puffing of cheeks; rapid or fine, worm-like movements of tongue; uncontrolled chewing movements; uncontrolled movements of arms or legs

Although not all of the side effects listed above have been reported for all of these medicines, they have been reported for at least one of them. However, since all of the phenothiazines are very similar, any of the above side effects may occur with any of these medicines.

Other side effects not listed above may also occur in some patients. If you notice any other effects, check with your doctor.

Additional Information

Once a medicine has been approved for marketing for a certain use, experience may show that it is also useful for other medical problems. Although these uses are not included in product labeling, phenothiazines are used in certain patients with the following medical conditions:

- Chronic neurogenic pain (certain continuing pain conditions)
- Huntington's chorea (hereditary movement disorder)

Other than the above information, there is no additional information relating to proper use, precautions, or side effects for these uses.

POTASSIUM SUPPLEMENTS   Systemic

This information applies to the following medicines:

> Potassium Acetate (poe-TAS-ee-um AS-a-tate)
> Potassium Bicarbonate (bi-KAR-bo-nate)
> Potassium Bicarbonate and Potassium Chloride (KLOR-ide)
> Potassium Bicarbonate and Potassium Citrate (SIH-trayt)
> Potassium Chloride
> Potassium Chloride, Potassium Bicarbonate, and Potassium Citrate
> Potassium Gluconate (GLOO-ko-nate)
> Potassium Gluconate and Potassium Chloride
> Potassium Gluconate and Potassium Citrate
> Trikates (TRI-kates)

Some commonly used brand names are:

For Potassium Acetate
  In the U.S.
> Generic name product is available.

  In Canada
> Generic name product is available.

For Potassium Bicarbonate
  In the U.S.

K+ Care ET	Klor-Con/EF
K-Ide	K-Lyte

  In Canada
> K-Lyte

For Potassium Bicarbonate and Potassium Chloride
  In the U.S.

Klorvess	K-Lyte/Cl
Klorvess Effervescent Granules	K-Lyte/Cl 50

In Canada
Neo-K
Potassium-Sandoz

For Potassium Bicarbonate and Potassium Citrate†
In the U.S.
Effer-K
K-Lyte DS

For Potassium Chloride
In the U.S.

Cena-K
Gen-K
K+ 10
Kaochlor 10%
Kaochlor S-F 10%
Kaon-Cl
Kaon-Cl-10
Kaon-Cl 20% Liquid
Kato
Kay Ciel
K+ Care
K-Dur
K-Ide
K-Lease
K-Lor
Klor-Con 8

Klor-Con 10
Klor-Con Powder
Klor-Con/25 Powder
Klorvess 10% Liquid
Klotrix
K-Lyte/Cl Powder
K-Norm
K-Tab
Micro-K
Micro-K 10
Micro-K LS
Potage
Potasalan
Rum-K
Slow-K
Ten-K

Generic name product may also be available.

In Canada

Apo-K
K-10
Kalium Durules
Kaochlor-10
Kaochlor-20
KCL 5%
K-Dur
K-Long
K-Lor

K-Lyte/Cl
Micro-K
Micro-K 10
Novolente-K
Roychlor-10%
Slow-K

Generic name product may also be available.

For Potassium Chloride, Potassium Bicarbonate, and Potassium Citrate†
In the U.S.
Kaochlor-Eff

For Potassium Gluconate
In the U.S.
Kaon   K-G Elixir
Kaylixir

Generic name product may also be available.

In Canada
Kaon
Potassium-Rougier

For Potassium Gluconate and Potassium Chloride†
  In the U.S.
    Kolyum

For Potassium Gluconate and Potassium Citrate†
  In the U.S.
    Twin-K

For Trikates†
  In the U.S.
    Tri-K

    Generic name product may also be available.

Another commonly used name for trikates is potassium triplex.

---

†Not commercially available in Canada.

Description

Potassium is needed to maintain good health. Although a balanced diet usually supplies all the potassium a person needs, potassium supplements may be needed by patients who do not have enough potassium in their regular diet or have lost too much potassium because of illness or treatment with certain medicines.

There is no evidence that potassium supplements are useful in the treatment of high blood pressure.

Lack of potassium may cause muscle weakness, irregular heartbeat, mood changes, or nausea and vomiting.

Some forms of potassium may be available in stores without a prescription. Since too much potassium may cause health problems, you should take potassium supplements only if directed by your doctor. Potassium supplements are available with your doctor's prescription in the following dosage forms:

  Oral

    Potassium Bicarbonate
      • Tablets for solution (U.S. and Canada)
    Potassium Bicarbonate and Potassium Chloride
      • Powder for solution (U.S. and Canada)
      • Tablets for solution (U.S. and Canada)
    Potassium Bicarbonate and Potassium Citrate
      • Tablets for solution (U.S.)

Potassium Chloride
- Extended-release capsules (U.S. and Canada)
- Solution (U.S. and Canada)
- Powder for solution (U.S. and Canada)
- Powder for suspension (U.S.)
- Extended-release tablets (U.S. and Canada)

Potassium Chloride, Potassium Bicarbonate, and Potassium Citrate
- Tablets for solution (U.S.)

Potassium Gluconate
- Elixir (U.S. and Canada)
- Tablets (U.S.)

Potassium Gluconate and Potassium Chloride
- Solution (U.S.)
- Powder for solution (U.S.)

Potassium Gluconate and Potassium Citrate
- Solution (U.S.)

Trikates
- Solution (U.S.)

Parenteral

Potassium Acetate
- Injection (U.S. and Canada)

Potassium Chloride
- Concentrate for injection (U.S. and Canada)

It is very important that you read and understand the following information. If any of it causes you special concern, check with your doctor. Also, *if you have any questions* or if you want more information about this medicine or your medical problem, *ask your doctor, nurse, or pharmacist.*

Importance of Diet

Many nutritionists recommend that, if possible, people get the potassium they need from the foods they eat. However, many people do not get enough potassium from their diets. For example, people on weight-loss diets may consume too little food to get enough potassium. Others may lose potassium from the body because of illness or treatment with certain medicines. For such people, a potassium supplement, given under a doctor's supervision, is important.

In order to get enough vitamins and minerals in your diet, it is important that you eat a balanced and varied diet.

Follow carefully any diet program your doctor may recommend. For your specific vitamin and/or mineral needs, ask your doctor for a list of appropriate foods.

The following table includes some potassium-rich foods.

Food (amount)	Milligrams of potassium	Milli-equivalents of potassium
Acorn squash, cooked (1 cup)	896	23
Potato with skin, baked (1 long)	844	22
Spinach, cooked (1 cup)	838	21
Lentils, cooked (1 cup)	731	19
Kidney beans, cooked (1 cup)	713	18
Split peas, cooked (1 cup)	710	18
White navy beans, cooked (1 cup)	669	17
Butternut squash, cooked (1 cup)	583	15
Watermelon ($1/16$)	560	14
Raisins (½ cup)	553	14
Yogurt, low-fat, plain (1 cup)	531	14
Orange juice, frozen (1 cup)	503	13
Brussel sprouts, cooked (1 cup)	494	13
Zucchini, cooked, sliced (1 cup)	456	12
Banana (medium)	451	12
Collards, frozen, cooked (1 cup)	427	11
Cantaloupe (¼)	412	11
Milk, low-fat 1% (1 cup)	348	9
Broccoli, frozen, cooked (1 cup)	332	9

Experts have developed a list of recommended dietary allowances (RDA) for most of the vitamins and some minerals. The RDA are not an exact number but a general idea of how much you need. They do not cover amounts needed for problems caused by a serious lack of vitamins or minerals. Because lack of potassium is rare, there are no RDA for this mineral. However, it is thought that 1600 to 2000 mg (40 to 50 mEq) per day for adults is adequate.

Remember:
- The total amount of potassium that you get every day includes what you get from food *and* what you may take as a supplement. Read the labels of processed foods. Many foods now have added potassium.
- Your total intake of potassium should not be greater than the recommended amounts, unless ordered by your doctor. In some cases, too much potassium may cause muscle weakness, confusion, irregular heartbeat, or difficult breathing.

Before Using This Medicine

In deciding to use a medicine, the risks of taking the medicine must be weighed against the good it will do. This is a decision you and your doctor will make. For potassium supplements, the following should be considered:

Allergies—Tell your doctor if you have ever had any unusual or allergic reaction to potassium preparations. Also tell your doctor and pharmacist if you are allergic to any other substances, such as foods, preservatives, or dyes.

Pregnancy—Potassium supplements have not been shown to cause problems in humans.

Breast-feeding—Potassium supplements pass into breast milk. However, this medicine has not been reported to cause problems in nursing babies.

Children—Although there is no specific information comparing use of potassium supplements in children with use in other age groups, they are not expected to cause different side effects or problems in children than they do in adults.

Older adults—Many medicines have not been studied specifically in older people. Therefore, it may not be known whether they work exactly the same way they do in younger adults. Although there is no specific information comparing use of potassium supplements in the elderly with use in other age groups, they are not expected to cause different side effects or problems in older people than they do in younger adults.

Older adults may be at a greater risk of developing high blood levels of potassium (hyperkalemia).

Other medicines—Although certain medicines should not be used together at all, in other cases two different medicines may be used together even if an interaction might occur. In these cases, your doctor may want to change the dose, or other precautions may be necessary. When you are taking potassium supplements, it is especially important that your doctor and pharmacist know if you are taking any of the following:

- Amantadine (e.g., Symmetrel) or
- Anticholinergics (medicine for abdominal or stomach spasms or cramps) or
- Antidepressants (medicine for depression) or
- Antidyskinetics (medicine for Parkinson's disease or other conditions affecting control of muscles) or
- Antihistamines or
- Antipsychotic medicine (medicine for mental illness) or
- Buclizine (e.g., Bucladin) or
- Carbamazepine (e.g., Tegretol) or
- Cyclizine (e.g., Marezine) or
- Cyclobenzaprine (e.g., Flexeril) or
- Disopyramide (e.g., Norpace) or
- Flavoxate (e.g., Urispas) or
- Ipratropium (e.g., Atrovent) or
- Meclizine (e.g., Antivert) or
- Methylphenidate (e.g., Ritalin) or
- Orphenadrine (e.g., Norflex) or
- Oxybutynin (e.g., Ditropan) or
- Procainamide (e.g., Pronestyl) or
- Promethazine (e.g., Phenergan) or
- Quinidine (e.g., Quinidex) or
- Trimeprazine (e.g., Temaril)—Use with potassium supplements may cause or worsen certain stomach or intestine problems
- Angiotensin-converting enzyme (ACE) inhibitors (benazepril [e.g., Lotensin], captopril [e.g., Capoten], enalapril [e.g., Vasotec], fosinopril [e.g., Monotril], lisinopril [e.g., Prinivil, Zestril], quinapril [e.g., Accupril], ramipril [e.g., Altace]) or

- Amiloride (e.g., Midamor) or
- Beta-adrenergic blocking agents (acebutolol [e.g., Sectral], atenolol [e.g., Tenormin], betaxolol [e.g., Kerlone], carteolol [e.g., Cartrol], labetalol [e.g., Normodyne], metoprolol [e.g., Lopressor], nadolol [e.g., Corgard], oxprenolol [e.g., Trasicor], penbutolol [e.g., Levatol], pindolol [e.g., Visken], propranolol [e.g., Inderal], sotalol [e.g., Sotacor], timolol [e.g., Blocadren]) or
- Heparin (e.g., Panheprin) or
- Inflammation or pain medicine (except narcotics) or
- Potassium-containing medicines (other) or
- Salt substitutes, low-salt foods, or milk or
- Spironolactone (e.g., Aldactone) or
- Triamterene (e.g., Dyrenium)—Use with potassium supplements may further increase potassium blood levels, which may cause or worsen heart problems
- Digitalis glycosides (heart medicine)—Use with potassium supplements may make heart problems worse
- Thiazide diuretics (water pills)—If you have been taking a potassium supplement and a thiazide diuretic together, stopping the thiazide diuretic may cause hyperkalemia (high blood levels of potassium)

Other medical problems—The presence of other medical problems may affect the use of potassium supplements. Make sure you tell your doctor if you have any other medical problems, especially:

- Addison's disease (underactive adrenal glands) or
- Dehydration (excessive loss of body water, continuing or severe)
- Diabetes mellitus or
- Kidney disease—Potassium supplements may increase the risk of hyperkalemia (high blood levels of potassium), which may worsen or cause heart problems in patients with these conditions
- Diarrhea (continuing or severe)—The loss of fluid in combination with potassium supplements may cause kidney problems, which may increase the risk of hyperkalemia (high blood levels of potassium)
- Heart disease—Potassium supplements may make this condition worse
- Intestinal or esophageal blockage—Potassium supplements may damage the intestines

- Stomach ulcer—Potassium supplements may make this condition worse

Before you begin using any new medicine (prescription or nonprescription) or if you develop any new medical problem while you are using this medicine, check with your doctor, nurse, or pharmacist.

Proper Use of This Medicine

For patients taking the *liquid form* of this medicine:

- This medicine *must be diluted* in at least one-half glass (4 ounces) of cold water or juice to reduce its possible stomach-irritating or laxative effect.
- If you are on a salt (sodium)-restricted diet, check with your doctor before using tomato juice to dilute your medicine. Tomato juice has a high salt content.

For patients taking the *soluble granule, soluble powder, or soluble tablet form* of this medicine:

- This medicine must be completely dissolved in at least one-half glass (4 ounces) of cold water or juice to reduce its possible stomach-irritating or laxative effect.
- Allow any "fizzing" to stop before taking the dissolved medicine.
- If you are on a salt (sodium)-restricted diet, check with your doctor before using tomato juice to dilute your medicine. Tomato juice has a high salt content.

For patients taking the *extended-release tablet form* of this medicine:

- Swallow the tablets whole with a full (8-ounce) glass of water. Do not chew or suck on the tablet.
- Some tablets may be broken or crushed and sprinkled on applesauce or other soft food. However, check with your doctor or pharmacist first, since this should not be done for most tablets.
- If you have trouble swallowing tablets or if they seem to stick in your throat, check with your doctor. When this medicine is not properly released, it can cause irritation that may lead to ulcers.

For patients taking the *extended-release capsule form* of this medicine:

- Do not crush or chew the capsule. Swallow the capsule whole with a full (8-ounce) glass of water.
- Some capsules may be opened and the contents sprinkled on applesauce or other soft food. However, check with your doctor or pharmacist first, since this should not be done for most capsules.

Take this medicine immediately after meals or with food to lessen possible stomach upset or laxative action.

Take this medicine only as directed by your doctor. Do not take more of it, do not take it more often, and do not take it for a longer time than your doctor ordered. *This is especially important if you are also taking both diuretics (water pills) and digitalis medicines for your heart.*

Missed dose—If you miss a dose of this medicine and remember within 2 hours, take the missed dose right away with food or liquids. Then go back to your regular dosing schedule. However, if you do not remember until later, skip the missed dose and go back to your regular dosing schedule. Do not double doses.

Storage—To store this medicine:

- Keep out of the reach of children.
- Store away from heat and direct light.
- Do not store in the bathroom, near the kitchen sink, or in other damp places. Heat or moisture may cause the medicine to break down.
- Keep the liquid form of this medicine from freezing.
- Do not keep outdated medicine or medicine no longer needed. Be sure that any discarded medicine is out of the reach of children.

Precautions While Using This Medicine

Your doctor should check your progress at regular visits to make sure the medicine is working properly and that possible side effects are avoided. Laboratory tests may be necessary.

Do not use salt substitutes, eat low-sodium foods, especially some breads and canned foods, or drink low-sodium milk unless you are told to do so by your doctor, since these products may contain potassium. It is important to read the labels carefully on all low-sodium food products.

Check with your doctor before starting any physical exercise program, especially if you are out of condition and are taking any other medicine. Exercise and certain medicines may increase the amount of potassium in the blood.

Check with your doctor at once if you notice blackish stools or other signs of stomach or intestinal bleeding. This medicine may cause such a condition to become worse, especially when taken in tablet form.

Side Effects of This Medicine

Along with its needed effects, a medicine may cause some unwanted effects. Although not all of these side effects may occur, if they do occur they may need medical attention.

Stop taking this medicine and check with your doctor immediately if any of the following side effects occur:

Less common

Confusion; irregular or slow heartbeat; numbness or tingling in hands, feet, or lips; shortness of breath or difficult breathing; unexplained anxiety; unusual tiredness or weakness; weakness or heaviness of legs

Also, check with your doctor if any of the following side effects occur:

Rare

Abdominal or stomach pain, cramping, or soreness (continuing); chest or throat pain, especially when swallowing; stools with signs of blood (red or black color)

Other side effects may occur that usually do not need medical attention. These side effects may go away during treatment as your body adjusts to the medicine. However, check with your doctor if any of the following side effects continue or are bothersome:

More common
  Diarrhea; nausea; stomach pain, discomfort, or gas (mild);
    vomiting

Sometimes you may see what appears to be a whole tablet
in the stool after taking certain extended-release potassium
chloride tablets. This is to be expected. Your body has absorbed the potassium from the tablet and the shell is then
expelled.

Other side effects not listed above may also occur in some
patients. If you notice any other effects, check with your
doctor.

PRAZOSIN Systemic

A commonly used brand name in the U.S. and Canada is Minipress.
Generic name product may also be available in the U.S.

Description

Prazosin (PRA-zoe-sin) belongs to the general class of medicines called antihypertensives. It is used to treat high blood
pressure (hypertension).

High blood pressure adds to the workload of the heart and
arteries. If it continues for a long time, the heart and arteries
may not function properly. This can damage the blood vessels of the brain, heart, and kidneys, resulting in a stroke,
heart failure, or kidney failure. High blood pressure may
also increase the risk of heart attacks. These problems may
be less likely to occur if blood pressure is controlled.

Prazosin works by relaxing blood vessels so that blood passes
through them more easily. This helps to lower blood pressure.

Prazosin may also be used for other conditions as determined
by your doctor.

Prazosin is available only with your doctor's prescription, in
the following dosage forms:

Oral
- Capsules (U.S.)
- Tablets (Canada)

It is very important that you read and understand the following information. If any of it causes you special concern, check with your doctor. Also, *if you have any questions* or if you want more information about this medicine or your medical problem, *ask your doctor, nurse, or pharmacist.*

Before Using This Medicine

In deciding to use a medicine, the risks of taking the medicine must be weighed against the good it will do. This is a decision you and your doctor will make. For prazosin, the following should be considered:

Allergies—Tell your doctor if you have ever had any unusual or allergic reaction to prazosin, doxazosin, or terazosin. Also tell your doctor and pharmacist if you are allergic to any other substance, such as foods, preservatives, or dyes.

Pregnancy—Limited use of prazosin to control high blood pressure in pregnant women has not shown that prazosin causes birth defects or other problems. Studies in animals given many times the highest recommended human dose of prazosin also have not shown that prazosin causes birth defects. However, in rats given many times the highest recommended human dose, lower birth weights were seen.

Breast-feeding—Prazosin passes into breast milk in small amounts. However, it has not been reported to cause problems in nursing babies.

Children—Studies on this medicine have been done only in adult patients, and there is no specific information comparing use of prazosin in children with use in other age groups.

Older adults—Dizziness, lightheadedness, or fainting (especially when getting up from a lying or sitting position) may be more likely to occur in the elderly, who are more sensitive to the effects of prazosin. In addition, prazosin may reduce tolerance to cold temperatures in elderly patients.

Other medicines—Although certain medicines should not be used together at all, in other cases two different medicines may be used together even if an interaction might occur. In these cases, your doctor may want to change the dose, or other precautions may be necessary. Tell your doctor and pharmacist if you are taking any other prescription or non-prescription (over-the-counter [OTC]) medicine.

Other medical problems—The presence of other medical problems may affect the use of prazosin. Make sure you tell your doctor if you have any other medical problems, especially:

- Angina (chest pain)—Prazosin may make this condition worse
- Heart disease (severe)—Prazosin may make this condition worse
- Kidney disease—Possible increased sensitivity to the effects of prazosin

Before you begin using any new medicine (prescription or nonprescription) or if you develop any new medical problem while you are using this medicine, check with your doctor, nurse, or pharmacist.

Proper Use of This Medicine

For patients *taking this medicine for high blood pressure:*

- In addition to the use of the medicine your doctor has prescribed, treatment for your high blood pressure may include weight control and care in the types of foods you eat, especially foods high in sodium. Your doctor will tell you which of these are most important for you. You should check with your doctor before changing your diet.

- Many patients who have high blood pressure will not notice any signs of the problem. In fact, many may feel normal. It is very important that you *take your medicine exactly as directed* and that you keep your appointments with your doctor even if you feel well.

- Remember that prazosin will not cure your high blood pressure but it does help control it. Therefore, you must continue to take it as directed if you expect to lower your blood pressure and keep it down. *You may have*

*to take high blood pressure medicine for the rest of
your life.* If high blood pressure is not treated, it can
cause serious problems such as heart failure, blood vessel disease, stroke, or kidney disease.

To help you remember to take your medicine, try to get into
the habit of taking it at the same time each day.

Missed dose—If you miss a dose of this medicine, take it
as soon as possible. However, if it is almost time for your
next dose, skip the missed dose and go back to your regular
dosing schedule. Do not double doses.

Storage—To store this medicine:
- Keep out of the reach of children.
- Store away from heat and direct light.
- Do not store in the bathroom, near the kitchen sink, or
  in other damp places. Heat or moisture may cause the
  medicine to break down.
- Do not keep outdated medicine or medicine no longer
  needed. Be sure that any discarded medicine is out of
  the reach of children.

Precautions While Using This Medicine

It is important that your doctor check your progress at regular visits to make sure that this medicine is working properly.

For patients *taking this medicine for high blood pressure:*
- *Do not take other medicines unless they have been
  discussed with your doctor.* This especially includes
  over-the-counter (nonprescription) medicines for appetite control, asthma, colds, cough, hay fever, or sinus
  problems, since they may tend to make prazosin less
  effective.

Dizziness, lightheadedness, or sudden fainting may occur
after you take this medicine, especially when you get up
from a lying or sitting position. These effects are more likely
to occur when you take the first dose of this medicine. Taking
the first dose at bedtime may prevent problems. However,

be especially careful if you need to get up during the night.
These effects may also occur with any doses you take after
the first dose. Getting up slowly may help lessen this problem. *If you feel dizzy, lie down so that you do not faint.*
Then sit for a few moments before standing to prevent the
dizziness from returning.

The dizziness, lightheadedness, or fainting is more likely to
occur if you drink alcohol, stand for a long time, exercise,
or if the weather is hot. *While you are taking this medicine,
be careful to limit the amount of alcohol you drink. Also,
use extra care during exercise or hot weather or if you must
stand for a long time.*

Prazosin may cause some people to become drowsy or less
alert than they are normally. *Make sure you know how you
react to this medicine before you drive, use machines, or
do anything else that could be dangerous if you are dizzy,
drowsy, or are not alert.* After you have taken several doses
of this medicine, these effects should lessen.

Side Effects of This Medicine

Along with its needed effects, a medicine may cause some
unwanted effects. Although not all of these side effects may
occur, if they do occur they may need medical attention.

Check with your doctor as soon as possible if any of the
following side effects occur:

More common

Dizziness or lightheadedness, especially when getting up from
a lying or sitting position; fainting (sudden)

Less common

Loss of bladder control; pounding heartbeat; swelling of feet
or lower legs

Rare

Chest pain; painful inappropriate erection of penis (continuing); shortness of breath

Other side effects may occur that usually do not need medical attention. These side effects may go away during treat-

ment as your body adjusts to the medicine. However, check with your doctor if any of the following side effects continue or are bothersome:

More common

Drowsiness; headache; lack of energy

Less common

Dryness of mouth; nervousness; unusual tiredness or weakness

Rare

Nausea; frequent urge to urinate

Other side effects not listed above may also occur in some patients. If you notice any other effects, check with your doctor.

Additional Information

Once a medicine has been approved for marketing for a certain use, experience may show that it is also useful for other medical problems. Although these uses are not included in product labeling, prazosin is used in certain patients with the following medical conditions:

- Congestive heart failure
- Ergot alkaloid poisoning
- Pheochromocytoma
- Raynaud's disease
- Benign enlargement of the prostate

Other than the above information, there is no additional information relating to proper use, precautions, or side effects for these uses.

PROBENECID   Systemic

Some commonly used brand names are:

In the U.S.

Benemid   Probalan

Generic name product may also be available.

In Canada

Benemid   Benuryl

Description

Probenecid (proe-BEN-e-sid) is used in the treatment of chronic gout or gouty arthritis. These conditions are caused by too much uric acid in the blood. The medicine works by removing the extra uric acid from the body. Probenecid does not cure gout, but after you have been taking it for a few months it will help prevent gout attacks. This medicine will help prevent gout attacks only as long as you continue to take it.

Probenecid is also used to prevent or treat other medical problems that may occur if too much uric acid is present in the body.

Probenecid is sometimes used with certain kinds of antibiotics to make them more effective in the treatment of infections.

Probenecid is available only with your doctor's prescription, in the following dosage form:

Oral
- Tablets (U.S. and Canada)

It is very important that you read and understand the following information. If any of it causes you special concern, check with your doctor. Also, *if you have any questions* or if you want more information about this medicine or your medical problem, *ask your doctor, nurse, or pharmacist.*

Before Using This Medicine

In deciding to use a medicine, the risks of taking the medicine must be weighed against the good it will do. This is a decision you and your doctor will make. For probenecid, the following should be considered:

Allergies—Tell your doctor if you have ever had any unusual or allergic reaction to probenecid. Also tell your doctor and pharmacist if you are allergic to any other substances, such as foods, preservatives, or dyes.

Pregnancy—Probenecid has not been shown to cause birth defects or other problems in humans.

Breast-feeding—Probenecid has not been reported to cause problems in nursing babies.

Children—Probenecid has been tested in children 2 to 14 years of age for use together with antibiotics. It has not been shown to cause different side effects or problems than it does in adults. Studies on the effects of probenecid in patients with gout have been done only in adults. Gout is very rare in children.

Older adults—Many medicines have not been studied specifically in older people. Therefore, it may not be known whether they work exactly the same way they do in younger adults. There is no specific information comparing use of probenecid in the elderly with use in other age groups.

Athletes—Probenecid is banned by the International Olympic Committee (IOC), the U.S. Olympic Committee (USOC), and the National Collegiate Athletic Association (NCAA). Probenecid use can change the amounts of other medicines in urine samples. This is considered tampering with urine samples, and can lead to disqualification of athletes in most athletic events.

Other medicines—Although certain medicines should not be used together at all, in other cases two different medicines may be used together even if an interaction might occur. In these cases, your doctor may want to change the dose, or other precautions may be necessary. When you are taking probenecid, it is especially important that your doctor and pharmacist know if you are taking any of the following:

- Antineoplastics (cancer medicine)—The chance of serious side effects may be increased
- Aspirin or other salicylates—These medicines may keep probenecid from working properly for treating gout, depending on the amount of aspirin or other salicylate that you take and how often you take it
- Heparin—Probenecid may increase the effects of heparin, which increases the chance of side effects
- Indomethacin (e.g., Indocin) or
- Ketoprofen (e.g., Orudis) or
- Methotrexate (e.g., Mexate)—Probenecid may increase the blood levels of these medicines, which increases the chance of side effects

- Medicine for infection, including tuberculosis or virus infection—Probenecid may increase the blood levels of many of these medicines. In some cases, this is a desired effect and probenecid may be used to help the other medicine work better. However, the chance of side effects is sometimes also increased
- Nitrofurantoin (e.g., Furadantin)—Probenecid may keep nitrofurantoin from working properly
- Zidovudine (e.g., AZT, Retrovir)—Probenecid increases the blood level of zidovudine and may allow lower doses of zidovudine to be used. However, the chance of side effects is also increased

Other medical problems—The presence of other medical problems may affect the use of probenecid. Make sure you tell your doctor if you have any other medical problems, especially:

- Blood disease or
- Cancer being treated by antineoplastics (cancer medicine) or radiation (x-rays) or
- Kidney disease or stones (or history of) or
- Stomach ulcer (history of)—The chance of side effects may be increased

Before you begin using any new medicine (prescription or nonprescription) or if you develop any new medical problem while you are using this medicine, check with your doctor, nurse, or pharmacist.

Proper Use of This Medicine

If probenecid upsets your stomach, it may be taken with food. If this does not work, an antacid may be taken. If stomach upset (nausea, vomiting, or loss of appetite) continues, check with your doctor.

For patients taking probenecid *for gout:*

- After you begin to take probenecid, gout attacks may continue to occur for a while. However, if you take this medicine regularly as directed by your doctor, the attacks will gradually become less frequent and less painful than before. After you have been taking probenecid for several months, they may stop completely.

- This medicine will help prevent gout attacks but it will not relieve an attack that has already started. *Even if you take another medicine for gout attacks, continue to take this medicine also.* If you have any questions about this, check with your doctor.

For patients taking probenecid *for gout or to help remove uric acid from the body:*

- When you first begin taking probenecid, the amount of uric acid in the kidneys is greatly increased. This may cause kidney stones or other kidney problems in some people. To help prevent this, your doctor may want you to drink at least 10 to 12 full glasses (8 ounces each) of fluids each day, or to take another medicine to make your urine less acid. It is important that you follow your doctor's instructions very carefully.

Dosing—The dose of probenecid will be different for different patients. *Follow your doctor's orders or the directions on the label.* The following information includes only the average doses of probenecid. *If your dose is different, do not change it* unless your doctor tells you to do so.

- *For treating gout or removing uric acid from the body:*

  —Adults: 250 mg (one-half of a 500-mg tablet) two times a day for about one week, then 500 mg (one tablet) two times a day for a few weeks. After this, the dose will depend on the amount of uric acid in your blood or urine. Most people need 2, 3, or 4 tablets a day, but some people may need higher doses.

  —Children: It is not likely that probenecid will be needed to treat gout or to remove uric acid from the body in children. If a child needs this medicine, however, the dose would have to be determined by the doctor.

- *For helping antibiotics work better:*

  —Adults: The amount of probenecid will depend on the condition being treated. Sometimes, only one dose of 2 tablets is needed. Other times, the dose will be 1 tablet four times a day.

  —Children: The dose will have to be determined by the doctor. It depends on the child's weight, as well as on the condition being treated. Older children and teenagers may need the same amount as adults.

Missed dose—If you are taking probenecid regularly and you miss a dose, take the missed dose as soon as possible. However, if you do not remember until it is almost time for the next dose, skip the missed dose and go back to your regular dosing schedule. Do not double doses.

Storage—To store this medicine:
- Keep out of the reach of children.
- Store away from heat and direct light.
- Do not store this medicine in the bathroom, near the kitchen sink, or in other damp places. Heat or moisture may cause the medicine to break down.
- Do not keep outdated medicine or medicine no longer needed. Be sure that any discarded medicine is out of the reach of children.

Precautions While Using This Medicine

If you will be taking probenecid for more than a few weeks, your doctor should check your progress at regular visits.

Before you have any medical tests, tell the person in charge that you are taking this medicine. The results of some tests may be affected by probenecid.

For *diabetic patients:*
- Probenecid may cause false test results with copper sulfate urine sugar tests (Clinitest®), but not with glucose enzymatic urine sugar tests (Clinistix®). If you have any questions about this, check with your doctor or pharmacist.

For patients taking probenecid *for gout or to help remove uric acid from the body:*
- Taking aspirin or other salicylates may lessen the effects of probenecid. This will depend on the dose of aspirin or other salicylate that you take, and on how often you take it. Also, drinking too much alcohol may increase the amount of uric acid in the blood and lessen

the effects of this medicine. Therefore, *do not take aspirin or other salicylates or drink alcoholic beverages while taking this medicine,* unless you have first checked with your doctor.

Side Effects of This Medicine

Along with its needed effects, a medicine may cause some unwanted effects. Although not all of these side effects may occur, if they do occur they may need medical attention.

The following side effects may mean that you are having an allergic reaction to this medicine. *Check with your doctor immediately* if any of the following side effects occur:

Rare

> Fast or irregular breathing; puffiness or swellings of the eyelids or around the eyes; shortness of breath, troubled breathing, tightness in chest, or wheezing; changes in the skin color of the face occurring together with any of the other side effects listed here; or skin rash, hives, or itching occurring together with any of the other side effects listed here

Also, check with your doctor as soon as possible if any of the following side effects occur:

Less common

> Bloody urine; difficult or painful urination; lower back or side pain (especially if severe or sharp); skin rash, hives, or itching (occurring without other signs of an allergic reaction)

Rare

> Cloudy urine; cough or hoarseness; fast or irregular breathing; fever; pain in back and/or ribs; sores, ulcers, or white spots on lips or in mouth; sore throat and fever with or without chills; sudden decrease in the amount of urine; swelling of face, fingers, feet, and/or lower legs; swollen and/or painful glands; unusual bleeding or bruising; unusual tiredness or weakness; yellow eyes or skin; weight gain

Other side effects may occur that usually do not need medical attention. These side effects may go away during treat-

ment as your body adjusts to the medicine. However, check with your doctor if any of the following side effects continue or are bothersome:

More common

Headache; joint pain, redness, or swelling; loss of appetite; nausea or vomiting (mild)

Less common

Dizziness; flushing or redness of face (occurring without any signs of an allergic reaction); frequent urge to urinate; sore gums

Other side effects not listed above may also occur in some patients. If you notice any other effects, check with your doctor.

PROBUCOL   Systemic

Some commonly used brand names are:

In the U.S.
Lorelco

In Canada
Lorelco

Other

Bifenabid	Panesclerina
Lesterol	Superlipid
Lurselle	

Description

Probucol (PROE-byoo-kole) is used to lower levels of cholesterol (a fat-like substance) in the blood. This may help prevent medical problems caused by cholesterol clogging the blood vessels.

Probucol is available only with your doctor's prescription, in the following dosage form:

Oral

• Tablets (U.S. and Canada)

It is very important that you read and understand the following information. If any of it causes you special concern,

check with your doctor. Also, *if you have any questions* or if you want more information about this medicine or your medical problem, *ask your doctor, nurse, or pharmacist.*

Before Using This Medicine

In deciding to use a medicine, the risks of taking the medicine must be weighed against the good it will do. This is a decision you and your doctor will make. For probucol, the following should be considered:

Allergies—Tell your doctor if you have ever had any unusual or allergic reaction to probucol. Also tell your doctor and pharmacist if you are allergic to any other substances, such as foods, preservatives, or dyes.

Diet—Before prescribing medicine for your condition, your doctor will probably try to control your condition by prescribing a personal diet for you. Such a diet may be low in fats, sugars, and/or cholesterol. Many people are able to control their condition by carefully following their doctor's orders for proper diet and exercise. Medicine is prescribed only when additional help is needed and is effective only when a schedule of diet and exercise is properly followed.

Also, this medicine is less effective if you are greatly overweight. It may be very important for you to go on a reducing diet. However, check with your doctor before going on any diet.

Make certain your doctor and pharmacist know if you are on a low-sodium, low-sugar, or any other special diet.

Pregnancy—Probucol has not been studied in pregnant women; however, it has not been shown to cause birth defects or other problems in rats or rabbits.

Breast-feeding—It is not known whether probucol passes into the breast milk. However, this medicine is not recommended for use during breast-feeding because it may cause unwanted effects in nursing babies.

Children—There is no specific information about the use of probucol in children. However, use is not recommended in children under 2 years of age since cholesterol is needed for normal development.

Older adults—Many medicines have not been studied specifically in older people. Therefore, it may not be known whether they work exactly the same way they do in younger adults or if they cause different side effects or problems in older people. There is no specific information comparing use of probucol in the elderly with use in other age groups.

Other medicines—Although certain medicines should not be used together at all, in other cases two different medicines may be used together even if an interaction might occur. In these cases, your doctor may want to change the dose, or other precautions may be necessary. Tell your doctor and pharmacist if you are taking any other prescription or non-prescription (over-the-counter [OTC]) medicine.

Other medical problems—The presence of other medical problems may affect the use of probucol. Make sure you tell your doctor if you have any other medical problems, especially:

- Gallbladder disease or gallstones or
- Heart disease—Probucol may make these conditions worse
- Liver disease—Higher blood levels of probucol may result, which may increase the chance of side effects

Before you begin using any new medicine (prescription or nonprescription) or if you develop any new medical problem while you are using this medicine, check with your doctor, nurse, or pharmacist.

Proper Use of This Medicine

Many patients who have high cholesterol levels will not notice any signs of the problem. In fact, many may feel normal. *Take this medicine exactly as directed by your doctor, even though you may feel well.* Try not to miss any doses and do not take more medicine than your doctor ordered.

Remember that this medicine will not cure your condition but it does help control it. Therefore, you must continue to take it as directed if you expect to keep your cholesterol levels down.

Follow carefully the special diet your doctor gave you. This is the most important part of controlling your condition, and is necessary if the medicine is to work properly.

This medicine works better when taken with meals.

Missed dose—If you miss a dose of this medicine, take it as soon as possible. However, if it is almost time for your next dose, skip the missed dose and go back to your regular dosing schedule. Do not double doses.

Storage—To store this medicine:
- Keep out of the reach of children.
- Store away from heat and direct light.
- Do not store in the bathroom, near the kitchen sink, or in other damp places. Heat or moisture may cause the medicine to break down.
- Do not keep outdated medicine or medicine no longer needed. Be sure that any discarded medicine is out of the reach of children.

Precautions While Using This Medicine

It is very important that your doctor check your progress at regular visits. This will allow your doctor to see if the medicine is working properly to lower your cholesterol levels and to decide if you should continue to take it.

Do not stop taking this medicine without first checking with your doctor. When you stop taking this medicine, your blood fat levels may increase again. Your doctor may want you to follow a special diet to help prevent this.

Side Effects of This Medicine

Along with its needed effects, a medicine may cause some unwanted effects. Although not all of these side effects may occur, if they do occur they may need medical attention.

Check with your doctor as soon as possible if any of the following side effects occur:

More common
    Dizziness or fainting

Rare

Fast or irregular heartbeat; swellings on face, hands, or feet, or in mouth; unusual bleeding or bruising; unusual tiredness or weakness

Other side effects may occur that usually do not need medical attention. These side effects may go away during treatment as your body adjusts to the medicine. However, check with your doctor if any of the following side effects continue or are bothersome:

More common

Bloating; diarrhea; nausea and vomiting; stomach pain

Less common

Dizziness; headache; numbness or tingling of fingers, toes, or face

Other side effects not listed above may also occur in some patients. If you notice any other effects, check with your doctor.

PROCAINAMIDE   Systemic

Some commonly used brand names are:

In the U.S.

Procan SR	Pronestyl
Promine	Pronestyl-SR

Generic name product may also be available.

In Canada

Procan SR	Pronestyl-SR
Pronestyl	

Generic name product may also be available.

Description

Procainamide (proe-KANE-a-mide) is used to correct irregular heartbeats to a normal rhythm and to slow an overactive heart. This allows the heart to work more efficiently. Procainamide produces its beneficial effects by slowing nerve impulses in the heart and reducing sensitivity of heart tissues.

Procainamide is available only with your doctor's prescription, in the following dosage forms:

Oral
- Capsules (U.S. and Canada)
- Tablets (U.S.)
- Extended-release tablets (U.S. and Canada)

Parenteral
- Injection (U.S. and Canada)

It is very important that you read and understand the following information. If any of it causes you special concern, check with your doctor. Also, *if you have any questions* or if you want more information about this medicine or your medical problem, *ask your doctor, nurse, or pharmacist.*

Before Using This Medicine

In deciding to use a medicine, the risks of taking the medicine must be weighed against the good it will do. This is a decision you and your doctor will make. For procainamide, the following should be considered:

Allergies—Tell your doctor if you have ever had any unusual or allergic reaction to procainamide, procaine, or any other "caine-type" medicine. Also tell your doctor and pharmacist if you are allergic to any other substance, such as foods, preservatives, or dyes.

Pregnancy—Although procainamide has not been shown to cause problems in humans, it is known to pass from the mother to the fetus.

Breast-feeding—Although procainamide passes into breast milk, it has not been reported to cause problems in nursing babies.

Children—Although there is no specific information about the use of procainamide in children, it is not expected to cause different side effects or problems in children than it does in adults.

Older adults—Dizziness or lightheadedness are more likely to occur in the elderly, who are usually more sensitive to the effects of this medicine.

Other medicines—Although certain medicines should not be used together at all, in other cases two different medicines may be used together even if an interaction might occur. In these cases, your doctor may want to change the dose, or other precautions may be necessary. When you are taking procainamide, it is especially important that your doctor and pharmacist know if you are taking any of the following:

- Antihypertensives (high blood pressure medicine)—Effects on blood pressure may be increased
- Antimyasthenics (ambenonium [e.g., Mytelase], neostigmine [e.g., Prostigmin], pyridostigmine [e.g., Mestinon])—Effects may be blocked by procainamide
- Pimozide (e.g., Orap)—Possible increased risk of heart rhythm problems

Other medical problems—The presence of other medical problems may affect the use of procainamide. Make sure you tell your doctor if you have any other medical problems, especially:

- Asthma—Possible allergic reaction
- Kidney disease or
- Liver disease—Effects may be increased because of slower removal of procainamide from the body
- Lupus erythematosus (history of)—Procainamide may cause the condition to become active
- Myasthenia gravis—Procainamide may increase muscle weakness

Before you begin using any new medicine (prescription or nonprescription) or if you develop any new medical problem while you are using this medicine, check with your doctor, nurse, or pharmacist.

Proper Use of This Medicine

Take procainamide exactly as directed by your doctor, even though you may feel well. Do not take more medicine than ordered.

Procainamide should be taken with a glass of water on an empty stomach 1 hour before or 2 hours after meals so that it will be absorbed more quickly. However, to lessen stomach upset, your doctor may want you to take the medicine with food or milk.

For patients taking the *extended-release tablets:*
- Swallow the tablet whole without breaking, crushing, or chewing it.

This medicine works best when there is a constant amount in the blood. *To help keep the amount constant, do not miss any doses. Also, it is best to take the doses at evenly spaced times day and night.* For example, if you are to take 6 doses a day, the doses should be spaced about 4 hours apart. If this interferes with your sleep or other daily activities, or if you need help in planning the best times to take your medicine, check with your doctor, nurse, or pharmacist.

Missed dose—If you do miss a dose of this medicine and remember within 2 hours (4 hours if you are taking the long-acting tablets), take it as soon as possible. However, if you do not remember until later, skip the missed dose and go back to your regular dosing schedule. Do not double doses.

Storage—To store this medicine:
- Keep out of the reach of children.
- Store away from heat and direct light.
- Do not store in the bathroom, refrigerator, near the kitchen sink, or in other damp places. Moisture usually present in these areas may cause the medicine to break down. Keep the container tightly closed and store in a dry place.
- Do not keep outdated medicine or medicine no longer needed. Be sure that any discarded medicine is out of the reach of children.

Precautions While Using This Medicine

It is important that your doctor check your progress at regular visits to make sure the medicine is working properly. This will allow necessary changes in the amount of medicine you are taking, which also may help reduce side effects.

Do not stop taking this medicine without first checking with your doctor. Stopping it suddenly may cause a serious change in the activity of your heart. Your doctor may want you to reduce gradually the amount you are taking before stopping completely.

Before having any kind of surgery (including dental surgery) or emergency treatment, tell the medical doctor or dentist in charge that you are taking this medicine.

Your doctor may want you to carry a medical identification card or bracelet stating that you are taking this medicine.

Dizziness or lightheadedness may occur, especially in elderly patients and when large doses are used. *Elderly patients should use extra care to avoid falling. Make sure you know how you react to this medicine before you drive, use machines, or do anything else that could be dangerous if you are dizzy or are not alert.*

Tell the doctor in charge that you are taking this medicine before you have any medical tests. The results of some tests may be affected by this medicine.

Side Effects of This Medicine

Along with its needed effects, a medicine may cause some unwanted effects. Although not all of these side effects may occur, if they do occur they may need medical attention.

Check with your doctor as soon as possible if any of the following side effects occur:

> *Less common*
>> Fever and chills; joint pain or swelling; pains with breathing; skin rash or itching

Rare

Confusion; fever or sore mouth, gums, or throat; hallucinations (seeing, hearing, or feeling things that are not there); mental depression; unusual bleeding or bruising; unusual tiredness or weakness

Signs and symptoms of overdose

Confusion; decrease in urination; dizziness (severe) or fainting; drowsiness; fast or irregular heartbeat; nausea and vomiting

Other side effects may occur that usually do not need medical attention. These side effects may go away during treatment as your body adjusts to the medicine. However, check with your doctor if any of the following side effects continue or are bothersome:

More common

Diarrhea; loss of appetite

Less common

Dizziness or lightheadedness

The medicine in the extended-release tablets is contained in a special wax form (matrix). The medicine is slowly released, after which the wax matrix passes out of the body. Sometimes it may be seen in the stool. This is normal and is no cause for concern.

Other side effects not listed above may also occur in some patients. If you notice any other effects, check with your doctor.

PROGESTINS   Systemic

This information applies to the following medicines:

Hydroxyprogesterone (hye-drox-ee-proe-JESS-te-rone)
Medroxyprogesterone (me-DROX-ee-proe-JESS-te-rone)
Megestrol (me-JESS-trole)
Norethindrone (nor-eth-IN-drone)
Norethindrone Acetate
Norgestrel (nor-JESS-trel)
Progesterone (proe-JESS-ter-one)

Some commonly used brand names or other names are:	Generic names:
Delalutin Duralutin Gesterol L.A. Hylutin Hyprogest Hyproval P.A. Pro-Depo Prodrox	Hydroxyprogesterone†
Amen Curretab Cycrin Depo-Provera Provera	Medroxyprogesterone†
Megace	Megestrol
Micronor Norethisterone Norlutin Nor-Q.D.	Norethindrone
Aygestin Norlutate	Norethindrone Acetate
Ovrette	Norgestrel
Femotrone Gesterol Progestaject Progestilin	Progesterone†

†Generic name product may be available in the U.S.

Description

Progestins (proe-JESS-tins) are sometimes called female hormones. They are produced by the body and are necessary during the childbearing years for the development of the milk-producing glands, and for the proper regulation of the menstrual cycle.

Progestins are prescribed for several reasons:

- for the proper regulation of the menstrual cycle.
- to treat a certain type of disorder of the uterus known as endometriosis.

- to prevent pregnancy, when used in birth-control pills.
- to help treat selected cases of cancer of the breast, kidney, or uterus.
- for testing the body's production of certain hormones.

Progestins may also be used for other conditions as determined by your doctor.

Progestins should not be used in pregnancy tests or in most cases of threatened miscarriage, since there have been some reports that these medications may cause harmful effects on the fetus. However, progesterone is sometimes used in a few patients to treat a certain type of infertility. These patients are given progesterone because their bodies do not produce enough natural progesterone to support a pregnancy. Progesterone is used if this problem has not responded well to other types of treatment.

To make the use of a progestin as safe and reliable as possible, you should understand how and when to take it and what effects may be expected. A paper with information for the patient may be given to you with your filled prescription, and will provide many details concerning most uses of this medicine. Read this paper carefully and ask your doctor, nurse, or pharmacist if you need additional information or explanation.

Progestins are available only with your doctor's prescription, in the following dosage forms:

Oral

Medroxyprogesterone
- Tablets

Megestrol
- Tablets

Norethindrone
- Tablets

Norgestrel
- Tablets

Parenteral

Hydroxyprogesterone
- Injection

Medroxyprogesterone
- Injection

Progesterone
- Injection

Rectal

Progesterone
- Suppositories

Vaginal

Progesterone
- Suppositories

It is very important that you read and understand the following information. If any of it causes you special concern, check with your doctor. Also, *if you have any questions* or if you want more information about this medicine or your medical problem, *ask your doctor, nurse, or pharmacist.*

Before Using This Medicine

In deciding to use a medicine, the risks of taking the medicine must be weighed against the good it will do. This is a decision you and your doctor will make. For progestins, the following should be considered:

Allergies—Tell your doctor if you have ever had any unusual or allergic reaction to progestins. Also tell your doctor and pharmacist if you are allergic to any other substances, such as foods, preservatives, or dyes.

Pregnancy—Progestins are not recommended for use during pregnancy since there have been some reports that these medications may cause harmful effects on the fetus. However, progesterone is sometimes used in a few patients to treat a certain type of infertility. These patients are given progesterone because their bodies do not produce enough natural progesterone to support a pregnancy. Progesterone is used if this problem has not responded well to other types of treatment.

Breast-feeding—Progestins pass into the breast milk and may cause unwanted effects in the nursing baby. It may be necessary for you to take another medicine or to stop breast-feeding during treatment.

Children—Studies on this medicine have been done only in adults, and there is no specific information about its use in children.

Older adults—This medicine has been tested and has not been shown to cause different side effects or problems in older people than it does in younger adults.

Other medicines—Although certain medicines should not be used together at all, in other cases two different medicines may be used together even if an interaction might occur. In these cases, your doctor may want to change the dose, or other precautions may be necessary. When you are taking a progestin, it is especially important that your doctor and pharmacist know if you are taking any of the following:
- Bromocriptine (e.g., Parlodel)

Other medical problems—The presence of other medical problems may affect the use of progestins. Make sure you tell your doctor if you have any other medical problems, especially:
- Asthma
- Blood clots (or history of)
- Cancer (or history of)
- Changes in vaginal bleeding
- Diabetes mellitus (sugar diabetes)
- Epilepsy
- Heart or circulation disease
- High blood cholesterol
- Kidney disease
- Liver or gallbladder disease
- Mental depression (or history of)
- Migraine headaches
- Stroke (or history of)

Before you begin using any new medicine (prescription or nonprescription) or if you develop any new medical problem while you are using this medicine, check with your doctor, nurse, or pharmacist.

Proper Use of This Medicine

Take this medicine only as directed by your doctor. Do not take more of it and do not take it for a longer time than your doctor ordered. To do so may increase the chance of side effects. Try to take the medicine at the same time each day to reduce the possibility of side effects and to allow it to work better. When used for birth control, this medicine should be taken every day of the year, with doses taken 24 hours apart without interruption.

For patients using the rectal suppository form of this medicine:

- If the suppository is too soft to insert, chill it in the refrigerator for 30 minutes.
- To insert the suppository: Moisten the suppository with cold water. Lie down on your side and use your finger to push the suppository well up into the rectum.

For patients using the vaginal suppository form of this medicine:

- Use as directed by your doctor.

Missed dose—If you miss a dose of this medicine:

- If you are *not* taking this medicine for birth control, take the missed dose as soon as possible. However, if it is almost time for your next dose, skip the missed dose and go back to your regular dosing schedule. Do not double doses.
- *If you are taking this medicine for birth control,* the safest thing to do when you miss 1 day's dose is to stop taking the medicine immediately and use another method of birth control until your period begins or until your doctor determines that you are not pregnant. This procedure is different from the one used after missed doses of birth control tablets that contain more than one hormone.

Storage—To store this medicine:

- Keep out of the reach of children.
- Store away from heat and direct light.

- Do not store in the bathroom medicine cabinet because the heat or moisture may cause the medicine to break down.
- Keep the injectable form of this medicine from freezing.
- Do not keep outdated medicine or medicine no longer needed. Be sure that any discarded medicine is out of the reach of children.

Precautions While Using This Medicine

It is very important that your doctor check your progress at regular visits. This will allow your dosage to be adjusted to your changing needs, and will allow any unwanted effects to be detected. These visits will usually be every 6 to 12 months, but some doctors require them more often.

Check with your doctor right away:

- if vaginal bleeding continues for an unusually long time.
- if your menstrual period has not started within 45 days of your last period.
- *if you suspect that you may have become pregnant. You should stop taking this medicine immediately,* since there have been some reports that these medications may cause harmful effects on the fetus when used during pregnancy. However, progesterone is sometimes used during early pregnancy to treat a certain type of infertility.

If you are scheduled for any laboratory tests, tell your doctor that you are taking a progestin.

In some patients, tenderness, swelling, or bleeding of the gums may occur. Brushing and flossing your teeth carefully and regularly and massaging your gums may help prevent this. See your dentist regularly to have your teeth cleaned. Check with your medical doctor or dentist if you have any questions about how to take care of your teeth and gums, or if you notice any tenderness, swelling, or bleeding of your gums.

If you are taking this medicine for birth control:

- *When you begin to use birth control tablets,* your body will require time to adjust before pregnancy will be prevented; therefore, you should *use a second method of birth control for at least the first 3 weeks to ensure full protection.*
- Since one of the most important factors in the proper use of birth control tablets is taking every dose exactly on schedule, you should make sure you never run out of tablets. Therefore, always keep 1 extra month's supply of tablets on hand. To keep the extra month's supply from becoming too old, use it next, after the pills now being used, and replace the extra supply each month on a regular schedule. The tablets will keep well when kept dry and at room temperature (light will fade some tablet colors but will not change the tablets' effect).
- Keep the tablets in the container in which you received them. Most containers aid you in keeping track of dosage schedule.
- Your doctor has prescribed this medicine only for you after studying your health record and the results of your physical examination. Use of the tablets by other persons may be dangerous because of differences in health and body make-up. Therefore, do not give your birth control tablets to anyone else, and do not take tablets prescribed for someone else. Also, check with your doctor before taking any leftover birth control tablets from an old prescription, especially after a pregnancy. This medicine may be dangerous if your health has changed since your last physical examination.

Side Effects of This Medicine

Along with their needed effects, progestins sometimes cause some unwanted effects such as blood clots, heart attacks, and strokes, and problems of the liver and eyes. Although these effects are rare, they can be very serious and may cause death.

The following side effects may be caused by blood clots. Although not all of these side effects may occur, if they do occur they need immediate medical attention. *Get emergency help immediately* if any of the following side effects occur:

Headache (severe or sudden); loss of coordination (sudden); loss of vision or change in vision (sudden); pains in chest, groin, or leg (especially in calf of leg); shortness of breath (sudden); slurred speech (sudden); weakness, numbness, or pain in arm or leg

Also, check with your doctor as soon as possible if any of the following side effects occur:

More common

Changes in vaginal bleeding (spotting, breakthrough bleeding, prolonged or complete stoppage of bleeding)

Less common or rare

Bulging eyes; discharge from breasts; double vision; loss of vision (gradual, partial, or complete); mental depression; pains in stomach, side, or abdomen; skin rash or itching; yellow eyes or skin

Other side effects may occur that usually do not need medical attention. These side effects may go away during treatment as your body adjusts to the medicine. However, check with your doctor if any of the following side effects continue or are bothersome:

More common

Changes in appetite; changes in weight; pain or irritation at injection site (with progesterone); swelling of ankles and feet; unusual tiredness or weakness

Less common or rare

Acne; brown, blotchy spots on exposed skin; fever; increased body and facial hair; increased breast tenderness; nausea; some loss of scalp hair; trouble in sleeping

Other side effects not listed above may also occur in some patients. If you notice any other effects, check with your doctor.

PROPAFENONE   Systemic

A commonly used brand name in the U.S. and Canada is Rythmol.

Description

Propafenone (proe-pa-FEEN-none) belongs to the group of medicines known as antiarrhythmics. It is used to correct irregular heartbeats to a normal rhythm.

Propafenone produces its helpful effects by slowing nerve impulses in the heart and making the heart tissue less sensitive.

There is a chance that propafenone may cause new or make worse existing heart rhythm problems when it is used. Since similar medicines have been shown to cause severe problems in some patients, propafenone is only used to treat serious heart rhythm problems. Discuss this possible effect with your doctor.

This medicine is available only with your doctor's prescription, in the following dosage form:

Oral
- Tablets (U.S. and Canada)

It is very important that you read and understand the following information. If any of it causes you special concern, check with your doctor. Also, *if you have any questions* or if you want more information about this medicine or your medical problem, *ask your doctor, nurse, or pharmacist.*

Before Using This Medicine

In deciding to use a medicine, the risks of taking the medicine must be weighed against the good it will do. This is a decision you and your doctor will make. For propafenone, the following should be considered:

Allergies—Tell your doctor if you have ever had any unusual or allergic reaction to propafenone. Also tell your doctor and pharmacist if you are allergic to any other substances, such as foods, preservatives, or dyes.

Pregnancy—Propafenone has not been studied in pregnant women. Although this medicine has not been shown to cause birth defects in animal studies, it has been shown to reduce fertility in monkeys, dogs, and rabbits. In addition, in rats it caused decreased growth in the infant and deaths of mothers and infants. Before taking propafenone, make sure your doctor knows if you are pregnant or if you may become pregnant.

Breast-feeding—Propafenone passes into breast milk. However, this medicine has not been reported to cause problems in nursing babies.

Children—Propafenone can cause serious side effects in any patient. Therefore, it is especially important that you discuss with the child's doctor the good that this medicine may do as well as the risks of using it.

Older adults—Many medicines have not been studied specifically in older people. Therefore, it may not be known whether they work exactly the same way they do in younger adults or if they cause different side effects or problems in older people. There is no specific information comparing use of propafenone in the elderly with use in other age groups.

Other medicines—Although certain medicines should not be used together at all, in other cases two different medicines may be used together even if an interaction might occur. In these cases, your doctor may want to change the dose, or other precautions may be necessary. When you are taking propafenone it is especially important that your doctor and pharmacist know if you are taking either of the following:
- Digoxin (e.g., Lanoxin) or
- Warfarin (e.g., Coumadin)—Effects of these medicines may be increased when used with propafenone

Other medical problems—The presence of other medical problems may affect the use of propafenone. Make sure you tell your doctor if you have any other medical problems, especially:
- Asthma or
- Bronchitis or
- Emphysema—Propafenone can increase trouble in breathing

- Bradycardia (unusually slow heartbeat)—There is a risk of further decreased heart function
- Congestive heart failure—Propafenone may make this condition worse
- Kidney disease or
- Liver disease—Effects of propafenone may be increased because of slower removal from the body
- Recent heart attack—Risk of irregular heartbeat may be increased
- If you have a pacemaker—Propafenone may interfere with the pacemaker and require more careful follow-up by the doctor

Before you begin using any new medicine (prescription or nonprescription) or if you develop any new medical problem while you are using this medicine, check with your doctor, nurse, or pharmacist.

Proper Use of This Medicine

Take propafenone exactly as directed by your doctor, even though you may feel well. Do not take more or less of it than your doctor ordered.

This medicine works best when there is a constant amount in the blood. *To help keep the amount constant, do not miss any doses. Also, it is best to take each dose at evenly spaced times day and night.* For example, if you are to take 3 doses a day, doses should be spaced about 8 hours apart. If you need help in planning the best times to take your medicine, check with your doctor or pharmacist.

Dosing—The dose of propafenone will be different for different patients. *Follow your doctor's orders or the directions on the label.* The following information includes only the average doses of propafenone. *If your dose is different, do not change it* unless your doctor tells you to do so:

- The number of tablets that you take depends on the strength of the medicine.
- For *oral* dosage forms (tablets):
  —Adults: 150 milligrams every eight hours; may be increased to 225 milligrams every eight hours or 300 mg every twelve hours; up to 300 mg every eight hours.

Missed dose—If you do miss a dose of propafenone and remember within 4 hours, take it as soon as possible. However, if you do not remember until later, skip the missed dose and go back to your regular dosing schedule. Do not double doses.

Storage—To store this medicine:

- Keep out of the reach of children.
- Store away from heat and direct light.
- Do not store in the bathroom, near the kitchen sink, or in other damp places. Heat or moisture may cause the medicine to break down.
- Do not keep outdated medicine or medicine no longer needed. Be sure that any discarded medicine is out of the reach of children.

Precautions While Using This Medicine

It is important that your doctor check your progress at regular visits to make sure the medicine is working properly. This will allow changes to be made in the amount of medicine you are taking, if necessary.

Your doctor may want you to carry a medical identification card or bracelet stating that you are using this medicine.

Before having any kind of surgery (including dental surgery) or emergency treatment, tell the medical doctor or dentist in charge that you are taking this medicine.

Propafenone may cause some people to become dizzy or lightheaded. Make sure you know how you react to this medicine before you drive, use machines, or do anything else that could be dangerous if you are dizzy.

Side Effects of This Medicine

Along with its needed effects, a medicine may cause some unwanted effects. Although not all of these side effects may occur, if they do occur they may need medical attention.

Check with your doctor as soon as possible if any of the following side effects occur:

More common
   Fast or irregular heartbeat

Less common
   Chest pain; shortness of breath; swelling of feet or lower legs

Rare
   Fever or chills; joint pain; low blood pressure; slow heartbeat; trembling or shaking

Other side effects may occur that usually do not need medical attention. These side effects may go away during treatment as your body adjusts to the medicine. However, check with your doctor if any of the following side effects continue or are bothersome:

More common
   Change in taste or bitter or metallic taste; dizziness

Less common
   Blurred vision; constipation or diarrhea; dryness of mouth; headache; nausea and/or vomiting; skin rash; unusual tiredness or weakness

Other side effects not listed above may also occur in some patients. If you notice any other effects, check with your doctor.

QUINIDINE   Systemic

Some commonly used brand names are:

In the U.S.

Cardioquin	Quinalan
Cin-Quin	Quinidex Extentabs
Duraquin	Quinora
Quinaglute Dura-tabs	

Generic name product may also be available.

Description

Quinidine (KWIN-i-deen) is most often used to correct certain irregular heartbeats to a normal rhythm and to slow an overactive heart. It is also sometimes used for other conditions as determined by your doctor.

Quinidine acts directly on the heart tissues to make them less responsive. It also slows impulses along special nerve networks to the heart. This allows the heart to work more efficiently.

Do not confuse this medicine with *quinine*, which, although related, has different medical uses.

Quinidine is available only with your doctor's prescription, in the following dosage forms:

Oral

- Capsules (U.S.)
- Tablets (U.S. and Canada)
- Extended-release tablets (U.S. and Canada)

Parenteral

- Injection (U.S. and Canada)

It is very important that you read and understand the following information. If any of it causes you special concern, check with your doctor. Also, *if you have any questions* or if you want more information about this medicine or your medical problem, *ask your doctor, nurse, or pharmacist.*

Before Using This Medicine

In deciding to use a medicine, the risks of taking the medicine must be weighed against the good it will do. This is a decision you and your doctor will make. For quinidine, the following should be considered:

Allergies—Tell your doctor if you have ever had any unusual or allergic reaction to quinidine or quinine. Also tell your doctor and pharmacist if you are allergic to any other substance, such as foods, preservatives, or dyes.

Pregnancy—Although studies have not been done in either humans or animals, a closely related medicine, quinine, has been shown to cause birth defects of the nervous system, fingers, and toes and decreased hearing in the infant. Quinine also may cause contractions of the uterus.

Breast-feeding—Although quinidine passes into the breast milk, it has not been reported to cause problems in nursing babies.

Children—There is no specific information about the use of quinidine in children. Use of the extended-release tablets in children is not recommended.

Older adults—Many medicines have not been tested in older people. Therefore, it may not be known whether they work exactly the same way they do in younger adults. Although there is no specific information about the use of quinidine in the elderly, it is not expected to cause different side effects or problems in older people than it does in younger adults.

Other medicines—Although certain medicines should not be used together at all, in other cases two different medicines may be used together even if an interaction might occur. In these cases, your doctor may want to change the dose, or other precautions may be necessary. When you are taking quinidine, it is especially important that your doctor and pharmacist know if you are taking any of the following:

- Anticoagulants (blood thinners)—Risk of bleeding may be increased
- Other heart medicine (especially digoxin)—Effects on the heart may be increased
- Pimozide (e.g., Orap)—Risk of heart rhythm problems may be increased
- Urinary alkalizers (medicine that makes the urine less acid, such as acetazolamide [e.g., Diamox], calcium- and/or magnesium-containing antacids, dichlorphenamide [e.g., Daranide], methazolamide [e.g., Neptazane], potassium or so-

dium citrate and/or citric acid, sodium bicarbonate [baking soda])—Effects may be increased because levels of quinidine in the body may be increased

Other medical problems—The presence of other medical problems may affect the use of quinidine. Make sure you tell your doctor if you have any other medical problems, especially:

- Asthma or emphysema—Possible allergic reaction
- Blood disease
- Infection
- Kidney disease or
- Liver disease—Effects may be increased because of slower removal of quinidine from the body
- Myasthenia gravis—Muscle weakness may be increased
- Overactive thyroid
- Psoriasis

Before you begin using any new medicine (prescription or nonprescription) or if you develop any new medical problem while you are using this medicine, check with your doctor, nurse, or pharmacist.

Proper Use of This Medicine

Take quinidine with a full glass (8 ounces) of water on an empty stomach 1 hour before or 2 hours after meals so that it will be absorbed more quickly. However, to lessen stomach upset, your doctor may want you to take the medicine with food or milk.

For patients taking the *extended-release tablet* form of this medicine:

- These tablets are to be swallowed whole.
- Do not break, crush, or chew before swallowing.

Take quinidine exactly as directed by your doctor even though you may feel well. Do not take more medicine than ordered and do not miss any doses.

Missed dose—If you do miss a dose of this medicine and remember within 2 hours of the missed dose, take it as soon as possible. However, if you do not remember until later, skip the missed dose and go back to your regular dosing schedule. Do not double doses.

Storage—To store this medicine:
- Keep out of the reach of children.
- Store away from heat and direct light.
- Do not store in the bathroom, near the kitchen sink, or in other damp places. Heat or moisture may cause the medicine to break down.
- Do not keep outdated medicine or medicine no longer needed. Be sure that any discarded medicine is out of the reach of children.

Precautions While Using This Medicine

It is very important that your doctor check your progress at regular visits to make sure that the quinidine is working properly and does not cause unwanted effects.

Do not stop taking this medicine without first checking with your doctor, to avoid possible worsening of your condition.

Before having any kind of surgery (including dental surgery) or emergency treatment, tell the medical doctor or dentist in charge that you are taking this medicine.

Your doctor may want you to carry a medical identification card or bracelet stating that you are using this medicine.

Some people who are unusually sensitive to this medicine may have side effects after the first dose or first few doses. Check with your doctor right away if the following side effects occur: breathing difficulty, changes in vision, dizziness, fever, headache, ringing in ears, or skin rash.

Side Effects of This Medicine

Along with its needed effects, a medicine may cause some unwanted effects. Although not all of these side effects may occur, if they do occur they may need medical attention.

Check with your doctor immediately if any of the following side effects occur:

Less common
> Blurred vision or any change in vision; dizziness, lightheadedness, or fainting; fever; headache (severe); ringing or buzzing in the ears or any loss of hearing; skin rash, hives, or itching; wheezing, shortness of breath, or troubled breathing

Rare
> Fast heartbeat; unusual bleeding or bruising; unusual tiredness or weakness

Other side effects may occur that usually do not need medical attention. These side effects may go away during treatment as your body adjusts to the medicine. However, check with your doctor if any of the following side effects continue or are bothersome:

More common
> Bitter taste; diarrhea; flushing of skin with itching; loss of appetite; nausea or vomiting; stomach pain or cramping

Less common
> Confusion

Other side effects not listed above may also occur in some patients. If you notice any other effects, check with your doctor.

Additional Information

Once a medicine has been approved for marketing for a certain use, experience may show that it is also useful for other medical problems. Although this use is not included in product labeling, quinidine is used in certain patients with the following medical condition:

- Malaria

Other than the above information, there is no additional information relating to proper use, precautions, or side effects for these uses.

RAUWOLFIA ALKALOIDS   Systemic

This information applies to the following medicines:
> Deserpidine (de-SER-pi-deen)
> Rauwolfia Serpentina (rah-WOOL-fee-a ser-pen-TEE-na)
> Reserpine (re-SER-peen)

Some commonly used brand names are:

For Deserpidine†
In the U.S.
    Harmonyl

For Rauwolfia Serpentina†
In the U.S.
    Raudixin   Rauverid
    Rauval   Wolfina
    Generic name product may also be available.

For Reserpine
In the U.S.
    Serpalan
    Generic name product may also be available.

In Canada
    Novoreserpine   Serpasil
    Reserfia
    Generic name product may also be available.

---

†Not commercially available in Canada.

Description

Rauwolfia alkaloids belong to the general class of medicines called antihypertensives. They are used to treat high blood pressure (hypertension).

High blood pressure adds to the workload of the heart and arteries. If it continues for a long time, the heart and arteries may not function properly. This can damage the blood vessels of the brain, heart, and kidneys, resulting in a stroke, heart failure, or kidney failure. High blood pressure may also increase the risk of heart attacks. These problems may be less likely to occur if blood pressure is controlled.

Rauwolfia alkaloids work by controlling nerve impulses along certain nerve pathways. As a result, they act on the heart and blood vessels to lower blood pressure.

Rauwolfia alkaloids may also be used to treat other conditions as determined by your doctor.

These medicines are available only with your doctor's prescription, in the following dosage forms:

Oral
   Deserpidine
      • Tablets (U.S.)
   Rauwolfia Serpentina
      • Tablets (U.S.)
   Reserpine
      • Tablets (U.S. and Canada)

It is very important that you read and understand the following information. If any of it causes you special concern, check with your doctor. Also, *if you have any questions* or if you want more information about this medicine or your medical problem, *ask your doctor, nurse, or pharmacist.*

Before Using This Medicine

In deciding to use a medicine, the risks of taking the medicine must be weighed against the good it will do. This is a decision you and your doctor will make. For rauwolfia alkaloids, the following should be considered:

Allergies—Tell your doctor if you have ever had any unusual or allergic reaction to rauwolfia alkaloids. Also tell your doctor and pharmacist if you are allergic to any other substance, such as foods, preservatives, or dyes.

Pregnancy—Rauwolfia alkaloids have not been studied in pregnant women. However, too much use of rauwolfia alkaloids during pregnancy may cause unwanted effects (difficult breathing, low temperature, loss of appetite) in the baby. In rats, use of rauwolfia alkaloids during pregnancy causes birth defects and in guinea pigs decreases newborn survival rates. Before taking this medicine, make sure your doctor knows if you are pregnant or if you may become pregnant.

Breast-feeding—Rauwolfia alkaloids pass into breast milk and may cause unwanted effects (difficult breathing, low temperature, loss of appetite) in infants of mothers taking large doses of this medicine. Be sure you have discussed this with your doctor before taking this medicine.

Children—Although there is no specific information comparing use of rauwolfia alkaloids in children with use in other age groups, rauwolfia alkaloids are not expected to cause different side effects or problems in children than they do in adults.

Older adults—Many medicines have not been studied specifically in older people. Therefore, it may not be known whether they work exactly the same way they do in younger adults. Although there is no specific information comparing use of rauwolfia alkaloids in the elderly with use in other age groups, dizziness or drowsiness may be more likely to occur in the elderly, who are more sensitive to the effects of rauwolfia alkaloids.

Other medicines—Although certain medicines should not be used together at all, in other cases two different medicines may be used together even if an interaction might occur. In these cases, your doctor may want to change the dose, or other precautions may be necessary. When you are taking rauwolfia alkaloids, it is especially important that your doctor and pharmacist know if you are taking any of the following:

- Monoamine oxidase (MAO) inhibitors (furazolidone [e.g., Furoxone], isocarboxazid [e.g., Marplan], phenelzine [e.g., Nardil], procarbazine [e.g., Matulane], selegiline [e.g., Eldepryl], tranylcypromine [e.g., Parnate])—Taking a rauwolfia alkaloid while you are taking or within 2 weeks of taking MAO inhibitors may increase the risk of central nervous system depression or may cause a severe high blood pressure reaction

Other medical problems—The presence of other medical problems may affect the use of rauwolfia alkaloids. Make sure you tell your doctor if you have any other medical problems, especially:

- Allergies or other breathing problems such as asthma—Rauwolfia alkaloids can cause breathing problems
- Epilepsy
- Gallstones or
- Stomach ulcer or
- Ulcerative colitis—Rauwolfia alkaloids increase activity of the stomach, which may make the condition worse
- Heart disease—Rauwolfia alkaloids can cause heart rhythm problems or slow heartbeat

- Kidney disease—Some patients may not do well when blood pressure is lowered by rauwolfia alkaloids
- Mental depression (or history of)—Rauwolfia alkaloids cause mental depression
- Parkinson's disease—Rauwolfia alkaloids can cause parkinsonism-like effects
- Pheochromocytoma

Before you begin using any new medicine (prescription or nonprescription) or if you develop any new medical problem while you are using this medicine, check with your doctor, nurse, or pharmacist.

Proper Use of This Medicine

For patients taking this medicine *for high blood pressure*:

- In addition to the use of the medicine your doctor has prescribed, treatment for your high blood pressure may include weight control and care in the types of foods you eat, especially foods high in sodium. Your doctor will tell you which of these are most important for you. You should check with your doctor before changing your diet.
- Many patients who have high blood pressure will not notice any signs of the problem. In fact, many may feel normal. It is very important that you *take your medicine exactly as directed* and that you keep your appointments with your doctor even if you feel well.
- Remember that this medicine will not cure your high blood pressure but it does help control it. Therefore, you must continue to take it as directed if you expect to lower your blood pressure and keep it down. *You may have to take high blood pressure medicine for the rest of your life.* If high blood pressure is not treated, it can cause serious problems such as heart failure, blood vessel disease, stroke, or kidney disease.

To help you remember to take your medicine, try to get into the habit of taking it at the same time each day.

This medicine is sometimes given together with certain other medicines. If you are using a combination of drugs, make sure that you take each medicine at the proper time and do not mix them. Ask your doctor, nurse, or pharmacist to help you plan a way to remember to take your medicines at the right times.

If this medicine upsets your stomach, it may be taken with meals or milk. If stomach upset (nausea, vomiting, stomach cramps or pain) continues or gets worse, check with your doctor.

Missed dose—If you miss a dose of this medicine, do not take the missed dose at all and do not double the next one. Instead, go back to your regular dosing schedule.

Storage—To store this medicine:
- Keep out of the reach of children.
- Store away from heat and direct light.
- Do not store in the bathroom, near the kitchen sink, or in other damp places. Heat or moisture may cause the medicine to break down.
- Do not keep outdated medicine or medicine no longer needed. Be sure that any discarded medicine is out of the reach of children.

Precautions While Using This Medicine

It is important that your doctor check your progress at regular visits to make sure that this medicine is working properly.

For patients taking this medicine *for high blood pressure*:
- *Do not take other medicines unless they have been discussed with your doctor.* This especially includes over-the-counter (nonprescription) medicines for appetite control, asthma, colds, cough, hay fever, or sinus problems, since they may tend to increase your blood pressure.

Before having any kind of surgery (including dental surgery) or emergency treatment, *tell the medical doctor or dentist in charge that you are taking this medicine.*

In some patients, this medicine may cause mental depression. *Tell your doctor right away:*

- if you or anyone else notices unusual changes in your mood.
- if you start having early-morning sleeplessness or unusually vivid dreams or nightmares.

This medicine will add to the effects of alcohol and other CNS depressants (medicines that slow down the nervous system, possibly causing drowsiness). Some examples of CNS depressants are antihistamines or medicine for hay fever, other allergies, or colds; sedatives, tranquilizers, or sleeping medicine; prescription pain medicine or narcotics; barbiturates; medicine for seizures; muscle relaxants; or anesthetics, including some dental anesthetics. *Check with your doctor before taking any of the above while you are using this medicine.*

This medicine may cause some people to become drowsy or less alert than they are normally. This is more likely to happen when you begin to take it or when you increase the amount of medicine you are taking. *Make sure you know how you react to this medicine before you drive, use machines, or do anything else that could be dangerous if you are not alert.*

This medicine may cause dryness of the mouth. For temporary relief, use sugarless candy or gum, melt bits of ice in your mouth, or use a saliva substitute. However, if dry mouth continues for more than 2 weeks, check with your medical doctor or dentist. Continuing dryness of the mouth may increase the chance of dental disease, including tooth decay, gum disease, and fungus infections.

This medicine often causes stuffiness in the nose. However, do not use nasal decongestant medicines without first checking with your doctor or pharmacist.

Side Effects of This Medicine

Suggestions that rauwolfia alkaloids may increase the risk of breast cancer occurring later have not been proven. However, rats and mice given 100 to 300 times the human dose had an increased number of tumors.

Along with its needed effects, a medicine may cause some unwanted effects. Although not all of these side effects may occur, if they do occur they may need medical attention.

Check with your doctor immediately if any of the following side effects occur:

> *Less common*
>> Drowsiness or faintness; impotence or decreased sexual interest; lack of energy or weakness; mental depression or inability to concentrate; nervousness or anxiety; vivid dreams or nightmares or early-morning sleeplessness

Check with your doctor as soon as possible if any of the following side effects occur:

> *More common*
>> Dizziness

> *Less common*
>> Black, tarry stools; bloody vomit; chest pain; headache; irregular heartbeat; shortness of breath; slow heartbeat; stomach cramps or pain

> *Rare*
>> Painful or difficult urination; skin rash or itching; stiffness; trembling and shaking of hands and fingers; unusual bleeding or bruising

> *Signs and symptoms of overdose*
>> Dizziness or drowsiness (severe); flushing of skin; pinpoint pupils of eyes; slow pulse

Other side effects may occur that usually do not need medical attention. These side effects may go away during treatment as your body adjusts to the medicine. However, check with your doctor if any of the following side effects continue or are bothersome:

> *More common*
>> Diarrhea; dryness of mouth; loss of appetite; nausea and vomiting; stuffy nose

> *Less common*
>> Swelling of feet and lower legs

After you stop using this medicine, it may still produce some side effects that need attention. During this period of time *check with your doctor immediately* if you notice any of the following side effects:

Drowsiness or faintness; impotence or decreased sexual interest; irregular or slow heartbeat; lack of energy or weakness; mental depression or inability to concentrate; nervousness or anxiety; vivid dreams or nightmares or early-morning sleeplessness

Other side effects not listed above may also occur in some patients. If you notice any other effects, check with your doctor.

Additional Information

Once a medicine has been approved for marketing for a certain use, experience may show that it is also useful for other medical problems. Although this use is not included in product labeling, reserpine is used in certain patients with the following medical condition:

• Raynaud's disease

Other than the above information, there is no additional information relating to proper use, precautions, or side effects for these uses.

SELEGILINE   Systemic

Some commonly used brand names are:

In the U.S.
Eldepryl

In Canada
Eldepryl   SD Deprenyl

Other
Jumex   Movergan
Jumexal   Procythol
Juprenil

Other commonly used names are deprenil and deprenyl.

Description

Selegiline (seh-LEDGE-ah-leen) is used in combination with levodopa or levodopa and carbidopa combination to treat Parkinson's disease, sometimes called shaking palsy or paralysis agitans. This medicine works to increase and extend the effects of levodopa, and may help to slow the progress of Parkinson's disease.

Selegiline is available only with your doctor's prescription, in the following dosage form:

Oral
- Tablets (U.S. and Canada)

It is very important that you read and understand the following information. If any of it causes you special concern, check with your doctor. Also, *if you have any questions* or if you want more information about this medicine or your medical problem, *ask your doctor, nurse, or pharmacist.*

Before Using This Medicine

In deciding to use a medicine, the risks of taking the medicine must be weighed against the good it will do. This is a decision you and your doctor will make. For selegiline, the following should be considered:

Allergies—Tell your doctor if you have ever had any unusual or allergic reaction to selegiline. Also tell your doctor and pharmacist if you are allergic to any other substances, such as foods, preservatives, or dyes.

Pregnancy—Selegiline has not been studied in pregnant women. However, this medicine has not been shown to cause birth defects or other problems in animal studies.

Breast-feeding—It is not known whether selegiline passes into the breast milk.

Children—Studies on this medicine have been done only in adult patients and there is no specific information about its use in children. Therefore, be sure to discuss with your doctor the use of this medicine in children.

Older adults—In studies done to date that included elderly people, selegiline did not cause different side effects or problems in older people than it did in younger adults.

Other medicines—Although certain medicines should not be used together at all, in other cases 2 different medicines may be used together even if an interaction might occur. In these cases, your doctor may want to change the dose, or other precautions may be necessary. When you are taking selegiline, it is especially important that your doctor and pharmacist know if you are taking any of the following:

- Fluoxetine (e.g., Prozac) or
- Meperidine (e.g., Demerol)—Using these medicines together may increase the chance of serious side effects

Other medical problems—The presence of other medical problems may affect the use of selegiline. Make sure you tell your doctor if you have any other medical problems, especially:

- Stomach ulcer (history of)—Selegiline may make the condition worse

Before you begin using any new medicine (prescription or nonprescription) or if you develop any new medical problem while you are using this medicine, check with your doctor, nurse, or pharmacist.

Proper Use of This Medicine

Take this medicine only as directed by your doctor. Do not take more of it, do not take it more often, and do not take it for a longer time than your doctor ordered.

Dosing—The dose of selegiline will be different for different patients. Your doctor will determine the proper dose of selegiline for you. *Follow your doctor's orders or the directions on the label.*

For the treatment of Parkinson's disease, the usual dose of selegiline is 5 mg two times a day, taken with breakfast and lunch. Some patients may need less than this.

Missed dose—If you miss a dose of this medicine, take it as soon as possible. However, if you do not remember the missed dose until late afternoon or evening, skip the missed dose and go back to your regular dosing schedule. Do not double doses.

Storage—To store this medicine:

- Keep out of the reach of children.
- Store away from heat and direct light.

- Do not store in the bathroom, near the kitchen sink, or in other damp places. Heat or moisture may cause the medicine to break down.
- Do not keep outdated medicine or medicine no longer needed. Be sure that any discarded medicine is out of the reach of children.

Precautions While Using This Medicine

When selegiline is taken at doses of 10 mg or less per day for the treatment of Parkinson's disease, there are no restrictions on food or beverages you eat or drink. However, the chance exists that dangerous reactions, such as sudden high blood pressure, may occur if doses higher than those used for Parkinson's disease are taken with certain foods, beverages, or other medicines. These foods, beverages, and medicines include:

- Foods that have a high tyramine content (most common in foods that are aged or fermented to increase their flavor), such as cheeses; fava or broad bean pods; yeast or meat extracts; smoked or pickled meat, poultry, or fish; fermented sausage (bologna, pepperoni, salami, summer sausage) or other fermented meat; sauerkraut; or any overripe fruit. If a list of these foods and beverages is not given to you, ask your doctor, nurse, or pharmacist to provide one.
- Alcoholic beverages or alcohol-free or reduced-alcohol beer and wine.
- Large amounts of caffeine-containing food or beverages such as coffee, tea, cola, or chocolate.
- Any other medicine unless approved or prescribed by your doctor. This especially includes nonprescription (over-the-counter [OTC]) medicine, such as that for colds (including nose drops or sprays), cough, asthma, hay fever, and appetite control; "keep awake" products; or products that make you sleepy.

Also, for at least 2 weeks after you stop taking this medicine, these foods, beverages, and other medicines may continue to react with selegiline if it was taken in doses higher than those usually used for Parkinson's disease.

Check with your doctor or hospital emergency room immediately if severe headache, stiff neck, chest pains, fast heartbeat, or nausea and vomiting occur while you are taking this medicine. These may be symptoms of a serious side effect that should have a doctor's attention.

Dizziness, lightheadedness, or fainting may occur, especially when you get up from a lying or sitting position. Getting up slowly may help. If the problem continues or gets worse, check with your doctor.

Selegiline may cause dryness of the mouth. For temporary relief, use sugarless candy or gum, melt bits of ice in your mouth, or use a saliva substitute. However, if your mouth continues to feel dry for more than 2 weeks, check with your medical doctor or dentist. Continuing dryness of the mouth may increase the chance of dental disease, including tooth decay, gum disease, and fungus infections.

Side Effects of This Medicine

When you start taking selegiline in addition to levodopa or carbidopa and levodopa combination, you may experience an increase in side effects. If this occurs, your doctor may gradually reduce the amount of levodopa or carbidopa and levodopa combination you take.

Along with its needed effects, a medicine may cause some unwanted effects. Although not all of these side effects may occur, if they do occur they may need medical attention.

Stop taking this medicine and get emergency help immediately if any of the following side effects occur:

> *Symptoms of unusually high blood pressure (caused by reaction of higher than usual doses of selegiline with restricted foods or medicines)*
>
> Chest pain (severe); enlarged pupils; fast or slow heartbeat; headache (severe); increased sensitivity of eyes to light; increased sweating (possibly with fever or cold, clammy skin); nausea and vomiting (severe); stiff or sore neck

Check with your doctor as soon as possible if any of the following side effects occur:

More common

> Increase in unusual movements of body; mood or other mental changes

Less common or rare

> Bloody or black, tarry stools; severe stomach pain; or vomiting of blood or material that looks like coffee grounds; difficulty in speaking; loss of balance control; uncontrolled movements, especially of face, neck, and back; restlessness or desire to keep moving; or twisting movements of body; difficult or frequent urination; dizziness or lightheadedness, especially when getting up from a lying or sitting position; hallucinations (seeing, hearing, or feeling things that are not there); irregular heartbeat; lip smacking or puckering, puffing of cheeks, rapid or worm-like movements of tongue, uncontrolled chewing movements, uncontrolled movements of arms and legs; swelling of feet or lower legs; wheezing, difficulty in breathing, or tightness in chest

Symptoms of overdose

> Agitation or irritability; chest pain; convulsions (seizures); difficulty opening mouth or lockjaw; dizziness (severe) or fainting; fast or irregular pulse (continuing); high fever; high or low blood pressure; increased sweating (possibly with fever or cold, clammy skin); severe spasm where the head and heels are bent backward and the body arched forward; troubled breathing

Other side effects may occur that usually do not need medical attention. These side effects may go away during treatment as your body adjusts to the medicine. However, check with your doctor if any of the following side effects continue or are bothersome:

More common

> Abdominal or stomach pain; dizziness or feeling faint; dryness of mouth; nausea or vomiting; trouble in sleeping

Less common or rare

> Anxiety, nervousness, or restlessness; blurred or double vision; body ache or back or leg pain; burning of lips, mouth, or throat; chills; constipation or diarrhea; drowsiness; headache; heartburn; high or low blood pressure; inability to move; slow or difficult urination; frequent urge to urinate; increased sensitivity of skin to light; increased sweating; irritability (temporary); loss of appetite or weight

loss; memory problems; muscle cramps or numbness of fingers or toes; pounding or fast heartbeat; red, raised, or itchy skin; ringing or buzzing in ears; slowed movements; uncontrolled closing of eyelids; taste changes; unusual feeling of well-being; unusual tiredness or weakness

With doses higher than 10 mg a day

Clenching, gnashing, or grinding teeth; sudden jerky movements of body

Other side effects not listed above may also occur in some patients. If you notice any other effects, check with your doctor.

SKELETAL MUSCLE RELAXANTS Systemic

This information applies to the following medicines:

Carisoprodol (kar-eye-soe-PROE-dole)
Chlorphenesin (klor-FEN-e-sin)
Chlorzoxazone (klor-ZOX-a-zone)
Metaxalone (me-TAX-a-lone)
Methocarbamol (meth-oh-KAR-ba-mole)

This information does *not* apply to the following medicines: Baclofen, cyclobenzaprine, dantrolene, diazepam, and orphenadrine.

Some commonly used brand names are:

For Carisoprodol
In the U.S.

Rela	Soprodol
Sodol	Soridol
Soma	

Generic name product may also be available.

In Canada
Soma

For Chlorphenesin
In the U.S.
Maolate

For Chlorzoxazone
In the U.S.

Paraflex	Parafon Forte DSC

Generic name product may also be available.

For Metaxalone
In the U.S.
    Skelaxin

For Methocarbamol
In the U.S.
Carbacot	Robamol
Delaxin	Robaxin
Marbaxin	Robomol

    Generic name product may also be available.

In Canada
    Robaxin

Description

Skeletal muscle relaxants are used to relax certain muscles in your body and relieve the pain and discomfort caused by strains, sprains, or other injury to your muscles. However, these medicines do not take the place of rest, exercise or physical therapy, or other treatment that your doctor may recommend for your medical problem. Methocarbamol also has been used to relieve some of the muscle problems caused by tetanus.

Skeletal muscle relaxants act in the central nervous system (CNS) to produce their muscle relaxant effects. Their actions in the CNS may also produce some of their side effects.

In the U.S., these medicines are available only with your doctor's prescription. In Canada, some of these medicines are available without a prescription.

These medicines are available in the following dosage forms:
Oral
    Carisoprodol
        • Tablets (U.S. and Canada)
    Chlorphenesin
        • Tablets (U.S.)
    Chlorzoxazone
        • Tablets (U.S.)
    Metaxalone
        • Tablets (U.S.)
    Methocarbamol
        • Tablets (U.S. and Canada)

Parenteral
Methocarbamol
- Injection (U.S. and Canada)

It is very important that you read and understand the following information. If any of it causes you special concern, check with your doctor. Also, *if you have any questions* or if you want more information about this medicine or your medical problem, *ask your doctor, nurse, or pharmacist.*

Before Using This Medicine

In deciding to use a medicine, the risks of taking the medicine must be weighed against the good it will do. This is a decision you and your doctor will make. For the skeletal muscle relaxants, the following should be considered:

Allergies—Tell your doctor if you have ever had any unusual or allergic reaction to any of the skeletal muscle relaxants or to carbromal, mebutamate, meprobamate (e.g., Equanil), or tybamate. Also tell your doctor and pharmacist if you are allergic to any other substances, such as foods, preservatives, or dyes.

Pregnancy—Although skeletal muscle relaxants have not been shown to cause birth defects or other problems, studies on birth defects have not been done in pregnant women. Studies in animals with metaxalone have not shown that it causes birth defects.

Breast-feeding—Carisoprodol passes into the breast milk and may cause drowsiness or stomach upset in nursing babies. Chlorphenesin, chlorzoxazone, metaxalone, and methocarbamol have not been shown to cause problems in nursing babies. However, methocarbamol passes into the breast milk in small amounts. It is not known whether chlorphenesin, chlorzoxazone, or metaxalone passes into the breast milk.

Children—Chlorzoxazone has been tested in children and has not been shown to cause different side effects or problems than it does in adults.

Although there is no specific information about the use of carisoprodol in children, it is not expected to cause different side effects or problems in children than it does in adults.

There is no specific information about the use of other skeletal muscle relaxants in children.

Older adults—Many medicines have not been tested in older people. Therefore, it may not be known whether they work exactly the same way they do in younger adults or if they cause different side effects or problems in older people. There is no specific information about the use of skeletal muscle relaxants in the elderly.

Athletes—Skeletal muscle relaxants are banned and tested for in shooters by the U.S. Olympic Committee (USOC) and the National Collegiate Athletic Association (NCAA). Use of a skeletal muscle relaxant can lead to disqualification of shooters in most events.

Other medicines—Although certain medicines should not be used together at all, in other cases two different medicines may be used together even if an interaction might occur. In these cases, your doctor may want to change the dose, or other precautions may be necessary. When you are taking a skeletal muscle relaxant, it is especially important that your doctor and pharmacist know if you are taking any of the following:
- Central nervous system (CNS) depressants or
- Tricyclic antidepressants (amitriptyline [e.g., Elavil], amoxapine [e.g., Asendin], clomipramine [e.g., Anafranil], desipramine [e.g., Pertofrane], doxepin [e.g., Sinequan], imipramine [e.g., Tofranil], nortriptyline [e.g., Aventyl], protriptyline [e.g., Vivactil], trimipramine [e.g., Surmontil])—The chance of side effects may be increased

Other medical problems—The presence of other medical problems may affect the use of a skeletal muscle relaxant. Make sure you tell your doctor if you have any other medical problems, especially:
- Allergies, history of, or
- Blood disease caused by an allergy or reaction to any other medicine, history of, or
- Drug abuse or dependence, or history of, or
- Kidney disease or
- Liver disease or
- Porphyria—Depending on which of the skeletal muscle relaxants you take, the chance of side effects may be increased;

your doctor can choose a muscle relaxant that is less likely
to cause problems

- Epilepsy—Convulsions may be more likely to occur if methocarbamol is given by injection

Before you begin using any new medicine (prescription or
nonprescription) or if you develop any new medical problem
while you are using this medicine, check with your doctor,
nurse, or pharmacist.

Proper Use of This Medicine

Chlorzoxazone, metaxalone, or methocarbamol tablets may
be crushed and mixed with a little food or liquid if needed
to make the tablets easier to swallow.

Missed dose—If you miss a dose of this medicine and remember within an hour or so of the missed dose, take it
right away. But if you do not remember until later, skip the
missed dose and go back to your regular dosing schedule.
Do not double doses.

Storage—To store this medicine:

- Keep out of the reach of children.
- Store away from heat and direct light.
- Do not store this medicine in the bathroom, near the
kitchen sink, or in other damp places. Heat or moisture
may cause the medicine to break down.
- Do not keep outdated medicine or medicine no longer
needed. Be sure that any discarded medicine is out of
the reach of children.

Precautions While Using This Medicine

If you will be taking this medicine for a long time (for
example, more than a few weeks), your doctor should check
your progress at regular visits.

This medicine will add to the effects of alcohol and other
CNS depressants (medicines that slow down the nervous
system, possibly causing drowsiness). Some examples of CNS
depressants are antihistamines or medicine for hay fever,
other allergies, or colds; sedatives, tranquilizers, or sleeping

medicine; prescription pain medicine or narcotics; barbiturates; medicine for seizures; other muscle relaxants; or anesthetics, including some dental anesthetics. *Do not drink alcoholic beverages, and check with your doctor before taking any of the medicines listed above, while you are using this medicine.*

Skeletal muscle relaxants may cause blurred vision or clumsiness or unsteadiness in some people. They may also cause some people to feel drowsy, dizzy, lightheaded, faint, or less alert than they are normally. *Make sure you know how you react to this medicine before you drive, use machines, or do anything else that could be dangerous if you are dizzy or are not alert, well-coordinated, and able to see well.*

For *diabetic patients:*
- Metaxalone (e.g., Skelaxin) may cause false test results with one type of test for sugar in your urine. If your urine sugar test shows an unusually large amount of sugar, or if you have any questions about this, check with your doctor, nurse, or pharmacist. This is especially important if your diabetes is not well controlled.

Side Effects of This Medicine

Along with its needed effects, a medicine may cause some unwanted effects. Although not all of these side effects may occur, if they do occur they may need medical attention.

Check with your doctor as soon as possible if any of the following side effects occur:

Less common

Fainting; fast heartbeat; fever; hive-like swellings (large) on face, eyelids, mouth, lips, and/or tongue; mental depression; shortness of breath, troubled breathing, tightness in chest, and/or wheezing; skin rash, hives, itching, or redness; slow heartbeat (methocarbamol injection only); stinging or burning of eyes; stuffy nose and red or bloodshot eyes

Rare

Blood in urine; bloody or black, tarry stools; convulsions (seizures) (methocarbamol injection only); cough or hoarseness; fast or irregular breathing; lower back or side pain;

muscle cramps or pain (not present before treatment or more painful than before treatment); painful or difficult urination; pain, tenderness, heat, redness, or swelling over a blood vessel (vein) in arm or leg (methocarbamol injection only); pinpoint red spots on skin; puffiness or swelling of the eyelids or around the eyes; sores, ulcers, or white spots on lips or in mouth; sore throat and fever with or without chills; swollen and/or painful glands; unusual bruising or bleeding; unusual tiredness or weakness; vomiting of blood or material that looks like coffee grounds; yellow eyes or skin

Other side effects may occur that usually do not need medical attention. These side effects may go away during treatment as your body adjusts to the medicine. However, check with your doctor if any of the following side effects continue or are bothersome:

More common

Blurred or double vision or any change in vision; dizziness or lightheadedness; drowsiness

Less common or rare

Abdominal or stomach cramps or pain; clumsiness or unsteadiness; confusion; constipation; diarrhea; excitement, nervousness, restlessness, or irritability; flushing or redness of face; headache; heartburn; hiccups; muscle weakness; nausea or vomiting; pain or peeling of skin at place of injection (methocarbamol only); trembling; trouble in sleeping; uncontrolled movements of eyes (methocarbamol injection only)

Although not all of the side effects listed above have been reported for all of these medicines, they have been reported for at least one of them. However, since all of these skeletal muscle relaxants have similar effects, it is possible that any of the above side effects may occur with any of these medicines.

In addition to the other side effects listed above, chlorzoxazone may cause your urine to turn orange or reddish purple. Methocarbamol may cause your urine to turn black, brown, or green. This effect is harmless and will go away when you stop taking the medicine. However, if you have any questions about this, check with your doctor.

Other side effects not listed above may also occur in some patients. If you notice any other effects, check with your doctor.

SUCRALFATE   Oral

Some commonly used brand names are:
In the U.S.
Carafate
In Canada
Sulcrate

Description

Sucralfate (soo-KRAL-fate) is used to treat and prevent duodenal ulcers. This medicine may also be used for other conditions as determined by your doctor.

Sucralfate works by forming a "barrier" or "coating" over the ulcer. This protects the ulcer from the acid of the stomach, allowing it to heal. Sucralfate contains an aluminum salt.

This medicine is available only with your doctor's prescription, in the following dosage form:
Oral
- Oral suspension (Canada)
- Tablets (U.S. and Canada)

It is very important that you read and understand the following information. If any of it causes you special concern, check with your doctor. Also, *if you have any questions* or if you want more information about this medicine or your medical problem, *ask your doctor, nurse, or pharmacist.*

Before Using This Medicine

In deciding to use a medicine, the risks of taking the medicine must be weighed against the good it will do. This is a decision you and your doctor will make. For sucralfate, the following should be considered:

Allergies—Tell your doctor if you have ever had any unusual or allergic reaction to sucralfate. Also, tell your doctor and pharmacist if you are allergic to any other substances, such as foods, preservatives, or dyes.

Pregnancy—Studies have not been done in humans. However, sucralfate has not been shown to cause birth defects or other problems in animal studies.

Breast-feeding—Sucralfate has not been shown to cause problems in nursing babies.

Children—This medicine has been tested in a limited number of children. In effective doses, the medicine has not been shown to cause different side effects or problems than it does in adults.

Older adults—Many medicines have not been studied specifically in older people. Therefore, it may not be known whether they work exactly the same way they do in younger adults. Although there is no specific information comparing the use of sucralfate in the elderly with use in other age groups, this medicine is not expected to cause different side effects or problems in older people than it does in younger adults.

Other medicines—Although certain medicines should not be used together at all, in other cases two different medicines may be used together even if an interaction might occur. In these cases, your doctor may want to change the dose, or other precautions may be necessary. When you are taking sucralfate, it is especially important that your doctor and pharmacist know if you are taking the following:

- Ciprofloxacin or
- Digoxin or
- Norfloxacin or
- Ofloxacin or
- Phenytoin or
- Theophylline—Sucralfate may prevent these medicines from working properly

Other medical problems—The presence of other medical problems may affect the use of sucralfate. Make sure you tell your doctor if you have any other medical problems, especially:

- Gastrointestinal tract obstruction disease—Sucralfate may bind with other foods and drugs and cause obstruction of the gastrointestinal tract
- Kidney failure—Use may lead to a toxic increase of aluminum blood levels

Before you begin using any new medicine (prescription or nonprescription) or if you develop any new medical problem while you are using this medicine, check with your doctor, nurse, or pharmacist.

Proper Use of This Medicine

Sucralfate is best taken with water on an empty stomach 1 hour before meals and at bedtime, unless otherwise directed by your doctor.

Take this medicine for the full time of treatment, even if you begin to feel better. Also, it is important that you keep your doctor's appointments for check-ups so that your doctor will be better able to tell you when to stop taking this medicine.

Missed dose—If you miss a dose of this medicine, take it as soon as possible. However, if it is almost time for your next dose, skip the missed dose and go back to your regular dosing schedule. Do not double doses.

Storage—To store this medicine:

- Keep out of the reach of children.
- Store away from heat and direct light.
- Do not store in the bathroom, near the kitchen sink, or in other damp places. Heat or moisture may cause the medicine to break down.
- Keep the liquid form of this medicine from freezing. Do not refrigerate.
- Do not keep outdated medicine or medicine no longer needed. Be sure that any discarded medicine is out of the reach of children.

Precautions While Using This Medicine

Antacids may be taken with sucralfate to help relieve any stomach pain, unless your doctor has told you not to use them. *However, antacids should not be taken within 30 minutes before or after sucralfate.* Taking these medicines too close together may keep sucralfate from working properly.

Side Effects of This Medicine

Along with its needed effects, a medicine may cause some unwanted effects. Some side effects may occur that usually do not need medical attention. These side effects may go away during treatment as your body adjusts to the medicine. *Check with your doctor immediately* if any of the following side effects occur:

Signs of aluminum toxicity
Drowsiness; convulsions (seizures)

Check with your doctor as soon as possible if any of the following side effects continue or are bothersome:

More common
Constipation

Less common or rare
Backache; diarrhea; dizziness or lightheadedness; dryness of mouth; indigestion; nausea; skin rash, hives, or itching; stomach cramps or pain

Other side effects not listed above may also occur in some patients. If you notice any other effects, check with your doctor.

Additional Information

Once a medicine has been approved for marketing for a certain use, experience may show that it is also useful for other medical problems. Although these uses are not included in product labeling, sucralfate is used in certain patients with the following medical conditions:

• Gastric ulcers
• Gastroesophageal reflux disease (a condition in which stomach acid washes back into the esophagus)

    • Stomach or intestinal ulcers resulting from stress or trauma damage or from damage caused by medication used to treat rheumatoid arthritis

Other than the above information, there is no additional information relating to proper use, precautions, or side effects for these uses.

SULFASALAZINE   Systemic

Some commonly used brand names are:

   In the U.S.
      Azulfidine   Azulfidine EN-Tabs
      Generic name product may also be available.

   In Canada
      PMS Sulfasalazine   Salazopyrin EN-Tabs
      PMS Sulfasalazine E.C.   S.A.S.-500
      Salazopyrin   S.A.S. Enteric-500

Other commonly used names are salazosulfapyridine and salicylazosulfapyridine.

Description

Sulfasalazine (sul-fa-SAL-a-zeen), a sulfa medicine, is used to prevent and treat inflammatory bowel disease, such as ulcerative colitis. It works inside the bowel by helping to reduce the inflammation and other symptoms of the disease. Sulfasalazine is sometimes given with other medicines to treat inflammatory bowel disease. However, this medicine will not work for all kinds of infection the way other sulfa medicines do.

Sulfasalazine is available only with your doctor's prescription, in the following dosage forms:

   Oral
      • Enteric-coated tablets (U.S. and Canada)
      • Oral suspension (U.S.)
      • Tablets (U.S. and Canada)

It is very important that you read and understand the following information. If any of it causes you special concern,

check with your doctor. Also, *if you have any questions* or if you want more information about this medicine or your medical problem, *ask your doctor, nurse, or pharmacist.*

Before Using This Medicine

In deciding to use a medicine, the risks of taking the medicine must be weighed against the good it will do. This is a decision you and your doctor will make. For sulfasalazine, the following should be considered:

Allergies—Tell your doctor if you have ever had any unusual or allergic reaction to any of the sulfa medicines, furosemide (e.g., Lasix) or thiazide diuretics (water pills), oral antidiabetics (diabetes medicine you take by mouth), glaucoma medicine you take by mouth (for example, acetazolamide [e.g., Diamox], dichlorphenamide [e.g., Daranide], methazolamide [e.g., Neptazane]), or salicylates (for example, aspirin). Also tell your doctor and pharmacist if you are allergic to any other substances, such as foods, preservatives, or dyes.

Pregnancy—Studies have not been done in humans. However, reports on women who took sulfasalazine during pregnancy have not shown that it causes birth defects or other problems. In addition, sulfasalazine has not been shown to cause birth defects in studies in rats and rabbits given doses of up to 6 times the human dose.

Breast-feeding—Sulfa medicines pass into the breast milk in small amounts. They may cause unwanted effects in nursing babies with glucose-6-phosphate dehydrogenase (G6PD) deficiency.

Children—Sulfasalazine should not be used in children up to 2 years of age because it may cause brain problems. However, sulfasalazine has not been shown to cause different side effects or problems in children over the age of 2 than it does in adults.

Older adults—Many medicines have not been studied specifically in older people. Therefore, it may not be known whether they work exactly the same way they do in younger adults or if they cause different side effects or problems in older people. There is no specific information comparing use of sulfasalazine in the elderly with use in other age groups.

Other medicines—Although certain medicines should not be used together at all, in other cases two different medicines may be used together even if an interaction might occur. In these cases, your doctor may want to change the dose, or other precautions may be necessary. When you are taking sulfasalazine, it is especially important that your doctor and pharmacist know if you are taking any of the following:

- Acetaminophen (e.g., Tylenol) (with long-term, high-dose use) or
- Amiodarone (e.g., Cordarone) or
- Anabolic steroids (nandrolone [e.g., Anabolin], oxandrolone [e.g., Anavar], oxymetholone [e.g., Anadrol], stanozolol [e.g., Winstrol]) or
- Androgens (male hormones) or
- Antithyroid agents (medicine for overactive thyroid) or
- Carbamazepine (e.g., Tegretol) or
- Carmustine (e.g., BiCNU) or
- Chloroquine (e.g., Aralen) or
- Dantrolene (e.g., Dantrium) or
- Daunorubicin (e.g., Cerubidine) or
- Disulfiram (e.g., Antabuse) or
- Divalproex (e.g., Depakote) or
- Estrogens (female hormones) or
- Etretinate (e.g., Tegison) or
- Gold salts (medicine for arthritis) or
- Hydroxychloroquine (e.g., Plaquenil) or
- Mercaptopurine (e.g., Purinethol) or
- Naltrexone (e.g., Trexan) (with long-term, high-dose use) or
- Oral contraceptives (birth control pills) containing estrogen or
- Other anti-infectives by mouth or by injection (medicine for infection) or
- Phenothiazines (acetophenazine [e.g., Tindal], chlorproma-zine [e.g., Thorazine], fluphenazine [e.g., Prolixin], meso-ridazine [e.g., Serentil], perphenazine [e.g., Trilafon], pro-chlorperazine [e.g., Compazine], promazine [e.g., Sparine], promethazine [e.g., Phenergan], thioridazine [e.g., Mellaril], trifluoperazine [e.g., Stelazine], triflupromazine [e.g., Ves-prin], trimeprazine [e.g., Temaril]) or

- Plicamycin (e.g., Mithracin) or
- Valproic acid (e.g., Depakene)—Use of sulfasalazine with these medicines may increase the chance of side effects affecting the liver

- Acetohydroxamic acid (e.g., Lithostat) or
- Dapsone or
- Furazolidone (e.g., Furoxone) or
- Nitrofurantoin (e.g., Furadantin) or
- Primaquine or
- Procainamide (e.g., Pronestyl) or
- Quinidine (e.g., Quinidex) or
- Quinine (e.g., Quinamm) or
- Sulfoxone (e.g., Diasone) or
- Vitamin K (e.g., AquaMEPHYTON, Synkayvite)—Use of sulfasalazine with these medicines may increase the chance of side effects affecting the blood

- Anticoagulants (blood thinners) or
- Ethotoin (e.g., Peganone) or
- Mephenytoin (e.g., Mesantoin)—Use of sulfasalazine with these medicines may increase the chance of side effects of these medicines

- Antidiabetics, oral (diabetes medicine you take by mouth)—Use of oral antidiabetics with sulfasalazine may increase the chance of side effects affecting the blood and/or the side effects or oral antidiabetics

- Methotrexate (e.g., Mexate)—Use of methotrexate with sulfasalazine may increase the chance of side effects affecting the liver and/or the side effects of methotrexate

- Methyldopa (e.g., Aldomet)—Use of methyldopa with sulfasalazine may increase the chance of side effects affecting the liver and/or the blood

- Phenytoin (e.g., Dilantin)—Use of phenytoin with sulfasalazine may increase the chance of side effects affecting the liver and/or the side effects of phenytoin

Other medical problems—The presence of other medical problems may affect the use of sulfasalazine. Make sure you tell your doctor if you have any other medical problems, especially:

- Blood problems or
- Glucose-6-phosphate dehydrogenase deficiency (lack of G6PD enzyme)—Patients with these problems may have an increase in side effects affecting the blood

- Kidney disease or
- Liver disease—Patients with kidney disease or liver disease may have an increased chance of side effects
- Porphyria—Use of sulfasalazine may cause an attack of porphyria

Before you begin using any new medicine (prescription or nonprescription) or if you develop any new medical problem while you are using this medicine, check with your doctor, nurse, or pharmacist.

Proper Use of This Medicine

Do not give sulfasalazine to infants up to 2 years of age, unless otherwise directed by your doctor. It may cause brain problems.

Sulfasalazine is best taken after meals or with food to lessen stomach upset. If stomach upset continues or is bothersome, check with your doctor.

Each dose of sulfasalazine should also be taken with a full glass (8 ounces) of water. Several additional glasses of water should be taken every day, unless otherwise directed by your doctor. Drinking extra water will help to prevent some unwanted effects (e.g., kidney stones) of the sulfa medicine.

For patients taking the *enteric-coated tablet form* of this medicine:

- Swallow tablets whole. Do not break or crush.

Keep taking this medicine for the full time of treatment, even if you begin to feel better after a few days. *Do not miss any doses.*

Missed dose—If you do miss a dose of this medicine, take it as soon as possible. However, if it is almost time for your next dose, skip the missed dose and go back to your regular dosing schedule. Do not double doses.

Storage—To store this medicine:

- Keep out of the reach of children.
- Store away from heat and direct light.

- Do not store the tablet form of this medicine in the bathroom, near the kitchen sink, or in other damp places. Heat or moisture may cause the medicine to break down.
- Keep the oral liquid form of this medicine from freezing.
- Do not keep outdated medicine or medicine no longer needed. Be sure that any discarded medicine is out of the reach of children.

Precautions While Using This Medicine

It is very important that your doctor check your progress at regular visits. This medicine may cause blood problems, especially if it is taken for a long time.

If your symptoms (including diarrhea) do not improve within a month or 2, or if they become worse, check with your doctor.

Sulfasalazine may cause blood problems. These problems may result in a greater chance of certain infections, slow healing, and bleeding of the gums. Therefore, you should be careful when using regular toothbrushes, dental floss, and toothpicks. Dental work should be delayed until your blood counts have returned to normal. Check with your medical doctor or dentist if you have any questions about proper oral hygiene (mouth care) during treatment.

Sulfasalazine may cause your skin to be more sensitive to sunlight than it is normally. Exposure to sunlight, even for brief periods of time, may cause a skin rash, itching, redness or other discoloration of the skin, or a severe sunburn. When you begin taking this medicine:

- Stay out of direct sunlight, especially between the hours of 10:00 a.m. and 3:00 p.m., if possible.
- Wear protective clothing, including a hat. Also, wear sunglasses.
- Apply a sun block product that has a skin protection factor (SPF) of at least 15. Some patients may require a product with a higher SPF number, especially if they have a fair complexion. If you have any questions about this, check with your doctor or pharmacist.

- Apply a sun block lipstick that has an SPF of at least 15 to protect your lips.
- Do not use a sunlamp or tanning bed or booth.

If you have a severe reaction from the sun, check with your doctor.

This medicine may also cause some people to become dizzy. *Make sure you know how you react to this medicine before you drive, use machines, or do anything else that could be dangerous if you are dizzy.* If this reaction is especially bothersome, check with your doctor.

Before you have any medical tests, tell the doctor in charge that you are taking this medicine. The results of the bentiromide (e.g., Chymex) test for pancreas function are affected by this medicine.

Side Effects of This Medicine

Along with its needed effects, a medicine may cause some unwanted effects. Although not all of these side effects may occur, if they do occur they may need medical attention.

Check with your doctor immediately if any of the following side effects occur:

More common

Aching of joints and muscles; headache (continuing); itching; skin rash

Less common

Back, leg, or stomach pains; difficulty in swallowing; fever and sore throat; pale skin; redness, blistering, peeling, or loosening of skin; unusual bleeding or bruising; unusual tiredness or weakness; yellow eyes or skin

Rare

Bloody diarrhea, fever, and rash; cough; difficult breathing

Also, check with your doctor as soon as possible if the following side effect occurs:

More common

Increased sensitivity of skin to sunlight

Other side effects may occur that usually do not need medical attention. These side effects may go away during treat-

ment as your body adjusts to the medicine. However, check with your doctor if any of the following side effects continue or are bothersome:

More common
    Abdominal or stomach pain or upset; diarrhea; dizziness; loss
        of appetite; nausea or vomiting

In some patients this medicine may also cause the urine or skin to become orange-yellow. This side effect does not need medical attention.

Other side effects not listed above may also occur in some patients. If you notice any other effects, check with your doctor.

Additional Information

Once a medicine has been approved for marketing for a certain use, experience may show that it is also useful for other medical problems. Although these uses are not included in product labeling, sulfasalazine is used in certain patients with the following medical conditions:

- Ankylosing spondylitis
- Rheumatoid arthritis

Other than the above information, there is no additional information relating to proper use, precautions, or side effects for these uses.

SULFONAMIDES   Systemic

This information applies to the following medicines:
    Sulfacytine (sul-fa-SYE-teen)
    Sulfadiazine (sul-fa-DYE-a-zeen)
    Sulfamethizole (sul-fa-METH-a-zole)
    Sulfamethoxazole (sul-fa-meth-OX-a-zole)
    Sulfisoxazole (sul-fi-SOX-a-zole)
Some commonly used brand names are:
For Sulfacytine†
    In the U.S.
        Renoquid

For Sulfadiazine†
> *In the U.S.*
>> Generic name product may be available.

For Sulfamethizole†
> *In the U.S.*
>> Thiosulfil Forte

For Sulfamethoxazole
> *In the U.S.*
>> Gantanol
>>
>> Generic name product may also be available.
>
> *In Canada*
>> Apo-Sulfamethoxazole   Gantanol

For Sulfisoxazole
> *In the U.S.*
>> Gantrisin
>>
>> Generic name product may be available.
>
> *In Canada*
>> Novosoxazole

Another commonly used name is sulfafurazole.

---

†Not commercially available in Canada.

Description

Sulfonamides (sul-FON-a-mides) or sulfa medicines are used to treat infections. They will not work for colds, flu, or other virus infections.

Sulfonamides are available only with your doctor's prescription, in the following dosage forms:

> *Oral*
>> Sulfacytine
>> • Tablets (U.S.)
>> Sulfadiazine
>> • Tablets (U.S.)
>> Sulfamethizole
>> • Tablets (U.S.)
>> Sulfamethoxazole
>> • Oral suspension (U.S.)
>> • Tablets (U.S. and Canada)
>> Sulfisoxazole
>> • Oral suspension (U.S.)
>> • Syrup (U.S.)
>> • Tablets (U.S. and Canada)

It is very important that you read and understand the following information. If any of it causes you special concern, check with your doctor. Also, *if you have any questions* or if you want more information about this medicine or your medical problem, *ask your doctor, nurse, or pharmacist.*

Before Using This Medicine

In deciding to use a medicine, the risks of taking the medicine must be weighed against the good it will do. This is a decision you and your doctor will make. For sulfonamides, the following should be considered:

Allergies—Tell your doctor if you have ever had any unusual or allergic reaction to sulfa medicines, furosemide (e.g., Lasix) or thiazide diuretics (water pills), oral antidiabetics (diabetes medicine you take by mouth), glaucoma medicine you take by mouth (for example, acetazolamide [e.g., Diamox], dichlorphenamide [e.g., Daranide], or methazolamide [e.g., Neptazane]). Also tell your doctor and pharmacist if you are allergic to any other substances, such as foods, preservatives, or dyes.

Pregnancy—Studies have not been done in pregnant women. However, studies in mice, rats, and rabbits have shown that some sulfonamides cause birth defects, including cleft palate and bone problems.

Breast-feeding—Sulfonamides pass into the breast milk. This medicine is not recommended for use during breast-feeding. It may cause liver problems, anemia, and other unwanted effects in nursing babies, especially those with glucose-6-phosphate dehydrogenase (G6PD) deficiency.

Children—Sulfonamides should not be given to infants under 2 months of age unless directed by the child's doctor, because they may cause brain problems. Sulfacytine should not be given to children up to the age of 14.

Older adults—Elderly people are especially sensitive to the effects of sulfonamides. Severe skin problems and blood problems may be more likely to occur in the elderly. These problems may also be more likely to occur in patients who are taking diuretics (water pills) along with this medicine.

Other medicines—Although certain medicines should not be used together at all, in other cases two different medicines may be used together even if an interaction might occur. In these cases, your doctor may want to change the dose, or other precautions may be necessary. When you are taking sulfonamides, it is especially important that your doctor and pharmacist know if you are taking any of the following:

- Acetaminophen (e.g., Tylenol) (with long-term, high-dose use) or
- Amiodarone (e.g., Cordarone) or
- Anabolic steroids (nandrolone [e.g., Anabolin], oxandrolone [e.g., Anavar], oxymetholone [e.g., Anadrol], stanozolol [e.g., Winstrol]) or
- Androgens (male hormones) or
- Antithyroid agents (medicine for overactive thyroid) or
- Carbamazepine (e.g., Tegretol) or
- Carmustine (e.g., BiCNU) or
- Chloroquine (e.g., Aralen) or
- Dantrolene (e.g., Dantrium) or
- Daunorubicin (e.g., Cerubidine) or
- Disulfiram (e.g., Antabuse) or
- Divalproex (e.g., Depakote) or
- Estrogens (female hormones) or
- Etretinate (e.g., Tegison) or
- Gold salts (medicine for arthritis) or
- Hydroxychloroquine (e.g., Plaquenil) or
- Mercaptopurine (e.g., Purinethol) or
- Naltrexone (e.g., Trexan) (with long-term, high-dose use) or
- Oral contraceptives (birth control pills) containing estrogens or
- Other anti-infectives by mouth or by injection (medicine for infection) or
- Phenothiazines (acetophenazine [e.g., Tindal], chlorpromazine [e.g., Thorazine], fluphenazine [e.g., Prolixin], mesoridazine [e.g., Serentil], perphenazine [e.g., Trilafon], prochlorperazine [e.g., Compazine], promazine [e.g., Sparine], promethazine [e.g., Phenergan], thioridazine [e.g., Mellaril], trifluoperazine [e.g., Stelazine], triflupromazine [e.g., Vesprin], trimeprazine [e.g., Temaril]) or
- Plicamycin (e.g., Mithracin) or
- Valproic acid (e.g., Depakene)—Use of sulfonamides with these medicines may increase the chance of side effects affecting the liver

- Acetohydroxamic acid (e.g., Lithostat) or
- Dapsone or
- Furazolidone (e.g., Furoxone) or
- Nitrofurantoin (e.g., Furadantin) or
- Primaquine or
- Procainamide (e.g., Pronestyl) or
- Quinidine (e.g., Quinidex) or
- Quinine (e.g., Quinamm) or
- Sulfoxone (e.g., Diasone)—Use of sulfonamides with these medicines may increase the chance of side effects affecting the blood
- Anticoagulants (blood thinners) or
- Ethotoin (e.g., Peganone) or
- Mephenytoin (e.g., Mesantoin)—Use of sulfonamides with these medicines may increase the chance of side effects of these medicines
- Antidiabetics, oral (diabetes medicine you take by mouth)— Use of oral antidiabetics with sulfonamides may increase the chance of side effects affecting the blood and/or the side effects of oral antidiabetics
- Methenamine (e.g., Mandelamine)—Use of this medicine with sulfonamides may increase the chance of side effects of sulfonamides
- Methyldopa (e.g., Aldomet)—Use of methyldopa with sulfonamides may increase the chance of side effects affecting the liver and/or the blood
- Methotrexate (e.g., Mexate) or
- Phenytoin (e.g., Dilantin)—Use of these medicines with sulfonamides may increase the chance of side effects affecting the liver and/or the side effects of these medicines

Other medical problems—The presence of other medical problems may affect the use of sulfonamides. Make sure you tell your doctor if you have any other medical problems, especially:

- Anemia or other blood problems or
- Glucose-6-phosphate dehydrogenase (G6PD) deficiency—Patients with these problems may have an increase in side effects affecting the blood
- Kidney disease or
- Liver disease—Patients with kidney and/or liver disease may have an increased chance of side effects
- Porphyria—This medicine may bring on an attack of porphyria

Before you begin using any new medicine (prescription or nonprescription) or if you develop any new medical problem while you are using this medicine, check with your doctor, nurse, or pharmacist.

Proper Use of This Medicine

Sulfonamides are best taken with a full glass (8 ounces) of water. Several additional glasses of water should be taken every day, unless otherwise directed by your doctor. Drinking extra water will help to prevent some unwanted effects (e.g., kidney stones) of sulfonamides.

For patients taking the *oral liquid form* of this medicine:

- Use a specially marked measuring spoon or other device to measure each dose accurately. The average household teaspoon may not hold the right amount of liquid.

To help clear up your infection completely, *keep taking this medicine for the full time of treatment,* even if you begin to feel better after a few days. If you stop taking this medicine too soon, your symptoms may return.

This medicine works best when there is a constant amount in the blood or urine. *To help keep the amount constant, do not miss any doses. Also, it is best to take the doses at evenly spaced times day and night.* For example, if you are to take 4 doses a day, the doses should be spaced about 6 hours apart. If this interferes with your sleep or other daily activities, or if you need help in planning the best times to take your medicine, check with your doctor, nurse, or pharmacist.

Missed dose—If you do miss a dose of this medicine, take it as soon as possible. This will help to keep a constant amount of medicine in the blood or urine. However, if it is almost time for your next dose, skip the missed dose and go back to your regular dosing schedule. Do not double doses.

Storage—To store this medicine:

- Keep out of the reach of children.
- Store away from heat and direct light.

- Do not store the tablet form of this medicine in the bathroom, near the kitchen sink, or in other damp places. Heat or moisture may cause the medicine to break down.
- Keep the oral liquid forms of this medicine from freezing.
- Do not keep outdated medicine or medicine no longer needed. Be sure that any discarded medicine is out of the reach of children.

Precautions While Using This Medicine

It is very important that your doctor check your progress at regular visits. This medicine may cause blood problems, especially if it is taken for a long time.

If your symptoms do not improve within a few days, or if they become worse, check with your doctor.

Sulfonamides may cause blood problems. These problems may result in a greater chance of certain infections, slow healing, and bleeding of the gums. Therefore, you should be careful when using regular toothbrushes, dental floss, and toothpicks. Dental work should be delayed until your blood counts have returned to normal. Check with your medical doctor or dentist if you have any questions about proper oral hygiene (mouth care) during treatment.

Sulfonamides may cause your skin to be more sensitive to sunlight than it is normally. Exposure to sunlight, even for brief periods of time, may cause a skin rash, itching, redness or other discoloration of the skin, or a severe sunburn. When you begin taking this medicine:

- Stay out of direct sunlight, especially between the hours of 10:00 a.m. and 3:00 p.m., if possible.
- Wear protective clothing, including a hat. Also, wear sunglasses.
- Apply a sun block product that has a skin protection factor (SPF) of at least 15. Some patients may require a product with a higher SPF number, especially if they have a fair complexion. If you have any questions about this, check with your doctor or pharmacist.

- Apply a sun block lipstick that has an SPF of at least 15 to protect your lips.
- Do not use a sunlamp or tanning bed or booth.

If you have a severe reaction from the sun, check with your doctor.

This medicine may also cause some people to become dizzy. *Make sure you know how you react to this medicine before you drive, use machines, or do anything else that could be dangerous if you are dizzy or are not alert.* If this reaction is especially bothersome, check with your doctor.

Side Effects of This Medicine

Along with its needed effects, a medicine may cause some unwanted effects. Although not all of these side effects may occur, if they do occur they may need medical attention.

Check with your doctor immediately if any of the following side effects occur:

More common
Itching; skin rash

Less common
Aching of joints and muscles; difficulty in swallowing; pale skin; redness, blistering, peeling, or loosening of skin; sore throat and fever; unusual bleeding or bruising; unusual tiredness or weakness; yellow eyes or skin

Rare
Blood in urine; greatly increased or decreased frequency of urination or amount of urine; increased thirst; lower back pain; pain or burning while urinating; swelling of front part of neck

Also, check with your doctor as soon as possible if the following side effect occurs:

More common
Increased sensitivity of skin to sunlight

Other side effects may occur that usually do not need medical attention. These side effects may go away during treatment as your body adjusts to the medicine. However, check with your doctor if any of the following side effects continue or are bothersome:

More common
> Diarrhea; dizziness; headache; loss of appetite; nausea or
> vomiting; tiredness

Other side effects not listed above may also occur in some
patients. If you notice any other effects, check with your
doctor.

TERAZOSIN Systemic

A commonly used brand name in the U.S. and Canada is Hytrin.

Description

Terazosin (ter-AY-zoe-sin) belongs to the general class of
medicines called antihypertensives. It is used to treat high
blood pressure (hypertension).

High blood pressure adds to the workload of the heart and
arteries. If it continues for a long time, the heart and arteries
may not function properly. This can damage the blood vessels of the brain, heart, and kidneys, resulting in a stroke,
heart failure, or kidney failure. High blood pressure may
also increase the risk of heart attacks. These problems may
be less likely to occur if blood pressure is controlled.

Terazosin works by relaxing blood vessels so that blood passes
through them more easily. This helps to lower blood pressure.

Terazosin is available only with your doctor's prescription,
in the following dosage form:

Oral
- Tablets (U.S. and Canada)

It is very important that you read and understand the following information. If any of it causes you special concern,
check with your doctor. Also, *if you have any questions* or
if you want more information about this medicine or your
medical problem, *ask your doctor, nurse, or pharmacist.*

Before Using This Medicine

In deciding to use a medicine, the risks of taking the medicine must be weighed against the good it will do. This is a decision you and your doctor will make. For terazosin, the following should be considered:

Allergies—Tell your doctor if you have ever had any unusual or allergic reaction to terazosin, prazosin, or doxazosin. Also tell your doctor and pharmacist if you are allergic to any other substances, such as foods, preservatives, or dyes.

Pregnancy—Studies have not been done in humans. Studies in animals given many times the highest recommended human dose have not shown that terazosin causes birth defects. However, these studies have shown a decrease in successful pregnancies.

Breast-feeding—It is not known whether terazosin passes into breast milk. However, this medicine has not been reported to cause problems in nursing babies.

Children—Studies on this medicine have been done only in adult patients, and there is no specific information comparing use of terazosin in children with use in other age groups.

Older adults—Dizziness, lightheadedness, or fainting (especially when getting up from a lying or sitting position) may be more likely to occur in the elderly, who are more sensitive to the effects of terazosin.

Other medicines—Although certain medicines should not be used together at all, in other cases two different medicines may be used together even if an interaction might occur. In these cases, your doctor may want to change the dose, or other precautions may be necessary. Tell your doctor and pharmacist if you are taking any other prescription or nonprescription (over-the-counter [OTC]) medicine.

Other medical problems—The presence of other medical problems may affect the use of terazosin. Make sure you

tell your doctor if you have any other medical problems, especially:

- Angina (chest pain)—Terazosin may make this condition worse
- Heart disease (severe)—Terazosin may make this condition worse
- Kidney disease—Possible increased sensitivity to the effects of terazosin

Before you begin using any new medicine (prescription or nonprescription) or if you develop any new medical problem while you are using this medicine, check with your doctor, nurse, or pharmacist.

Proper Use of This Medicine

For patients *taking this medicine for high blood pressure:*

- In addition to the use of the medicine your doctor has prescribed, treatment for your high blood pressure may include weight control and care in the types of foods you eat, especially foods high in sodium. Your doctor will tell you which of these are most important for you. You should check with your doctor before changing your diet.
- Many patients who have high blood pressure will not notice any signs of the problem. In fact, many may feel normal. It is very important that you *take your medicine exactly as directed* and that you keep your appointments with your doctor even if you feel well.
- Remember that terazosin will not cure your high blood pressure but it does help control it. Therefore, you must continue to take it as directed if you expect to lower your blood pressure and keep it down. *You may have to take high blood pressure medicine for the rest of your life.* If high blood pressure is not treated, it can cause serious problems such as heart failure, blood vessel disease, stroke, or kidney disease.

To help you remember to take your medicine, try to get into the habit of taking it at the same time each day.

Missed dose—If you miss a dose of this medicine, take it as soon as possible the same day. However, if you do not remember the missed dose until the next day, skip the missed dose and go back to your regular dosing schedule. Do not double doses.

Storage—To store this medicine:
- Keep out of the reach of children.
- Store away from heat and direct light.
- Do not store in the bathroom, near the kitchen sink, or in other damp places. Heat or moisture may cause the medicine to break down.
- Do not keep outdated medicine or medicine no longer needed. Be sure that any discarded medicine is out of the reach of children.

Precautions While Using This Medicine

It is important that your doctor check your progress at regular visits to make sure that this medicine is working properly.

For patients *taking this medicine for high blood pressure:*
- *Do not take other medicines unless they have been discussed with your doctor.* This especially includes over-the-counter (nonprescription) medicines for appetite control, asthma, colds, cough, hay fever, or sinus problems, since they may tend to increase your blood pressure.

Dizziness, lightheadedness, or sudden fainting may occur after you take this medicine, especially when you get up from a lying or sitting position. These effects are more likely to occur when you take the first dose of this medicine. Taking the first dose at bedtime may prevent problems. However, *be especially careful if you need to get up during the night*. These effects may also occur with any doses you take after the first dose. Getting up slowly may help lessen this problem. *If you feel dizzy, lie down so that you do not faint*. Then sit for a few moments before standing to prevent the dizziness from returning.

The dizziness, lightheadedness, or fainting is more likely to occur if you drink alcohol, stand for long periods of time, exercise, or if the weather is hot. *While you are taking this medicine, be careful to limit the amount of alcohol you drink. Also, use extra care during exercise or hot weather or if you must stand for long periods of time.*

Terazosin may cause some people to become drowsy or less alert than they are normally. *Make sure you know how you react to this medicine before you drive, use machines, or do anything else that could be dangerous if you are dizzy, drowsy, or are not alert.* After you have taken several doses of this medicine, these effects should lessen.

Side Effects of This Medicine

Along with its needed effects, a medicine may cause some unwanted effects. Although not all of these side effects may occur, if they do occur they may need medical attention.

Check with your doctor as soon as possible if any of the following side effects occur:

More common
> Dizziness

Less common
> Chest pain; dizziness or lightheadedness, when getting up from a lying or sitting position; fainting (sudden); fast or irregular heartbeat; pounding heartbeat; shortness of breath; swelling of feet or lower legs

Rare
> Weight gain

Other side effects may occur that usually do not need medical attention. These side effects may go away during treatment as your body adjusts to the medicine. However, check with your doctor if any of the following side effects continue or are bothersome:

More common
> Headache; unusual tiredness or weakness

Less common
> Back or joint pain; blurred vision; drowsiness; nausea and vomiting; stuffy nose

Other side effects not listed above may also occur in some patients. If you notice any other effects, check with your doctor.

Additional Information

Once a medicine has been approved for marketing for a certain use, experience may show that it is also useful for other medical problems. Although this use is not included in product labeling, terazosin is used in certain patients with the following medical condition:

• Benign enlargement of the prostate

Other than the above information, there is no additional information relating to proper use, precautions, or side effects for this use.

TETRACYCLINES Systemic

This information applies to the following medicines:

Demeclocycline (dem-e-kloe-SYE-kleen)
Doxycycline (dox-i-SYE-kleen)
Minocycline (mi-noe-SYE-kleen)
Oxytetracycline (ox-i-te-tra-SYE-kleen)
Tetracycline (te-tra-SYE-kleen)

Some commonly used brand names are:

For Demeclocycline
In the U.S.
Declomycin

In Canada
Declomycin

For Doxycycline
In the U.S.

Doryx	Monodox
Doxy	Vibramycin
Doxy-Caps	Vibra-Tabs

Generic name product may also be available.

In Canada

Apo-Doxy	Novodoxylin
Doryx	Vibramycin
Doxycin	Vibra-Tabs

For Minocycline
In the U.S.
Minocin

Generic name product may also be available.

In Canada
　　Minocin

For Oxytetracycline
In the U.S.
　　Terramycin　　　　　　　　　Tija
　　Generic name product may also be available.

For Tetracycline
In the U.S.
　　Achromycin　　　　　　　　Robitet
　　Achromycin V　　　　　　　Sumycin
　　Panmycin　　　　　　　　　Tetracyn
　　Generic name product may also be available.

In Canada
　　Achromycin　　　　　　　　Novotetra
　　Achromycin V　　　　　　　Nu-Tetra
　　Apo-Tetra　　　　　　　　　Tetracyn

Description

Tetracyclines are used to treat infections and to help control acne. Demeclocycline and doxycycline may also be used for other problems as determined by your doctor. Tetracyclines will not work for colds, flu, or other virus infections.

Tetracyclines are available only with your doctor's prescription, in the following dosage forms:

Oral
　Demeclocycline
　　• Capsules (U.S.)
　　• Tablets (U.S. and Canada)
　Doxycycline
　　• Capsules (U.S. and Canada)
　　• Delayed-release capsules (U.S. and Canada)
　　• Oral suspension (U.S.)
　　• Tablets (U.S. and Canada)
　Minocycline
　　• Capsules (U.S. and Canada)
　　• Oral suspension (U.S.)
　　• Tablets (U.S.)
　Oxytetracycline
　　• Capsules (U.S.)
　Tetracycline
　　• Capsules (U.S. and Canada)
　　• Oral suspension (U.S. and Canada)
　　• Tablets (U.S. and Canada)

Parenteral

Doxycycline
- Injection (U.S. and Canada)

Minocycline
- Injection (U.S.)

Oxytetracycline
- Injection (U.S.)

Tetracycline
- Injection (U.S. and Canada)

It is very important that you read and understand the following information. If any of it causes you special concern, check with your doctor. Also, *if you have any questions* or if you want more information about this medicine or your medical problem, *ask your doctor, nurse, or pharmacist.*

Before Using This Medicine

In deciding to use a medicine, the risks of taking the medicine must be weighed against the good it will do. This is a decision you and your doctor will make. For tetracyclines, the following should be considered:

Allergies—Tell your doctor if you have ever had any unusual or allergic reaction to any of the tetracyclines or combination medicines containing a tetracycline. Also tell your doctor and pharmacist if you are allergic to any other substances, such as foods, preservatives, or dyes. In addition, if you are going to be given oxytetracycline or tetracycline by injection, tell your doctor if you have ever had an unusual or allergic reaction to "caine-type" anesthetics.

Pregnancy—Use is not recommended during the last half of pregnancy. Tetracyclines may cause the unborn infant's teeth to become discolored and may slow down the growth of the infant's teeth and bones if they are taken during that time. In addition, liver problems may occur in pregnant women, especially those receiving high doses by injection into a vein.

Breast-feeding—Use is not recommended since tetracyclines pass into the breast milk. They may cause the nursing baby's teeth to become discolored and may slow down the growth of the baby's teeth and bones. They may also cause increased sensitivity of nursing babies' skin to sunlight and fungus infections of the mouth and vagina. In addition, minocycline may cause dizziness, lightheadedness, or unsteadiness in nursing babies.

Children—Tetracyclines may cause permanent discoloration of teeth and slow down the growth of bones. These medicines should not be given to children up to 8 years of age unless directed by the child's doctor.

Older adults—Many medicines have not been studied specifically in older people. Therefore, it may not be known whether they work exactly the same way they do in younger adults or if they cause different side effects or problems in older people. There is no specific information comparing use of tetracyclines in the elderly with use in other age groups.

Other medicines—Although certain medicines should not be used together at all, in other cases two different medicines may be used together even if an interaction might occur. In these cases, your doctor may want to change the dose, or other precautions may be necessary. When you are taking tetracyclines, it is especially important that your doctor and pharmacist know if you are taking any of the following:

- Antacids or
- Calcium supplements such as calcium carbonate or
- Cholestyramine (e.g., Questran) or
- Choline and magnesium salicylates (e.g., Trilisate) or
- Colestipol (e.g., Colestid) or
- Iron-containing medicine or
- Laxatives (magnesium-containing) or
- Magnesium salicylate (e.g., Magan)—Use of these medicines with tetracyclines may decrease the effect of tetracyclines
- Oral contraceptives (birth control pills) containing estrogen— Use of birth control pills with tetracyclines may decrease the effect of the birth control pills and increase the chance of unwanted pregnancy

Other medical problems—The presence of other medical problems may affect the use of tetracyclines. Make sure you tell your doctor if you have any other medical problems, especially:

- Diabetes insipidus (water diabetes)—Demeclocycline may make the condition worse

- Kidney disease (does not apply to doxycycline or minocycline)—Patients with kidney disease may have an increased chance of side effects
- Liver disease—Patients with liver disease may have an increased chance of side effects if they use doxycycline or minocycline

Before you begin using any new medicine (prescription or nonprescription) or if you develop any new medical problem while you are using this medicine, check with your doctor, nurse, or pharmacist.

Proper Use of This Medicine

Do not give tetracyclines to infants or children up to 8 years of age unless directed by your doctor. Tetracyclines may cause permanently discolored teeth and other problems in this age group.

Do not take milk, milk formulas, or other dairy products within 1 to 2 hours of the time you take tetracyclines (except doxycycline and minocycline) by mouth. They may keep this medicine from working properly.

If this medicine has changed color or tastes or looks different, has become outdated (old), has been stored incorrectly (too warm or too damp area or place), do not use it. To do so may cause *serious side effects.* Discard the medicine. If you have any questions about this, check with your doctor or pharmacist.

Tetracyclines should be taken with a full glass (8 ounces) of water to prevent irritation of the esophagus (tube between the throat and stomach) or stomach. In addition, most tetracyclines (except doxycycline and minocycline) are best taken on an empty stomach (either 1 hour before or 2 hours after meals). However, if this medicine upsets your stomach, your doctor may want you to take it with food.

For patients taking the *oral liquid form* of this medicine:

- Use a specially marked measuring spoon or other device to measure each dose accurately. The average household teaspoon may not hold the right amount of liquid.

- Do not use after the expiration date on the label since the medicine may not work properly after that date. Check with your pharmacist if you have any questions about this.

For patients taking *doxycycline or minocycline:*
- These medicines may be taken with food or milk if they upset your stomach.
- Swallow the capsule (with enteric-coated pellets) form of doxycycline whole. Do not break or crush.

To help clear up your infection completely, *keep taking this medicine for the full time of treatment*, even if you begin to feel better after a few days. If you stop taking this medicine too soon, your symptoms may return.

This medicine works best when there is a constant amount in the blood or urine. *To help keep the amount constant, do not miss any doses. Also, it is best to take the doses at evenly spaced times day and night*. For example, if you are to take 4 doses a day, the doses should be spaced about 6 hours apart. If this interferes with your sleep or other daily activities, or if you need help in planning the best times to take your medicine, check with your doctor, nurse, or pharmacist.

Missed dose—If you do miss a dose of this medicine, take it as soon as possible. This will help to keep a constant amount of medicine in the blood or urine. However, if it is almost time for your next dose, skip the missed dose and go back to your regular dosing schedule. Do not double doses.

Storage—To store this medicine:
- Keep out of the reach of children.
- Store away from heat and direct light.
- Do not store the capsule or tablet form of this medicine in the bathroom, near the kitchen sink, or in other damp places. Heat or moisture may cause the medicine to break down.
- Keep the oral liquid forms of this medicine from freezing.

- Do not keep outdated medicine or medicine no longer needed. Be sure that any discarded medicine is out of the reach of children.

Precautions While Using This Medicine

If your symptoms do not improve within a few days (or a few weeks or months for acne patients), or if they become worse, check with your doctor.

Do not take antacids; calcium supplements such as calcium carbonate; *choline and magnesium salicylates combination (e.g., Trilisate); magnesium salicylate (e.g., Magan); magnesium-containing laxatives* such as Epsom salt; *or sodium bicarbonate* (baking soda) within 1 to 2 hours of the time you take any of the tetracyclines by mouth. In addition, *do not take iron preparations* (including vitamin preparations that contain iron) within 2 to 3 hours of the time you take tetracyclines by mouth. To do so may keep this medicine from working properly.

Oral contraceptives (birth control pills) containing estrogen may not work properly if you take them while you are taking tetracyclines. Unplanned pregnancies may occur. You should use a different or additional means of birth control while you are taking tetracyclines. If you have any questions about this, check with your doctor or pharmacist.

Before having surgery (including dental surgery) with a general anesthetic, tell the medical doctor or dentist in charge that you are taking a tetracycline. This does not apply to doxycycline, however.

Tetracyclines may cause your skin to be more sensitive to sunlight than it is normally. Exposure to sunlight, even for brief periods of time, may cause a skin rash, itching, redness or other discoloration of the skin, or a severe sunburn. When you begin taking this medicine:

- Stay out of direct sunlight, especially between the hours of 10:00 a.m. and 3:00 p.m., if possible.
- Wear protective clothing, including a hat. Also, wear sunglasses.

- Apply a sun block product that has a skin protection factor (SPF) of at least 15. Some patients may require a product with a higher SPF number, especially if they have a fair complexion. If you have any questions about this, check with your doctor or pharmacist.
- Apply a sun block lipstick that has an SPF of at least 15 to protect your lips.
- Do not use a sunlamp or tanning bed or booth.

You may still be more sensitive to sunlight or sunlamps for 2 weeks to several months or more after stopping this medicine. *If you have a severe reaction, check with your doctor.*

For patients taking *minocycline:*

- Minocycline may also cause some people to become dizzy, lightheaded, or unsteady. *Make sure you know how you react to this medicine before you drive, use machines, or do anything else that could be dangerous if you are dizzy or are not alert.* If these reactions are especially bothersome, check with your doctor.

Side Effects of This Medicine

Along with its needed effects, a medicine may cause some unwanted effects. In some infants and children, tetracyclines may cause the teeth to become discolored. Even though this may not happen right away, check with your doctor as soon as possible if you notice this effect or if you have any questions about it.

For all tetracyclines
  More common
    Increased sensitivity of skin to sunlight (rare with minocycline)
  Rare
    Abdominal pain; bulging fontanel (soft spot on head) of infants; headache; loss of appetite; nausea and vomiting; yellowing skin; visual changes

For demeclocycline only
  Less common
    Greatly increased frequency of urination or amount of urine; increased thirst; unusual tiredness or weakness

For minocycline only
   Less common
      Pigmentation (darker color or discoloration) of skin and
       mucous membranes

Other side effects may occur that usually do not need medical attention. These side effects may go away during treatment as your body adjusts to the medicine. However, check with your doctor if any of the following side effects continue or are bothersome:

For all tetracyclines
   More common
      Cramps or burning of the stomach; diarrhea; nausea or
       vomiting

   Less common
      Itching of the rectal or genital (sex organ) areas; sore
       mouth or tongue

For minocycline only
   More common
      Dizziness, lightheadedness, or unsteadiness

In some patients tetracyclines may cause the tongue to become darkened or discolored. This effect is only temporary and will go away when you stop taking this medicine.

Other side effects not listed above may also occur in some patients. If you notice any other effects, check with your doctor.

Additional Information

Once a medicine has been approved for marketing for a certain use, experience may show that it is also useful for other medical problems. Although these uses are not included in product labeling, tetracyclines are used in certain patients with the following medical conditions:

- Syndrome of inappropriate antidiuretic hormone (SIADH) (for demeclocycline)
- Traveler's diarrhea (for doxycyline)

For patients taking this medicine for *SIADH:*

- Some doctors may prescribe demeclocycline for certain patients who retain (keep) more body water than usual.

Although demeclocycline works like a diuretic (water pill) in these patients, it will not work that way in other patients who may need a diuretic.

For patients taking this medicine for *Traveler's diarrhea:*
- Some doctors may prescribe doxycycline by mouth to help prevent or treat traveler's diarrhea. It is usually given daily for three weeks to prevent traveler's diarrhea. If you have any questions about this, check with your doctor.

Other than the above information, there is no additional information relating to proper use, precautions, or side effects for these uses.

THIOXANTHENES   Systemic

This information applies to the following medicines:
    Chlorprothixene (klor-proe-THIX-een)
    Flupenthixol (floo-pen-THIX-ole)
    Thiothixene (thye-oh-THIX-een)
Some commonly used brand names are:

For Chlorprothixene
    In the U.S.
        Taractan

    In Canada
        Tarasan

For Flupenthixol*
    In Canada
        Fluanxol
        Fluanxol Depot

For Thiothixene
    In the U.S.
        Navane
        Generic name product may also be available.

    In Canada
        Navane

---

*Not commercially available in the U.S.

Description

This medicine belongs to the family of medicines known as thioxanthenes (thye-oh-ZAN-theens). It is used in the treatment of nervous, mental, and emotional conditions. Improvement in such conditions is thought to result from the effect of the medicine on nerve pathways in specific areas of the brain.

Thioxanthene medicines are available only with your doctor's prescription, in the following dosage forms:

Oral

Chlorprothixene
- Suspension (U.S.)
- Tablets (U.S. and Canada)

Flupenthixol
- Tablets (Canada)

Thiothixene
- Capsules (U.S. and Canada)
- Solution (U.S.)

Parenteral

Chlorprothixene
- Injection (U.S.)

Flupenthixol
- Injection (Canada)

Thiothixene
- Injection (U.S.)

It is very important that you read and understand the following information. If any of it causes you special concern, check with your doctor. Also, *if you have any questions* or if you want more information about this medicine or your medical problem, *ask your doctor, nurse, or pharmacist*.

Before Using This Medicine

In deciding to use a medicine, the risks of taking the medicine must be weighed against the good it will do. This is a decision you and your doctor will make. For thioxanthenes, the following should be considered:

Allergies—Tell your doctor if you have ever had any unusual or allergic reaction to thioxanthene or to phenothiazine medicines. Also tell your doctor and pharmacist if you are allergic to any other substances, such as foods, preservatives, or dyes.

Pregnancy—Studies have not been done in pregnant women. Although animal studies have not shown thioxanthenes to cause birth defects, the studies have shown that these medicines cause a decrease in fertility and fewer successful pregnancies.

Breast-feeding—It is not known if thioxanthenes pass into the breast milk, and thioxanthenes have not been reported to cause problems in nursing babies. However, similar medicines for nervous, mental, or emotional conditions do pass into breast milk and may cause drowsiness and increase the risk of other problems in the nursing baby. Be sure you have discussed the risks and benefits of this medicine with your doctor.

Children—Certain side effects, such as muscle spasms of the face, neck, and back, tic-like or twitching movements, inability to move the eyes, twisting of the body, or weakness of the arms and legs, are more likely to occur in children, who are usually more sensitive than adults to the side effects of thioxanthenes.

Older adults—Constipation, dizziness or fainting, drowsiness, dryness of mouth, trembling of the hands and fingers, and symptoms of tardive dyskinesia (such as rapid, worm-like movements of the tongue or any other uncontrolled movements of the mouth, tongue, or jaw, and/or arms and legs) are especially likely to occur in elderly patients, who are usually more sensitive than younger adults to the effects of thioxanthenes.

Athletes—Thioxanthenes are banned and, in some cases, tested for in shooters by the U.S. Olympic Committee (USOC) and the National Collegiate Athletic Association (NCAA).

Other medicines—Although certain medicines should not be used together at all, in other cases 2 different medicines may be used together even if an interaction might occur. In these cases, your doctor may want to change the dose, or other

precautions may be necessary. When you are taking thioxanthenes, it is especially important that your doctor and pharmacist know if you are taking any of the following:

- Amoxapine (e.g., Asendin) or
- Methyldopa (e.g., Aldomet) or
- Metoclopramide (e.g., Reglan) or
- Metyrosine (e.g., Demser) or
- Other antipsychotics (medicine for mental illness) or
- Pemoline (e.g., Cylert) or
- Pimozide (e.g., Orap) or
- Promethazine (e.g., Phenergan) or
- Rauwolfia alkaloids (alseroxylon [e.g., Rauwiloid], deserpidine [e.g., Harmonyl], rauwolfia serpentina [e.g., Raudixin], reserpine [e.g., Serpasil]) or
- Trimeprazine (e.g., Temaril)—Taking these medicines with thioxanthenes may increase the chance and severity of certain side effects
- Central nervous system (CNS) depressants—Taking these medicines with thioxanthenes may add to the CNS depressant effects
- Epinephrine (e.g., Adrenalin)—Severe low blood pressure (hypotension) and fast heartbeat may occur if epinephrine is used with thioxanthenes
- Levodopa (e.g., Sinemet)—Thioxanthenes may keep levodopa from working properly in the treatment of Parkinson's disease
- Quinidine (e.g., Quinidex)—Unwanted effects on your heart may occur

Other medical problems—The presence of other medical problems may affect the use of thioxanthenes. Make sure you tell your doctor if you have any other medical problems, especially:

- Alcohol abuse—Drinking alcohol will add to the central nervous system (CNS) depressant effects of thioxanthenes
- Blood disease or
- Enlarged prostate or
- Glaucoma or
- Heart or blood vessel disease or
- Lung disease or
- Parkinson's disease or
- Stomach ulcers or
- Urination problems—Thioxanthenes may make the condition worse

- Liver disease—Higher blood levels of thioxanthenes may occur, increasing the chance of side effects
- Seizure disorders—The risk of seizures may be increased

Before you begin using any new medicine (prescription or nonprescription) or if you develop any new medical problem while you are using this medicine, check with your doctor, nurse, or pharmacist.

Proper Use of This Medicine

This medicine may be taken with food or a full glass (8 ounces) of water or milk to reduce stomach irritation.

For patients taking *thiothixene oral solution:*
- This medicine must be diluted before you take it. Just before taking, measure the dose with the specially marked dropper. Mix the medicine with a full glass of water, milk, tomato or fruit juice, soup, or carbonated beverage.

Do not take more of this medicine or take it more often than your doctor ordered. This is particularly important when this medicine is given to children, since they may react very strongly to its effects.

Sometimes this medicine must be taken for several weeks before its full effect is reached.

Missed dose—If you miss a dose of this medicine, take it as soon as possible. However, if it is within 2 hours of your next dose, skip the missed dose and go back to your regular dosing schedule. Do not double doses.

Storage—To store this medicine:
- Keep out of the reach of children.
- Store away from heat and direct light.
- Do not store the capsule or tablet form of this medicine in the bathroom, near the kitchen sink, or in other damp places. Heat or moisture may cause the medicine to break down.
- Keep the liquid form of this medicine from freezing.

- Do not keep outdated medicine or medicine no longer needed. Be sure that any discarded medicine is out of the reach of children.

Precautions While Using This Medicine

Your doctor should check your progress at regular visits. This will allow the dosage of the medicine to be adjusted when necessary and also will reduce the possibility of side effects.

Do not stop taking this medicine without first checking with your doctor. Your doctor may want you to gradually reduce the amount you are taking before stopping completely. This is to prevent side effects and to prevent your condition from becoming worse.

This medicine will add to the effects of alcohol and other CNS depressants (medicines that slow down the nervous system, possibly causing drowsiness). Some examples of CNS depressants are antihistamines or medicine for hay fever, other allergies, or colds; sedatives, tranquilizers, or sleeping medicine; prescription pain medicine or narcotics; barbiturates; medicine for seizures; muscle relaxants; or anesthetics, including some dental anesthetics. *Check with your doctor before taking any such depressants while you are using this medicine.*

Do not take this medicine within an hour of taking antacids or medicine for diarrhea. Taking them too close together may make this medicine less effective.

Before having any kind of surgery, dental treatment, or emergency treatment, tell the medical doctor or dentist in charge that you are using this medicine.

This medicine may cause some people to become drowsy or less alert than they are normally, especially during the first few weeks the medicine is being taken. Even if you take this medicine only at bedtime, you may feel drowsy or less alert on arising. *Make sure you know how you react to this medicine before you drive, use machines, or do anything else that could be dangerous if you are not alert.*

Dizziness, lightheadedness, or fainting may occur while you are taking this medicine, especially when you get up from a lying or sitting position. Getting up slowly may help. If the problem continues or gets worse, check with your doctor.

This medicine may make you sweat less, causing your body temperature to increase. *Use extra care not to become overheated during exercise or hot weather while you are taking this medicine,* since overheating may result in heat stroke. Also, hot baths or saunas may make you feel dizzy or faint while you are taking this medicine.

Thioxanthenes may cause your skin to be more sensitive to sunlight than it is normally. Exposure to sunlight, even for brief periods of time, may cause a skin rash, itching, redness or other discoloration of the skin, or a severe sunburn. When you begin taking this medicine:

- Stay out of direct sunlight, especially between the hours of 10:00 a.m. and 3:00 p.m., if possible.
- Wear protective clothing, including a hat. Also, wear sunglasses.
- Apply a sun block product that has a skin protection factor (SPF) of at least 15. Some patients may require a product with a higher SPF number, especially if they have a fair complexion. If you have any questions about this, check with your doctor or pharmacist.
- Apply a sun block lipstick that has an SPF of at least 15 to protect your lips.
- Do not use a sunlamp or tanning bed or booth.

If you have a severe reaction from the sun, check with your doctor.

This medicine may cause dryness of the mouth. For temporary relief, use sugarless gum or candy, melt bits of ice in your mouth, or use a saliva substitute. However, if your mouth continues to feel dry for more than 2 weeks, check with your medical doctor or dentist. Continuing dryness of the mouth may increase the chance of dental disease, including tooth decay, gum disease, and fungus infections.

If you are taking a liquid form of this medicine, *try to avoid spilling it on your skin or clothing*. Skin rash and irritation have been caused by similar medicines.

If you are receiving this medicine by injection:

- The effects of the long-acting injection form of this medicine may last for up to 3 weeks. *The precautions and side effects information for this medicine applies during this period of time.*

Side Effects of This Medicine

Along with their needed effects, thioxanthenes can sometimes cause serious side effects. Tardive dyskinesia (a movement disorder) may occur and may not go away after you stop using the medicine. Signs of tardive dyskinesia include fine, worm-like movements of the tongue, or other uncontrolled movements of the mouth, tongue, cheeks, jaw, or arms and legs. Other serious but rare side effects may also occur. These include severe muscle stiffness, fever, unusual tiredness or weakness, fast heartbeat, difficult breathing, increased sweating, loss of bladder control, and seizures (neuroleptic malignant syndrome). *You and your doctor should discuss the good this medicine will do as well as the risks of taking it.*

Although not all of these side effects may occur, if they do occur they may need medical attention.

Stop taking this medicine and get emergency help immediately if any of the following side effects occur:

Rare

Convulsions (seizures); difficulty in breathing; fast heartbeat; high fever; high or low (irregular) blood pressure; increased sweating; loss of bladder control; muscle stiffness (severe); unusually pale skin; unusual tiredness

Also, check with your doctor as soon as possible if any of the following side effects occur:

More common

Difficulty in talking or swallowing; inability to move eyes; lip smacking or puckering; loss of balance control; mask-like face; muscle spasms, especially of the neck and back;

puffing of cheeks; rapid or worm-like movements of tongue; restlessness or need to keep moving (severe); shuffling walk; stiffness of arms and legs; trembling and shaking of fingers and hands; twisting movements of body; uncontrolled chewing movements; uncontrolled movements of the arms and legs

Less common

Blurred vision or other eye problems; difficult urination; fainting; skin discoloration; skin rash

Rare

Hot, dry skin or lack of sweating; muscle weakness; sore throat and fever; unusual bleeding or bruising; yellow eyes or skin

Symptoms of overdose

Difficulty in breathing (severe); dizziness (severe); drowsiness (severe); muscle trembling, jerking, stiffness, or uncontrolled movements (severe); small pupils; tiredness or weakness (severe); unusual excitement

Other side effects may occur that usually do not need medical attention. These side effects may go away during treatment as your body adjusts to the medicine. However, check with your doctor if any of the following side effects continue or are bothersome:

More common

Constipation; decreased sweating; dizziness, lightheadedness, or fainting; drowsiness (mild); dryness of mouth; increased appetite and weight; increased sensitivity of skin to sunlight (skin rash, itching, redness or other discoloration of skin, or severe sunburn); stuffy nose

Less common

Changes in menstrual period; decreased sexual ability; swelling of breasts (in males and females); unusual secretion of milk

After you stop taking this medicine your body may need time to adjust, especially if you took this medicine in high doses or for a long time. If you stop taking it too quickly, the following withdrawal effects may occur and should be reported to your doctor:

Dizziness; nausea and vomiting; stomach pain; trembling of fingers and hands; uncontrolled, continuing movements of mouth, tongue, or jaw

Although not all of the side effects listed above have been reported for all thioxanthenes, they have been reported for at least one of them. However, since these medicines are very similar, any of the above side effects may occur with any of them.

Other side effects not listed above may also occur in some patients. If you notice any other effects, check with your doctor.

THYROID HORMONES   Systemic

This information applies to the following medicines:

Levothyroxine (lee-voe-thye-ROX-een)
Liothyronine (lye-oh-THYE-roe-neen)
Liotrix (LYE-oh-trix)
Thyroglobulin (thye-roe-GLOB-yoo-lin)
Thyroid (THYE-roid)

Note: This information does *not* apply to Thyrotropin.

Some commonly used brand names are:

For Levothyroxine
In the U.S.

Levoid	Levoxine
Levothroid	Synthroid

Generic name product may also be available.

In Canada
Eltroxin
Synthroid

For Liothyronine
In the U.S.
Cytomel

Generic name product may also be available.

In Canada
Cytomel

For Liotrix
In the U.S.
Euthroid
Thyrolar

In Canada
Thyrolar

For Thyroglobulin*
In Canada
Proloid

For Thyroid
In the U.S. and Canada
Generic name product available.

---

*Not commercially available in the U.S.

Description

Thyroid medicines belong to the general group of medicines called hormones. They are used when the thyroid gland does not produce enough hormone. They are also used to help decrease the size of enlarged thyroid glands (known as goiter) and to treat thyroid cancer.

These medicines are available only with your doctor's prescription, in the following dosage forms:

Oral
Levothyroxine
• Tablets (U.S. and Canada)
Liothyronine
• Tablets (U.S. and Canada)
Liotrix
• Tablets (U.S. and Canada)
Thyroglobulin
• Tablets (Canada)
Thyroid
• Tablets (U.S. and Canada)
• Enteric-coated tablets (U.S.)

Parenteral
Levothyroxine
• Injection (U.S. and Canada)

It is very important that you read and understand the following information. If any of it causes you special concern, check with your doctor. Also, *if you have any questions* or if you want more information about this medicine or your medical problem, *ask your doctor, nurse, or pharmacist.*

Before Using This Medicine

In deciding to use a medicine, the risks of taking the medicine must be weighed against the good it will do. This is a decision you and your doctor will make. For thyroid hormones, the following should be considered:

Allergies—Tell your doctor if you have ever had any unusual or allergic reaction to thyroid hormones. Also tell your doctor and pharmacist if you are allergic to any other substances, such as foods, preservatives, or dyes.

Pregnancy—It is essential that your baby receive the right amount of thyroid for normal development. You may need to take different amounts while you are pregnant. In addition, you may respond differently than usual to some tests. Your doctor should check your progress at regular visits while you are pregnant.

Breast-feeding—Use of proper amounts of thyroid hormones by mothers has not been shown to cause problems in nursing babies.

Children—Thyroid hormones have been tested in children and have not been shown to cause different side effects or problems in children than they do in adults.

Older adults—This medicine has been tested and has not been shown to cause different side effects or problems in older people than it does in younger adults. However, a different dose may be needed in the elderly. Therefore, it is important to take the medicine only as directed by the doctor.

Other medical problems—The presence of other medical problems may affect the use of thyroid hormones. Make sure you tell your doctor if you have any other medical problems, especially:
- Diabetes mellitus (sugar diabetes)
- Hardening of the arteries
- Heart disease
- High blood pressure
- Overactive thyroid (history of)

- Underactive adrenal gland
- Underactive pituitary gland

Other medicines—Although certain medicines should not be used together at all, in other cases two different medicines may be used together even if an interaction might occur. In these cases, your doctor may want to change the dose, or other precautions may be necessary. When you are taking thyroid hormones, it is especially important that your doctor and pharmacist know if you are taking any of the following:

- Amphetamines
- Anticoagulants (blood thinners)
- Appetite suppressants (diet pills)
- Cholestyramine (e.g., Questran)
- Colestipol (e.g., Colestid)
- Medicine for asthma or other breathing problems
- Medicine for colds, sinus problems, or hay fever or other allergies (including nose drops or sprays)

Before you begin using any new medicine (prescription or nonprescription) or if you develop any new medical problem while you are using this medicine, check with your doctor, nurse, or pharmacist.

Proper Use of This Medicine

Use this medicine only as directed by your doctor. Do not use more or less of it, and do not use it more often than your doctor ordered. Your doctor has prescribed the exact amount your body needs and if you take different amounts, you may experience symptoms of an overactive or underactive thyroid. Take it at the same time each day to make sure it always has the same effect.

If your condition is due to a lack of thyroid hormone, you may have to take this medicine for the rest of your life. It is very important that you *do not stop taking this medicine without first checking with your doctor.*

Missed dose—If you miss a dose of this medicine, take it as soon as possible. However, if it is almost time for your next dose, skip the missed dose and go back to your regular dosing schedule. Do not double doses. If you miss 2 or more doses in a row or if you have any questions about this, check with your doctor.

Storage—To store this medicine:
- Keep out of the reach of children.
- Store away from heat and direct light.
- Do not store in the bathroom, near the kitchen sink, or in other damp places. Heat or moisture may cause the medicine to break down.
- Do not keep outdated medicine or medicine no longer needed. Be sure that any discarded medicine is out of the reach of children.

Precautions While Using This Medicine

It is very important that your doctor check your progress at regular visits, to make sure that this medicine is working properly.

If you have certain kinds of heart disease, this medicine may cause chest pain or shortness of breath when you exert yourself. If these occur, do not overdo exercise or physical work. If you have any questions about this, check with your doctor.

Before having any kind of surgery (including dental surgery) or emergency treatment, *tell the medical doctor or dentist in charge that you are taking this medicine.*

Do not take any other medicine unless prescribed by your doctor. Some medicines may increase or decrease the effects of thyroid on your body and cause problems in controlling your condition. Also, thyroid hormones may change the effects of other medicines.

Side Effects of This Medicine

Along with its needed effects, a medicine may cause some unwanted effects. Although not all of these side effects may occur, if they do occur they may need medical attention.

Check with your doctor as soon as possible if any of the following side effects occur since they may indicate an overdose or an allergic reaction:

Rare

Headache (severe) in children; skin rash or hives

Signs and symptoms of overdose

Chest pain; fast or irregular heartbeat; shortness of breath

For patients taking this medicine for underactive thyroid:

- This medicine usually takes several weeks to have a noticeable effect on your condition. Until it begins to work, you may experience no change in your symptoms. Check with your doctor if the following symptoms continue:

Clumsiness; coldness; constipation; dry, puffy skin; listlessness; muscle aches; sleepiness; tiredness; weakness; weight gain

Other effects may occur if the dose of the medicine is not exactly right. These side effects will go away when the dose is corrected. Check with your doctor if any of the following symptoms occur:

Changes in appetite; changes in menstrual periods; diarrhea; fever; hand tremors; headache; increased sensitivity to heat; irritability; leg cramps; nervousness; sweating; trouble in sleeping; vomiting; weight loss

Other side effects not listed above may also occur in some patients. If you notice any other effects, check with your doctor.

TICLOPIDINE   Systemic

A commonly used brand name in the U.S. and Canada is Ticlid.

Description

Ticlopidine (tye-KLOE-pi-deen) is used to lower the chance of having a stroke. It is given to people who have already had a stroke and to people with certain medical problems that may lead to a stroke. Because ticlopidine can cause serious side effects, especially during the first 3 months of treatment, it is used mostly for people who cannot take aspirin to prevent strokes.

A stroke may occur when a blood vessel in the brain is blocked by a blood clot. Ticlopidine lessens the chance that a harmful blood clot will form, by preventing certain cells in the blood from clumping together. This effect of ticlopidine may also increase the chance of serious bleeding in some people.

This medicine is available in the following dosage forms:

> *Oral*
> - Tablets (U.S. and Canada)

It is very important that you read and understand the following information. If any of it causes you special concern, check with your doctor. Also, *if you have any questions* or if you want more information about this medicine or your medical problem, *ask your doctor, nurse, or pharmacist*.

Before Using This Medicine

In deciding to use a medicine, the risks of taking the medicine must be weighed against the good it will do. This is a decision you and your doctor will make. For ticlopidine, the following should be considered:

Allergies—Tell your doctor if you have ever had any unusual or allergic reaction to ticlopidine. Also tell your doctor and pharmacist if you are allergic to any other substances, such as foods, preservatives, or dyes.

Pregnancy—Studies with ticlopidine have not been done in pregnant women. This medicine did not cause birth defects in animal studies. However, it caused other unwanted effects in animal studies when it was given in amounts that were large enough to cause harmful effects in the mother.

Breast-feeding—It is not known whether ticlopidine passes into the breast milk.

Children—There is no specific information comparing use of ticlopidine in children with use in other age groups.

Older adults—This medicine has been tested and has not been shown to cause different side effects or problems in older people than it does in younger adults.

Other medicines—Although certain medicines should not be used together at all, in other cases two different medicines may be used together even if an interaction might occur. In these cases, your doctor may want to change the dose, or other precautions may be necessary. When you are taking ticlopidine, it is especially important that your doctor and pharmacist know if you are taking any of the following:

- Anticoagulants (blood thinners) or
- Aspirin or
- Heparin (e.g., Hepalean, Liquaemin)—The chance of serious bleeding may be increased

Other medical problems—The presence of other medical problems may affect the use of ticlopidine. Make sure you tell your doctor if you have any other medical problems, especially:

- Blood disease—The chance of serious side effects may be increased
- Blood clotting problems, such as hemophilia, or
- Liver disease (severe) or
- Stomach ulcers—The chance of serious bleeding may be increased
- Kidney disease (severe)—Ticlopidine is removed from the body more slowly when the kidneys are not working properly. This may increase the chance of side effects.

Before you begin using any new medicine (prescription or nonprescription) or if you develop any new medical problem while you are using this medicine, check with your doctor, nurse, or pharmacist.

Proper Use of This Medicine

Ticlopidine should be taken with food. This increases the amount of medicine that is absorbed into the body. It may also lessen the chance of stomach upset.

Take this medicine only as directed by your doctor. Ticlopidine will not work properly if you take less of it than
directed. Taking more ticlopidine than directed may increase
the chance of serious side effects without increasing the
helpful effects.

Dosing—*Follow your doctor's orders or the directions on
the label*. The following dose was used, and found effective,
in studies. However, some people may need a different dose.
If your dose is different, do not change it unless your doctor
tells you to do so:

- For adults—1 tablet (250 mg) two times a day, with
  food.
- For children—It is not likely that ticlopidine would be
  used to help prevent strokes in children. If a child needs
  this medicine, however, the dose would have to be determined by the doctor.

Missed dose—If you miss a dose of this medicine, take it
as soon as possible. However, if it is almost time for your
next dose, skip the missed dose and go back to your regular
dosing schedule. Do not double doses.

Storage—To store this medicine:
- Keep out of the reach of children.
- Store away from heat and direct light.
- Do not store in the bathroom, near the kitchen sink, or
  in other damp places. Heat or moisture may cause the
  medicine to break down.
- Do not keep outdated medicine or medicine no longer
  needed. Be sure that any discarded medicine is out of
  the reach of children.

Precautions While Using This Medicine

*It is very important that blood tests be done every 2 weeks
for the first 3 months of treatment with ticlopidine*. The
tests are needed to find out whether certain side effects are
occurring. Finding these side effects early helps to prevent
them from becoming serious. Your doctor will arrange for
the blood tests to be done. *Be sure that you do not miss*

any appointments for these tests. You will probably not need to have your blood tested so often after the first 3 months of treatment, because the side effects are less likely to occur after that time.

Tell all medical doctors, dentists, nurses, and pharmacists you go to that you are taking this medicine. Ticlopidine may increase the risk of serious bleeding during an operation or some kinds of dental work. Therefore, treatment may have to be stopped about 10 days to 2 weeks before the operation or dental work is done.

Ticlopidine may cause serious bleeding, especially after an injury. Sometimes, bleeding inside the body can occur without your knowing about it. Ask your doctor whether there are certain activities you should avoid while taking this medicine (for example, sports that can cause injuries). *Also, check with your doctor immediately if you are injured while being treated with this medicine.*

Check with your doctor immediately if you notice any of the following side effects:

- Bruising or bleeding, especially bleeding that is hard to stop.
- Any sign of infection, such as fever, chills, or sore throat.
- Sores, ulcers, or white spots in the mouth.

After you stop taking ticlopidine, the chance of bleeding may continue for 1 or 2 weeks. During this period of time, continue to follow the same precautions that you followed while you were taking the medicine.

Side Effects of This Medicine

Along with its needed effects, a medicine may cause some unwanted effects. Although not all of these side effects may occur, if they do occur they may need medical attention.

Check with your doctor immediately if any of the following side effects occur:

> *Less common or rare*
>> Abdominal or stomach pain (severe) or swelling; back pain; blood in eyes; blood in urine; bloody or black, tarry stools; bruising or purple areas on skin; coughing up blood; de-

creased alertness; dizziness; fever, chills, or sore throat; headache (severe or continuing); joint pain or swelling; nosebleeds; pinpoint red spots on skin; sores, ulcers, or white spots in mouth; paralysis or problems with coordination; stammering or other difficulty in speaking; unusually heavy bleeding or oozing from cuts or wounds; unusually heavy or unexpected menstrual bleeding; vomiting of blood or material that looks like coffee grounds

Also, check with your doctor as soon as possible if any of the following side effects occur:

More common
Skin rash

Less common or rare
Hives or itching of skin; ringing or buzzing in ears; yellow eyes or skin

Other side effects may occur that usually do not need medical attention. These side effects may go away during treatment as your body adjusts to the medicine. However, check with your doctor if any of the following side effects continue or are bothersome:

More common
Abdominal or stomach pain (mild); bloating or gas; diarrhea; nausea

Less common
Indigestion; vomiting

Other side effects not listed above may also occur in some patients. If you notice any other effects, check with your doctor.

TRAZODONE   Systemic

Some commonly used brand names are:

In the U.S.
Desyrel   Trialodine
Trazon
Generic name product may also be available.

In Canada
Desyrel

Description

Trazodone (TRAZ-oh-done) belongs to the group of medicines known as antidepressants or "mood elevators." It is used to relieve mental depression and depression that sometimes occurs with anxiety.

Trazodone is available only with your doctor's prescription, in the following dosage form:

Oral
- Tablets (U.S. and Canada)

It is very important that you read and understand the following information. If any of it causes you special concern, check with your doctor. Also, *if you have any questions* or if you want more information about this medicine or your medical problem, *ask your doctor, nurse, or pharmacist.*

Before Using This Medicine

In deciding to use a medicine, the risks of taking the medicine must be weighed against the good it will do. This is a decision you and your doctor will make. For trazodone, the following should be considered:

Allergies—Tell your doctor if you have ever had any unusual or allergic reaction to trazodone. Also tell your doctor and pharmacist if you are allergic to any other substances, such as foods, preservatives, or dyes.

Pregnancy—Studies have not been done in pregnant women. However, studies in animals have shown that trazodone causes birth defects and a decrease in the number of successful pregnancies when given in doses many times larger than human doses.

Breast-feeding—Trazodone passes into breast milk. However, this medicine has not been reported to cause problems in nursing babies.

Children—Studies on this medicine have been done only in adult patients, and there is no specific information about its use in children.

Older adults—Drowsiness, dizziness, confusion, vision problems, dryness of mouth, and constipation may be more likely to occur in the elderly, who are usually more sensitive to the effects of trazodone.

Other medicines—Although certain medicines should not be used together at all, in other cases 2 different medicines may be used together even if an interaction might occur. In these cases, your doctor may want to change the dose, or other precautions may be necessary. When you are taking trazodone, it is especially important that your doctor and pharmacist know if you are taking any of the following:

- Antihypertensives (high blood pressure medicine)—Taking these medicines with trazodone may result in low blood pressure (hypotension); the amount of medicine you need to take may change
- Central nervous system (CNS) depressants—Taking these medicines with trazodone may add to the CNS depressant effects

Other medical problems—The presence of other medical problems may affect the use of trazodone. Make sure you tell your doctor if you have any other medical problems, especially:

- Alcohol abuse (or history of)—Drinking alcohol with trazodone will increase the central nervous system (CNS) depressant effects
- Heart disease—Trazodone may make the condition worse
- Kidney disease or
- Liver disease—Higher blood levels of trazodone may occur, increasing the chance of side effects

Before you begin using any new medicine (prescription or nonprescription) or if you develop any new medical problem while you are using this medicine, check with your doctor, nurse, or pharmacist.

Proper Use of This Medicine

To lessen stomach upset and to reduce dizziness and light-headedness, take this medicine with or shortly after a meal or light snack, even for a daily bedtime dose, unless your doctor has told you to take it on an empty stomach.

Take trazodone only as directed by your doctor, to benefit your condition as much as possible.

Sometimes trazodone must be taken for up to 4 weeks before you begin to feel better, although most people notice improvement within 2 weeks.

Missed dose—If you miss a dose of this medicine, take it as soon as possible. However, if it is within 4 hours of your next dose, skip the missed dose and go back to your regular dosing schedule. Do not double doses.

Storage—To store this medicine:
- Keep out of the reach of children.
- Store away from heat and direct light.
- Do not store in the bathroom, near the kitchen sink, or in other damp places. Heat or moisture may cause the medicine to break down.
- Do not keep outdated medicine or medicine no longer needed. Be sure that any discarded medicine is out of the reach of children.

Precautions While Using This Medicine

It is very important that your doctor check your progress at regular visits. This will allow your doctor to check the medicine's effects and to change the dose if needed.

Do not stop taking this medicine without first checking with your doctor. Your doctor may want you to reduce gradually the amount you are using before stopping completely, to prevent a possible return of your medical problem.

Before having any kind of surgery, dental treatment, or emergency treatment, tell the medical doctor or dentist in charge that you are using this medicine.

This medicine will add to the effects of alcohol and other CNS depressants (medicines that slow down the nervous system, possibly causing drowsiness). Some examples of CNS depressants are antihistamines or medicine for hay fever, other allergies, or colds; sedatives, tranquilizers, or sleeping medicine; prescription pain medicine or narcotics; barbiturates; medicine for seizures; muscle relaxants; or anesthetics, including some dental anesthetics. *Check with your doctor before taking any of the above while you are using this medicine.*

This medicine may cause some people to become drowsy or less alert than they are normally. *Make sure you know how you react to this medicine before you drive, use machines, or do anything else that could be dangerous if you are not alert.*

Dizziness, lightheadedness, or fainting may occur, especially when you get up from a lying or sitting position. Getting up slowly may help. If this problem continues or gets worse, check with your doctor.

Trazodone may cause dryness of the mouth. For temporary relief, use sugarless gum or candy, melt bits of ice in your mouth, or use a saliva substitute. However, if your mouth continues to feel dry for more than 2 weeks, check with your medical doctor or dentist. Continuing dryness of the mouth may increase the chance of dental disease, including tooth decay, gum disease, and fungus infections.

Side Effects of This Medicine

Along with its needed effects, a medicine may cause some unwanted effects. Although not all of these side effects may occur, if they do occur they may need medical attention.

Stop taking this medicine and check with your doctor immediately if the following side effect occurs:

> *Rare*
> Painful, inappropriate erection of the penis, continuing

Also, check with your doctor as soon as possible if any of the following side effects occur:

> *Less common*
> Confusion; muscle tremors
>
> *Rare*
> Fainting; fast or slow heartbeat; skin rash; unusual excitement

Symptoms of overdose

Drowsiness; loss of muscle coordination; nausea and vomiting

Other side effects may occur that usually do not need medical attention. These side effects may go away during treatment as your body adjusts to the medicine. However, check with your doctor if any of the following side effects continue or are bothersome:

More common

Dizziness or lightheadedness; drowsiness; dryness of mouth (usually mild); headache; nausea and vomiting; unpleasant taste

Less common

Blurred vision; constipation; diarrhea; muscle aches or pains; unusual tiredness or weakness

Other side effects not listed above may also occur in some patients. If you notice any other effects, check with your doctor.

ZIDOVUDINE   Systemic

Some commonly used brand names are:

In the U.S.
    Retrovir

In Canada
    Apo-Zidovudine   Retrovir
    Novo-AZT

Another commonly used name is AZT.

Description

Zidovudine (zye-DOE-vue-deen) (also known as AZT) is used in the treatment of the infection caused by the human immunodeficiency virus (HIV). HIV is the virus responsible for acquired immune deficiency syndrome (AIDS). Zidovudine is also used to slow the progression of disease in patients infected with HIV who have early symptoms or no symptoms at all.

Zidovudine will not cure or prevent HIV infection or AIDS. It appears to slow down the destruction of the immune system caused by HIV. This may help delay the development of symptoms related to advanced HIV disease. However, it will not keep you from spreading the virus to other people. People who receive this medicine may continue to have the problems usually related to AIDS or HIV disease.

HIV infection can result in a very serious, usually fatal, disease. An estimated 1 to 1.5 million persons in the United States are currently infected with HIV. It has become one of the leading causes of death in men and women under the age of 45 and in children between 1 and 5 years of age.

HIV primarily attacks certain white blood cells in the body and slowly, over several years, breaks down the body's immune system. When this happens, the person may get other serious infections as well. These include serious fungus infections, *Pneumocystis* (noo-moe-SISS-tis) *carinii* pneumonia (PCP), and cytomegalovirus (CMV) infections, which can affect the retina of the eyes, the lungs, and the stomach and intestines. The person may also develop certain kinds of cancer, such as non-Hodgkin's lymphoma or Kaposi's sarcoma, a form of cancer usually involving purplish tumors of the skin or mouth. AZT may be given with other medicines to treat these problems.

Although most cases of HIV infection in the U.S. have occurred in homosexual and bisexual men, HIV infection has increased most rapidly in people exposed to the virus through heterosexual contact. Other people at risk of contracting HIV are intravenous drug users, their sexual partners and people who received transfusions with blood or blood products contaminated with the AIDS virus and their sexual partners. Children born to mothers infected with HIV are also at risk of getting the virus.

This virus is spread from person to person by infected body fluids, such as blood, semen, vaginal fluids (including menstrual blood), and breast milk. HIV is almost always spread by the intimate exchange of these fluids that occurs during unprotected sex (vaginal, anal, and possibly oral) with someone who is infected with the virus, and/or by sharing contaminated needles and syringes when injecting drugs. HIV is also spread from an infected mother to her fetus during pregnancy or childbirth, and, rarely, through breast-feeding. It is not spread by casual contact, such as touching, shaking hands, coughing, sneezing, or routine everyday contact, such as working in the same office, going to the same school, or eating in the same restaurant.

HIV can infect people of any age, sex, race, or sexual orientation. Because symptoms may take months, or more often years, to appear, an infected person may look and feel fine. During this time a person may spread the infection to others without knowing it.

The early symptoms of HIV infection may include fever; night sweats; swollen glands in the neck, armpit, and/or groin; unexplained weight loss; profound tiredness; yeast infections in the mouth; diarrhea; continuing cough; weakness; loss of appetite; or in women, vaginal yeast infections.

Zidovudine may cause some serious side effects, including bone marrow problems. Symptoms of bone marrow problems include fever, chills, or sore throat; pale skin; and unusual tiredness or weakness. These problems may require blood transfusions or temporarily stopping treatment with zidovudine. *Check with your doctor if any new health problems or symptoms occur while you are taking zidovudine.*

Zidovudine is available only with your doctor's prescription, in the following dosage forms:

   Oral
   • Capsules (U.S. and Canada)
   • Syrup (U.S. and Canada)
   Parenteral
   • Injection (U.S. and Canada)

It is very important that you read and understand the following information. If any of it causes you special concern, check with your doctor. Also, *if you have any questions* or if you want more information about this medicine or your medical problem, *ask your doctor, nurse, or pharmacist.*

Before Using This Medicine

In deciding to use a medicine, the risks of taking the medicine must be weighed against the good it will do. This is a decision you and your doctor will make. For zidovudine, the following should be considered:

Allergies—Tell your doctor if you have ever had any unusual or allergic reaction to zidovudine. Also tell your doctor and pharmacist if you are allergic to any other substances, such as foods, preservatives, or dyes.

Pregnancy—Zidovudine crosses the placenta. Studies in pregnant women have not been completed. However, zidovudine has not been shown to cause birth defects in studies in rats and rabbits given this medicine by mouth in doses many times larger than the human dose.

Breast-feeding—It is not known whether zidovudine passes into the breast milk. However, if your baby does not have the AIDS virus, there is a chance that you could pass it to your baby by breast-feeding. Talk to your doctor first if you are thinking about breast-feeding your baby.

Children—Zidovudine can cause serious side effects in any patient. Therefore, it is especially important that you discuss with your child's doctor the good that this medicine may do as well as the risks of using it. Your child must be carefully followed, and frequently seen, by the doctor while he or she is taking zidovudine.

Older adults—Zidovudine has not been studied specifically in older people. Therefore, it is not known whether it causes different side effects or problems in the elderly than it does in younger adults.

Other medicines—Although certain medicines should not be used together at all, in other cases 2 different medicines may be used together even if an interaction might occur. In these cases, your doctor may want to change the dose, or other precautions may be necessary. When you are taking zidovudine, it is especially important that your doctor and pharmacist know if you are taking any of the following:

- Amphotericin B by injection (e.g., Fungizone) or
- Antineoplastics (cancer medicine) or

- Antithyroid agents (medicine for overactive thyroid) or
- Azathioprine (e.g., Imuran) or
- Chloramphenicol (e.g., Chloromycetin) or
- Colchicine or
- Cyclophosphamide (e.g., Cytoxan) or
- Flucytosine (e.g., Ancobon) or
- Ganciclovir (e.g., Cytovene) or
- Interferon (e.g., Intron A, Roferon-A) or
- Mercaptopurine (e.g., Purinethol) or
- Methotrexate (e.g., Mexate) or
- Plicamycin (e.g., Mithracin)—Caution should be used if these medicines and zidovudine are used together; taking zidovudine while you are using or receiving these medicines may make anemia and other blood problems worse
- Clarithromycin (e.g., Biaxin)—Clarithromycin may decrease the amount of zidovudine in the blood
- Probenecid (e.g., Benemid)—Probenecid may increase the blood levels of zidovudine, increasing the chance of side effects

Other medical problems—The presence of other medical problems may affect the use of zidovudine. Make sure you tell your doctor if you have any other medical problems, especially:

- Anemia or other blood problems—Zidovudine may make these conditions worse
- Liver disease—Patients with liver disease may have an increase in side effects from zidovudine
- Low amounts of folic acid or vitamin B_{12} in the blood—Zidovudine may worsen anemia caused by a decrease of folic acid or vitamin B_{12}

Before you begin using any new medicine (prescription or nonprescription) or if you develop any new medical problem while you are using this medicine, check with your doctor, nurse, or pharmacist.

Proper Use of This Medicine

Patient information sheets about zidovudine are available. Read this information carefully.

Take this medicine exactly as directed by your doctor. Do not take more of it, do not take it more often, and do not take it for a longer time than your doctor ordered. Also, do not stop taking this medicine without checking with your doctor first.

Keep taking zidovudine for the full time of treatment, even if you begin to feel better.

For patients using *zidovudine syrup:*
- Use a specially marked measuring spoon or other device to measure each dose accurately. The average household teaspoon may not hold the right amount of liquid.

This medicine works best when there is a constant amount in the blood. *To help keep the amount constant, do not miss any doses.* If you need help in planning the best times to take your medicine, check with your doctor, nurse, or pharmacist.

Missed dose—If you do miss a dose of this medicine, take it as soon as possible. However, if it is almost time for your next dose, skip the missed dose and go back to your regular dosing schedule. Do not double doses.

Storage—To store this medicine:
- Keep out of the reach of children.
- Store away from heat and direct light.
- Do not store in the bathroom, near the kitchen sink, or in other damp places. Heat or moisture may cause the medicine to break down.
- Do not keep outdated medicine or medicine no longer needed. Be sure that any discarded medicine is out of the reach of children.

Precautions While Using This Medicine

It is very important that your doctor check your progress at regular visits. This medicine may cause blood problems.

Do not take any other medicines without checking with your doctor first. To do so may increase the chance of side effects from zidovudine.

Zidovudine may cause blood problems. These problems may result in a greater chance of certain infections and slow healing. Therefore, you should be careful when using regular toothbrushes, dental floss, and toothpicks not to damage your gums. Check with your medical doctor or dentist if you have any questions about proper oral hygiene (mouth care) during treatment.

HIV may be acquired from or spread to other people through infected body fluids, including blood, vaginal fluid, or semen. *If you are infected, it is best to avoid any sexual activity involving an exchange of body fluids with other people. If you do have sex, always wear (or have your partner wear) a condom ("rubber").* Only use condoms made of latex, and *use them every time you have vaginal, anal, or oral sex.* The use of a spermicide (such as nonoxynol-9) may also help prevent transmission of HIV if it is not irritating to the vagina, rectum, or mouth. Spermicides have been shown to kill HIV in lab tests. Do not use oil-based jelly, cold cream, baby oil, or shortening as a lubricant—these products can cause the rubber to break. Lubricants without oil, such as *K-Y Jelly*, are recommended. Women may wish to carry their own condoms. Birth control pills and diaphragms will help protect against pregnancy, but they will not prevent someone from giving or getting the AIDS virus. *If you inject drugs, get help to stop. Do not share needles with anyone.* In some cities, more than half of the drug users are infected and sharing even 1 needle can spread the virus. If you have any questions about this, check with your doctor, nurse, or pharmacist.

Side Effects of This Medicine

Along with its needed effects, a medicine may cause some unwanted effects. Although not all of these side effects may occur, if they do occur they may need medical attention.

Check with your doctor immediately if any of the following side effects occur:

> *More common*
>> Fever, chills, or sore throat; pale skin; unusual tiredness or weakness
>> Note: The above side effects may also occur up to weeks or months after you stop taking this medicine.

Rare

> Abdominal discomfort; confusion; convulsions (seizures); general feeling of discomfort; loss of appetite; mania; muscle tenderness and weakness; nausea

Other side effects may occur that usually do not need medical attention. These side effects may go away during treatment as your body adjusts to the medicine. However, check with your doctor if any of the following side effects continue or are bothersome:

More common

> Headache (severe); muscle soreness; nausea; trouble in sleeping

Less common

> Bluish-brown colored bands on nails

Other side effects not listed above may also occur in some patients. If you notice any other effects, check with your doctor.

Additional Information

Once a medicine has been approved for marketing for a certain use, experience may show that it is also useful for other medical problems. Although this use is not included in product labeling, zidovudine is used in certain patients with the following medical condition:

- Human immunodeficiency virus (HIV) infection due to occupational exposure (possible prevention of)

Other than the above information, there is no additional information relating to proper use, precautions, or side effects for this use.

Glossary

Abdomen—The body cavity between the chest and pelvis.

Abortifacient—Medicine that causes abortion.

Abrade—Scrape or rub away the outer cover or layer of a part.

Absorption—Passing into the body; incorporation of substances into or across tissues of the body, for example, digested food into the blood from the small intestine, or poisons through the skin.

Achlorhydria—Absence of acid in the stomach.

Acidifier, urinary—Medicine that makes the urine more acidic.

Acidosis—Build-up of too much acid in the blood, body fluids, and tissues.

Acromegaly—Enlargement of the face, hands, and feet because of too much growth hormone.

Acute—Describing a condition lasting a short length of time that begins suddenly and has severe symptoms; sharp or intense.

Addison's disease—Disease caused by not enough secretion of hormones by the adrenal glands.

Adhesion—The union by connective tissue of two parts that are normally separate (such as parts of a joint).

Adjunct—An additional or secondary treatment that is helpful but is not necessary to treatment of a particular condition; not effective for that condition if used alone.

Adjuvant—1. A substance added to or used with another substance to assist its action. 2. Something that assists or enhances the effectiveness of medical treatment.

Adrenal cortex—Outer layer of tissue of the adrenal gland, which produces hormones.

Adrenal glands—Two triangle-shaped organs located next to the kidneys. They produce adrenaline and hormones related to metabolism and sexual development and functioning.

Adrenaline—See epinephrine.

Adrenal medulla—Inner part of the adrenal gland, which produces adrenaline.

Adrenocorticoids—See corticosteroids.

Aerosol—Suspension of very small liquid or solid particles in compressed gas; drugs in aerosol form are dispensed in the form of a mist by releasing the gas.

African sleeping sickness—See Trypanosomiasis, African.

Agoraphobia—Fear of public places or open spaces.

AIDS (acquired immunodeficiency syndrome)—Disease caused by human immunodeficiency virus (HIV) which results in a breakdown of the body's immune system. The disease makes a person more susceptible to other infections and some forms of cancer.

Alcohol-abuse deterrent—Medicine used to help alcoholics avoid the use of alcohol.

Alkaline—Having a pH of more than 7. Opposite of acidic.

Alkalizer, urinary—Medicine used to make the urine more alkaline.

Altitude sickness agent—Medicine used to prevent or lessen some of the effects of high altitude on the body.

Alzheimer's disease—Progressive disorder of thinking and other mental processes, usually associated with age.

Aminoglycosides—A class of chemically related antibiotics used to treat some serious types of bacterial infections.

Anabolic steroids—Synthetic forms of androgens.

Analgesic—Medicine that relieves pain without causing unconsciousness.

Anaphylaxis—Sudden, severe allergic reaction.

Androgens—Male hormones, such as testosterone.

Anemia—Too little hemoglobin in the blood, resulting in tiredness, breathlessness, and low resistance to infection.

Anesthesiologist—A physician who is qualified to give an anesthetic and other medicines to a patient before and during surgery.

Anesthetic—Medicine that causes a loss of sensation of pain, sometimes through loss of consciousness.

Angina—Pain, tightness, or feeling of heaviness in the chest, due mostly to lack of oxygen passing into the heart wall; sometimes accompanied by trouble in breathing. The pain may be felt in the left shoulder and arm instead of or in addition to the chest. These symptoms often occur during exercise.

Angioedema—Allergic condition marked by continuing swelling and severe itching of areas of the skin.

Antacid—Medicine used to neutralize excess acid in the stomach.

Antagonist—Drug or other substance that blocks or works against the action of another.

Anthelmintic—Medicine used to treat infections caused by worms.

Antiacne agent—Medicine used to treat acne.

Antiadrenal—Medicine used to prevent an overactive adrenal gland (adrenal cortex) from producing too much cortisone-like hormone.

Antianemic—Medicine to treat anemia.

Antianginal—Medicine used to prevent or treat angina attacks.

Antianxiety agent—Medicine used for the treatment of nervousness, tension, or excessive anxiety.

Antiarrhythmic—Medicine used to treat irregular heartbeats.

Antiasthmatic—Medicine used to treat asthma.

Antibacterial—Medicine that destroys bacteria or suppresses their growth.

Antibiotic—Medicine produced by microorganisms and used to treat various types of infections.

Antibody—Special kind of blood protein that helps the body fight infection.

Anticholelithic—Medicine that dissolves gallstones.

Anticoagulant—Medicine that prevents blood clots from being formed in the blood vessels.

Anticonvulsant—Medicine used to prevent or treat convulsions (seizures).

Antidepressant—Medicine used to treat mental depression.

Antidiabetic agent—Medicine used to control blood sugar levels in patients with diabetes mellitus (sugar diabetes).

Antidiarrheal—Medicine used to treat diarrhea.

Antidiuretic—Medicine used to help hold water in the body (for example, in patients with diabetes insipidus [water diabetes]).

Antidote—Medicine used to prevent or treat harmful effects of another medicine or a poison.

Antidyskinetic—Medicine used to help treat the loss of muscle control caused by certain diseases or some other medicines.

Antidysmenorrheal—Medicine used to treat menstrual cramps.

Antiemetic—Medicine used to prevent or treat nausea and vomiting.

Antiendometriotic—Medicine used to treat endometriosis.

Antienuretic—Medicine used to help prevent bedwetting.

Antifibrotic—Medicine used to treat fibrosis.

Antiflatulent—Medicine used to help relieve excess gas in the stomach or intestines.

Antifungal—Medicine used to treat infections caused by a fungus.

Antiglaucoma agent—Medicine used to treat glaucoma.

Antigout agent—Medicine used to prevent or relieve gout attacks.

Antihemorrhagic—Medicine used to prevent or help stop serious bleeding.

Antihistamine—Medicine used to prevent or relieve the symptoms of allergies (such as hay fever).

Antihypercalcemic—Medicine used to help lower the amount of calcium in the blood.

Antihyperlipidemic—Medicine used to help lower the amount of cholesterol or other fat-like substances in the blood.

Antihyperphosphatemic—Medicine used to help lower the amount of phosphate in the blood.

Antihypertensive—Medicine used to treat high blood pressure.

Antihyperuricemic—Medicine used to prevent or treat gout or other medical problems caused by too much uric acid in the blood.

Antihypocalcemic—Medicine used to increase calcium levels in patients with too little calcium.

Antihypoglycemic—Medicine used to increase blood sugar levels in patients with low blood sugar.

Antihypokalemic—Medicine used to increase potassium levels in patients with too little potassium.

Antihypoparathyroid—Medicine used to treat the effects of an underactive parathyroid gland.

Anti-infective—Medicine that fights infection.

Anti-inflammatory—Medicine used to relieve pain, swelling, and other symptoms caused by inflammation.

Anti-inflammatory, nonsteroidal—An anti-inflammatory medicine that is not a cortisone-like medicine.

Anti-inflammatory, steroidal—A cortisone-like anti-inflammatory medicine.

Antimanic—Medicine used to treat manic-depressive mental illness.

Antimetabolite—Medicine that interferes with the normal processes within cells, preventing their growth.

Antimuscarinic—Medicine used to block the effects of a certain chemical in the body; often used to reduce smooth muscle spasms, especially abdominal or stomach cramps or spasms. It is also used to help reduce the amount of stomach acid.

Antimyasthenic—Medicine used in the treatment of myasthenia gravis.

Antimyotonic—Medicine used to prevent or relieve nighttime leg cramps or muscle spasms.

Antineoplastic—Medicine used to treat cancer.

Antineuralgic—Medicine used to treat neuralgia.

Antiprotozoal—Medicine used to treat infections caused by protozoa (tiny, one-celled animals).

Antipsoriatic—Medicine used to treat psoriasis.

Antipsychotic—Medicine used to treat certain nervous, mental, and emotional conditions.

Antipyretic—Medicine used to reduce high fever.

Antirheumatic—Medicine used to treat arthritis (rheumatism).

Antiseborrheic—Medicine used to treat dandruff and seborrhea.

Antiseptic—Medicine that stops the growth of germs. Used on the surface of the skin to prevent the development of infections in cuts, scrapes, and wounds.

Antispasmodic—Medicine used to reduce smooth muscle spasms (for example, stomach, intestinal, or urinary tract spasms).

Antispastic—Medicine used to treat muscle spasms.

Antithyroid agent—Medicine used to treat an overactive thyroid gland.

Antitremor agent—Medicine used to treat tremors (trembling or shaking).

Antitubercular—Medicine used to treat tuberculosis (TB).

Antitussive—Medicine used to relieve cough.

Antiulcer agent—Medicine used in the treatment of stomach and duodenal ulcers.

Antivertigo agent—Medicine used to prevent dizziness.

Antiviral—Medicine used to treat infections caused by a virus.

Anxiety—An emotional state in which there is an abnormal anticipation of unreal or imagined danger to a situation. May be accompanied by feelings of powerlessness, apprehension, tension, and fear and may include signs such as sweating, increased pulse, trembling, weakness, and fatigue.

Apoplexy—See Stroke.

Appendicitis—Inflammation of the appendix.

Appetite stimulant—Medicine used to help increase the appetite.

Appetite suppressant—Medicine used in weight control programs to help decrease the desire for food.

ARC (AIDS-related complex)—Thought to be a forerunner of AIDS. Refers to certain conditions caused by human immunodeficiency virus (HIV). Although not AIDS itself, the symptoms of ARC are usually the same as those of AIDS.

Arteritis, temporal—Inflammatory disease of the blood vessels, usually of the scalp, occurring in the elderly.

Arthritis, rheumatoid—Chronic disease of the joints, marked by pain and swelling at the sites.

Asthma—Lung condition marked by spasms of the bronchial tubes (air passages). During an attack, normal breathing is difficult and air exchange is incomplete.

Atherosclerosis—Common disease of the arteries in which fat deposits thicken and harden the artery walls.

Avoid—To keep away from deliberately.

Bacterium—Tiny, one-celled organism. Many types of bacteria are responsible for a number of diseases and infections.

Bancroft's filariasis—Disease transmitted by mosquitos in which an infection with the filarial worm occurs. Affects the lymph system, producing inflammation.

Beriberi—Disorder caused by too little vitamin B_1 (thiamine), marked by an accumulation of fluid in the body, extreme weight loss, inflammation of nerves, or paralysis.

Bile—Thick fluid produced by the liver and stored in the gallbladder. Bile helps in the digestion of food.

Bile duct—Tubular passage through which bile passes from the liver to the gallbladder.

Bilharziasis—See Manson's schistosomiasis.

Biliary—Relating to bile, the bile duct, or the gallbladder.

Bipolar disorder—Also called manic-depressive illness. Severe mental illness marked by repeated episodes of depression, mania, or both.

Bisexual—One whose sexual attraction is toward persons of both sexes.

Black fever—See Leishmaniasis, visceral.

Blackwater fever—Fever associated with a severe complication of malaria.

Blood fluke—See Manson's schistosomiasis.

Bone marrow—Soft material contained within the cavities of bones. One form produces red blood cells.

Bone resorption inhibitor—Medicine used to prevent or treat certain types of bone disorders, such as Paget's disease of the bone.

Bowel disease, inflammatory, suppressant—Medicine used to treat certain intestinal disorders, such as colitis.

Bradycardia—Slowing of the heart rate to fewer than 50 beats per minute.

Bronchitis—Inflammation of the bronchial tubes (air passages) of the lungs.

Bronchodilator—Medicine used to open up the bronchial tubes (air passages) of the lungs to increase the flow of air through them.

Buccal—Relating to the cheek. A buccal medicine is taken by placing it in the cheek pocket and letting it slowly dissolve.

Bursa—Small sac of tissue present where body parts move over one another (such as a joint) to help reduce friction.

Bursitis—Inflammation of a bursa.

Candidiasis of the mouth—See Thrush.

Cardiac—Relating to the heart.

Cardiac load–reducing agent—Medicine used to ease the workload of the heart by allowing the blood to flow through the blood vessels more easily.

Cardiotonic—Medicine used to improve the strength and efficiency of the heart.

Caries, dental—Also called "cavities." Tooth decay, sometimes causing pain, and leading to the crumbling of the tooth.

Cataract—An opacity (cloudiness) in the eye or lens that impairs vision or causes blindness.

Catheter—Tube inserted into a small opening in the body so that fluids can be put in or taken out.

Caustic—Burning or corrosive agent. Medicine applied to the skin to remove calluses, corns, and warts.

Cavities—See Caries, dental.

Central nervous system—Part of the nervous system that is composed of the brain and spinal cord.

Cerebral palsy—Brain condition resulting in weakness and poor coordination of the limbs.

Cervix—Lower end or necklike part of the uterus.

Chemotherapy—Treatment of illness or disease by chemical agents. The term most commonly refers to the use of drugs to treat cancer.

Chickenpox—See Varicella.

Chlamydia—A family of microorganisms that cause a variety of diseases in humans. One form is transmitted by sexual contact.

Cholesterol—Fat-like substance found in the blood and most tissues. Too much cholesterol is associated with several potential health risks, especially atherosclerosis (hardening of the arteries).

Chronic—Describing a condition of long duration, involving very slow changes, and often of gradual onset. Note that the term "chronic" has nothing to do with how serious the condition is.

Cirrhosis—Liver disease marked by abnormal cell growth, which may in turn lead to other serious conditions.

Clitoris—Small elongated, erectile organ, not connected with the urethra; female counterpart of the penis.

CNS—See Central nervous system.

Cold sores—See Herpes simplex.

Colitis—Inflammation of the colon (bowel).

Colostomy—Operation in which part of the colon (bowel) is brought through the abdominal wall to create an artificial opening. The contents of the intestine are discharged through the opening, bypassing the rest of the intestines.

Coma—State of unconsciousness from which the patient cannot be aroused.

Coma, hepatic—Disturbances in mental function and the nervous system caused by severe liver disease.

Condom—Thin sheath or cover worn over the penis during sexual intercourse to prevent pregnancy or infection.

Congestive heart failure—Inability of the heart to pump strongly enough, causing blood to back up in veins and body organs.

Conjunctiva—Delicate mucous membrane covering the front of the eye and the inside of the eyelid.

Conjunctivitis—Inflammation of the conjunctiva.

Constriction—Squeezing together and becoming narrower or smaller, such as blood vessels or eye pupils.

Contamination—To make impure or unclean, especially by introducing germs or unclean material into or on normally sterile substances or objects.

Contraceptive—Medicine or device used to prevent pregnancy.

Corticosteroids—Group of cortisone-like hormones that are secreted by the adrenal cortex, critical to the body. The two major groups of corticosteroids are glucocorticoids, which affect fat and body metabolism, and mineralocorticoids, which regulate salt/water balance. Also known as adrenocorticoids.

Cortisol—Natural hormone produced by the adrenal cortex, important for carbohydrate, protein, and fat metabolism and for the normal response to stress; synthetic (hydrocortisone) is used to treat inflammations, allergies, collagen diseases, rheumatic disorders, and adrenal failure.

Cot death—See Sudden infant death syndrome (SIDS).

Cowpox—See Vaccinia.

Creutzfeldt-Jakob disease—Rare disease, probably caused by a slow-acting virus that affects the brain and nervous system.

Crib death—See Sudden infant death syndrome (SIDS).

Crohn's disease—Condition in which parts of the digestive tract become thick and inflamed.

Croup—Inflammation and blockage of the larynx (voice box) in young children.

Cushing's syndrome—Condition in which the adrenal gland produces too much cortisone-like hormone, leading to weight gain, round face, and high blood pressure.

Cycloplegia—Paralysis of certain eye muscles, which can be useful in resting the muscles.

Cycloplegic—Medicine used to induce cycloplegia.

Cyst—Abnormal sac or closed cavity filled with liquid or semisolid matter.

Cystic—Marked by cysts.

Cystine—An amino acid. It is a part of most proteins and is produced by the digestion of them.

Cystitis, interstitial—Inflammation of the bladder, predominantly in women, with frequent urge to urinate and painful urination.

Cytomegalovirus—One of a group of viruses. One form is sexually transmitted and can cause blindness and be fatal in immunocompromised patients.

Cytotoxic agent—Chemical that kills cells or stops cell division.

Decongestant, nasal—Medicine used to help relieve nasal congestion (stuffy nose).

Decongestant, ophthalmic—Medicine used in the eye to relieve redness, burning, itching, or other irritation.

Dental—Related to the teeth or gums.

Depression, mental—Deep sadness and difficulty in performing day-to-day tasks. Other symptoms include disturbances in sleep, appetite, and concentration.

Dermatitis herpetiformis—Skin disease marked by sores and itching.

Dermatitis, seborrheic—Type of eczema found on the scalp and face.

Dermatomyositis—Inflammatory disorder of the skin and underlying tissues, including breakdown of muscle fibers.

Diabetes insipidus—Disorder in which the patient produces large amounts of urine and is constantly thirsty. Also called "water diabetes."

Diabetes mellitus—Disorder in which the body cannot process sugars to produce energy, due to lack of the hormone called insulin or because the body cannot use the insulin that it has. This leads to too much sugar in the blood (hyperglycemia). Also called "sugar diabetes."

Diagnose—Find out the cause or nature of a disorder by an examination or laboratory tests.

Diagnostic procedure—A process carried out to determine the cause or nature of a condition, disease, or disorder.

Dialysis, renal—Artificial technique for removing waste materials or poisons from the blood when the kidneys are not working properly.

Digestant—Medicine used to help the stomach digest food.

Diuretic—Also called "water pill." Medicine that increases the amount of urine produced by helping the kidneys get rid of water and salt.

Diverticulitis—Inflammation of a diverticulum (sac or pouch formed at weak points in the digestive tract).

Down's syndrome—Also called "mongolism." Mental retardation caused by a defect in the genes. Patients with Down's syndrome are marked physically by a round head, flat nose, slightly slanted eyes, and short stature.

Dumdum fever—See Leishmaniasis, visceral.

Duodenal ulcer—Open sore in that part of the small intestine closest to the stomach.

Duodenum—First of the three parts of the small intestine.

Eczema—Inflammation of the skin, marked by itching and rash.

Edema—Swelling of body tissue due to accumulation of fluids, usually first noticed in the feet or lower legs.

Eighth-cranial-nerve disease—Disease of the eighth cranial (brain) nerve, resulting in dizziness, loss of balance, loss of hearing, nausea, or vomiting.

Electrolyte—Substance which can, when in solution, conduct an electric current. In medical use, these substances are needed for normal functioning of the body. Body electrolytes include bicarbonate, chloride, sodium, potassium, etc.

Embryo—In humans, a developing fertilized egg within the womb from about two weeks to the eighth week after fertilization.

Emergency—Extremely serious unexpected or sudden happening or situation that calls for immediate action.

Emollient—Substance that soothes and softens an irritated surface, such as the skin.

Emphysema—Lung condition in which too much air accumulates in lung tissue because of blockage or narrowing of the bronchial tubes (air passages), leading to troubled breathing and heart problems.

Encephalitis—Inflammation of the brain.

Encephalopathy—Any of a group of diseases that affect the brain.

Endocarditis—Inflammation of the lining of the heart, leading to fever, heart murmurs, and heart failure.

Endometriosis—Condition in which material similar to the lining of the womb appears at other sites within the pelvic cavity, causing pain and bleeding.

Enteric coating—Coating on tablets which allows them to pass through the stomach unchanged before being broken up in the intestine and being absorbed. Used to protect the stomach from the medicine and/or the medicine from the stomach's acid.

Enteritis—Inflammation of the small intestine, usually causing diarrhea.

Enuresis—Urinating while asleep (bedwetting).

Enzyme—Type of protein produced by living cells that is important for normal chemical reactions in the body.

Epidural space—Area in the spinal column into which medicines (usually for pain) can be administered.

Epilepsy—Any of a group of brain disorders featuring sudden attacks of seizures and other symptoms.

Epinephrine—Hormone secreted by the adrenal medulla. It stimulates the heart, constricts blood vessels, and relaxes muscles. Also known as adrenaline.

EPO—See erythropoietin.

Ergot alkaloids—Medicines that cause narrowing of blood vessels; used to treat migraine headaches, and to reduce bleeding in childbirth.

Erythropoietin—Hormone secreted by the kidney. It controls the production of red blood cells by the bone marrow.

Esophagus—The muscular tube extending from the pharynx to the stomach.

Estrogen—Female hormone necessary for the normal sexual development of the female and for the regulation of the menstrual cycle during the childbearing years.

Expectorant—Medicine used to relieve cough by loosening and thinning the mucus or phlegm in the lungs so that it may be coughed up.

Familial Mediterranean fever—Also called polyserositis. Inherited condition involving inflammation of the lining of the chest, abdomen, and joints.

Favism—Inherited allergy to broad (fava) beans.

Fertility—Capacity to bring about the start of pregnancy.

Fetus—In humans, a developing baby within the womb from about the beginning of the third month of pregnancy until birth.

Fibrocystic—Having benign (noncancerous) tumors of connective tissue.

Fibroid tumor—A noncancerous tumor in the uterus formed of fibrous or fully developed connective tissue.

Fibrosis—Condition in which the skin and underlying tissues tighten and become less flexible.

Fibrosis, cystic—Disease in which abnormally thick mucus is produced, which interferes with a number of important organs, and often leads to infections of the lungs.

Flu—See Influenza.

Flushing—Temporary redness of the face and/or neck.

Fungus infection—Infection caused by a fungus, such as a mold or yeast. Some common fungus infections are tinea pedis (athlete's foot), tinea capitis (ringworm of the scalp), tinea cruris (ringworm of the groin, or jock itch, and vaginal candidiasis (yeast infections).

Gait—Manner of walk.

Gamma globulin—Type of protein found in the blood that is important in the body's immunity to infection.

Gastric—Relating to the stomach.

Gastric acid secretion inhibitor—Medicine used to decrease the amount of acid produced by the stomach.

Gastroenteritis—Inflammation of the stomach and intestine.

Gastroesophageal reflux—Backward flow into the esophagus of the contents of the stomach and duodenum. The condition is often characterized by "heartburn."

Gastroparesis, diabetic—Condition brought on by diabetes in which the stomach does not function as it should.

Generic—General in nature; relating to an entire group or class. In relation to medicines, the general name of a drug substance; not owned by one specific group as would be true for a trademark or brand name.

Genital—1. Relating to the organs concerned with reproduction; the sexual organs. 2. Relating to reproduction.

Genital warts—Small, hard growths found on the genitals or around the anus. The disease may be transmitted by sexual contact.

Gilles de la Tourette syndrome—See Tourette's disorder.

Gingiva—Gums.

Gingival hyperplasia—Enlargement of the gums.

Gingivitis—Inflammation of the gums.

Glandular fever—See Mononucleosis.

Glaucoma—Condition in which loss of vision may occur because of abnormally high pressure in the eye.

Glucose-6-phosphate dehydrogenase (G6PD) deficiency—Lack of or reduced amounts of an enzyme (glucose-6-phosphate dehydrogenase) that breaks down certain sugar compounds in the body.

Gluten—Type of protein found primarily in wheat and rye.

Goiter—Enlargement of the thyroid gland that causes the neck to swell. Condition results from a lack of iodine or thyroid hormone.

Gonadotropin—Hormone that stimulates the actions of the sex organs.

Gonorrhea—An infectious disease, usually transmitted by sexual contact. It causes infection in the genital mucous membranes in both men and women.

Gout—Disease in which too much uric acid builds up in the blood and joints, leading to painful swelling.

Graves' disease—Disorder in which too much thyroid hormone is present in the blood.

Groin—The area between the abdomen and thigh.

Guillain-Barré syndrome—Nerve disease marked by sudden numbness and weakness in the limbs that may progress to complete paralysis.

Hair follicle—Sheath of tissue surrounding a hair root.

Hansen's disease—See Leprosy.

Hartnup disease—Hereditary disease in which the body has trouble processing certain chemicals, leading to mental retardation, rough skin, and problems with muscle coordination.

Heart attack—See Myocardial infarction.

Hemoglobin—Iron-containing substance found in red blood cells that transports oxygen from the lungs to the tissues of the body.

Hemolytic anemia—Type of anemia caused by destruction of red blood cells.

Hemophilia—Hereditary blood disease in males in which blood clotting is delayed, leading to excessive and uncontrolled bleeding even after minor injuries.

Hemorrhoids—Also called "piles." Enlarged veins in the walls of the anus.

Hepatic—Relating to the liver.

Hepatitis—Inflammation of the liver.

Hernia, hiatal—Condition in which the stomach passes partly into the chest through the opening for the esophagus in the diaphragm.

Herpes simplex—The virus that causes "cold sores." These are an inflammation of the skin resulting in small, painful blisters. They may occur either around the mouth or, in the case of genital herpes, around the genitals (sex organs).

Herpes zoster—The virus that causes "shingles," an inflammation usually marked by pain and blisters along one nerve, often on the face, chest, or stomach. The virus also causes chickenpox.

Heterosexual—One whose sexual attraction is toward persons of the opposite sex.

High blood pressure—See Hypertension.

HIV (human immunodeficiency virus)—Virus that causes AIDS and ARC.

Hodgkin's disease—Malignant condition marked by swelling of the lymph glands, with weight loss and fever.

Homosexual—One whose sexual attraction is toward persons of the same sex.

Hormone—Substance produced in one part of the body (such as a gland) which then passes into the bloodstream and travels to other organs or tissues, where it carries out its effect.

Hot flashes—Sensations of heat of the face, neck, and upper body, often accompanied by sweating and flushing.

Hydrocortisone—See cortisol.

Hyperactivity—Abnormally increased activity.

Hyperammonemia—Elevated concentration of ammonia or its compounds in the blood.

Hypercalcemia—Too much calcium in the blood.

Hypercalciuria—Too much calcium in the urine.

Hyperglycemia—High blood sugar.

Hyperphosphatemia—Too much phosphate in the blood.

Hypertension—Also called "high blood pressure." Blood pressure in the arteries (blood vessels) that is higher than normal for the patient's age group. Hypertension often shows no outward signs or symptoms but may lead to a number of serious health problems.

Hyperthermia—Very high body temperature.

Hypocalcemia—Too little calcium in the blood.

Hypoglycemia—Low blood sugar.

Hypothalamus—Area of the brain that controls a number of body functions, including temperature, thirst, hunger, sexual and emotional activity, and sleep.

Hypothermia—Very low body temperature.

Ileostomy—Operation in which the ileum is brought through the abdominal wall to create an artificial opening. The contents of the intestine are discharged through the opening, bypassing the colon (bowel).

Ileum—Lowest of the three portions of the small intestine.

Immune deficiency condition—Lack of immune response to protect against infectious disease.

Immune system—Defense network of the body, designed to destroy anything "foreign" in the body.

Immunizing agent, active—Agent that causes the body to produce its own antibodies for protection against certain infections.

Immunocompromised—Having natural immunity decreased because of irradiation, certain medicine or diseases, and other conditions.

Immunosuppressant—Medicine that reduces the body's natural immunity.

Implant—1. Special form of medicine, often a small pellet or rod, that is inserted into the body or beneath the skin so that the medicine will be released continuously over a period of time. 2. To insert or graft material or an object into a body site. 3. Material or an object inserted into a body site, such as a lens implant or a breast implant. 4. Action of a fertilized ovum becoming attached or embedded in the uterus.

Impotence—Difficulty or inability in the male to have or maintain an erection of the penis.

Infertility—Medical condition which results in the difficulty or inability of a woman to become pregnant or of a man to cause pregnancy.

Inflammation—Pain, redness, swelling, and heat in a part of the body, usually in response to injury or illness.

Influenza—Also called "flu." Highly contagious virus infection of the lungs, marked by coughing and sneezing, headache, chills, fever, muscle pain, and general weakness.

Ingredient—One of the parts or substances that make up a mixture or compound.

Inhalation—Medicine used by being breathed (inhaled) into the lungs. Some inhalations work locally in the lungs, while others produce their effects elsewhere in the body.

Inhibitor—Substance that prevents a process or reaction.

Insomnia—Inability to sleep or remain asleep.

Insulin—Hormone that enables the body to use sugar. Used in the treatment and control of diabetes mellitus (sugar diabetes).

Interstitial plasma cell pneumonia—See Pneumocystis pneumonia.

Intra-amniotic—Within the sac that contains the fetus and amniotic fluid.

Intra-arterial—Into an artery.

Intracavernosal—Into the corpus cavernosa (cavities in the penis that, when filled with blood, produce an erection).

Intracavitary—Into a body cavity (for example, the chest cavity or bladder).

Intramuscular—Into a muscle.

Intrauterine device (IUD)—Small plastic or metal device placed in the uterus (womb) to prevent pregnancy.

Intravenous—Into a vein.

Irrigation—Washing out a body cavity or wound with a solution of a medicine.

Jaundice—Yellowing of the eyes and skin due to too much of a certain pigment in the bile.

Jock itch—Ringworm of the groin.

Kala-azar—See Leishmaniasis, visceral.

Kaposi's sarcoma—Malignant skin tumor. One form occurs in immunocompromised patients, for example, transplant recipients and AIDS patients.

Keratolytic—Medicine used to soften hardened areas of the skin (e.g., warts).

Ketoacidosis—Type of acidosis associated with diabetes.

Lactation—Secretion of milk by the mammary glands (breasts).

Larvae—Young or immature insects.

Larynx—Organ that serves as a passage for air from the pharynx to the lungs; it contains the vocal cords.

Laxative—Medicine taken to encourage bowel movements.

Laxative, bulk-forming—Laxative that acts by absorbing liquid in the intestines and swelling to form a soft, bulky stool. The bowel is then stimulated normally by the presence of the bulky mass.

Laxative, hyperosmotic—Laxative that acts by drawing water into the bowel from surrounding body tissues. This provides a soft stool mass and increased bowel action.

Laxative, lubricant—Laxative that acts by coating the bowel and the stool mass with a waterproof film. This keeps moisture in the stool. The stool remains soft and its passage is made easier.

Laxative, stimulant—Also called contact laxative. Laxative that acts directly on the intestinal wall. The direct stimulation increases the muscle contractions that move the stool mass along.

Laxative, stool softener—Also called emollient laxative. Laxative that acts by helping liquids mix into the stool and prevent dry, hard stool masses. The stool remains soft and its passage is made easier.

Legionnaires' disease—Lung infection caused by a certain bacterium.

Leishmaniasis, visceral—Also called "black fever," "Dum-dum fever," or "kala-azar." Tropical disease, transmitted by sandfly bites, which causes liver and spleen enlargement, anemia, weight loss, and fever.

Leprosy—Also called "Hansen's disease." Chronic disease affecting the skin, mucous membranes, and nerves. Symptoms include severe numbness, weakness, and paralysis leading to disfigurement and deformity.

Leukemia—Disease of the blood and bone marrow in which too many white blood cells are produced, resulting in anemia, bleeding, and low resistance to infections.

Leukoderma—See Vitiligo.

Local effect—Affecting only the area to which something is being applied.

Loiasis—The state of being infected by a roundworm.

Lugol's solution—Transparent, deep brown liquid containing iodine and potassium iodide, which may be given before a radiopharmaceutical medicine.

Lupus—See Lupus erythematosus, systemic.

Lupus erythematosus, systemic—Also called "lupus" or "SLE (systemic lupus erythematosus)." Chronic inflammatory disease affecting the skin and various internal organs.

Lymph—Fluid that bathes the tissues. It is derived from blood and circulated by the lymphatic system.

Lymphatic system—Network of vessels that conveys lymph from the tissue fluids to the bloodstream.

Lymph node—Small, rounded body found at intervals along the lymphatic system. They act as filters for the lymph keeping bacteria and other foreign particles from entering the bloodstream. They also produce lymphocytes.

Lymphocyte—Any of a number of white blood cells found in the blood, lymph, and lymphatic tissues. They are involved in immunity.

Lymphoma—Malignant tumor of lymph nodes or tissue.

Lyse—To cause breakdown. In cells, damage or rupture of the membrane results in destruction of the cell.

Macrobiotic—Vegetarian diet consisting mostly of whole grains.

Malignant—Describing a condition that becomes continually worse if untreated; also used to mean cancerous.

Malnutrition—Condition caused by unbalanced or insufficient diet.

Mammogram—X-ray picture of the breast, usually taken to check for abnormal growths.

Mania—Mental state of unusual cheerfulness and activity, but marked by illogical thought and speech, and overbearing, often violent behavior.

Manson's schistosomiasis—Also called "blood fluke" or "bilharziasis." Tropical infection in which worms enter the body from contaminated water and settle in the intestines, causing anemia and inflammation.

Mast cell—Large cell that releases substances that cause allergic reactions.

Mastocytosis—Accumulation of too many mast cells in the tissues in infants, resulting in a distinctive skin rash.

Megavitamin therapy—Taking very large doses of vitamins to prevent or treat certain medical problems. Studies have not proven this to be useful.

Melanoma—Highly malignant cancer tumor, usually occurring on the skin.

Meningitis—Inflammation of the tissues that surround the brain and spinal cord.

Menopause—The time in a woman's life when the ovaries no longer produce an egg cell at regular times and menstruation stops.

Migraine—Throbbing headache caused by enlarged blood vessels, usually affecting one side of the head.

Miotic—Medicine used in the eye that causes the pupil to constrict (become smaller).

Mongolism—See Down's syndrome.

Mono—See Mononucleosis.

Monoclonal—Derived from a single cell; related to production of drugs by genetic engineering (e.g., monoclonal antibodies).

Mononucleosis—Also called "mono" or "glandular fever." Infectious viral disease occurring mostly in adolescents and young adults, marked by swelling of the lymph nodes in the neck, armpits, and groin, and by severe fatigue.

Motility—Ability to move without outside aid, force, or cause.

Mucolytic—Medicine that breaks down or dissolves mucus.

Mucosal—Relating to the mucous membrane.

Mucous membrane—Moist layer of tissue surrounding or lining many body structures and cavities, including the mouth, lips, and inside of nose.

Mucus—Thick fluid produced by the body as a protective barrier, as a lubricant, and as a carrier of enzymes.

Multiple sclerosis (MS)—Chronic, progressive nerve disease marked by unsteadiness, shakiness, and problems in speech.

Myasthenia gravis—Chronic disease marked by abnormal weakness, and sometimes paralysis, of certain muscles.

Mydriatic—Medicine used in the eye that causes the pupil to dilate (become larger).

Myelogram—X-ray picture of the spinal cord.

Myeloma, multiple—Cancerous bone marrow disease that affects the body's ability to fight infections.

Myocardial infarction—Also called "heart attack." Interruption of blood supply to the heart, leading to sudden, severe chest pain, and damage to the heart muscle.

Myocardial reinfarction prophylactic—Medicine used to help prevent additional heart attacks in patients who have already had one attack.

Myotonia congenita—Hereditary muscle disorder marked by difficulty in relaxing a muscle or releasing a grip after any strong effort.

Narcolepsy—Extreme tendency to fall asleep suddenly.

Nasal—Relating to the nose.

Nasogastric (NG) tube—Tube that is inserted through the nose, down the throat, and into the stomach, so that medicine, food, or nutrients may be administered to patients who cannot swallow.

Nebulizer—Instrument that applies liquid in the form of a fine spray.

Neoplasm—Also called tumor. New and abnormal growth of tissue in or on a part of the body, in which the multiplication of cells is uncontrolled and progressive.

Neuralgia—Pain along the course of one or more nerves, occurring suddenly and intensely.

Neuralgia, trigeminal—Also called "tic douloureux." Severe burning or stabbing pain along the nerves in the face.

Neuritis, optic—Disease of the nerves in the eye.

Nicotinamide adenine dinucleotide (NADH) methemoglobin reductase deficiency—Reduced ability of the blood to carry oxygen caused by the lack of or reduced amount of a specific enzyme.

Nonsuppurative—Not discharging pus.

NSAIDs (nonsteroidal anti-inflammatory drugs)—Refers to a group of medicines used to treat inflammation and pain.

Obesity—Excess accumulation of fat in the body along with an increase in body weight exceeding the healthy range of the body's frame.

Obstetrics—Area of medicine concerned with the care of women during pregnancy and childbirth.

Occlusive dressing—Dressing (such as plastic kitchen wrap) that completely cuts off air to the skin.

Occult—Concealed, hidden, or of unknown cause; cannot be seen by the human eye; detectable only by microscope or chemical testing, as for occult blood in the stools or feces.

Ophthalmic—Relating to the eye.

Opioid—1. Any synthetic narcotic with opium-like actions; not derived from opium. 2. Natural chemicals that produce opium-like effects by acting at the same cell sites where opium exerts action.

Oral—Relating to the mouth.

Orchitis—Inflammation of the testis.

Osteitis deformans—See Paget's disease.

Osteomalacia—Softening of the bones due to lack of vitamin D.

Osteoporosis—Loss of bone tissue, resulting in bones that are brittle and easily fractured.

Otic—Relating to the ear.

Ovary—Female reproductive organ that produces egg cells and sex hormones. There are two ovaries, one on each side of the uterus.

Overactive thyroid—A condition in which the thyroid gland produces extra thyroxine, causing cells to burn up glucose and fat at a faster than normal rate, resulting in an increase in respiration, heart rate, and nervous and muscular activity.

Ovulation—Process by which an ovum is released from the ovary. In human adult females, this occurs once a month.

Ovum—Mature female reproductive cell, or egg cell. It is capable of developing into a new organism if fertilized.

Paget's disease—Also called "osteitis deformans." Chronic bone disease, marked by thickening of the bones and severe pain.

Pancreatitis—Inflammation of the pancreas.

Paralysis agitans—See Parkinson's disease.

Parathyroid gland—Two pairs of small bodies situated beside the thyroid gland; secrete parathyroid hormone and are associated with absorption and metabolism of calcium and phosphorus.

Parenteral—Injecting a medicine into the body using a needle and syringe.

Parkinsonism—See Parkinson's disease.

Parkinson's disease—Also called "Parkinsonism," "paralysis agitans," or "shaking palsy." Brain disease marked by tremor (shaking), stiffness, and difficulty in moving.

Patent ductus arteriosus (PDA)—Condition in newborn babies in which an important blood vessel in the heart fails to close as it should, resulting in faulty circulation and serious health problems.

Pediculicide—Medicine that kills lice.

Pellagra—Disease caused by too little vitamin B_3 (niacin), resulting in scaly skin, diarrhea, and mental depression.

Pemphigus—Skin disease marked by successive outbreaks of blisters.

Peptic ulcer—Open sore in esophagus, stomach, or duodenum, caused by acidic gastric juice.

Peritoneum—Sac that contains the liver, stomach, and intestines.

Peyronie's disease—Dense, fiber-like growth in the penis, which can be felt as an irregular hard lump, and which usually causes bending and pain when the penis is erect.

Pharynx—Space just behind the mouth that serves as a passageway for food from the mouth to the esophagus and for air from the nose and mouth to the larynx.

Phenol—Substance used as a preservative for injections.

Pheochromocytoma (PCC)—Small tumor of the adrenal gland.

Phlebitis—Inflammation of a vein.

Phlegm—Thick mucus produced in the respiratory passages.

Piles—See Hemorrhoids.

Pituitary gland—Pea-sized body located at the base of the skull. It produces a number of hormones that are essential to normal body growth and functioning.

Placebo—Also called "sugar pill." Medicine that has no actual effect on the patient but may help to relieve a condition because the patient believes it will.

Plaque—Mixture of saliva, bacteria, and carbohydrates that forms on the teeth, leading to caries (cavities) and other dental problems.

Platelet—Disc-shaped structure in the blood which performs several functions relating to blood clotting.

Platelet aggregation inhibitor—Medicine used to help prevent the platelets in the blood from clumping together. This effect reduces the chance of heart attack or stroke in certain patients.

Pleura—Membrane covering the lungs.

Pneumococcal—Relating to certain bacteria that cause pneumonia.

Pneumocystis pneumonia—Also called "interstitial plasma cell pneumonia." A very serious type of pneumonia usually affecting infants and patients in a weakened condition.

Polymorphous light eruption—A skin problem in certain people resulting from exposure to sunlight.

Polymyalgia rheumatica—Rheumatic disease, most common in elderly patients, that causes aching and stiffness in the shoulders and hips.

Polyp—Swollen or tumorous tissue which may or may not be cancerous.

Porphyria—Rare, inherited blood disease in which there is a disturbance of porphyrin metabolism.

Prevent—To stop or to keep from happening.

Priapism—Prolonged abnormal, painful erection of the penis.

Proctitis—Inflammation of the rectum.

Progestin—Female hormone necessary during the childbearing years for the development of the milk-producing glands, and for the proper regulation of the menstrual cycle.

Prolactin—Hormone secreted by cells of the anterior pituitary gland that stimulates and maintains milk flow in women following childbirth.

Prolactinoma—Pituitary tumor.

Prophylactic—1. Used to prevent the occurrence of a specific condition. 2. Condom.

Prostate—Gland surrounding the neck of the male urethra just below the base of the bladder. It secretes a fluid producing a major portion of the semen.

Prosthesis—Any artificial substitute for a missing body part.

Protozoa—Tiny, one-celled animals, some of which are important disease-causing parasites in man.

Psoralen—Chemical found in plants and used in certain perfumes and medicines. Exposure to a psoralen and then to sunlight may increase the risk of severe burning.

Psoriasis—Chronic skin disease marked by itchy, scaly, red patches.

Psychosis—Severe mental illness marked by loss of contact with reality, often involving delusions, hallucinations, and disordered thinking.

PUVA—The combination of a psoralen, such as methoxsalen or trioxsalen, and ultraviolet light A; used to treat psoriasis and some other skin conditions.

Rachischisis—See Spina bifida.

Radiopaque agent—Substance that makes it easier to see an area of the body with x-rays. Radiopaque agents are used to help diagnose a variety of medical problems.

Radiopharmaceutical—Radioactive agent used to diagnose certain medical problems or treat certain diseases.

Raynaud's syndrome—Condition marked by paleness, numbness, and discomfort in the fingers when they are exposed to cold.

Rectal—Relating to the rectum.

Renal—Relating to the kidneys.

Reye's syndrome—Serious disease affecting the liver and brain that sometimes occurs after a virus infection such as influenza or chickenpox. It occurs most often in young children and teenagers. The first sign of Reye's syndrome is usually severe, prolonged vomiting.

Rheumatic heart disease—Heart disease marked by scarring and chronic inflammation of the heart and its valves, occurring after rheumatic fever.

Rhinitis—Inflammation of the mucous membrane inside the nose.

Rickets—Bone disease caused by too little vitamin D, resulting in soft and malformed bones.

Ringworm—See Tinea.

Risk—The possibility of injury or of suffering harm.

River blindness—Disease in which one is infected with worms of the Onchocera type. The condition can progress to different eye nerve conditions or even blindness. Also called Roble's disease, blinding filarial disease, and craw-craw.

Sarcoidosis—Chronic disorder in which the lymph nodes in many parts of the body are enlarged, and small fleshy swellings develop in the lungs, liver, and spleen.

Scabicide—Medicine used to treat scabies (itch mite) infection.

Scabies—Skin infection caused by a mite, resulting in severe itching and redness.

Schizophrenia—Severe mental disorder marked by a breakdown of the thinking process, of contact with reality, and of normal emotional responses.

Scintigram—Image obtained by detecting radiation emitted from a radiopharmaceutical introduced into the body.

Scleroderma—Persistent hardening and shrinking of the body's connective tissue.

Scrotum—Sac that holds the testes (male sex glands).

Scurvy—Disease caused by too little vitamin C (ascorbic acid), marked by bleeding gums, bleeding beneath the skin, and impaired healing of wounds.

Seborrhea—Skin condition caused by the excess release of a thick, semi-fluid substance from the sebaceous glands.

Secretion—1. Process in which a gland releases a substance into the body for use. 2. The substance released by the gland.

Sedative-hypnotic—Medicine used to treat nervousness, restlessness, or insomnia.

Sedation—A relaxed or calmed state.

Seizure—Sudden, unnatural involuntary contraction or series of contractions of the muscles.

Semen—Fluid released from the penis at sexual climax. It is made up of sperm suspended in secretions from the reproductive tract.

Severe—Of a great degree, such as very serious pain or distress.

Shaking palsy—See Parkinson's disease.

Shingles—See Herpes zoster.

Shock—Severe condition associated with reduced blood volume and blood pressure too low to supply adequate blood to the tissues.

Shunt—Surgical tube used to transfer blood or other fluid from one part of the body to another.

SIADH (secretion of inappropriate antidiuretic hormone) syndrome—Disease in which the body retains (keeps) more fluid and loses more sodium than normal.

Sickle cell anemia—Hereditary blood disease that predominantly affects blacks; name comes from the sickle-shaped red blood cells found in the blood of patients.

Sinusitis—Inflammation of a sinus.

Sjögren's syndrome—Condition marked by swollen salivary glands and dryness of the mouth.

Skeletal muscle relaxant—Medicine used to relax certain muscles and help relieve the pain and discomfort caused by strains, sprains, or other injury to the muscles.

SLE—See Lupus erythematosus, systemic.

Spastic paralysis—Weakness of a limb because of too much reflex response.

Spermicide—Substance that kills sperm.

Spina bifida—Also called "rachischisis." Birth defect in which the infant's spinal cord is partially exposed through a hole in the backbone.

Sterility—1. Inability to produce children. 2. The state of being free of living microorganisms.

Stimulant, respiratory—Medicine used to stimulate breathing.

Streptokinase—Enzyme that dissolves blood clots.

Stroke—Also called "apoplexy." Sudden weakness or paralysis, usually affecting one side of the body. Stroke occurs when the flow of blood to an area of the brain is interrupted.

Stye—Infection of one or more sebaceous glands of the eyelid, marked by swelling.

Subcutaneous—Under the skin.

Sublingual—Under the tongue. A sublingual medicine is taken by placing it under the tongue and letting it slowly dissolve.

Sudden infant death syndrome (SIDS)—Also called "crib death" or "cot death." Death of an infant, usually while asleep, from an unknown cause.

Sugar diabetes—See Diabetes mellitus.

Sugar pill—See Placebo.

Sulfite—Type of preservative; causes allergic reactions, such as asthma, in some sensitive patients.

Sulfone—Medicine that acts against the bacteria that cause leprosy and tuberculosis.

Sunscreen—Substance, usually an ointment, cream, or lotion, that blocks light rays and helps prevent sunburn when applied to the skin.

Suppository—Mass of medicated material shaped for insertion into the rectum, vagina, or urethra. Suppository is solid at room temperature but melts at body temperature.

Suppressant—Medicine that stops an action or condition.

Suspension—A liquid in which the drug is not dissolved. When left standing for a period of time, particles settle at the bottom of the liquid and the top portion turns clear. When shaken it is ready for use.

Syphilis—An infectious disease, usually transmitted by sexual contact. The three stages of the disease may be separated by months or years.

Syringe—Device used to inject liquids into the body, remove material from a part of the body, or wash out a body cavity.

Systemic—For general effects throughout the body; applies to most medicines when taken by mouth or given by injection.

Temporomandibular joint (TMJ)—Hinge that connects the lower jaw to the skull.

Tendinitis—Inflammation of a tendon.

Testosterone—Principal male sex hormone.

Therapeutic—Relating to the treatment of a specific condition.

Thimerosal—Chemical used as a preservative in some medicines, and as an antiseptic and disinfectant.

Thrombocytopenic purpura—Blood disease marked by skin rash.

Thrombolytic agent—Substance that dissolves blood clots.

Thrush—Also called "white mouth" or "candidiasis of the mouth." Mild fungal infection of the mouth marked by white patches on the tongue or insides of cheeks.

Thyroid gland—Large gland in the base of the neck. It releases thyroid hormone, which controls body metabolism.

Tic—Repeated involuntary movement or spasm of a muscle.

Tic douloureux—See Neuralgia, trigeminal.

Tinea—Also called "ringworm." Fungus infection of the surface of the skin, particularly the scalp, feet, and nails.

Topical—For local effects when applied directly to the skin.

Tourette's disorder—Also called "Gilles de la Tourette syndrome." Condition of severe tics, including vocal tics and involuntary obscene speech.

Toxemia—Blood poisoning caused by bacteria growth at the site of infection.

Toxemia of pregnancy—Disease occurring in pregnant women in which there are metabolic disturbances which may result in hypertension, edema, excess proteins in the urine, convulsions, and coma.

Toxic—Poisonous; potentially deadly.

Toxoplasmosis—Disease caused by a protozoan; generally the symptoms are mild but a severe lymph node infection can result.

Tracheostomy—A surgical opening through the throat into the trachea (main passage from the lungs to the mouth) to permit a patient to breathe easily.

Tranquilizer—Medicine that produces a calming effect. It is used to relieve anxiety and tension.

Transdermal disk—Patch applied to the skin as a means of administering medicine; medicine contained in the patch is absorbed into the body through the skin.

Trichomoniasis—Infection of the vagina resulting in inflammation of genital tissues and discharge. It can be passed on to males.

Triglyceride—Substance formed in the body from fat in foods, and used to store fats in blood and tissues.

Trypanosome fever—See Trypanosomiasis, African.

Trypanosomiasis, African—Also called "trypanosome fever" or "African sleeping sickness." Tropical disease, transmitted by tsetse fly bites, which causes fever, headache, and chills, followed by enlarged lymph nodes, anemia, and painful limbs and joints. Months or even years later, the disease affects the central nervous system, causing drowsiness and lethargy.

Tuberculosis (TB)—Infectious disease, usually of the lungs, marked by fever, night sweats, weight loss, and spitting up blood.

Tumor—Abnormal swelling or enlargement in or on a part of the body.

Tyramine—Chemical present in many foods and beverages. Its structure and action in the body are similar to epinephrine.

Ulcer—Open sore or break in the skin or mucous membrane; often fails to heal and is accompanied by inflammation.

Underactive thyroid—A condition occurring when the thyroid does not produce enough hormone, thus causing cell metabolism to slow down.

Ureters—Pair of tubes through which urine passes from the kidneys to the bladder.

Urethra—Tube through which urine passes from the bladder to the outside of the body.

Vaccine—Medicine given by mouth or by injection to produce immunity to a certain infection.

Vaccinia—Also called "cowpox." Mild virus infection causing symptoms similar to smallpox.

Vaginal—Relating to the vagina.

Varicella—Also called "chickenpox." Very infectious virus disease marked by fever and itchy rash that develops into blisters and then scabs.

Vascular—Relating to the blood vessels.

Vasodilator—Medicine that dilates the blood vessels, which permits increased blood flow.

Veterinary—Relating to the medical care of animals.

Vitiligo—Also called "leukoderma." Condition in which some areas of skin lose their color and turn white.

von Willebrand's disease—Hereditary blood disease in which blood clotting is delayed, leading to excessive and uncontrolled bleeding even after minor injuries.

Water diabetes—See Diabetes insipidus.

Water pill—See Diuretic.

Wheezing—A whistling sound made when there is difficulty in breathing.

White mouth—See Thrush.

Wilson's disease—Inborn defect in the body's ability to process copper. Too much copper may lead to jaundice, cirrhosis, mental retardation, or symptoms like those of Parkinson's disease.

Zollinger-Ellison syndrome—Disorder in which the stomach produces too much acid, leading to ulcers.

Index

Brand names are in *italics*. There are many brands and different manufacturers of drugs and the listing of selected American and Canadian brand names is intended only for ease of reference. There are additional brands that have not been included. The inclusion of a brand name does not mean the USPC has any particular knowledge that the brand listed has properties different from other brands of the same drug, nor should it be interpreted as an endorsement by the USPC. Similarly, the fact that a particular brand has not been included does not indicate that the product has been judged to be unsatisfactory or unacceptable.

A

C

E

H

I

M

Q

R

T

U